New Frontiers in Medical Science

New Frontiers in Medical Science

Edited by Gretchen Flammer

hayle
medical

New York

Hayle Medical,
750 Third Avenue, 9th Floor,
New York, NY 10017, USA

Visit us on the World Wide Web at:
www.haylemedical.com

ISBN: 978-1-63241-475-5

Cataloging-in-Publication Data

New frontiers in medical science / edited by Gretchen Flammer.
    p. cm.
Includes bibliographical references and index.
ISBN 978-1-63241-475-5
1. Medical sciences. 2. Medicine. I. Flammer, Gretchen.
R708 .N49 2018
610--dc23

Table of Contents

Preface

Medicine studies practices that diagnose, treat and prevent diseases and disorders. It is divided into many sub-branches like epidemiology, immunology, microbiology, pharmacology, pathology and physiology to name a few. This book discusses the fundamentals as well as modern approaches of medicine. It elaborates on the various crucial theories, concepts and applications of the subject. The topics covered in the text provide detailed insights into this field of medicine. It aims to present researches that have transformed this discipline and aided its advancement. For all those who are interested in medicine, this text can prove to be an essential guide.

This book is the end result of constructive efforts and intensive research done by experts in this field. The aim of this book is to enlighten the readers with recent information in this area of research. The information provided in this profound book would serve as a valuable reference to students and researchers in this field.

At the end, I would like to thank all the authors for devoting their precious time and providing their valuable contribution to this book. I would also like to express my gratitude to my fellow colleagues who encouraged me throughout the process.

Editor

Advances in Proteomic Technologies and Its Contribution to the Field of Cancer

Mehdi Mesri

Office of Cancer Clinical Proteomics Research, National Cancer Institute, NIH, Bethesda, MD 20892, USA

Correspondence should be addressed to Mehdi Mesri; mesrim@mail.nih.gov

Academic Editor: Runjan Chetty

Systematic studies of the cancer genome have generated a wealth of knowledge in recent years. These studies have uncovered a number of new cancer genes not previously known to be causal targets in cancer. Genetic markers can be used to determine predisposition to tumor development, but molecularly targeted treatment strategies are not widely available for most cancers. Precision care plans still must be developed by understanding and implementing basic science research into clinical treatment. Proteomics is continuing to make major strides in the discovery of fundamental biological processes as well as more recent transition into an assay platform capable of measuring hundreds of proteins in any biological system. As such, proteomics can translate basic science discoveries into the clinical practice of precision medicine. The proteomic field has progressed at a fast rate over the past five years in technology, breadth and depth of applications in all areas of the bioscience. Some of the previously experimental technical approaches are considered the gold standard today, and the community is now trying to come to terms with the volume and complexity of the data generated. Here I describe contribution of proteomics in general and biological mass spectrometry in particular to cancer research, as well as related major technical and conceptual developments in the field.

1. Introduction

Although remarkable advances in cancer research have extended our understanding of how cancer develops, grows, and metastasizes, it is projected that close to 600,000 Americans will die from one of more than 200 types of cancer in 2013. Moreover, because an excess of 75 percent of cancer diagnoses occur in those aged 55 and older and this segment of the population is increasing in size, the number of cancer-related deaths will increase dramatically in the future. As a result, cancer is projected to soon become the number one disease-related killer of Americans. This trend is also observed globally, and it is estimated that, in 2030, more than 13 million people worldwide will die of cancer [1]. While significant amounts of resources are devoted to cancer research, the complexity and multifaceted nature of cancers reflect the obstacles to unravel the etiology of cancer and control and ultimately cure this debilitating disease. The heterogeneity and complexity of cancer progression originate from the complex interplay of genomic aberrations and immunological, hormonal, environmental, and other factors, acting individually or in concert which constitute the hallmarks of cancer.

The proteome is the operating machinery for nearly all biological functions; its abundance and interactions are precisely controlled and it is the link between the genome and phenotypes. Proteins can be present at vastly different abundances, expressed in various sizes, shapes, and charges, and have more complex twenty amino acid forms in contrast to the four nucleotides of the genome itself. It undergoes dynamic changes in different cells, tissues, and organs during development, in response to environmental stimuli and in disease processes. Understanding the dynamics of protein interactions with other proteins, nucleic acids, and metabolites is the key to delineating biological mechanisms and understanding disease including cancer. Genomic sequencing has been the focus of attention in recent decades and has produced a wealth of information. However, proteins are the component that functionally governs cellular processes. Moreover, variation in levels of DNA or transcripts does not correlate well with protein abundance [2]. Thus, proteomics bridges the gap between genomic information and functional proteins and translates this information. The possibility to systematically quantify protein abundances positions proteomics to monitor heterogeneous alterations in multiple pathways and mechanisms that drive the transformation of the malignant phenotype. Proteomics can be considered as an integral part of cancer research to identify biomarkers to detect patients at the early stage, monitor drug response of tumors, understand mechanisms that lead to cancer pathogenesis, and design new therapeutics. Scientists and oncologists thus use the various proteomics tools, design experiments, and interpret results of proteomics to determine the causative mechanisms, guide prognostication, and even develop precision medicine for cancer treatment.

2. Genomics

A key role of proteins in realizing the full potential of the human genome project (HGP) is linking the genome to normal and disease phenotypes. The HGP has changed many aspects of human biology and medical research including cancer. Despite many skeptics, the HGP became a reality by daring goals and new technology platforms [3]. Advanced technology platforms for sequencing dramatically changed the study of genes and gene regulation in all organisms [4]. The HGP has made all genes accessible to biologists by providing a part list of genes and putative protein products and stimulated a new perspective in studying biological processes through systems biology. Furthermore, the HGP has helped the creation of whole new commercial sector with high throughput instruments, reagents, and services and opened the door for large data sets, open-source data along with large-scale application of bioinformatics. The field has transformed our thinking about cancer diagnostics and targeted therapies. Despite all of these achievements skeptics are still concerned about the slow progress in transforming public health.

Both endogenous and exogenous stimuli may result in evading the normal regulatory mechanisms of the cells with ultimate aberrant phenotypes enabling cancer cell to proliferate, invade, and metastasize. Tumors contain endogenous aberrations that are largely caused by somatic alterations of genome that result in mutations of oncogenes and/or tumor suppressors [5]. For example, deletions, insertion, copy number variations, and mutations can drive initiation and progression of cancer [6]. Genomics, the comprehensive large scale analysis of gene expression in biological specimens to determine their associations with disease or treatment, has particularly been growing since 2005. New types of sequencing instruments that permit amazing acceleration of data-collection rates for DNA sequencing were introduced by commercial manufacturers including platforms such as massively parallel sequencing (MPS). For example, single instruments can generate data to decipher an entire human genome within only 2 weeks. It is anticipated that instruments that will further accelerate this whole genome sequencing data production timeline to days or hours will be a reality in the near future [7].

The main challenge in genomics today is to understand the role of molecular aberrations in various diseases such as cancer [8]. The Cancer Genome Atlas (TCGA) project (http://cancergenome.nih.gov/) and the International Cancer Genome Consortium (http://www.icgc.org/) aim to determine the genomic aberrations in human cancer types and their roles in pathophysiology of cancers. TCGA launched as a three-year pilot in 2006 by the National Cancer Institute (NCI) and National Human Genome Research Institute (NHGRI) in the United States. TCGA pilot project confirmed that an atlas of changes could be created. It also proved that a network of research and technology teams could pool the results of their efforts and develop an infrastructure for making the data publicly accessible. Moreover, it proved that public availability of data would enable researchers to validate important discoveries. The success of the pilot led the National Institutes of Health (NIH) to commit major resources to TCGA to collect and characterize more than 20 additional tumor types (http://cancergenome.nih.gov/). The ultimate goal is to translate genomics data into clinical applications such as routine clinical screening and precision medicine.

Classification of cancer and diagnosis has been based on cellular morphology and histological architecture. However, patients with similar histopathology, cancer staging, and treatments have shown variable clinical outcomes. Such methods are subjective and prone to interpretation variability, and pathologists do not always agree on the diagnosis. Therefore, diagnostic tools for cancers have evolved from histology to methods such as genomic testing with FISH, microarrays, and chromosome karyotype analysis. For example, gene expression profiles can be used as unique molecular signatures to aid diagnosis and classify histopathologically similar tumors into biologically distinct subtypes [9]. Molecular signatures can be used to identify patients with high risk for occurrence and poor survival and receive targeted therapies. Mammaprint is a Food and Drug Administration (FDA) approved breast cancer recurrence microarray-based test [10]. The Oncotype DX assay is used to predict risk for distant recurrence among invasive breast cancers [11]. A recent example of genomic signature for prognosis prediction of stages II and III colorectal cancer is ColoPrint [12]. In addition to biomarkers, genomics has led to discovery of new genes not previously known to play a causal role in cancer and leads to cancer therapeutics [3]. Some of the first sequencing attempts were focused in receptor tyrosine kinases (RTKs) in early 2000s. The studies indicated mutations in BRAF in 50% of melanomas [13], PIK3CA in 25%–30% of breast and colorectal cancers [14], and EFGR in 10%–15% of non-small cell lung cancers [15–17]. Interestingly some of the findings have resulted in a major impact on drug development and clinical treatment, including the development of selective RAF and MEK inhibitors that have produced dramatic remissions in melanoma and the ability to target the use of EGFR inhibitors to the subset of lung cancer patients who derive benefit.

3. Proteomic Challenge

By analogy, democratization of protein studies by generating a broader and deeper parts list to enable systems biology as well as deciphering protein interactions and biological signaling that mediate physiological and pathological conditions can have a major impact on medicine parallel to genome project [4]. This can take the form of cataloging all of the components, functionalization of the individual proteins, and putting the parts into relevant networks and circuitries and learning how these networks collectively process and execute their activities. The genome project identified all the genes and by inference all proteins. The challenge now is how these entities are integrated into molecular mechanisms resulting in phenotypes. An integral component of this system approach is requirement for technologies that can systematically identify and quantify all proteins, protein isoforms, and protein interactions. Proteins can take many different forms, for example, posttranslational modifications (PTMs), single-nucleotide polymorphisms (SNPs), and alternative splicing of proteins, resulting in numerous different structures of individual primary products, making the dimensions of proteome much larger than the human genome. Genomics alone cannot inform and delineate this protein diversity and its functional consequences.

Mass spectrometry platforms are the workhorse of experimental proteomics for protein analyses and in the last five years there has been significant progress in sensitivity, throughput, type, and depth of proteome analysis. The goals of innovation are concentrated on increasing signal/noise in identifying and sequencing peptides, detecting and quantifying specific peptides with PTMs, SNPs, or splicing, and enhancing the throughput to make assays useful for clinical and population studies. Another area is to be able to study the dynamics of how proteomes change (in concentration and in structure) in response to exogenous signals and disease. There are two main proteomic platforms: discovery-based versus targeted proteomics workflows. Discovery-based proteomics, which detect a mixture of hundreds to thousands of proteins, has been the standard approach in research to profile protein content in a biological sample which could lead to the discovery of protein candidates with diagnostic, prognostic, and therapeutic values. In practice, this approach requires significant resources and time and does not necessarily represent the goal of the researcher who would rather study a subset of such discovered proteins under different biological conditions. In this context, targeted proteomics is playing an increasingly important role in the accurate measurement of protein targets in biological samples with the expectation of elucidating the molecular mechanism of cellular function via the understanding of intricate protein networks and pathways (Figure 1).

4. Advances in Discovery-Based Proteomics in Cancer

Proteomic technologies encompass a whole array of methods such as electrospray ionization-liquid chromatography tandem mass spectroscopy (ESI-LC-MS), matrix assisted laser desorption ionization time of flight (MALDI-TOF), surface enhanced laser desorption ionization time of flight (SELDI-TOF), MALDI MS imaging (MALDI-MSI), two-dimensional

gel electrophoresis (2-DE), laser capture microdissection-MS (LCM-MS), and protein microarray, which can be used to derive important biological information to aid scientists and clinicians in understanding the dynamic biology of their system of interest such as in cancer [18–20].

4.1. ESI-LC-MS. ESI-LC-MS is a technology which produces gaseous ions carrying analytes byapplication of an electric potential to a flowing liquid in thepresence of heat. This causes formation of a spray upon high voltage, causing droplets tobecome electrically charged. Droplets eventually become unstable andexplode into even finer droplets and subsequently cause desorption of the analyte ions, which are then passed to themass spectrometer [21]. Most types of mass detection systems can be used with ESI including TOFs, ion traps (ITs), and quadrupoles. This technology can adopt various forms such as label-free or isotope labeling (metabolic labeling, ^{18}O labeling), and chemical labeling (isotope coded affinity tag (ICAT), isobaric tags (iTRAQ), tandem mass tag (TMT), and dimethyl labeling).

4.1.1. Label-Free. Quantitation method is relatively inexpensive and much easier to perform. This method uses spectral counting by measuring the frequency with which the peptide of interest has been sequenced by the MS, that is, the number of spectra for each peptide or protein being proportional to the amount of protein in the sample. This method can be used for biomarker discovery which normally requires high sample throughput by comparing peak intensity from multiple LC-MS data [22, 23]. Many studies have used label-free proteomics in cancer such as comparative proteomic analysis of non-small cell lung cancer [24] and proteins associated with metastasis in paraffin-embedded archival melanomas [25]. Application of this method for the analysis of changes in protein abundances in complex biological samples has certain limitations. For instance measuring small changes in the quantity of low-abundance proteins, which is often masked by sampling error, can be difficult. However, the method has an excellent linear dynamic range of about three orders of magnitude. Additionally, run to run analysis of the samples can exhibit differences in the peak intensities of the peptides as a result of sample processing requiring normalization. Additional issues may include experimental drifts in retention time and m/z (mass-to-charge ratio) complicating accurate comparison of multiple LC-MS data sets, chromatographic shifts as a result of multiple sample injections onto the same reversed-phase HPLC column, and unaligned peak comparison resulting in large variability and inaccuracy in quantitation. Also, large volume of data acquisition during LC-MS/MS requires the data analysis of these spectra to be automated. Computer algorithms have been developed to solve these issues and automatically compare the peak intensity data between LC-MS samples at a comprehensive scale [26, 27].

4.1.2. Isotopic Labeling. Isotopic labeling can be either *in vivo* or *in vitro* by incorporating stable isotope into proteins or peptides for comparative analysis. Labeling techniques allow

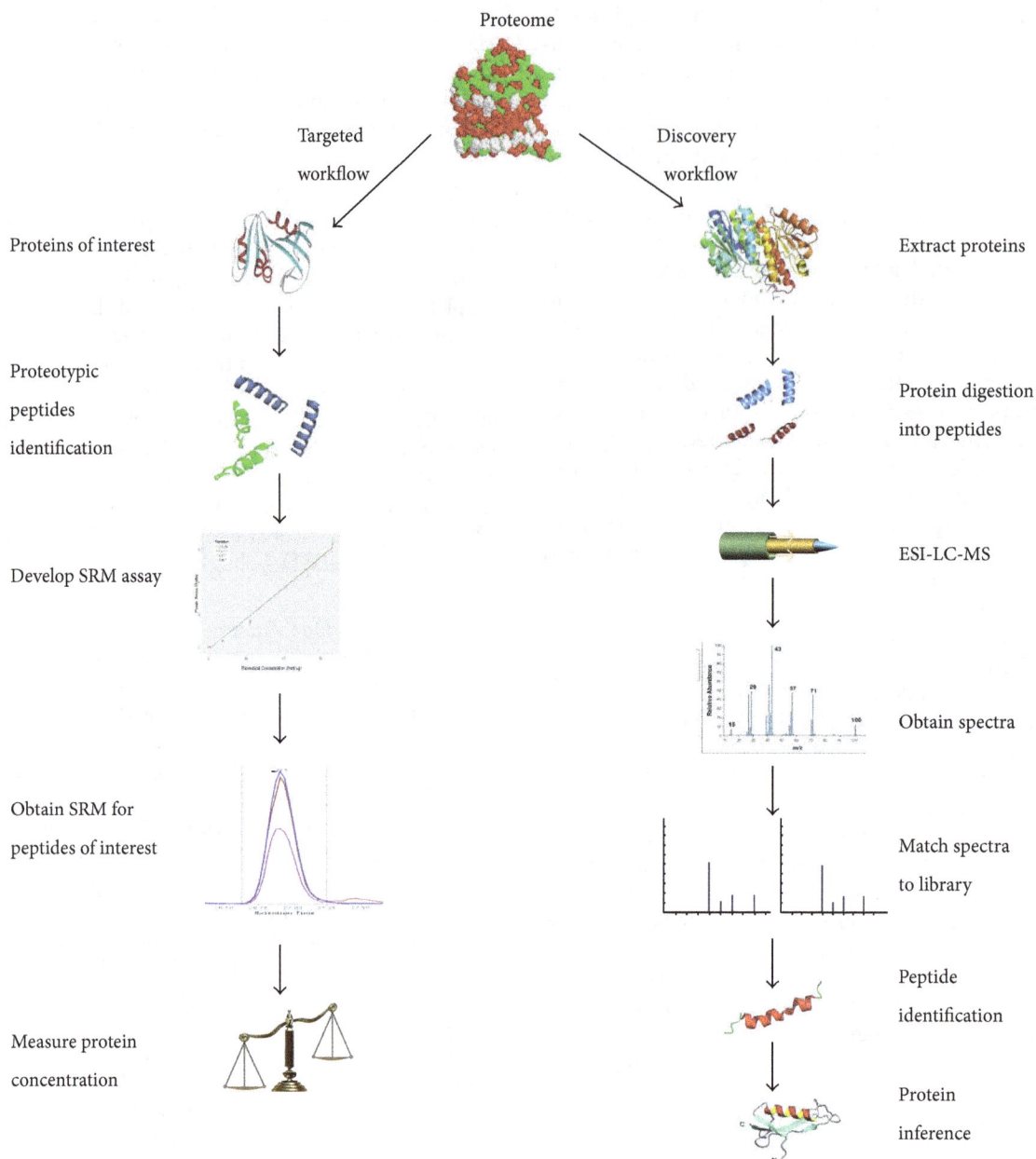

FIGURE 1: Discovery-based versus targeted proteomics workflows using mass spectrometry.

for multiplexing several samples to be analyzed and mitigate experimental variability inherent in sample processing.

(i) *Metabolic Labeling.* In this *in vivo* method cells are cultured with media containing isotopically labeled amino acids (13C and 15N) which are incorporated into the proteome during cell growth. In this method which requires metabolically active cells, samples grown with different labeled amino acids can be pooled for analysis [28]. More recently a stable isotope labeling with amino acids in cell culture (SILAC) mouse with a diet containing either the natural or the 13C6-substituted version of lysine was introduced

[29]. With no effect on growth or behavior, MS analysis of incorporation levels allowed for the determination of incorporation rates of proteins from blood cells and organs. Mann's group has also introduced super-SILAC method by combining a mixture of five SILAC-labeled cell lines with human carcinoma tissue. This generated hundreds of thousands of isotopically labeled peptides in appropriate amounts to serve as internal standards for mass spectrometry-based analysis [30]. Super-SILAC can play a role in expanding the use of relative proteomic quantitation methods to further enhance our understanding of cancer biology and a tool for biomarker discovery [31]. Some of the disadvantages of metabolic labeling include

incomplete labeling in cell culture medium which will affect accurate relative quantitation, labeling of all proteins necessitating purification, metabolic lability of amino acid precursors, and protein turnover [32].

(ii) *Proteolytic ^{18}O Labeling.* In this technique ^{18}O is incorporated during proteolytic digestion [33]. Differential $^{16}O/^{18}O$ coding relies on the ^{18}O exchange where two ^{16}O atoms are typically replaced by two ^{18}O atoms by enzyme-catalyzed oxygen-exchange in the presence of $H_2^{18}O$. The resulting 2–4 Da mass shift between differentially labeled peptide ions permits identification, characterization, and quantitation of proteins from which the peptides are proteolytically generated [34]. ^{18}O labeling bears at least two potential shortcomings: inhomogeneous ^{18}O incorporation and inability to compare multiple samples within a single experiment. Unlike chemical labeling method such as ICAT, ^{18}O labeling is simple with limited sample manipulations. It is much cheaper than ICAT and SILAC, comparing the price of reagents needed to label proteins. SILAC may be the method of choice for labeling of cultured cells, while ^{18}O labeling may be used for samples with limited availability such as human tissue specimens [34]. In contrast to ICAT, ^{18}O labeling does not favor peptides containing certain amino acids (e.g., cysteine) nor does it require an additional affinity step to enrich these peptides. Unlike iTRAQ, ^{18}O labeling does not require a specific MS platform nor does it depend on fragmentation spectra (MS^2) for quantitative peptide measurements. It is amenable to the labeling of human specimens (e.g., plasma, serum, and tissues), which represents a limitation of metabolic labeling approaches (e.g., SILAC). Taken together, recent advancements in the homogeneity of ^{18}O incorporation, improvements made on algorithms employed for calculating $^{16}O/^{18}O$ ratios, and the inherent simplicity of this technique make this method a reasonable choice for proteomic profiling of human specimens (e.g., plasma, serum, and tissues) in the field of biomarker discovery.

(iii) *Chemical Labeling.* At least three methods of chemical labeling have been in use: ICAT, TMT, and iTRAQ. The ICAT reagent consists of three elements: an affinity tag (biotin), which is used to isolate ICAT-labeled peptides; a linker that can incorporate stable isotopes; and a reactive group with specificity toward thiol groups (cysteines). The reagent exists in two forms, heavy (contains eight deuteriums) and light (contains no deuteriums), leading to a difference in molecular weight of 8 Da between the two different forms of the tag. For quantifying differential protein expression, the protein mixtures are combined and proteolyzed to peptides and ICAT-labeled peptides are isolated utilizing the biotin tag. These peptides are separated by liquid chromatography. The pair of light and heavy ICAT-labeled peptides co-elute, and

the 8 Da mass difference is measured in a scanning mass spectrometer. The ratios of the original amounts of proteins from the two cell states are strictly maintained in the peptide fragments. The relative quantification is determined by the ratio of the peptide pairs. The protein is identified by computer-searching the recorded sequence information against large protein databases [35–37]. The main disadvantage of ICAT labeling technique is that it only binds to cysteine residues, which constitutes approximately 1% of the protein composition. Similar to ^{18}O labeling, ICAT has the limitation of having only two labels available, resulting in frequent experimentation and high cost if multiple samples need to be compared.

Multiplexed sets of reagents for quantitative protein analysis have been developed which enable comparing of a larger number of treatments including the development of the 4- or 8-plex isobaric tag (iTRAQ) [38] and the 2- or 6-plex TMT [39] labeling techniques. The former can compare up to eight and the latter up to six samples in a single analysis. In these methods, both N-termini and lysine peptides are labeled with different isobaric mass reagents such that all derivative peptides are isobaric and indistinguishable. The different mass tags can only be distinguished upon peptide fragmentation. As each tag adds an identical mass to a given peptide, each peptide produces only a single peak during liquid chromatography and therefore only a single m/z will be isolated for fragmentation. The different mass tags only separate upon fragmentation, when reporter ions that are typical for each of the different labels are generated. The intensity ratio of the different reporter ions is used as a quantitative readout. One drawback of these methods is that only a single fragmentation spectrum per peptide may be available, while in quantitation-based MS1 scan, multiple data points are sampled resulting in a lower overall sensitivity. Some additional disadvantages of these techniques are the inconsistencies in labeling efficiencies and the high cost of the reagents. Use of standard operating protocols (SOPs) is recommended to achieve reproducible and reliable results with iTRAQ and therefore alleviating potential variability as a consequence of multistep sample preparations [40]. iTRAQ may also have limitations in dynamic range; experiments typically report fold changes of less than 2 orders of magnitude. From a purely technical point of view, this may be perceived as a limitation of iTRAQ for quantitative proteomics [41–43].

It is clear that both labeled and unlabeled MS analyses will continue to have their uses. Stable isotope labeling provides higher quality data at the analysis end. And with labeling methods, such as iTRAQ, the labels are introduced so late in the process that the experiment can be performed much faster than in earlier labeling methods. Even so, it is a lot more challenging technically than label-free techniques and also prone to systematic errors. The choice of isotope labeling technique is highly dependent upon experimental design, the scope of a particular analysis, and the sample or system being analyzed.

At the technology level, there is still room for progress. Performance in proteomics can be characterized by three factors: ion injection efficiency, cycling speed, and detector sensitivity. While the detectors are sensitive already at the level of detecting a single ion, the process of funneling the ions to the detector can be improved. Despite improvements in electrospray ionization injection, the majority of ions are still lost on their way to the detector. In addition, irrelevant molecules cannot be filtered out which result in generating a lot of noise. Improvements in these areas can enhance the signal/noise ratio. Furthermore, speeding up the cycling rate (the number of spectra per second) can increase the measurement depth. Given the wide dynamic range, this can in turn result in quantifying maximum proteins present in the sample [44].

4.2. MALDI-TOF. MALDI-TOF is a MS platform in which time of flight mass analyzer is usually coupled with MALDI. Ions are accelerated by an electric field followed by ion separation according to their m/z ratios by measuring the time it takes for ions to travel through flight tube. Specifically, the m/z ratio of an ion is proportional to the square of its drift time with heavier ions taking longer to travel. The sample for MALDI is uniformly mixed in a large quantity of matrix. The matrix absorbs the ultraviolet light and converts it to heat energy. A small part of the matrix heats rapidly and is vaporized, together with the sample [45]. MALDI-TOF-MS has become a widespread and versatile method to analyze a range of macromolecules in a wide range of samples. Its ability to desorb high-molecular-weight molecules and its high accuracy and sensitivity, combined with its wide mass range (1–300 kDa), make MALDI-TOF-MS a method of choice for the clinical chemistry laboratory for the identification of biomolecules in complex samples, including peptides, proteins, oligosaccharides, and oligonucleotides [46, 47]. The first reports of MALDI-TOF-MS biochemical analysis were published in the late 1980s from Karas and Hillenkamp lab [45]. Although being relatively young compared to other analytical techniques using mass spectrometry, there has been an enormous increase in the publication of MALDI-TOF-MS methods and applications in the literature. While ESI can efficiently be interfaced with separation techniques enhancing its role in the life and health sciences, MALDI, however, has the advantage of producing singly charged ions of peptides and proteins, minimizing spectral complexity.

4.3. SELDI-TOF-MS. SELDI-TOF-MS technique was introduced in 1993 by Hutchens and Yip [48] and later commercialized by Ciphergen Biosystems in 1997. SELDI-TOF-MS is a variation of MALDI that uses a target modified to reach biochemical affinity with the sample proteins. There are some differences between the two techniques. In MALDI, the sample is mixed with the matrix molecule in solution, and a small amount of the mixture is deposited on a surface to dry. This makes the sample and matrix cocrystallized after the solvent evaporated. On the other hand, in SELDI, the mixture is spotted on a surface modified with a chemical functionality such as binding affinity. There are different types of chemicals and substances bound to the protein arrays, including antibodies, receptors, ligands, nucleic acids, carbohydrates, or chromatographic surfaces (i.e., cationic, anionic, hydrophobic, or hydrophilic). Still wet, some proteins in the samples would bind to the modified surface, while the others will be washed off. Then the matrix is applied to the surface for crystallization with the sample peptides. In the binding and washing off steps the surface-bound proteins are left for analyses. Samples spotted on an SELDI surface are analyzed with TOF mass spectrometry (TOF-MS) [49, 50]. The strength of this technology is the integration of on-chip selective capture, relative quantitation, and partial characterization of proteins and peptides. The differential expression data obtained from this technology has been used for identification of biomarker candidates for various cancer types, such as prostate [51, 52], pancreas [53–55], lung [56–58], breast [59–61], melanoma [62], colon [63, 64], ovarian [65–67], and liver cancers [68, 69].

4.4. MALDI-MSI. MALDI-MSI is a powerful technique which allows investigating the distribution of proteins and biomolecules directly from a tissue section [70, 71]. This technique also permits investigation of the spatial and temporal distribution of biomolecules such as phospholipids without the need for extraction, purification, and separation procedures of tissue sections [72]. MALDI-MSI can help in molecular diagnosis on tissue directly in the environment of the tumors and can detect the tumor boundary or infiltration of adjacent normal tissue. It could also help to detect the early stage of pathology that presents no histological modifications and to prevent tumor recurrence at the site of surgical resection. One of the advances of MSI is the correlation of the MALDI images with histological information. MALDI-MSI software [73] superimposes the MALDI images over a macroscopic or microscopic optical image of the sample taken before MALDI measurement. MALDI-MSI has been used in clinical proteomics for biomarker discovery in a variety of diseases including cancer [74–78]. Development of SOPs and standardization of protocols for sample collection, storage, data acquisition, and enhancement of imaging resolutions and 3D tumor mapping are still needed to further improve its utility [79, 80]. Also the present levels of sensitivity allow the detection of a small group of cells but are not sufficient to detect discrete modification at a single cell level. A major advance for MALDI-MSI will be its coupling with positron emission tomography, X-ray, computed tomography instrumentation, and MRI for both preclinical and clinical research. The complementarities between noninvasive techniques and molecular data obtained from MALDI MS imaging will result in a more precise diagnosis [81]. Ultimately comparing the MRI image of a tumor and the image generated by MALDI-MSI at a molecular level will provide a comprehensive data set for diagnosis and treatment selection.

4.5. 2-DE. 2-DE or two-dimensional gel electrophoresis technology was a pivotal turning point in the field of separation and has been shown to be a reliable and efficient method for separation of proteins based on mass and charge [82]. High resolution two-dimensional polyacrylamide gel electrophoresis (2D-PAGE) can resolve up to 10,000 protein spots per gel. This technique has been used in human tissue, plasma, and serum proteome analysis with or without prior fractionation [83–86]. Visualization of resolved proteins in the gel can be performed by staining methods such as Coomassie blue and silver staining [87, 88]. Some of the recent advances in silver staining products make it compatible with MS analysis too. To enable direct comparison of different mixtures of proteins, differential in-gel electrophoresis (DIGE) has been developed which permits simultaneous comparison of labeled proteins in different mixtures. In a typical experiment, two samples are labeled with different fluorescence dyes (Cy3 and Cy5) and mixed prior to electrophoresis and run in parallel with an internal standard labeled with a third dye (Cy2) for quantitative analysis [89, 90].

For identification purposes, gel-separated proteins can be digested into peptides. Analysis of the peptides can then provide a peptide mass fingerprint (PMF), which can be searched against theoretical fingerprints of sequences in protein databases. Alternatively, peptides can be sprayed into a tandem mass spectrometer (ESI) as they elute off a liquid chromatography (LC) column. The data can be searched for protein sequence and analyzed by the application of algorithms and comparison with theoretical production spectra of proteins in databases [91, 92].

2D-PAGE is a low throughput technology, labor intensive with low dynamic range, and prone to gel-to-gel variability. Although DIGE has shown improved accuracy, it is still a relatively low throughput method. It can be used in areas such as biomarker discovery, where high throughput processing of samples is not required [93].

4.6. LCM-MS. LCM-MS has proven an effective technique to harvest pure cell populations from tissue sections. Because proteome varies in different cells, the advent of laser capture microdissection has expanded the analytical capabilities of microproteomics by enabling protein analysis from extremely small samples. A typical protocol uses nanoscale liquid chromatography/tandem mass spectrometry (nano-LC-MS/MS) to simultaneously identify and quantify hundreds of proteins from LCMs of tissue sections from small tissue samples containing as few as 1000 cells. The LCM-dissected tissues are subjected to protein extraction, reduction, alkylation, and digestion, followed by injection into a nano-LC-MS/MS system for chromatographic separation and protein identification. The approach can be validated by secondary screening using immunological techniques such as immunohistochemistry or immunoblots [94].

LCM has significantly improved the analytical capabilities of comparative proteomic technologies to the extent that 2D-DIGE and quantitative gel-free mass spectrometry approaches have been coupled to LCM for proteomic analyses

of distinct, pure cell populations [95–101]. The LCM technology allows for miniaturization of extraction and isolation and detection of hundreds of proteins (100–300 proteins) from different cell populations containing as few as 1000 cells. Additionally, it can detect and verify robust protein expression differences between different cell populations. Unlike traditional proteomic technologies, the LCM procedure requires as little as 1-2 μg of protein. However, each step of the procedure requires greater care as the sample size decreases. Protein losses during extraction and separation become more significant as the protein detection limit (<0.75 μg) is approached [94]. Other methods such as punch biopsy can be used to microdissect tissues for proteomic analyses [102], but because the three-dimensional view of boundaries of tissue structures is limited, punch biopsies can sample adjacent regions that are not of interest. In a recent paper published by Mueller et al. [103], the authors claimed that data derived from nonmicrodissected glioblastoma multiforme (GBM) can result in inaccurate correlations between genomic and proteomic data and subsequent false classifications. This is because molecular signals could be masked where sample tumor content is low or where the signal is strong in the stromal cells. Mueller et al. investigated 39 glioblastoma samples taken from tissue previously analyzed by the TCGA project. Using reverse phase protein array (RPPA) they measured the levels of 133 proteins and phosphoproteins, comparing LCM and non-LCM samples, finding differences in 44 percent of the analytes between the two types. They specifically investigated in more depth the genomic and proteomic data for epidermal growth factor receptor (EGFR) and phosphatase and tensin homolog (PTEN), two clinically important proteins in glioblastoma. While the researchers observed in both sample types increased EGFR protein and phosphoprotein levels in patients with increased EGFR gene copy number, they observed the increase in EGFR phosphorylation expected in carriers of EGFR mutations only in the LCM samples. In the case of PTEN, the researchers observed the expected decrease in PTEN levels in tumors with deep loss of PTEN or PTEN mutations only in the LCM samples. Additionally, they found the expected correlation between EGRF phosphorylation, PTEN levels, and phosphorylation of AKT only in the LCM samples which is regulated by the former two proteins. Mueller et al. also examined proteomic glioblastoma data previously generated by TCGA using non-LCM samples, again failing to observe the expected correlation between PTEN copy number or mutational status and PTEN protein levels. The authors recommend careful upfront cellular enrichment in biospecimens that form the basis for targeted therapy selection [103]. Further developments in LCM technology should facilitate effective sampling of specific cellular subtypes from tissue in a high throughput manner.

4.7. Protein Microarray. Protein microarray is a high throughput tool for studying the biochemical activities of proteins, tracking their interactions, and determining their function on a large scale [104]. Its main strength is that large numbers of proteins can be tracked in parallel. The chip usually consists of a support surface such as a glass slide, nitrocellulose membrane, bead, or microtiter plate, to which an array of capture proteins is bound. The commonest type of protein microarray may contain a large number of spots of either proteins or their ligands arranged in a predefined pattern, arrayed by robots onto coated glass slides, microplates, or membranes. The array may consist of antibodies to bind proteins of interest [105], enzymes that will interact with substrates, or substrates or ligands that will interact with applied proteins. Therefore, protein microarray formats can be divided into two major classes depending on what is immobilized on the support surface. In forward-phase protein array (FPPA) the capture antibody is first immobilized on a solid surface to capture the corresponding antigen in a test sample. The captured analyte is then directly detected with a fluorescent dye-conjugated detection antibody or detected indirectly with the detection antibody followed by a fluorescent dye-conjugated second antibody [106]. In this method, identification of a capture and a detection affinity reagent can be time-consuming. To bypass the requirement for two affinity reagents, reverse phase protein array (RPPA) may provide an alternative solution. In RPPA, test samples that could run into thousands are printed on the slide directly and detected with dye-conjugated antibodies [107]. RPPA assays are commonly used in tissue microarray and cell and tissue lysate microarray. While RPPA provides a high throughput platform, the specificity might be compromised to some degree owing to the use of single detection antibodies.

One technical downside to producing a reliable array is shelf-life. Most protein arrays use antibodies to deposit and be immobilized on the support surface which can denature the antibody and affect its recognition properties. Another bottleneck that chip manufacturers face is getting good quality and specific antibody against every protein in the human proteome which is a gigantic task. In addition to limited inventory of specific antibodies to PTMs (such as phosphorylation and glycosylation), generation of high throughput protein expression systems and purification including those with PTMs required for spotting the complete proteome under study is another challenge or may suffer from lack of reproducibility. Establishing standard criteria for array production and data normalization using noise models, variance estimation and differential expression analysis techniques would improve interpretation of microarray results [108].

The challenges in producing proteins to spot on the arrays fueled the development of a novel approach to protein microarrays technology called nucleic acid programmable protein array (NAPPA) which uses cell-free extracts to transcribe and translate cDNAs encoding target proteins directly onto glass slides. This approach eliminates the need to purify proteins, avoids protein stability problems during storage, and captures sufficient protein for functional studies [109, 110]. In recent studies NAPPA was coupled with MS and used for several applications, including the identification of peptide sequences for potential phosphorylation as well as a high throughput method for the detection of protein-protein interactions [111]. Moreover, the challenges of constructing solid-surface arrays holding thousands of proteins

with different properties raised interest in protein-interaction assays in solution. Suspension-bead assays are particularly flexible and as a result suspension platforms were developed such as the Bio-Plex system from Bio-Rad Laboratories which uses Luminex's bead-based xMAP technology [112] as does the LiquiChip system from Qiagen Instruments. Suspension-bead arrays are flexible enough to tackle any sort of protein-ligand interaction by simply coupling the required proteins or ligands to different bead populations. Luminex beads, for example, enable simultaneous quantitation of up to 100 different biomolecules in a single microplate well. Rather than a flat surface, Bio-Plex assays make use of differentially detectable bead sets as a substrate capturing analytes in solution and employ fluorescent methods for detection [113].

5. Advances in Targeted-Based Proteomics in Cancer

The field of biomarkers, in particular, has benefited significantly from application of proteomic platforms over the last decade or more, with the goal of identifying simple noninvasive tests that can indicate cancer risk, allow early cancer detection, classify tumors so that the patient can receive the most appropriate therapy, and monitor disease progression, regression, and recurrence. A variety of biospecimens such as tissue, proximal fluids, and blood have been interrogated for protein or peptide markers identification. Thousands of publications have explored the potential use of individual proteins or collections of proteins as cancer biomarkers and have produced promising results [114, 115]. One study by Polanski and Anderson [116] has identified >1261 protein biomarker candidates for cancer alone. However, only 23 protein plasma biomarkers have cleared the US Food and Drug Administration (FDA) since 2003 as clinical biomarkers averaging <2 proteins per year over the last 12 years, while assays for at least 96 analytes have been developed and used as laboratory-developed tests (LDTs) [115]. Despite recent technical advances, there are still huge analytical challenges for clinically relevant identification of biomarkers in serum or plasma. This is compounded by the lack of analytical validation of a platform(s) for the precise and accurate measurements of identified analytes in a smaller set of clinical samples prior to proceeding to costly and time-consuming large-scale clinical trials (Figure 2). The Clinical Proteomic Technology Assessment for Cancer (CPTAC 1) of the NCI developed the innovative concept of biomarker "verification" which bridges discovery and validation. This pipeline has the potential to enable delivery of highly credentialed protein biomarker candidates for clinical validation (Figure 3). Targeted proteomic technologies such as multiplexed MS, protein arrays, and enzyme-linked immunosorbent assays (ELISAs) can fill this bridging space. Verification of candidates relies upon specific, multiplex quantitative assays optimized for selective detection of biomarker candidates and is increasingly viewed as a critical step in the protein biomarker development pipeline that bridges unbiased biomarker discovery to clinical qualification [117, 118].

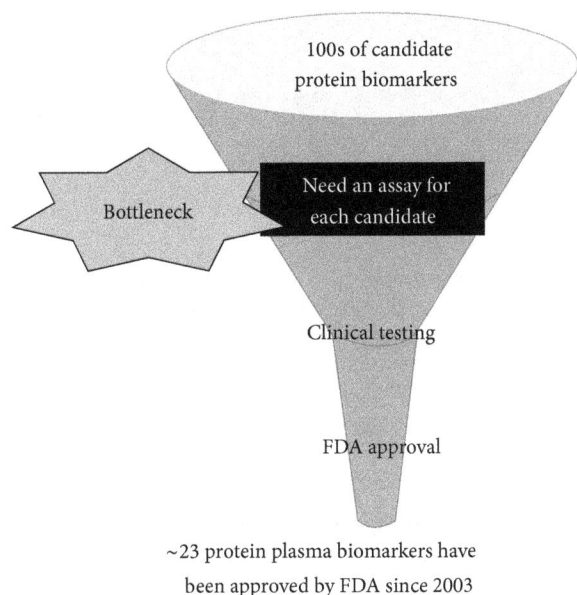

~23 protein plasma biomarkers have
been approved by FDA since 2003

Figure 2: The assay bottleneck prevents potential protein diagnostics from becoming clinically useful.

5.1. Selected Reaction Monitoring-MS (SRM-MS) and Multiple Reaction Monitoring-MS (MRM-MS).

SRM-MS is a targeted technique that is completely different from the mass spectrometry approaches widely used in discovery proteomics. SRM is performed on specialized instruments that enable targeting of specific analyte peptides of interest and provides exquisite specificity and sensitivity [119–121]. SRM-MS is a nonscanning mass spectrometry technique, performed on triple quadrupole-like instruments (QQQ-MS) and in which collision-induced dissociation (CID) is used as a means to increase selectivity. In SRM experiments two mass analyzers are used as static mass filters, to monitor a particular fragment ion of a selected precursor ion. Unlike common MS-based proteomics, no mass spectra are recorded in a SRM analysis. Instead, the detector acts as counting device for the ions matching the selected transition thereby returning an intensity value over time. In MRM, multiple SRM transitions can be measured within the same experiment on the chromatographic time scale by alternating between the different precursor/fragment pairs. Typically, the triple quadrupole instrument cycles through a series of transitions and records the signal of each transition as a function of the elution time. The method allows for additional selectivity by monitoring the chromatographic coelution of multiple transitions for a given analyte [122, 123]. A schematic representation of MRM-MS-based assay workflows (± immunoaffinity enrichment of proteins or peptides) is depicted in Figure 4 and described in the following sections.

5.2. MRM-MS-Based Assay Development for Protein Verification.

MRM-MS method for quantification of biomolecules has been long in use (e.g., drug metabolites [124, 125], hormones [126], protein degradation products [127], and pesticides [128]) with great precision (CV < 5%) but has only

recently been adopted for protein and peptide measurements. Stable isotope dilution (SID) multiple reaction monitoring MS (SID-MRM-MS) has emerged as one of the powerful targeted proteomic tools in the past few years. MRM mass spectrometry is being rapidly adopted by the biomedical research community as shown by increase in the number of publications in this area over the past decade (Figure 5). It has the advantage of accurately calculating protein concentrations in a multiplexed and high throughput manner, while avoiding many of the issues associated with antibody-based protein quantification [117]. SID-MRM-MS protein assays are based upon the quantitation of signature tryptic peptides as surrogates that uniquely represent the protein candidates of interest [129, 130]. To improve the specificity of the quantitative measurement for targeted analytes in MRM-based assays, a selection of three to five peptides per protein is selected [131]. Moreover, known quantities of synthetic stable isotope-labeled peptides (heavy peptides), corresponding to each endogenous peptide, are used as internal standard peptides (i.e., stable isotope-labeled internal standards or SIS). These SISs are identical to their endogenous analyte peptide counterparts with the exception of their masses (usually 6–10 Da more). For quantitation, specific fragment ion signals derived from the endogenous unlabeled peptides are compared to those from the spike-in SISs as ratios and are used to calculate the concentration of that protein [130, 131]. In SID-MRM-MS, the presence of SIS can calculate more accurate ratios with high sensitivity and across a wide dynamic range. The absence of an endogenous peptide signal typically means that the concentration of the peptide in the sample is below the detection limit of the instrument. Additionally the amount of SIS added should be optimized empirically in a preliminary study as this depends on the protein's individual relative abundance within a sample. High sensitivity and precision, combined with specific quantitation in a multiplex fashion, make MRM assays attractive for translational and clinical research [132, 133]. Targeted proteomics has also been recognized by the journal *Nature Methods* as the method of the year in 2012 [134].

There are many advantages to MRM-based assays which overcome major limitations of conventional protein assay technologies such as Western blot, IHC, and ELISA. Such advantages include moderate-to-high throughput capability, readily multiplexed assays, standards being readily synthesized, interferences being avoidable, use of internal standards for high interlaboratory reproducibility, and quantitation. Additionally, MRM assays have high molecular specificity, which does not require immunoassay-grade antibodies (those proteins for which no affinity reagent has been developed are accessible for routine quantification including isoforms and PTM analytes), and there is a large deployed instrument base. However, MRM assays are not easy to generate *de novo* and require expertise in addition to lack of validated reagents for most proteins [135, 136]. Over the past few years, the methods used to quantify proteins by MRM have steadily evolved and have been widely deployed. It has also been suggested recently that, considering the vast majority of protein identifications claimed from biological samples are still derived from Western blotting, it may be time

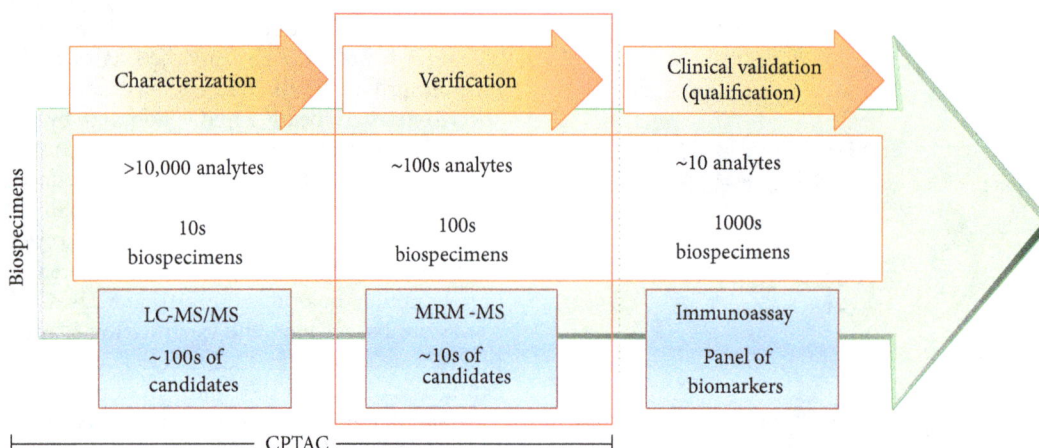

FIGURE 3: The incorporation of verification step into the NCI-CPTC pipeline bridging discovery and qualification.

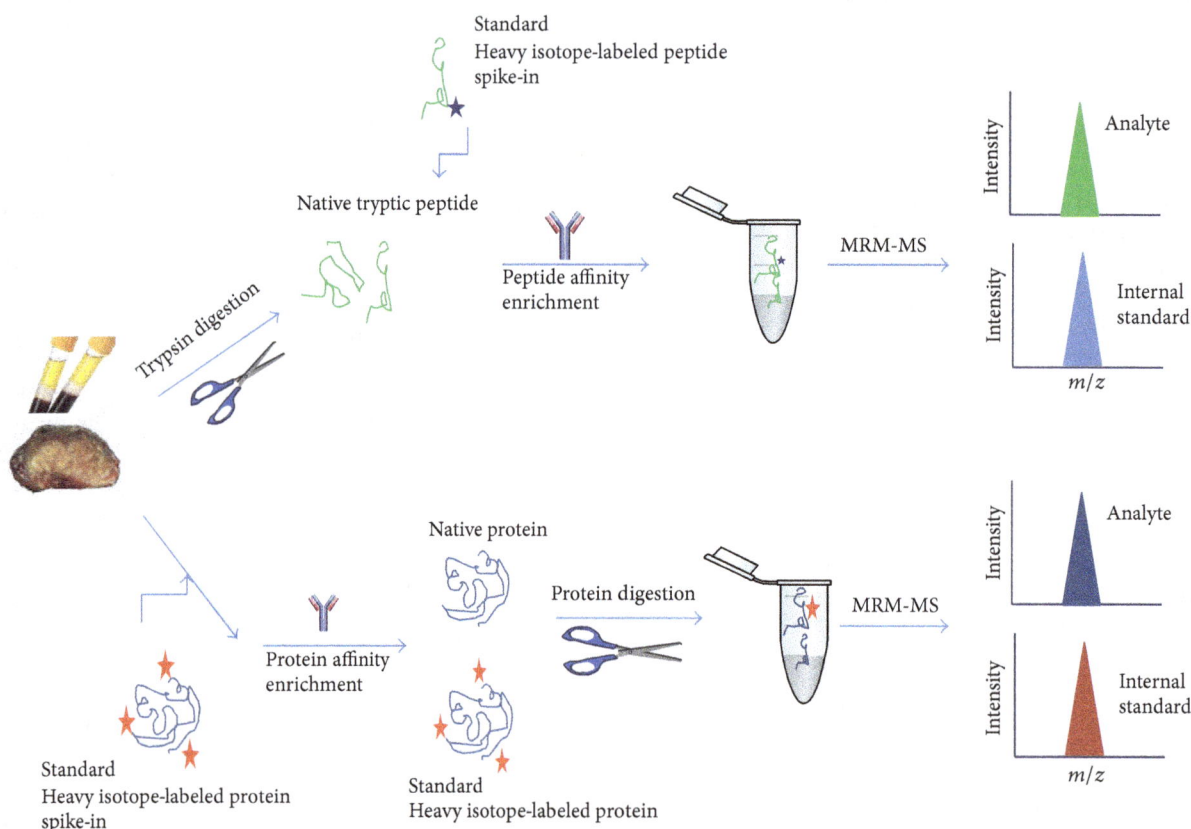

FIGURE 4: MRM-MS-based assay workflows (± immunoaffinity enrichment of proteins or peptides). SISCAPA workflow using proteolytic peptides as surrogates for their respective proteins, as illustrated in the top panel of the schematic, is a sensitive approach to measure protein concentrations using immunoaffinity enrichment of surrogate peptides prior to MRM-MS. To achieve quantitation of the targeted protein(s), they are digested to component peptides using an enzyme such as trypsin. A stable isotope standard (SIS, blue asterisk) is added to the sample at a known concentration for quantitative analysis. The selected peptides are then enriched using anti-peptide antibodies immobilized on a solid support. Following washing and elution from the anti-peptide antibody, the amount of surrogate peptide is measured relative to the stable isotope standard using targeted mass spectrometry. Alternatively, an assay can start with immunoaffinity enrichment of intact target proteins from biospecimens using an internal stable isotope-labeled protein standard (red asterisk, such as PSAQ approach) and an antibody, as illustrated in the bottom panel, followed by proteolysis and final quantitation of the target.

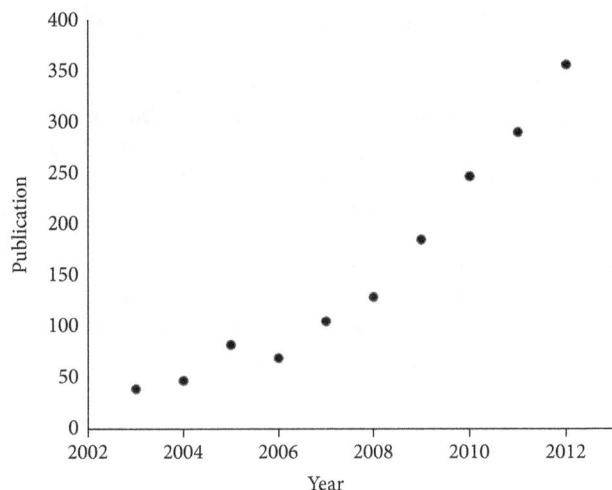

FIGURE 5: Increase in number of MRM publications in PubMed over the past decade.

that journal reviewers request that Western blotting results, or at least the assays that support these results, be validated by MS [136].

Recently in a landmark paper in *Nature Methods*, researchers have demonstrated the feasibility of both the development and application of MRM to reproducibly measure human proteins in breast cancer cell lysate across three labs in two countries in two continents. The international research collaboration, representing investigators from Fred Hutchinson Cancer Research Center (Seattle, Washington, USA), Broad Institute (Cambridge, Massachusetts, USA), and a team composed of researchers from the Korea Institute of Science and Technology and the Seoul National University College of Medicine (both Seoul, Republic of Korea), reported the development and application of 645 assays representing 319 proteins. The assays were deployed in multiplexed fashion in groups of at least 150 peptides to quantify proteins in a panel of breast cancer-related cell lines. Researchers were able to show that targeted mass spectrometry-based proteomic assay can be easily implemented anywhere, with minimal adjustments, while maintaining a high level of performance (accuracy, precision, and reproducibility), all essential for clinical implementation. Analyses of the results were able to recapitulate known molecular subtypes ascribed to breast cancer and also showed the added value of integrative analysis in identifying putative disease genes. This study demonstrates the tremendous promise on targeted proteomics to meet the interest of biologists and medical researchers and addresses the ability to replicate results from labs [137].

While adoption of targeted MS approaches such as MRM to study biological and biomedical questions is well underway in the proteomics community, there is no consensus on what criteria are acceptable and little understanding of the impact of variable criteria on the quality of the results generated. There is a wide range of criteria being applied to say that an assay has been successfully developed. Publications

describing targeted MS assays for peptides frequently do not contain sufficient information for readers to establish confidence that the tests work as intended or to be able to apply the tests described in their own labs. To address these issues, a workshop was held recently at the NIH with representatives from the multiple communities developing and employing targeted MS assays. Participants discussed the analytical goals of their experiments and the experimental evidence needed to establish that the assays they develop work as intended and are achieving the required levels of performance. Using this fit-for-purpose approach, the group defined three tiers of assays distinguished by their performance and extent of analytical characterization. Participants also detailed the information that authors need to provide in their manuscripts to enable reviewers and readers to clearly understand what procedures were performed and to evaluate the reliability of the peptide or protein quantification measurements reported [138].

5.3. Enriching Analytes to Increase the Sensitivity of MRM-MS Assays. Many analytes require enrichment for MRM-based quantification of endogenous levels such as most proteins in plasma, regulatory and signaling proteins in cells and tissues, and PTMs. Many clinically relevant biomarkers, such as prostate-specific antigen (PSA) and the troponins (Tns), are expressed in low ng/mL level in plasma below the lower limit of detection of a QQQ-MS. There have been reports of improving sensitivities by abundant protein depletion strategy combined with minimal fractionation or instrument modification which could further improve the LOD/LOQ of MRM measurements. For instance, antibody-based depletion columns combined with minimal fractionation of tryptic peptides have been shown to improve sensitivity for proteins in plasma [131, 139, 140]. Furthermore, enhanced sensitivity for SRM-MS targeted proteomics through enhanced ion transmission efficiency using a dual stage electrodynamic ion funnel interface has been reported [141]. In another development, Fortin et al. used MRM cubed (MRM^3), which enabled targeting protein biomarkers in the low nanogram/milliliter range in nondepleted human serum using a simple two-step workflow. This strategy takes advantage of the capability of a hybrid QQQ-MS/linear IT (LIT) mass spectrometer to further fragment the product ions monitored in Q3 [142].

5.4. PRISM. PRISM, reported very recently by Shi et al. [143], is an antibody-free strategy that involves high pressure, high resolution separations coupled with intelligent selection and multiplexing (PRISM) for sensitive selected reaction monitoring- (SRM-) based targeted protein quantification. The strategy uses high resolution reversed-phase liquid chromatographic separations for analyte enrichment, intelligent selection of target fractions via online SRM monitoring of internal standards, and fraction multiplexing before nanoliquid chromatography-SRM quantification [143]. This method has shown a major advance in the sensitivity of targeted protein quantification without the need for specific-affinity reagents. Applying this method to human plasma/serum demonstrated accurate and reproducible quantification of proteins at concentrations in the 50–100 pg/mL range. Excellent correlation between PRISM-SRM assay and those from clinical immunoassay for the prostate-specific antigen level was also noted [143]. A disadvantage of PRISM-SRM relative to SISCAPA (see Section 5.7) is reduced analytical throughput as a result of fractionation. However, even with limited fraction concatenation, moderate throughput (~50 sample analyses per week depending upon experimental details) can be achieved. For example, when quantifying a relatively large number of proteins (i.e., 100), all 96 fractions may contain target peptides; however, these fractions can still be carefully combined into 12 multiplexed fractions based on peptide elution times to achieve moderate throughput [143].

5.5. Parallel Reaction Monitoring (PRM).

PRM is a new targeted proteomics paradigm centered on the use of next generation, quadrupole-equipped high resolution and accurate mass instruments [144]. In PRM, made possible by the Q Exactive, the laborious development of SRM assays may be avoided. This instrument is similar to QQQ except that the third quadrupole is replaced with a high resolution, high mass accuracy Orbitrap mass analyzer. Whereas in SRM all transitions are monitored one at a time, the Q Exactive allows parallel detection of all transitions in a single analysis. Because all transitions can be monitored with PRM, one does not need to carry out laborious optimizations to generate idealized assays for selected transitions [145]. This will bring additional specificity because all potential product ions of a peptide, instead of just 3–5 transitions, are available to confirm the identity of the peptide [146] and that because PRM monitors all transitions, one need not have prior knowledge of, or preselect, target transitions before analysis. Also because many ions would be available, the presence of interfering ions in a full mass spectrum would be less problematic to overall spectral quality than interference in a narrow mass range [144]. In addition, the Q Exactive instrument is very flexible. Since one instrument can do both discovery and targeted analysis, this will allow researchers to use a discovery-based approach to identify a shortlist of interesting proteins and then use a targeted approach to follow those targets with high sensitivity under various conditions, all in a single experiment [145].

5.6. SWATH Acquisition.

SWATH (sequential window acquisition of all theoretical mass spectra) acquisition is a novel technique that is based on data-independent acquisition (DIA) which aims to complement traditional discovery MS-based proteomics techniques and SRM methods [147]. In this strategy systematic queries of sample sets are made for the presence and quantity of any protein of interest. It consists of using the information available in fragment ion spectral libraries to mine the complete fragment ion maps generated using a data-independent acquisition method. In SWATH acquisition, the first quadrupole sequentially cycles 25 Da precursor isolation windows (swaths) across the mass range of interest and time-resolves fragment ion spectra for all the analytes detectable [147, 148] and therefore the potential to perform a significant larger number of SRM-like experiments concurrently. In SWATH-MS approach, the instrumental scanning speed has to be fast enough to allow acquiring an adequate number of data points across the typical chromatographic peak such that ion chromatography can be reconstructed with acceptable signal-to-noise ratio. SWATH acquisition, however, has a major drawback in that the data is incompatible with conventional database searching, and it seems a deconvolution algorithm to process the SWATH-MS data for database searching has not been achieved. There are a number of challenges in designing a deconvolution algorithm to process such complex data [148].

5.7. Protein Capture Enrichment.

An alternative approach to immunoaffinity depletion (negative enrichment) and fractionation strategies is positive enrichment strategies which have also been extensively explored in proteomics for better detection of low-abundance peptides or proteins. These strategies include affinity enrichment of peptides or proteins and chemical enrichment of different subsets of the proteome including PTMs such as N-linked glycopeptides and phosphopeptides. Many of the enrichment strategies reported for general proteomics are also applicable to SRM applications.

Immunoaffinity capture of target proteins is probably the most effective method for sensitive detection of low-abundance proteins in complex samples [149, 150]. The immunoaffinity enrichment method coupled with MS has provided quantification of proteins in the low ng/mL range [151–153]. Nicol et al. [151] have demonstrated the immunoaffinity-SRM approach for the quantification of protein biomarkers for which ELISA assays are not available from lung cancer patients by using antibodies to enrich proteins, followed by digestion of captured proteins and subsequent SRM analysis. This approach enabled the quantification of multiple protein biomarkers in lung cancer and normal human sera in the low ng/mL range. In a different study, Kulasingam et al. reported the enrichment of endogenous PSA protein from 5 μL of serum with a monoclonal antibody (mAb) followed by product ion monitoring using a linear ion-trap mass spectrometer [152] demonstrating quantification of PSA down to less than 1 ng/mL level with acceptable CVs. Recently, Niederkofler et al. [154] developed an assay that incorporates a novel sample preparation method for dissociating IGF1 from its binding proteins. The workflow also includes an immunoaffinity step using antibody-derivatized pipette tips, followed by elution, trypsin digestion, and LC-MS/MS separation and detection of the signature peptides in SRM mode. The resulting quantitative mass spectrometric immunoassay (MSIA) exhibited good linearity in the range of 1 to 1,500 ng/mL IGF1, intra- and interassay precision with CVs of less than 10%, and lowest limits of detection of 1 ng/mL [154]. Additionally, intact protein targets from samples, along with their recombinant heavy isotope-labeled internal protein standards, such as protein standard absolute quantification (PSAQ) approach [155–157] can be immunoprecipitated with antibodies prior to proteolysis and SID-MRM-MS. In 2004, Nelson et al. described an immunoaffinity-based MALDI-TOF MS method for quantification of IGF1 from human plasma samples [158]. The limit of detection for the IGF-1 MSIA was evaluated and established to be approximately 15 pM.

An important application of protein enrichment method could be in detection and measurement of mutant proteins. Genome-wide analysis has shown that solid tumors typically contain 20–100 protein-encoding genes that are mutated [159]. A small fraction of these changes are "drivers" as cancer causing events; the remainder is "passengers," providing no selective growth advantage [160]. These proteins could be source of unique biomarker candidates. Unlike wild type protein biomarkers the mutant proteins are produced only by tumor cells. Moreover, they are not simply associated with tumors, but in the case of driver gene mutations are directly responsible for tumor generation [161]. A large number of disease-causing mutations are missense mutations that alter the encoded proteins only subtly, the detection of which can be very complicated mainly because there are few antibodies that can reliably distinguish mutant from normal versions of proteins. Because many different mutations can occur in a single cancer-related gene, it is necessary to develop a specific antibody for each possible mutant epitope which can be costly and time-consuming. Another approach measures the activity of mutant proteins but it is not generally applicable because no activity-based assays are available for most proteins. MS has been previously used to detect and quantify somatic mutations at the DNA level but not at the protein level [162]. To address this need, Vogelstein lab [161] developed an MS approach that could identify and quantify somatically mutant proteins in a generally applicable fashion. Using Ras and its mutants (most mutations clustered at residues 12 or 13 of the protein), they immunoprecipitated the Ras protein from human colorectal cancer cell line SW480 and it was then eluted and concentrated. More than 90% of the total cellular K-Ras protein was captured successfully from the lysates and eluted from the beads. Upon digestion and inclusion of heavy isotope-labeled synthetic peptides as internal controls, SRM was performed. The list of parent and product ions that were used for SRM included those representing trypsinized normal (WT) Ras protein as well as the two most common mutants of Ras in pancreatic cancers, K-Ras G12V and G12D. The summed peak intensities for the ions corresponding to the heavy and light versions of peptides representing WT and mutant proteins showed that they were related linearly to abundance across more than two orders of magnitude (10–2,000 fmol; $^2R > 0.99$ for WT and mutant proteins) [161]. Similarly, they found that mutant Ras proteins could be detected and quantified in clinical specimens such as colorectal and pancreatic tumor tissues as well as in premalignant pancreatic cyst fluids. In addition to answering basic questions about the relative levels of genetically abnormal proteins in tumors, this approach could prove useful for diagnostic applications. One potential limitation of this method is its sensitivity. Results from Vogelstein report estimated that SRM can be used to detect mutant proteins reliably when they are present at levels as low as 25 fmol/mg of total protein (~6,000 cells). However, this sensitivity may be inadequate to detect mutant proteins

in some clinical samples, such as sputum, serum, or urine [161]. As indicated above while the affinity MS approaches can improve the sensitivity for quantification of low-abundance proteins or mutants, the major drawback of protein capture method is that antibodies are typically not available for newly discovered biomarker candidates. The need for different antibodies for individual proteins inherently limits the multiplexing power and the throughput for quantifying a large number of target proteins when employing affinity MS approaches.

5.8. Peptide Capture Enrichment. An alternative for protein enrichment is to affinity capture for target peptides using anti-peptide antibodies, in which target peptides act as surrogates for protein quantification. Anderson et al. [163] introduced this method in 2004 using immobilized anti-peptide polyclonal rabbit antibodies to capture and, subsequently, elute the target peptides of four blood plasma proteins along with isotope-labeled peptide standards for MS quantification. This strategy, termed stable isotope standards and capture by anti-peptide antibodies (SISCAPA), and recent studies suggested that more than a 1000-fold enrichment can be achieved for plasma-digested peptides [164] with low ng/mL LOQs in plasma with CVs < 20% [141]. If stable isotope-labeled recombinant protein standard is available, it can be added to the biofluid in the beginning of the assay workflow to control for proteolytic efficiency. Upon digestion of the biospecimens and addition of known amounts of SIS, both spike-in and endogenous peptides are specifically enriched and their relative amounts are quantitated by MRM-MS. MS detector provides quantitation through peak areas for targeted m/z values. The SISCAPA strategy has been further optimized using a magnetic-bead-based platform, which can be performed in an automated fashion using 96-well plates [164, 165]. This strategy was implemented in a nine-target peptide multiplexed SISCAPA assay in which more sensitive detection in the 50–100 pg/mL range of protein concentration was reported when plasma volume was increased from 10 μL to 1 mL for SISCAPA enrichment [166].

One advantage of mAbs over polyclonal antibodies in SISCAPA assays is their higher specificity and as such Schoenherr et al. demonstrated that mAbs can be configured in SISCAPA assays and reported a platform for automated screening of mAbs [167]. In another more recent report, MALDI immunoscreening (MiSCREEN) was developed, enabling rapid screening and selection of high affinity anti-peptide mAbs [168]. In other studies immuno-MALDI (iMALDI) was used where affinity-bound peptides on a MALDI utilize MALDI matrix solvents to elute the bound peptides from the beads and the resultant peak height or peak area of the peptide from an MS spectrum is used for quantitation [169, 170]. While iMALDI can be performed with only a MALDI-MS instrument, it can also be used in the MRM mode on a MALDI-MS/MS instrument (iMALDI$^+$) [171].

Despite sensitivity, multiplexing, and throughput, some limitations of SISCAPA include a relatively high cost of Ab generation; long lead time (~24 weeks for assay generation) for SRM assay development [172]; success rate for producing potent antibodies as well as the potentially low peptide capture rate [166]; and background bead nonspecific binding.

The SISCAPA strategy has been also deployed in a clinical setting where the potential of the SISCAPA-SRM assays was illustrated by Hoofnagle et al., who implemented SISCAPA assays for quantification of low-abundance serum thyroglobulin, and simultaneous measurement of apolipoprotein A–I and apolipoprotein B [133, 173].

In collaboration with the Fred Hutchinson Cancer Research Center, Bio-Rad Laboratories has developed a SISCAPA training/QC kit which is currently in beta testing. The kit enables researchers who are new to the SISCAPA technique to implement an assay in their lab and gain experience with the process. Based on an assay for a murine osteopontin (OPN) peptide in a human plasma matrix, the kit provides researchers with the reagents and information needed for carrying out an assay, including a detailed standard operating procedure, antibody, heavy and light peptides, magnetic beads, and other necessary buffers and reagents. Results will be comparable to expected values, making the kit a valuable resource for quality control of the SISCAPA process.

5.9. MRM Reference Libraries. Access to reference spectral fragmentation libraries of proteotypic peptides and chromatographic retention time would be extremely useful for the generation of maximal product ion signal and the proteomics community in MRM-MS assay development. Skyline [174] and MRMer [175] are two open source software for developing MRM-MS-based assays by the proteomics community. Skyline (downloadable from https://brendanx-uwl.gs.washington.edu/labkey/project/home/software/Skyline/begin .view can be integrated with all major instrument platforms and has been used to design MRM-MS assays and support data analysis including SIS. Skyline supports all major publicly available spectral libraries such as the GPM, National Institute of Standards and Technology (NIST), and the Institute for Systems Biology. Library files from these sources can be downloaded and searched with the Skyline Spectral Library Explorer, to help choose peptide precursor and product ions to monitor specific proteins of interest [174]. MRMer was developed for organizing highly complex MRM-MS experiments, including quantitative analyses using heavy/light isotopic peptide pairs, and has the capability of importing data in a platform-independent mzXML format. MRMer extracts and infers precursor-product ion transition pairings, computes integrated ion intensities, and permits rapid visual curation for analyses exceeding 1000 precursor-product pairs [175].

Automated and targeted analysis with quantitative SRM (ATAQS) [176] is another open source software which supports MRM assay development (http://tools.proteomecenter.org/ATAQS/ATAQS.html). ATAQS is an integrated software platform that supports all stages of targeted, SRM-based proteomics experiments including target selection, transition optimization, and postacquisition data analysis. This software has the potential to significantly facilitate the use of targeted proteomic techniques and contribute to the generation of highly sensitive, reproducible, and complete datasets that are particularly critical for the discovery and validation of targets

in hypothesis-driven studies in systems biology. ATAQS also provides software API (application program interface) documentation that enables the addition of new algorithms to each of the workflow steps [176]. mProphet is another fully automated system that computes accurate error rates for the identification of targeted peptides in SRM data sets and maximizes specificity and sensitivity by combining relevant features in the data into a statistical model [177].

Another important source of targeted proteomic assays is SRMAtlas, which enables detection and quantification of proteins in complex proteomes (http://www.mrmatlas.org/) [178]. The information in this database results from MRM-MS measurements of natural and synthetic peptides performed on a QQQ-MS. Currently, this database allows users to query transitions from peptides from yeast, human, and mouse species obtained from QQQ-MS instruments, supplemented with ion trap (IT) observations and predictions where QQQ spectra are unavailable. An algorithm called automated detection of inaccurate and imprecise transitions (AuDIT) has been developed that can assist in MRM by automatically identifying inaccurate transition data based on the observation of interfering signal or inconsistent recovery among replicates [179]. This algorithm evaluates MRM-MS data by comparing the relative product ion intensities of the analyte peptide to those of the SIS peptides, followed by a t-test to determine any significant difference. The algorithm has already demonstrated the capability of identifying problematic transitions and achieving accuracies of 94–100% for the correct identification of errant transitions [179].

5.10. Assay Portal Community Resource. While many MRM-based assays have been published, the information is dispersed throughout the literature, and protocols for characterization of assay performances have not been standardized. Furthermore the use of MRM and its potential utility have not been realized by the biological and clinical research communities. To address these issues, the Clinical Proteomic Tumor Analysis Consortium (CPTAC 2) of the NCI has launched an assay portal to serve as a public resource of well-characterized quantitative mass spectrometry-based proteomic assays with associated SOPs, reagents, and assay validation data (http://assays.cancer.gov/). The portal database is tied to Panorama, an open source platform allowing for efficient collection and sharing of data in a vendor-neutral format. SOPs describing sample preparations are also available for download for each assay. Data quality is a major emphasis of the portal. Guidelines for MRM assay "fit-for-purpose" validation have also been established within the NCI-funded CPTAC 2, with input from the outside community solicited via a workshop [138]. To ensure uniform presentation and adequate data for establishing the accepted performance of the assays, a guidance document describing the minimal characterization data required for assay inclusion in the CPTAC assay portal has been made available for download on the portal. Five experiments of assay validation are described. Experiments 1 and 2 contain information on the assay sensitivity and linear range (determined through a response curve) and the repeatability (determined by analyzing validation samples on multiple days) and are the minimal validation requirement to qualify for inclusion in the CPTAC assay portal. A higher level of validation contains additional experiments to measure the selectivity, stability, and detection of endogenous analyte. At the time of launch, the portal contains ~462 assays with characterization data and SOPs. The CPTAC program will add several hundred more assays over the next 2-3 years, and, in the near future, the portal will be open for contributions from the community at large. The portal is able to accept data from any targeted mass spectrometry-based quantification method.

6. Proteomic Reproducibility and Standardization

Resistance about the validity of proteomics analyses persisted for several years in the late 90s and early 2000s. This stemmed partly from some questionable work in the pioneering years of large-scale protein identification. Many of the early landmark papers in the last 10–15 years were obtained on low-resolution instruments and without proper statistical analysis [44]. It was later found that a large proportion of the identifications obtained from such studies were false positives [180]. Many of the early problems were ascribed to the use of SELDI resulting from poor analytical technique with significant reproducibility issues. Some high profile papers were later shown to be invalid, which tainted the whole field for a while. For example a method for early ovarian cancer diagnosis was reported by a group of outstanding investigators that used mass spectrometry to detect proteomic patterns from serum samples in 2002. The reported sensitivities and specificities were approximately 100%, even for serum from patients with early-stage ovarian cancer [181]. This paper has received a few thousand citations since its publications [182]. The combination of quality investigators, the high profile journal that published the data, and a powerful editorial generated widespread media coverage and euphoria that a new era in cancer diagnostics has started. However, reports of methodological shortcomings of this method and questions about its validity were published soon after its publication [183–185]. Subsequently, others have identified bioinformatic artifacts and issues regarding variations in sample collection and storage that compromised the conclusions of the paper [184]. Despite positive publications that used similar approaches for other cancer types [186, 187], an independent validation study of this method for prostate cancer diagnosis, sponsored by Early Detection Research Network, has shown that the method does not reliably detect prostate cancer [188].

The issue of reproducibility was further exacerbated when Bergeron and colleagues published a study in 2009 [189]. The researchers sent standardized samples containing 20 known proteins to 27 labs for proteomics analysis. Each protein contained one or more unique tryptic peptides, which should have shown up in MS analysis. Only 7 out of the 27 labs initially reported all 20 proteins correctly, and only one saw all the proteotypic peptides. Yet centralized analysis of the raw data revealed that all 20 proteins and most of the peptides had been detected in all 27 labs. The message of this study was that, irrespective of instrumental method, the technology delivers high quality MS data. In contrast, this centralized

analysis determined missed identifications (false negatives), environmental contamination, database matching, and curation of protein identifications as sources of problems. One suggestion was that improved search engines and databases were needed for mass spectrometry-based proteomics [189].

In a separate study, the proteomics research group of the Association of Biomolecular Resource Facilities (ABRF) sponsored a number of research studies designed to enable participants to try new techniques and assess their capabilities relative to other laboratories analyzing the same samples. This study was designed to explore the use of different approaches for determining quantitative differences for several target proteins in human plasma that were centrally prepared. These results provide a cross-sectional view of current methodologies as well as a vehicle for sharing information regarding experimental protocols and education for the proteomics community and highlight that establishing good laboratory practices is important [190]. ABRF effort to assess individual laboratory's platforms, methods, and results was one of the first attempts to address variability in sample preparation and processing on different proteomic platforms.

To address many of the critical challenges in proteomics including the lack of an ability to accurately and reproducibly measure a meaningful number of proteins in biospecimens across laboratories, the National Cancer Institute (NCI) launched the Clinical Proteomic Technologies for Cancer (CPTC) in 2006 (http://proteomics.cancer.gov/). The overall goals of CPTC were focused on removing several of the major barriers in proteomics research to enable the accurate, efficient, and reproducible identification and quantification of meaningful numbers of proteins that could drive high value protein quantitation and qualification studies. Achieving this goal would provide a firm foundation for the field of discovery proteomics and enable the rational development of clinical biomarkers to address various needs in cancer drug development, diagnostics, and clinical management. CPTC took a multidisciplinary, multi-institutional approach through its CPTAC 1 network in addressing the long-standing problems of variability issues in proteomics resulting in large measurement noise from analytical platforms rather than assessing real biological differences. CPTAC 1 carried out the first quantitative assessment of discovery proteomics technology platforms across laboratories defining a set of performance standards for identifying the sources of variability [191–193], developed a standard yeast proteome reference material available to the community through NIST for investigators to benchmark their own performance [191, 194], and developed a quality control tool to monitor and troubleshoot instrument performance (http://peptide.nist.gov/software/nist_msqc_pipeline/NIST_MSQC_Pipeline.html). The yeast protein extract (RM8323) developed by NIST under the auspices of NCI's CPTC initiative is currently available to the public (https://www-s.nist.gov/srmors/view_detail.cfm?srm=8323) and offers researchers a unique biological reference material. RM8323 is the most extensively characterized complex biological proteome and the only one associated with several large-scale studies to estimate protein abundance across a wide concentration range. The yeast protein extract and its associated reference datasets [191, 194] can be used by the research community for benchmarking instrument detection efficiency for analysis of complex biological proteomes, to improve upon current methods and to evaluate new platforms when developed.

To address the issue of reproducibility in targeted proteomics, CPTAC 1 also spearheaded a multi-institutional study composed of three substudies designed to increase the level of complexity in sample preparation at eight individual sites [135]. Intralaboratory variability and reproducibility in all three substudies were evaluated by comparing the measured concentrations of seven target proteins (human C-reactive protein, PSA, aprotinin, leptin, myoglobin, myelin basic protein, and peroxidase) to the actual concentrations across the range of spiked-in analytes (a total of nine concentration points with LOQ at 2.92 nM, that is, 73.3 ng/mL for C-reactive protein) and by determining the CVs for these quantitative measurements. The results showed that the reproducibility and precision of these quantitative measurements for nine of ten peptides tested across eight laboratories ranged from 4 to 14%, 4 to 13%, and 10 to 23% interlaboratory CVs at or near the estimated LOQ of 2.92 nM for studies I, II, and III, respectively. Intralaboratory CVs were usually <15% and <25% at the identical concentration for studies I, II, and III. The incremental increases in CVs indicate that sample handling contributes more to assay variability than instrumental variability. Robotic automation of sample handling can furthermore improve analytical variability. Very recently, CPTAC 1 teams developed a system suitability protocol (SSP), which employs a predigested mixture of six proteins, to facilitate performance evaluation of LC-SID-MRM-MS instrument platforms, configured with nanoflow-LC systems interfaced to triple quadrupole mass spectrometers [195]. The SSP was designed for use with low multiplex analyses as well as high multiplex approaches when software-driven scheduling of data acquisition is required. Performance was assessed by monitoring of a range of chromatographic and mass spectrometric metrics including peak width, chromatographic resolution, peak capacity, and the variability in peak area and analyte retention time (RT) stability. The SSP, which was evaluated in 11 laboratories on a total of 15 different instruments, enabled early diagnoses of LC and MS anomalies that indicated suboptimal LC-MRM-MS performance. Robust LC-SID-MRM-MS-based assays that can be replicated across laboratories and ultimately in clinical laboratory settings require standardized protocols to demonstrate that the analysis platforms are performing adequately and therefore use of a SSP helps to ensure that analyte quantification measurements can be replicated with good precision within and across multiple laboratories and should facilitate more widespread use of MRM-MS technology by the basic biomedical and clinical laboratory research communities.

7. Clearance of MS-Based Platforms for Clinical Use

As indicated previously a typical protein biomarker discovery pipeline has three phases: discovery, verification, and clinical validation. The discovery work often uses research-grade samples from underpowered cohorts with limited sample numbers. Promising candidates from the discovery phase are verified by analyzing their performance in medium-sized clinical cohorts ($n > 100$) using standardized analytical platforms. Assays are then developed to validate the top performing candidates in larger clinical cohorts ($n > 200$). Ultimately, the utility of the validated candidates for routine clinical use is demonstrated in a clinical setting (improvement over gold standard diagnosis, cost, clinical outcomes, etc.) [196]. The path from development of biomarkers to clinical practices could take many possible steps. However, it is unequivocal that, prior to clinical use, any biomarkers have to prove their safety and efficacy in independent clinical trials using an appropriate study population for a clearly defined intended use. Three issues that are the key links in the path from discovered candidates to actual clinical diagnostics include generation of sufficient and portable evidence in preliminary validation studies; defining clinical utility for regulatory approval; and selecting/developing assays with analytical performance suitable for clinical deployment [197].

While proteomic methods may not yet be ready for implementation in routine clinical chemistry laboratories, the goal seems attainable in the near future [20]. Currently, LC-MS instruments are widely used in clinical laboratories for diagnosis of inborn errors of metabolism or for therapeutic drug monitoring and toxicology. MALDI-TOF-MS profiling methods have been recently implemented very successfully in clinical microbiology laboratories for simpler samples such as microbial colonies for identification of microorganisms, thus proving the validity of the approach [20]. BioMérieux recently announced US FDA clearance for VITEK MS, an evolutionary technology which reduces microbial identification from days to minutes (http://www.biomerieux-usa.com). VITEK MS is the first clinical mass spectrometry MALDI-TOF-based system available in the US for rapid identification of disease-causing bacteria and yeast. VITEK MS accuracy was compared to 16S ribosomal RNA gene sequencing, the gold standard, for a number of microbial categories. The overall accuracy of VITEK MS compared to nucleic acid sequencing for these organisms was 93.6 percent.

In addition, Bruker Corporation recently announced that it has been granted US FDA clearance under section 510(k) to market its MALDI Biotyper CA System in the United States for the identification of Gram negative bacterial colonies cultured from human specimens (http://www.bruker.com/). The *MALDI Biotyper* enables molecular identification and taxonomical classification or dereplication of microorganisms like bacteria, yeasts, and fungi. This is achieved using proteomic fingerprinting by high throughput MALDI-TOF mass spectrometry. The *MALDI Biotyper* uses specific proteomic fingerprints from bacterial strains. However, human protein analysis represents a level of complexity over drugs or bacterial proteins, thereby imposing particular constraints.

Another proteomic test that has been recently cleared by FDA is OVA1. OVA1 test is an *in vitro* Diagnostic Multivariate Index Assay (IVDMIA) for assessing ovarian cancer risk in women diagnosed with ovarian tumor prior to a planned surgery. OVA1 analyzes 5 proteomic biomarkers in serum and the results are combined through an algorithm to yield a single-valued index within the range of 0–10. OVA1 provides additional information to assist in identifying patients for referral to a gynecologic oncologist. In a prospective multiple-center clinical study, the addition of OVA1 in preoperative clinical assessment was found to improve sensitivity in the prediction of malignancy for ovarian tumor. OVA1 is intended to assess preoperatively the risk of ovarian cancer in women scheduled for surgery due to suspected ovarian cancer. The test result aids in the decision to refer the patient to a gynecologic oncologist for surgery for better long-term outcome [197].

To empower the scientific community with the right tools and to serve as a preview of the regulatory mindset and direction for multiplex protein assays, NCI's CPTAC 1 submitted 2 protein-based multiplex assay descriptions to the Office of In Vitro Diagnostic Device Evaluation and Safety of the FDA. The objective was to evaluate the analytical measurement criteria and studies needed to validate protein-based multiplex assays. Each submission described a different protein-based platform: a multiplex immunoaffinity mass spectrometry platform for protein quantification and an immunological array platform quantifying glycoprotein isoforms. Submissions provided a mutually beneficial way for members of the proteomics and regulatory communities to identify the analytical issues that the field should address when developing protein-based multiplex clinical assays. The goal of these submissions was to demonstrate the process and interactions between the sponsor and the FDA in a fashion similar to how they would proceed generally. Additionally, the feedback provided by the FDA generates some insight into the review issues that are relevant to these types of tests. Because the sponsors of the 2 mock submissions did not submit full responses and appropriate data, and because they submitted hypothetical data in large part, many issues and problems were not mentioned and discussed. For these reasons, this document is not meant to be inclusive of all the requirements for any future submission that would be made to the FDA [198].

To propel the adaptation of proteomics in clinical chemistry, important developments in workflows and instrumentation are necessary before various proteomic methods can compete with protein immunoassays performed on high throughput immunoanalyzers. The best chance for short-term application of proteomic methods in clinical chemistry laboratories will most likely be to capitalize on specific aspects of proteomic analysis such as targeting new types of biomarkers [199, 200] and offering new diagnostic solutions for orphan clinical problems [201]. In this context, SRM appears as potential alternative to classical immunoassays by combining analytical specificity and reliable quantification as described before. Among the advantages of SRM methods over classical immunoassays is the possibility of applying multiple protein tests on a single instrument without relying on commercial reagents. SRM thus can offer opportunities for measuring biomarkers in specific clinical areas that do not represent large markets for diagnostic industries. It might also be a way to reduce reagent costs such as antibodies borne by clinical laboratories. Therefore, the project for developing reliable SRM assays for a large set of human proteins is clearly of great interest [202]. It could promote broader access to this technology and, in turn, greatly facilitate application to clinical studies and increased use within clinical chemistry laboratories.

8. Proteogenomics

Proteogenomics, the integration of proteomic and genomic data, has recently emerged as a significant area of activity in proteomics as a promising potential approach to Omics research. The notion is based on the premise that protein data can shed light on the consequence of various genomic features, allowing researchers to determine, for example, whether or not a specific genetic variant may actually become a functional protein. Independently or as part of large-scale initiatives, a number of researchers are pursuing such studies including CPTAC 2, TCGA, and the National Human Genome Research Institute's Encyclopedia of DNA Elements Consortium (ENCODE). To a large degree, this surge in activity on the proteogenomics studies originates from advances within proteomics that have made it feasible to obtain coverage comparable to that achieved by genomics and transcriptomics. A requirement for good systems biology studies is the need to have good enough coverage in proteomics. In the last few years, obtaining coverage in the range of 10,000 to 12,000 proteins has become routine for some labs [203, 204]. In their recent work, for instance, Lehtiö and his colleagues identified 13,078 human and 10,637 mouse proteins including 39,941 peptides not previously present in the Peptide Atlas' human dataset. They also identified 224 novel human and 122 novel mouse peptides, which mapped to 164 and 101 genomic loci, respectively [205]. Using high resolution isoelectric focusing (HiRIEF) at the peptide level in the 3.7–5.0 pH range and accurate peptide isoelectric point (pI) prediction, Lehtiö probed the six-reading-frame translation of the human and mouse genomes and identified 98 and 52 previously undiscovered protein-coding loci, respectively [205].

In a separate study, Heck and his colleagues have completed a proteogenomics study of rat liver tissue, integrating whole genome sequencing, RNA-seq, and mass spec-based proteomics [206]. In this study the researchers identified 13,088 proteins, making it one of the most comprehensive proteome analyses performed to date. Integrating their genomics data, they were also able to validate 1,195 gene predictions, 83 splice events, 120 proteins with nonsynonymous variants, and 20 protein isoforms with nonsynonymous RNA editing. The effort also provided several biological insights such as the question of RNA editing—a process in which modifications are made to the sequence of an RNA molecule after it has been generated. While they indicate that RNA editing may occur, they may not often lead to a stable protein [206]. Enhancing mass spec sequence coverage as well as robust data analysis pipeline may further improve our protein variant detection.

Leveraging large-scale cancer genomics datasets, NCI is leveraging its investment in genomics through CPTAC 2, which is applying proteomic technologies to systematically identify proteins from genomically characterized tumors, such as those from TCGA program. The goal of the CPTAC 2 program is to illuminate the complex proteogenomic relationship between genomic (DNA, RNA) and proteomic (protein) abnormalities, thus producing a deeper understanding of cancer biology. The CPTAC 2 program is analyzing more than 300 samples from colorectal, breast, and ovarian cancer. A key component of the consortium is developing novel methods to integrate and visualize proteomic and genomic data to better comprehend the biological processes of the cell. The integration of terabytes of genomic and proteomic data is catalyzing the development of new computational tools and also leveraging findings from other fields such as machine learning and computer science to better understand biological processes. After this analysis, proteins of interest are selected as targets for highly reproducible and transportable assays. All of the data and resulting assays are made publicly available to help advance research in cancer biology and improve patient care. The first set of proteogenomic data were released in September 2013 (http://proteomics.cancer.gov/).

Technological advances in both the proteomics and genomics now provide the ability to discriminate genetic and posttranscriptional polymorphisms at the proteome level. The synergistic use of genomic, transcriptomic, and proteomic technologies significantly improves the data that can be gained from proteomics as well as genomics efforts. By matching deep MS-based proteomics to a personalized database built from a sample-specific genome and transcriptome, thousands of peptides that would otherwise escape identification can be identified. Such powerful tools and data demonstrate the power of and need for integrative proteogenomic analysis for understanding genetic control of molecular dynamics and phenotypic diversity in a system-wide manner which appears to be the future direction [206].

9. Concluding Remarks

The acceleration of biological knowledge through the mapping of HGP has resulted in the development of new high throughput next-generation sequencing (NGS) techniques. NGS analyses such as whole genome sequencing (WGS) and total RNA sequencing (RNA-seq) cannot however predict with high confidence the effects on the proteins and their variations including composition, function, and expression levels. Therefore, the completion of the HGP has also presented the new challenge of human proteome characterization using MS-based proteomics. Each of these technologies is capable of comprehensive measurements of gene products at a system level [207, 208]. Although MS and NGS are highly complementary, they have not yet effectively been integrated in large-scale studies [209] and sparsely performed in organisms with smaller genomes [210]. To correctly delineate the effects of genomic and transcriptomic variation on molecular processes and cellular functioning, integrative analyses of different data types, ideally derived from the same samples,

are required [211]. The integration and interrogation of the proteomic and genomic data will provide potential biomarker candidates which will be prioritized for downstream targeted proteomic analysis. These biomarker targets will be used to create multiplex, quantitative assays for verification and prescreening to test the relevance of the targets in clinically relevant and unbiased samples. The outcomes from this approach will provide the community with verified biomarkers which could be used for clinical qualification studies; high quality and publicly accessible datasets; and analytically validated, multiplex, quantitative protein/peptide assays and their associated high quality reagents for the research and clinical community.

State-of-the-art MS approaches can routinely identify over 10,000 proteins in a single experiment [203, 204] which suggests that the analysis of complete proteomes is within reach [212]. The comprehensive human proteome project however still faces challenges including very large number of proteins with PTMs, mutations, splice variants, the variety of technology platforms, and sensitivity limitations in detecting proteins and aberrations present in low abundances. Future proteomic undertakings should continue to support technology development, optimization, and standardization. Incorporation of the most up-to-date and efficient technologies is critical in successfully advancing the translation of proteomic findings into clinically relevant biomarkers. Meanwhile, rigorous assessment of biospecimen and data quality through quality assessment criteria at each step of the biomarker development pipeline should continue to be supported. These efforts, combined with continued collaborations with regulatory agencies and clinical chemists, will expedite the development of individualized patient care through clinical proteomics.

Abbreviations

SRM-MS:	Selected reaction monitoring-MS
MRM-MS:	Multiple reaction monitoring-MS
TCGA:	The Cancer Genome Atlas
CPTC:	Clinical Proteomic Technologies for Cancer
CPTAC 1:	Clinical Proteomic Technology Assessment for Cancer
CPTAC 2:	Clinical Proteomic Tumor Analysis Consortium
PTMs:	Posttranslational modifications
ESI-LC-MS:	Electrospray ionization-liquid chromatography tandem mass spectroscopy
MALDI-TOF:	Matrix assisted laser desorption ionization time of flight
SELDI-TOF:	Surface enhanced laser desorption ionization time of flight
MALDI-MSI:	MALDI MS imaging
2-DE:	Two-dimensional gel electrophoresis
LCM-MS:	Laser capture microdissection-MS
SILAC:	Stable isotope labeling with amino acids in cell culture

SISCAPA: Stable isotope standards and capture by anti-peptide antibodies
PSAQ: Protein standard absolute quantification
SID: Stable isotope dilution
SIS: Stable isotope-labelled internal standard
QQQ-MS: Triple quadrupole mass spectrometer
HGP: Human genome project
FDA: Food and Drug Administration
PRM: Parallel reaction monitoring.

Disclaimer

The views expressed in this paper are the employee's and do not represent the National Institutes of Health.

Conflict of Interests

The author declares that there is no conflict of interests regarding the publication of this paper.

References

[1] J. Potash and K. C. Anderson, "Announcing the AACR cancer progress report 2013," *Clinical Cancer Research*, vol. 19, p. 5545, 2013.

[2] B. Pradet-Balade, F. Boulmé, H. Beug, E. W. Müllner, and J. A. Garcia-Sanz, "Translation control: bridging the gap between genomics and proteomics?" *Trends in Biochemical Sciences*, vol. 26, no. 4, pp. 225–229, 2001.

[3] L. A. Garraway and E. S. Lander, "Lessons from the cancer genome," *Cell*, vol. 153, no. 1, pp. 17–37, 2013.

[4] L. Hood, "A personal journey of discovery: developing technology and changing biology," *Annual Review of Analytical Chemistry*, vol. 1, pp. 1–43, 2008.

[5] B. Weir, X. Zhao, and M. Meyerson, "Somatic alterations in the human cancer genome," *Cancer Cell*, vol. 6, no. 5, pp. 433–438, 2004.

[6] D. Hanahan and R. A. Weinberg, "Hallmarks of cancer: the next generation," *Cell*, vol. 144, no. 5, pp. 646–674, 2011.

[7] E. R. Mardis, "Next-generation sequencing platforms," *Annual Review of Analytical Chemistry*, vol. 6, pp. 287–303, 2013.

[8] R. D. Hawkins, G. C. Hon, and B. Ren, "Next-generation genomics: an integrative approach," *Nature Reviews Genetics*, vol. 11, no. 7, pp. 476–486, 2010.

[9] C. M. Perou, T. Sørile, M. B. Eisen et al., "Molecular portraits of human breast tumours," *Nature*, vol. 406, no. 6797, pp. 747–752, 2000.

[10] A. M. Glas, A. Floore, L. J. M. J. Delahaye et al., "Converting a breast cancer microarray signature into a high-throughput diagnostic test," *BMC Genomics*, vol. 7, article 278, 2006.

[11] L. A. Habel, S. Shak, M. K. Jacobs et al., "A population-based study of tumor gene expression and risk of breast cancer death among lymp node-negative patients," *Breast Cancer Research*, vol. 8, no. 3, article R25, 2006.

[12] R. Salazar, P. Roepman, G. Capella et al., "Gene expression signature to improve prognosis prediction of stage II and III colorectal cancer," *Journal of Clinical Oncology*, vol. 29, no. 1, pp. 17–24, 2011.

[13] H. Davies, G. R. Bignell, C. Cox et al., "Mutations of the BRAF gene in human cancer," *Nature*, vol. 417, no. 6892, pp. 949–954, 2002.

[14] Y. Samuels, Z. Wang, A. Bardelli et al., "High frequency of mutations of the PIK3CA gene in human cancers," *Science*, vol. 304, no. 5670, p. 554, 2004.

[15] T. J. Lynch, D. W. Bell, R. Sordella et al., "Activating mutations in the epidermal growth factor receptor underlying responsiveness of non-small-cell lung cancer to gefitinib," *The New England Journal of Medicine*, vol. 350, no. 21, pp. 2129–2139, 2004.

[16] J. G. Paez, P. A. Jänne, J. C. Lee et al., "EGFR mutations in lung, cancer: correlation with clinical response to gefitinib therapy," *Science*, vol. 304, no. 5676, pp. 1497–1500, 2004.

[17] W. Pao, V. Miller, M. Zakowski et al., "EGF receptor gene mutations are common in lung cancers from "never smokers" and are associated with sensitivity of tumors to gefitinib and erlotinib," *Proceedings of the National Academy of Sciences of the United States of America*, vol. 101, no. 36, pp. 13306–13311, 2004.

[18] E. Boja, T. Hiltke, R. Rivers et al., "Evolution of clinical proteomics and its role in medicine," *Journal of Proteome Research*, vol. 10, no. 1, pp. 66–84, 2011.

[19] M. Bantscheff and B. Kuster, "Quantitative mass spectrometry in proteomics," *Analytical and Bioanalytical Chemistry*, vol. 404, no. 4, pp. 937–938, 2012.

[20] P. Lescuyer, A. Farina, and D. F. Hochstrasser, "Proteomics in clinical chemistry: will it be long?" *Trends in Biotechnology*, vol. 28, no. 5, pp. 225–229, 2010.

[21] J. B. Fenn, M. Mann, C. K. Meng, S. F. Wong, and C. M. Whitehouse, "Electrospray ionization for mass spectrometry of large biomolecules," *Science*, vol. 246, no. 4926, pp. 64–71, 1989.

[22] J. Lengqvist, J. Andrade, Y. Yang, G. Alvelius, R. Lewensohn, and J. Lehtiö, "Robustness and accuracy of high speed LC-MS separations for global peptide quantitation and biomarker discovery," *Journal of Chromatography B: Analytical Technologies in the Biomedical and Life Sciences*, vol. 877, no. 13, pp. 1306–1316, 2009.

[23] N. M. Griffin, J. Yu, F. Long et al., "Label-free, normalized quantification of complex mass spectrometry data for proteomic analysis," *Nature Biotechnology*, vol. 28, no. 1, pp. 83–89, 2010.

[24] J. Pan, H. Chen, Y. Sun, J. Zhang, and X. Luo, "Comparative proteomic analysis of non-small-cell lung cancer and normal controls using serum label-free quantitative shotgun technology," *Lung*, vol. 186, no. 4, pp. 255–261, 2008.

[25] S. K. Huang, M. M. Darfler, M. B. Nicholl et al., "LC/MS-based quantitative proteomic analysis of paraffin-embedded archival melanomas reveals potential proteomic biomarkers associated with metastasis," *PLoS ONE*, vol. 4, no. 2, Article ID e4430, 2009.

[26] M. C. Wiener, J. R. Sachs, E. G. Deyanova, and N. A. Yates, "Differential mass spectrometry: a label-free LC-MS method for finding significant differences in complex peptide and protein mixtures," *Analytical Chemistry*, vol. 76, no. 20, pp. 6085–6096, 2004.

[27] R. E. Higgs, M. D. Knierman, V. Gelfanova, J. P. Butler, and J. E. Hale, "Comprehensive label-free method for the relative quantification of proteins from biological samples," *Journal of Proteome Research*, vol. 4, no. 4, pp. 1442–1450, 2005.

[28] S. E. Ong, B. Blagoev, I. Kratchmarova et al., "Stable isotope labeling by amino acids in cell culture, SILAC, as a simple and accurate approach to expression proteomics," *Molecular & Cellular Proteomics*, vol. 1, no. 5, pp. 376–386, 2002.

[29] M. Krüger, M. Moser, S. Ussar et al., "SILAC mouse for quantitative proteomics uncovers kindlin-3 as an essential factor for red blood cell function," *Cell*, vol. 134, no. 2, pp. 353–364, 2008.

[30] T. Geiger, J. Cox, P. Ostasiewicz, J. R. Wisniewski, and M. Mann, "Super-SILAC mix for quantitative proteomics of human tumor tissue," *Nature Methods*, vol. 7, no. 5, pp. 383–385, 2010.

[31] T. A. Neubert and P. Tempst, "Super-SILAC for tumors and tissues," *Nature Methods*, vol. 7, no. 5, pp. 361–362, 2010.

[32] G. W. Becker, "Stable isotopic labeling of proteins for quantitative proteomic applications," *Briefings in Functional Genomics and Proteomics*, vol. 7, no. 5, pp. 371–382, 2008.

[33] M. Schnölzer, P. Jedrzejewski, and W. D. Lehmann, "Protease-catalyzed incorporation of ^{18}O into peptide fragments and its application for protein sequencing by electrospray and matrix-assisted laser desorption/ionization mass spectrometry," *Electrophoresis*, vol. 17, no. 5, pp. 945–953, 1996.

[34] X. Ye, B. Luke, T. Andresson, and J. Blonder, "^{18}O stable isotope labeling in MS-based proteomics," *Briefings in Functional Genomics and Proteomics*, vol. 8, no. 2, pp. 136–144, 2009.

[35] S. P. Gygi, B. Rist, S. A. Gerber, F. Turecek, M. H. Gelb, and R. Aebersold, "Quantitative analysis of complex protein mixtures using isotope-coded affinity tags," *Nature Biotechnology*, vol. 17, no. 10, pp. 994–999, 1999.

[36] Y. Shiio and R. Aebersold, "Quantitative proteome analysis using isotope-coded affinity tags and mass spectrometry," *Nature Protocols*, vol. 1, no. 1, pp. 139–145, 2006.

[37] M. Mesri, C. Birse, J. Heidbrink et al., "Identification and characterization of angiogenesis targets through proteomic profiling of endothelial cells in human cancer tissues," *PLoS ONE*, vol. 8, no. 11, Article ID e78885, 2013.

[38] P. L. Ross, Y. N. Huang, J. N. Marchese et al., "Multiplexed protein quantitation in *Saccharomyces cerevisiae* using amine-reactive isobaric tagging reagents," *Molecular and Cellular Proteomics*, vol. 3, no. 12, pp. 1154–1169, 2004.

[39] A. Thompson, J. Schäfer, K. Kuhn et al., "Tandem mass tags: a novel quantification strategy for comparative analysis of complex protein mixtures by MS/MS," *Analytical Chemistry*, vol. 75, no. 8, pp. 1895–1904, 2003.

[40] M. M. Savitski, F. Fischer, T. Mathieson, G. Sweetman, M. Lang, and M. Bantscheff, "Targeted data acquisition for improved reproducibility and robustness of proteomic mass spectrometry assays," *Journal of the American Society for Mass Spectrometry*, vol. 21, no. 10, pp. 1668–1679, 2010.

[41] N. A. Karp, W. Huber, P. G. Sadowski, P. D. Charles, S. V. Hester, and K. S. Lilley, "Addressing accuracy and precision issues in iTRAQ quantitation," *Molecular and Cellular Proteomics*, vol. 9, no. 9, pp. 1885–1897, 2010.

[42] Y. O. Saw, M. Salim, J. Noirel, C. Evans, I. Rehman, and P. C. Wright, "iTRAQ underestimation in simple and complex mixtures: 'The good, the bad and the ugly'," *Journal of Proteome Research*, vol. 8, no. 11, pp. 5347–5355, 2009.

[43] L. V. DeSouza, A. D. Romaschin, T. J. Colgan, and K. W. M. Siu, "Absolute quantification of potential cancer markers in clinical tissue homogenates using multiple reaction monitoring on a hybrid triple quadrupole/linear ion trap tandem mass spectrometer," *Analytical Chemistry*, vol. 81, no. 9, pp. 3462–3470, 2009.

[44] P. Mitchell, "Proteomics retrenches," *Nature Biotechnology*, vol. 28, no. 7, pp. 665–670, 2010.

[45] M. Karas and F. Hillenkamp, "Laser desorption ionization of proteins with molecular masses exceeding 10,000 daltons," *Analytical Chemistry*, vol. 60, no. 20, pp. 2299–2301, 1988.

[46] L. F. Marvin, M. A. Roberts, and L. B. Fay, "Matrix-assisted laser desorption/ionization time-of-flight mass spectrometry in clinical chemistry," *Clinica Chimica Acta*, vol. 337, no. 1-2, pp. 11–21, 2003.

[47] G. L. Hortin, "The MALDI-TOF mass spectrometric view of the plasma proteome and peptidome," *Clinical Chemistry*, vol. 52, no. 7, pp. 1223–1237, 2006.

[48] T. W. Hutchens and T. T. Yip, "New desorption strategies for the mass spectrometric analysis of macromolecules," *Rapid Communications in Mass Spectrometry*, vol. 7, no. 7, pp. 576–580, 1993.

[49] M. Zhou and T. D. Veenstra, "Mass spectrometry: m/z 1983–2008," *Biotechniques*, vol. 44, no. 5, pp. 667–670, 2008.

[50] N. Tang, P. Tornatore, and S. R. Weinberger, "Current developments in SELDI affinity technology," *Mass Spectrometry Reviews*, vol. 23, no. 1, pp. 34–44, 2004.

[51] J. Zou, G. Hong, X. Guo et al., "Reproducible cancer biomarker discovery in SELDI-TOF MS using different pre-processing algorithms," *PLoS ONE*, vol. 6, no. 10, Article ID e26294, 2011.

[52] J. Li, N. White, Z. Zhang et al., "Detection of prostate cancer using serum proteomics pattern in a histologically confirmed population," *The Journal of Urology*, vol. 171, no. 5, pp. 1782–1787, 2004.

[53] A. Xue, R. C. Gandy, L. Chung, R. C. Baxter, and R. C. Smith, "Discovery of diagnostic biomarkers for pancreatic cancer in immunodepleted serum by SELDI-TOF MS," *Pancreatology*, vol. 12, no. 2, pp. 124–129, 2012.

[54] F. Navaglia, P. Fogar, D. Basso et al., "Pancreatic cancer biomarkers discovery by surface-enhanced laser desorption and ionization time-of-flight mass spectrometry," *Clinical Chemistry and Laboratory Medicine*, vol. 47, no. 6, pp. 713–723, 2009.

[55] H. Gao, Z. Zheng, Z. Yue, F. Liu, L. Zhou, and X. Zhao, "Evaluation of serum diagnosis of pancreatic cancer by using surface-enhanced laser desorption/ionization time-of-flight mass spectrometry," *International Journal of Molecular Medicine*, vol. 30, no. 5, pp. 1061–1068, 2012.

[56] Q. Song, W. Hu, P. Wang, Y. Yao, and H. Zeng, "Identification of serum biomarkers for lung cancer using magnetic bead-based SELDI-TOF-MS," *Acta Pharmacologica Sinica*, vol. 32, no. 12, pp. 1537–1542, 2011.

[57] C. Şimşek, Ó. Sónmez, A. S. Yurdakul et al., "Importance of serum SELDI-TOF-MS analysis in the diagnosis of early lung cancer," *Asian Pacific Journal of Cancer Prevention*, vol. 14, no. 3, pp. 2037–2042, 2013.

[58] X. Xiao, X. Wei, and D. He, "Proteomic approaches to biomarker discovery in lung cancers by SELDI technology," *Science in China C: Life Sciences*, vol. 46, no. 5, pp. 531–537, 2003.

[59] L. Lei, X. Wang, Z. Zheng et al., "Identification of serum protein markers for breast cancer relapse with SELDI-TOF MS," *Anatomical Record*, vol. 294, no. 6, pp. 941–944, 2011.

[60] A. W. van Winden, M.-C. W. Gast, J. H. Beijnen et al., "Validation of previously identified serum biomarkers for breast cancer with SELDI-TOF MS: a case control study," *BMC Medical Genomics*, vol. 2, article 4, 2009.

[61] M. W. Gast, C. H. van Gils, L. F. A. Wessels et al., "Serum protein profiling for diagnosis of breast cancer using SELDI-TOF MS," *Oncology Reports*, vol. 22, no. 1, pp. 205–213, 2009.

[62] L. L. Wilson, L. Tran, D. L. Morton, and D. S. B. Hoon, "Detection of differentially expressed proteins in early-stage melanoma patients using SELDI-TOF mass spectrometry," *Annals of the New York Academy of Sciences*, vol. 1022, pp. 317–322, 2004.

[63] Z. Wang, K. Ding, J. Yu et al., "Proteomic analysis of primary colon cancer-associated fibroblasts using the SELDI-ProteinChip platform," *Journal of Zhejiang University: Science B*, vol. 13, no. 3, pp. 159–167, 2012.

[64] N. Fan, C. Gao, and X. Wang, "Identification of regional lymph node involvement of colorectal cancer by serum SELDI proteomic patterns," *Gastroenterology Research and Practice*, vol. 2011, Article ID 784967, 6 pages, 2011.

[65] I. Cadron, T. Van Gorp, P. Moerman, E. Waelkens, and I. Vergote, "Proteomic analysis of laser microdissected ovarian cancer tissue with SELDI-TOF MS," *Methods in Molecular Biology*, vol. 755, pp. 155–163, 2011.

[66] H. Zhang, B. Kong, X. Qu, L. Jia, B. Deng, and Q. Yang, "Biomarker discovery for ovarian cancer using SELDI-TOF-MS," *Gynecologic Oncology*, vol. 102, no. 1, pp. 61–66, 2006.

[67] S.-P. Wu, Y.-W. Lin, H.-C. Lai, T.-Y. Chu, Y.-L. Kuo, and H.-S. Liu, "SELDI-TOF MS profiling of plasma proteins in ovarian cancer," *Taiwanese Journal of Obstetrics and Gynecology*, vol. 45, no. 1, pp. 26–32, 2006.

[68] C. Liu, "The application of SELDI-TOF-MS in clinical diagnosis of cancers," *Journal of Biomedicine and Biotechnology*, vol. 2011, Article ID 245821, 6 pages, 2011.

[69] C. Melle, R. Kaufmann, M. Hommann et al., "Proteomic profiling in microdissected hepatocellular carcinoma tissue using ProteinChip technology," *International Journal of Oncology*, vol. 24, no. 4, pp. 885–891, 2004.

[70] M. Wisztorski, R. Lemaire, J. Stauber et al., "New developments in MALDI imaging for pathology proteomic studies," *Current Pharmaceutical Design*, vol. 13, no. 32, pp. 3317–3324, 2007.

[71] R. M. Caprioli, T. B. Farmer, and J. Gile, "Molecular imaging of biological samples: localization of peptides and proteins using MALDI-TOF MS," *Analytical Chemistry*, vol. 69, no. 23, pp. 4751–4760, 1997.

[72] K. E. Burnum, D. S. Cornett, S. M. Puolitaival et al., "Spatial and temporal alterations of phospholipids determined by mass spectrometry during mouse embryo implantation," *Journal of Lipid Research*, vol. 50, no. 11, pp. 2290–2298, 2009.

[73] O. Jardin-Mathé, D. Bonnel, J. Franck et al., "MITICS (MALDI Imaging Team Imaging Computing System): a new open source mass spectrometry imaging software," *Journal of Proteomics*, vol. 71, no. 3, pp. 332–345, 2008.

[74] A. Mangé, P. Chaurand, H. Perrochia, P. Roger, R. M. Caprioli, and J. Solassol, "Liquid chromatography-tandem and MALDI imaging mass spectrometry analyses of RCL2/CS100-fixed, paraffin-embedded tissues: proteomics evaluation of an alternate fixative for biomarker discovery," *Journal of Proteome Research*, vol. 8, no. 12, pp. 5619–5628, 2009.

[75] Y. Kimura, K. Tsutsumi, Y. Sugiura, and M. Setou, "Medical molecular morphology with imaging mass spectrometry," *Medical Molecular Morphology*, vol. 42, no. 3, pp. 133–137, 2009.

[76] R. Mirnezami, K. Spagou, P. A. Vorkas et al., "Chemical mapping of the colorectal cancer microenvironment via MALDI imaging mass spectrometry (MALDI-MSI) reveals novel cancer-associated field effects," *Molecular Oncology*, vol. 8, no. 1, pp. 39–49, 2014.

[77] G. Marko-Varga, T. E. Fehniger, M. Rezeli, B. Döme, T. Laurell, and Á. Végvári, "Drug localization in different lung cancer phenotypes by MALDI mass spectrometry imaging," *Journal of Proteomics*, vol. 74, no. 7, pp. 982–992, 2011.

[78] X. Liu, J. L. Ide, I. Norton et al., "Molecular imaging of drug transit through the blood-brain barrier with MALDI mass

[79] S. C. C. Wong, C. M. L. Chan, B. B. Y. Ma et al., "Advanced proteomic technologies for cancer biomarker discovery," *Expert Review of Proteomics*, vol. 6, no. 2, pp. 123–134, 2009.

[80] M. Andersson, M. R. Groseclose, A. Y. Deutch, and R. M. Caprioli, "Imaging mass spectrometry of proteins and peptides: 3D volume reconstruction," *Nature Methods*, vol. 5, no. 1, pp. 101–108, 2008.

[81] J. Franck, K. Arafah, M. Elayed et al., "MALDI imaging mass spectrometry: state of the art technology in clinical proteomics," *Molecular and Cellular Proteomics*, vol. 8, no. 9, pp. 2023–2033, 2009.

[82] G. L. Wright Jr., "Two dimensional acrylamide gel electrophoresis of cancer patient serum proteins," *Annals of Clinical and Laboratory Science*, vol. 4, no. 4, pp. 281–293, 1974.

[83] D. Hariharan, M. E. Weeks, and T. Crnogorac-Jurcevic, "Application of proteomics in cancer gene profiling: two-dimensional difference in gel electrophoresis (2D-DIGE)," *Methods in Molecular Biology*, vol. 576, pp. 197–211, 2010.

[84] R. Deng, Z. Lu, Y. Chen, L. Zhou, and X. Lu, "Plasma proteomic analysis of pancreatic cancer by 2-dimensional gel electrophoresis," *Pancreas*, vol. 34, no. 3, pp. 310–317, 2007.

[85] P. Alfonso, A. Núñez, J. Madoz-Gurpide, L. Lombardia, L. Sánchez, and J. I. Casal, "Proteomic expression analysis of colorectal cancer by two-dimensional differential gel electrophoresis," *Proteomics*, vol. 5, no. 10, pp. 2602–2611, 2005.

[86] P. Gromov, I. Gromova, J. Bunkenborg et al., "Up-regulated proteins in the fluid bathing the tumour cell microenvironment as potential serological markers for early detection of cancer of the breast," *Molecular Oncology*, vol. 4, no. 1, pp. 65–89, 2010.

[87] J. Sasse and S. R. Gallagher, "Chapter 8: Unit 8.9. Staining proteins in gels," in *Current Protocols in Immunology*, 2004.

[88] T. H. Steinberg, "Chapter 31 protein gel staining methods: an introduction and overview," *Methods in Enzymology*, vol. 463, pp. 541–563, 2009.

[89] T. Kondo and S. Hirohashi, "Application of 2D-DIGE in cancer proteomics toward personalized medicine," *Methods in Molecular Biology*, vol. 577, pp. 135–154, 2009.

[90] J. Koo, K. Kim, B. Min, and G. M. Lee, "Differential protein expression in human articular chondrocytes expanded in serum-free media of different medium osmolalities by DIGE," *Journal of Proteome Research*, vol. 9, no. 5, pp. 2480–2487, 2010.

[91] Z. Ma, S. Dasari, M. C. Chambers et al., "IDPicker 2.0: improved protein assembly with high discrimination peptide identification filtering," *Journal of Proteome Research*, vol. 8, no. 8, pp. 3872–3881, 2009.

[92] R. Ummanni, F. Mundt, H. Pospisil et al., "Identification of clinically relevant protein targets in prostate cancer with 2D-DIGE coupled mass spectrometry and systems biology network platform," *PLoS ONE*, vol. 6, no. 2, Article ID e16833, 2011.

[93] J. L. López, "Two-dimensional electrophoresis in proteome expression analysis," *Journal of Chromatography B: Analytical Technologies in the Biomedical and Life Sciences*, vol. 849, no. 1-2, pp. 190–202, 2007.

[94] P. L. Roulhac, J. M. Ward, J. W. Thompson et al., "Microproteomics: quantitative proteomic profiling of small numbers of laser-captured cells," *Cold Spring Harbor Protocols*, vol. 6, no. 2, 2011.

[95] Y. Zhang, Y. Ye, D. Shen et al., "Identification of transgelin-2 as a biomarker of colorectal cancer by laser capture microdissection

and quantitative proteome analysis," *Cancer Science*, vol. 101, no. 2, pp. 523–529, 2010.

[96] H. Yao, Z. Zhang, Z. Xiao et al., "Identification of metastasis associated proteins in human lung squamous carcinoma using two-dimensional difference gel electrophoresis and laser capture microdissection," *Lung Cancer*, vol. 65, no. 1, pp. 41–48, 2009.

[97] L. F. Waanders, K. Chwalek, M. Monetti, C. Kumar, E. Lammert, and M. Mann, "Quantitative proteomic analysis of single pancreatic islets," *Proceedings of the National Academy of Sciences of the United States of America*, vol. 106, no. 45, pp. 18902–18907, 2009.

[98] M. S. Scicchitano, D. A. Dalmas, R. W. Boyce, H. C. Thomas, and K. S. Frazier, "Protein extraction of formalin-fixed, paraffin-embedded tissue enables robust proteomic profiles by mass spectrometry," *Journal of Histochemistry and Cytochemistry*, vol. 57, no. 9, pp. 849–860, 2009.

[99] Y. Nan, S. Yang, Y. Tian et al., "Analysis of the expression protein profiles of lung squamous carcinoma cell using shotgun proteomics strategy," *Medical Oncology*, vol. 26, no. 2, pp. 215–221, 2009.

[100] Z. Daohai and E. S. Koay, "Analysis of laser capture microdissected cells by 2-dimensional gel electrophoresis," *Methods in Molecular Biology*, vol. 428, pp. 77–91, 2007.

[101] D. J. Johann, S. Mukherjee, D. A. Prieto, T. D. Veenstra, and J. Blonder, "Profiling solid tumor heterogeneity by LCM and biological MS of fresh-frozen tissue sections," *Methods in Molecular Biology*, vol. 755, pp. 95–106, 2011.

[102] K. Uleberg, A. C. Munk, C. Brede et al., "Discrimination of grade 2 and 3 cervical intraepithelial neoplasia by means of analysis of water soluble proteins recovered from cervical biopsies," *Proteome Science*, vol. 9, article 36, 2011.

[103] C. Mueller, A. C. deCarvalho, T. Mikkelsen et al., "Glioblastoma cell enrichment is critical for analysis of phosphorylated drug targets and proteomic-genomic correlations," *Cancer Research*, vol. 74, no. 3, pp. 818–828, 2014.

[104] L. Melton, "Proteomics in multiplex," *Nature*, vol. 429, no. 6987, pp. 101–107, 2004.

[105] P. Moore and J. Clayton, "To affinity and beyond," *Nature*, vol. 426, no. 6967, pp. 725–731, 2003.

[106] L. A. Liotta, V. Espina, A. I. Mehta et al., "Protein microarrays: meeting analytical challenges for clinical applications," *Cancer Cell*, vol. 3, no. 4, pp. 317–325, 2003.

[107] C. P. Pjaweletz, L. Charboneau, V. E. Bichsel et al., "Reverse phase protein microarrays which capture disease progression show activation of pro-survival pathways at the cancer invasion front," *Oncogene*, vol. 20, no. 16, pp. 1981–1989, 2001.

[108] S. Sundaresh, D. L. Doolan, S. Hirst et al., "Identification of humoral immune responses in protein microarrays using DNA microarray data analysis techniques," *Bioinformatics*, vol. 22, no. 14, pp. 1760–1766, 2006.

[109] H. Chandra and S. Srivastava, "Cell-free synthesis-based protein microarrays and their applications," *Proteomics*, vol. 10, no. 4, pp. 717–730, 2010.

[110] N. Ramachandran, J. V. Raphael, E. Hainsworth et al., "Next-generation high-density self-assembling functional protein arrays," *Nature Methods*, vol. 5, no. 6, pp. 535–538, 2008.

[111] R. Spera, J. Labaer, and C. Nicolini, "MALDI-TOF characterization of NAPPA-generated proteins," *Journal of Mass Spectrometry*, vol. 46, no. 9, pp. 960–965, 2011.

[112] L. Melton, "Pharmacogenetics and genotyping: on the trail of SNPs," *Nature*, vol. 422, no. 6934, pp. 917–923, 2003.

[113] B. Houser, "Bio-rad's Bio-Plex suspension array system, xMAP technology overview," *Archives of Physiology and Biochemistry*, vol. 118, no. 4, pp. 192–196, 2012.

[114] S. M. Hanash, S. J. Pitteri, and V. M. Faca, "Mining the plasma proteome for cancer biomarkers," *Nature*, vol. 452, no. 7187, pp. 571–579, 2008.

[115] G. Poste, "Bring on the biomarkers," *Nature*, vol. 469, no. 7329, pp. 156–157, 2011.

[116] M. Polanski and N. L. Anderson, "A list of candidate cancer biomarkers for targeted proteomics," *Biomark Insights*, vol. 1, pp. 1–48, 2007.

[117] S. Ohtsuki, Y. Uchida, Y. Kubo, and T. Terasaki, "Quantitative targeted absolute proteomics-based ADME research as a new path to drug discovery and development: methodology, advantages, strategy, and prospects," *Journal of Pharmaceutical Sciences*, vol. 100, no. 9, pp. 3547–3559, 2011.

[118] E. S. Boja and H. Rodriguez, "Mass spectrometry-based targeted quantitative proteomics: achieving sensitive and reproducible detection of proteins," *Proteomics*, vol. 12, no. 8, pp. 1093–1110, 2012.

[119] D. C. Liebler and L. J. Zimmerman, "Targeted quantitation of proteins by mass spectrometry," *Biochemistry*, vol. 52, no. 22, pp. 3797–3806, 2013.

[120] P. Picotti and R. Aebersold, "Selected reaction monitoring-based proteomics: workflows, potential, pitfalls and future directions," *Nature Methods*, vol. 9, no. 6, pp. 555–566, 2012.

[121] S. Pan, R. Aebersold, R. Chen et al., "Mass spectrometry based targeted protein quantification: methods and applications," *Journal of Proteome Research*, vol. 8, no. 2, pp. 787–797, 2009.

[122] H. Rodriguez, R. Rivers, C. Kinsinger et al., "Reconstructing the pipeline by introducing multiplexed multiple reaction monitoring mass spectrometry for cancer biomarker verification: an NCI-CPTC initiative perspective," *Proteomics: Clinical Applications*, vol. 4, no. 12, pp. 904–914, 2010.

[123] B. Domon and R. Aebersold, "Mass spectrometry and protein analysis," *Science*, vol. 312, no. 5771, pp. 212–217, 2006.

[124] H. Schupke, R. Hempel, R. Eckardt, and T. Kronbach, "Identification of talinolol metabolites in urine of man, dog, rat and mouse after oral administration by high-performance liquid chromatography-thermospray tandem mass spectrometry," *Journal of Mass Spectrometry*, vol. 31, pp. 1371–1381, 1996.

[125] R. Kostiainen, T. Kotiaho, T. Kuuranne, and S. Auriola, "Liquid chromatography/atmospheric pressure ionization-mass spectrometry in drug metabolism studies," *Journal of Mass Spectrometry*, vol. 38, no. 4, pp. 357–372, 2003.

[126] S. S.-C. Tai, D. M. Bunk, E. White V, and M. J. Welch, "Development and evaluation of a reference measurement procedure for the determination of total 3,3′,5-triiodothyronine in human serum using isotope-dilution liquid chromatography-tandem mass spectrometry," *Analytical Chemistry*, vol. 76, no. 17, pp. 5092–5096, 2004.

[127] N. Ahmed and P. J. Thornalley, "Quantitative screening of protein biomarkers of early glycation, advanced glycation, oxidation and nitrosation in cellular and extracellular proteins by tandem mass spectrometry multiple reaction monitoring," *Biochemical Society Transactions*, vol. 31, no. 6, pp. 1417–1422, 2003.

[128] A. Sannino, L. Bolzoni, and M. Bandini, "Application of liquid chromatography with electrospray tandem mass spectrometry

to the determination of a new generation of pesticides in processed fruits and vegetables," *Journal of Chromatography A*, vol. 1036, no. 2, pp. 161–169, 2004.

[129] M. A. Kuzyk, D. Smith, J. Yang et al., "Multiple reaction monitoring-based, multiplexed, absolute quantitation of 45 proteins in human plasma," *Molecular and Cellular Proteomics*, vol. 8, no. 8, pp. 1860–1877, 2009.

[130] Z. Meng and T. D. Veenstra, "Targeted mass spectrometry approaches for protein biomarker verification," *Journal of Proteomics*, vol. 74, no. 12, pp. 2650–2659, 2011.

[131] H. Keshishian, T. Addona, M. Burgess, E. Kuhn, and S. A. Carr, "Quantitative, multiplexed assays for low abundance proteins in plasma by targeted mass spectrometry and stable isotope dilution," *Molecular and Cellular Proteomics*, vol. 6, no. 12, pp. 2212–2229, 2007.

[132] H. Keshishian, T. Addona, M. Burgess et al., "Quantification of cardiovascular biomarkers in patient plasma by targeted mass spectrometry and stable isotope dilution," *Molecular and Cellular Proteomics*, vol. 8, no. 10, pp. 2339–2349, 2009.

[133] A. N. Hoofnagle, J. O. Becker, M. H. Wener, and J. W. Heinecke, "Quantification of thyroglobulin, a low-abundance serum protein, by immunoaffinity peptide enrichment and tandem mass spectrometry," *Clinical Chemistry*, vol. 54, no. 11, pp. 1796–1804, 2008.

[134] "Method of the year 2012," *Nature Methods*, vol. 10, no. 1, 2013.

[135] T. A. Addona, S. E. Abbatiello, B. Schilling et al., "Multi-site assessment of the precision and reproducibility of multiple reaction monitoring-based measurements of proteins in plasma," *Nature Biotechnology*, vol. 27, pp. 633–641, 2009.

[136] R. Aebersold, A. L. Burlingame, and R. A. Bradshaw, "Western blots versus selected reaction monitoring assays: time to turn the tables?" *Molecular & Cellular Proteomics*, vol. 12, no. 9, pp. 2381–2382, 2013.

[137] J. J. Kennedy, S. E. Abbatiello, K. Kim, and et al, "Demonstrating the feasibility of large-scale development of standardized assays to quantify human proteins," *Nature Methods*, vol. 11, pp. 149–155, 2014.

[138] S. A. Carr, S. E. Abbatiello, B. L. Ackermann et al., "Targeted peptide measurements in biology and medicine: best practices for mass spectrometry-based assay development using a fit-for-purpose approach," *Molecular & Cellular Proteomics*, vol. 13, no. 3, pp. 907–917, 2014.

[139] E. Kuhn, T. Addona, H. Keshishian et al., "Developing multiplexed assays for troponin I and interleukin-33 in plasma by peptide immunoaffinity enrichment and targeted mass spectrometry," *Clinical Chemistry*, vol. 55, no. 6, pp. 1108–1117, 2009.

[140] T. Fortin, A. Salvador, J. P. Charrier et al., "Clinical quantitation of prostate-specific antigen biomarker in the low nanogram/milliliter range by conventional bore liquid chromatography-tandem mass spectrometry (multiple reaction monitoring) coupling and correlation with ELISA tests," *Molecular and Cellular Proteomics*, vol. 8, no. 5, pp. 1006–1015, 2009.

[141] M. Hossain, D. T. Kaleta, E. W. Robinson et al., "Enhanced sensitivity for selected reaction monitoring mass spectrometry-based targeted proteomics using a dual stage electrodynamic ion funnel interface," *Molecular & Cellular Proteomics*, vol. 10, no. 2, Article ID M000062-MCP201, 2011.

[142] T. Fortin, A. Salvador, J. P. Charrier et al., "Multiple reaction monitoring cubed for protein quantification at the low nanogram/milliliter level in nondepleted human serum," *Analytical Chemistry*, vol. 81, no. 22, pp. 9343–9352, 2009.

[143] T. Shi, T. L. Fillmore, X. Sun et al., "Antibody-free, targeted mass-spectrometric approach for quantification of proteins at low picogram per milliliter levels in human plasma/serum," *Proceedings of the National Academy of Sciences of the United States of America*, vol. 109, no. 38, pp. 15395–15400, 2012.

[144] A. C. Peterson, J. D. Russell, D. J. Bailey, M. S. Westphall, and J. J. Coon, "Parallel reaction monitoring for high resolution and high mass accuracy quantitative, targeted proteomics," *Molecular and Cellular Proteomics*, vol. 11, no. 11, pp. 1475–1488, 2012.

[145] A. Doerr, "Targeting with PRM," *Nature Methods*, vol. 9, no. 10, p. 950, 2012.

[146] J. Sherman, M. J. McKay, K. Ashman, and M. P. Molloy, "How specific is my SRM?: the issue of precursor and product ion redundancy," *Proteomics*, vol. 9, no. 5, pp. 1120–1123, 2009.

[147] L. C. Gillet, P. Navarro, S. Tate et al., "Targeted data extraction of the MS/MS spectra generated by data-independent acquisition: a new concept for consistent and accurate proteome analysis," *Molecular & Cellular Proteomics*, vol. 11, no. 6, 2012.

[148] K. P. Law and Y. P. Lim, "Recent advances in mass spectrometry: data independent analysis and hyper reaction monitoring," *Expert Review of Proteomics*, vol. 10, pp. 551–566, 2013.

[149] N. Rifai, M. A. Gillette, and S. A. Carr, "Protein biomarker discovery and validation: the long and uncertain path to clinical utility," *Nature Biotechnology*, vol. 24, no. 8, pp. 971–983, 2006.

[150] D. Nedelkov, "Mass spectrometry-based protein assays for in vitro diagnostic testing," *Expert Review of Molecular Diagnostics*, vol. 12, no. 3, pp. 235–239, 2012.

[151] G. R. Nicol, M. Han, J. Kim et al., "Use of an immunoaffinity-mass spectrometry-based approach for the quantification of protein biomarkers from serum samples of lung cancer patients," *Molecular & Cellular Proteomics*, vol. 7, no. 10, pp. 1974–1982, 2008.

[152] V. Kulasingam, C. R. Smith, I. Batruch, A. Buckler, D. A. Jeffery, and E. P. Diamandis, "'Product ion monitoring' assay for prostate-specific antigen in serum using a linear ion-trap," *Journal of Proteome Research*, vol. 7, no. 2, pp. 640–647, 2008.

[153] M. J. Berna, Y. Zhen, D. E. Watson, J. E. Hale, and B. L. Ackermann, "Strategic use of immunoprecipitation and LC/MS/MS for trace-level protein quantification: myosin light chain 1, a biomarker of cardiac necrosis," *Analytical Chemistry*, vol. 79, no. 11, pp. 4199–4205, 2007.

[154] E. E. Niederkofler, D. A. Phillips, B. Krastins et al., "Targeted selected reaction monitoring mass spectrometric immunoassay for insulin-like growth factor 1," *PLoS ONE*, vol. 8, Article ID e81125, 2013.

[155] V. Brun, C. Masselon, J. Garin, and A. Dupuis, "Isotope dilution strategies for absolute quantitative proteomics," *Journal of Proteomics*, vol. 72, no. 5, pp. 740–749, 2009.

[156] D. Lebert, A. Dupuis, J. Garin, C. Bruley, and V. Brun, "Production and use of stable isotope-labeled proteins for absolute quantitative proteomics," *Methods in Molecular Biology*, vol. 753, pp. 93–115, 2011.

[157] G. Picard, D. Lebert, M. Louwagie et al., "PSAQ standards for accurate MS-based quantification of proteins: from the concept to biomedical applications," *Journal of Mass Spectrometry*, vol. 47, no. 10, pp. 1353–1363, 2012.

[158] R. W. Nelson, D. Nedelkov, K. A. Tubbs, and U. A. Kiernan, "Quantitative mass spectrometric immunoassay of insulin like

growth factor 1," *Journal of Proteome Research*, vol. 3, no. 4, pp. 851–855, 2004.

[159] M. R. Stratton, P. J. Campbell, and P. A. Futreal, "The cancer genome," *Nature*, vol. 458, no. 7239, pp. 719–724, 2009.

[160] G. R. Bignell, C. D. Greenman, H. Davies et al., "Signatures of mutation and selection in the cancer genome," *Nature*, vol. 463, no. 7283, pp. 893–898, 2010.

[161] Q. Wang, R. Chaerkady, J. Wu et al., "Mutant proteins as cancer-specific biomarkers," *Proceedings of the National Academy of Sciences of the United States of America*, vol. 108, no. 6, pp. 2444–2449, 2011.

[162] D. P. Little, A. Braun, M. J. O'Donnell, and H. Koster, "Mass spectrometry from miniaturized arrays for full comparative DNA analysis," *Nature Medicine*, vol. 3, no. 12, pp. 1413–1416, 1997.

[163] N. L. Anderson, N. G. Anderson, L. R. Haines, D. B. Hardie, R. W. Olafson, and T. W. Pearson, "Mass spectrometric quantitation of peptides and proteins using Stable Isotope Standards and Capture by Anti-Peptide Antibodies (SISCAPA)," *Journal of Proteome Research*, vol. 3, no. 2, pp. 235–244, 2004.

[164] J. R. Whiteaker, L. Zhao, H. Y. Zhang et al., "Antibody-based enrichment of peptides on magnetic beads for mass-spectrometry-based quantification of serum biomarkers," *Analytical Biochemistry*, vol. 362, no. 1, pp. 44–54, 2007.

[165] N. L. Anderson, A. Jackson, D. Smith, D. Hardie, C. Borchers, and T. W. Pearson, "SISCAPA peptide enrichment on magnetic beads using an in-line bead trap device," *Molecular & Cellular Proteomics*, vol. 8, no. 5, pp. 995–1005, 2009.

[166] J. R. Whiteaker, L. Zhao, L. Anderson, and A. G. Paulovich, "An automated and multiplexed method for high throughput peptide immunoaffinity enrichment and multiple reaction monitoring mass spectrometry-based quantification of protein biomarkers," *Molecular and Cellular Proteomics*, vol. 9, no. 1, pp. 184–196, 2010.

[167] R. M. Schoenherr, L. Zhao, J. R. Whiteaker et al., "Automated screening of monoclonal antibodies for SISCAPA assays using a magnetic bead processor and liquid chromatography-selected reaction monitoring-mass spectrometry," *Journal of Immunological Methods*, vol. 353, no. 1-2, pp. 49–61, 2010.

[168] M. Razavi, M. E. Pope, M. V. Soste et al., "MALDI Immunoscreening (MiSCREEN): a method for selection of anti-peptide monoclonal antibodies for use in immunoproteomics," *Journal of Immunological Methods*, vol. 364, no. 1-2, pp. 50–64, 2011.

[169] J. D. Reid, D. T. Holmes, D. R. Mason, B. Shah, and C. H. Borchers, "Towards the development of an immuno MALDI (iMALDI) mass spectrometry assay for the diagnosis of hypertension," *Journal of the American Society for Mass Spectrometry*, vol. 21, no. 10, pp. 1680–1686, 2010.

[170] J. Jiang, C. E. Parker, K. A. Hoadley, C. M. Perou, G. Boysen, and C. H. Borchers, "Development of an immuno tandem mass spectrometry (iMALDI) assay for EGFR diagnosis," *Proteomics: Clinical Applications*, vol. 1, no. 12, pp. 1651–1659, 2007.

[171] M. H. Elliott, D. S. Smith, C. E. Parker, and C. Borchers, "Current trends in quantitative proteomics," *Journal of Mass Spectrometry*, vol. 44, no. 12, pp. 1637–1660, 2009.

[172] J. R. Whiteaker, C. Lin, J. Kennedy et al., "A targeted proteomics-based pipeline for verification of biomarkers in plasma," *Nature Biotechnology*, vol. 29, no. 7, pp. 625–634, 2011.

[173] S. A. Agger, L. C. Marney, and A. N. Hoofnagle, "Simultaneous quantification of apolipoprotein A-I and apolipoprotein B by liquid-chromatography-multiple-reaction-monitoring mass spectrometry," *Clinical Chemistry*, vol. 56, no. 12, pp. 1804–1813, 2010.

[174] B. MacLean, D. M. Tomazela, N. Shulman et al., "Skyline: an open source document editor for creating and analyzing targeted proteomics experiments," *Bioinformatics*, vol. 26, no. 7, pp. 966–968, 2010.

[175] D. B. Martin, T. Holzman, D. May et al., "MRMer, an interactive open source and cross-platform system for data extraction and visualization of multiple reaction monitoring experiments," *Molecular and Cellular Proteomics*, vol. 7, no. 11, pp. 2270–2278, 2008.

[176] M.-Y. K. Brusniak, S.-T. Kwok, M. Christiansen et al., "ATAQS: a computational software tool for high throughput transition optimization and validation for selected reaction monitoring mass spectrometry," *BMC Bioinformatics*, vol. 12, article 78, 2011.

[177] L. Reiter, O. Rinner, P. Picotti et al., "MProphet: automated data processing and statistical validation for large-scale SRM experiments," *Nature Methods*, vol. 8, no. 5, pp. 430–435, 2011.

[178] P. Picotti, H. Lam, D. Campbell et al., "A database of mass spectrometric assays for the yeast proteome," *Nature Methods*, vol. 5, no. 11, pp. 913–914, 2008.

[179] S. E. Abbatiello, D. R. Mani, H. Keshishian, and S. A. Carr, "Automated detection of inaccurate and imprecise transitions in peptide quantification by multiple reaction monitoring mass spectrometry," *Clinical Chemistry*, vol. 56, no. 2, pp. 291–305, 2010.

[180] M. Mann, "Comparative analysis to guide quality improvements in proteomics," *Nature Methods*, vol. 6, no. 10, pp. 717–719, 2009.

[181] E. F. Petricoin III, A. M. Ardekani, and B. A. Hitt, "Use of proteomic patterns in serum to identify ovarian cancer," *The Lancet*, vol. 364, no. 9434, p. 582, 2004.

[182] E. P. Diamandis, "Cancer biomarkers: can we turn recent failures into success?" *Journal of the National Cancer Institute*, vol. 102, no. 19, pp. 1462–1467, 2010.

[183] E. P. Diamandis, "Proteomic patterns in biological fluids: do they represent the future of cancer diagnostics?" *Clinical Chemistry*, vol. 49, no. 8, pp. 1272–1275, 2003.

[184] E. P. Diamandis, "Mass spectrometry as a diagnostic and a cancer biomarker discovery tool: opportunities and potential limitations," *Molecular and Cellular Proteomics*, vol. 3, no. 4, pp. 367–378, 2004.

[185] E. P. Diamandis, "Analysis of serum proteomic patterns for early cancer diagnosis: drawing attention to potential problems," *Journal of the National Cancer Institute*, vol. 96, no. 5, pp. 353–356, 2004.

[186] E. F. Petricoin, K. C. Zoon, E. C. Kohn, J. C. Barrett, and L. A. Liotta, "Clinical proteomics: translating benchside promise into bedside reality," *Nature Reviews Drug Discovery*, vol. 1, no. 9, pp. 683–695, 2002.

[187] K. Chapman, "The ProteinChip biomarker system from ciphergen biosystems: a novel proteomics platform for rapid biomarker discovery and validation," *Biochemical Society Transactions*, vol. 30, no. 2, pp. 82–87, 2002.

[188] D. McLerran, W. E. Grizzle, Z. Feng et al., "SELDI-TOF MS whole serum proteomic profiling with IMAC surface does not reliably detect prostate cancer," *Clinical Chemistry*, vol. 54, no. 1, pp. 53–60, 2008.

[189] A. W. Bell, E. W. Deutsch, C. E. Au et al., "A HUPO test sample study reveals common problems in mass spectrometry-based proteomics," *Nature Methods*, vol. 6, no. 6, pp. 423–430, 2009.

[190] D. B. Friedman, T. M. Andacht, M. K. Bunger et al., "The ABRF Proteomics Research Group Studies: Educational exercises for qualitative and quantitative proteomic analyses," *Proteomics*, vol. 11, no. 8, pp. 1371–1381, 2011.

[191] A. G. Paulovich, D. Billheimer, A. L. Ham et al., "Interlaboratory study characterizing a yeast performance standard for benchmarking LC-MS platform performance," *Molecular and Cellular Proteomics*, vol. 9, no. 2, pp. 242–254, 2010.

[192] P. A. Rudnick, K. R. Clauser, L. E. Kilpatrick et al., "Performance metrics for liquid chromatography-tandem mass spectrometry systems in proteomics analyses," *Molecular and Cellular Proteomics*, vol. 9, no. 2, pp. 225–241, 2010.

[193] D. L. Tabb, L. Vega-Montoto, P. A. Rudnick et al., "Repeatability and reproducibility in proteomic identifications by liquid chromatography-tandem mass spectrometry," *Journal of Proteome Research*, vol. 9, no. 2, pp. 761–776, 2010.

[194] A. Beasley-Green, D. Bunk, P. Rudnick, L. Kilpatrick, and K. Phinney, "A proteomics performance standard to support measurement quality in proteomics," *Proteomics*, vol. 12, no. 7, pp. 923–931, 2012.

[195] S. E. Abbatiello, D. R. Mani, B. Schilling et al., "Design, implementation and multisite evaluation of a system suitability protocol for the quantitative assessment of instrument performance in liquid chromatography-multiple reaction monitoring-MS (LC-MRM-MS)," *Molecular & Cellular Proteomics*, vol. 12, pp. 2623–2639, 2013.

[196] J. D. Theis, S. Dasari, J. A. Vrana, P. J. Kurtin, and A. Dogan, "Shotgun-proteomics-based clinical testing for diagnosis and classification of amyloidosis," *Journal of Mass Spectrometry*, vol. 48, pp. 1067–1077, 2013.

[197] Z. Zhang and D. W. Chan, "The road from discovery to clinical diagnostics: lessons learned from the first FDA-cleared in vitro diagnostic multivariate index assay of proteomic biomarkers," *Cancer Epidemiology Biomarkers and Prevention*, vol. 19, no. 12, pp. 2995–2999, 2010.

[198] F. E. Regnier, S. J. Skates, M. Mesri et al., "Protein-based multiplex assays: Mock presubmissions to the US food and drug administration," *Clinical Chemistry*, vol. 56, no. 2, pp. 165–171, 2010.

[199] H. A. Yeong, Y. L. Ji, Y. L. Ju, Y. Kim, H. K. Jeong, and S. Y. Jong, "Quantitative analysis of an aberrant glycoform of TIMP1 from colon cancer serum by L-PHA-enrichment and SISCAPA with MRM mass spectrometry," *Journal of Proteome Research*, vol. 8, no. 9, pp. 4216–4224, 2009.

[200] B. Wollscheid, D. Bausch-Fluck, C. Henderson et al., "Mass-spectrometric identification and relative quantification of N-linked cell surface glycoproteins," *Nature Biotechnology*, vol. 27, no. 4, pp. 378–386, 2009.

[201] S. Decramer, S. Wittke, H. Mischak et al., "Predicting the clinical outcome of congenital unilateral ureteropelvic junction obstruction in newborn by urinary proteome analysis," *Nature Medicine*, vol. 12, no. 4, pp. 398–400, 2006.

[202] N. L. Anderson, N. G. Anderson, T. W. Pearson et al., "A human proteome detection and quantitation project," *Molecular and Cellular Proteomics*, vol. 8, no. 5, pp. 883–886, 2009.

[203] J. Munoz, T. Y. Low, Y. J. Kok et al., "The quantitative proteomes of human-induced pluripotent stem cells and embryonic stem cells," *Molecular Systems Biology*, vol. 7, article 550, 2011.

[204] N. Nagaraj, J. R. Wisniewski, T. Geiger et al., "Deep proteome and transcriptome mapping of a human cancer cell line," *Molecular Systems Biology*, vol. 7, article 548, 2011.

[205] R. M. Branca, L. M. Orre, H. J. Johansson et al., "HiRIEF LC-MS enables deep proteome coverage and unbiased proteogenomics," *Nature Methods*, vol. 11, pp. 59–62, 2014.

[206] T. Y. Low, S. van Heesch, H. van den Toorn, and et al, "Quantitative and qualitative proteome characteristics extracted from in-depth integrated genomics and proteomics analysis," *Cell Reports*, vol. 5, pp. 1469–1478, 2013.

[207] A. F. M. Altelaar, J. Munoz, and A. J. R. Heck, "Next-generation proteomics: towards an integrative view of proteome dynamics," *Nature Reviews Genetics*, vol. 14, no. 1, pp. 35–48, 2013.

[208] W. W. Soon, M. Hariharan, and M. P. Snyder, "High-throughput sequencing for biology and medicine," *Molecular Systems Biology*, vol. 9, article 640, 2013.

[209] K. Ning, D. Fermin, and A. I. Nesvizhskii, "Comparative analysis of different label-free mass spectrometry based protein abundance estimates and their correlation with RNA-Seq gene expression data," *Journal of Proteome Research*, vol. 11, no. 4, pp. 2261–2271, 2012.

[210] E. Venter, R. D. Smith, and S. H. Payne, "Proteogenomic analysis of bacteria and archaea: a 46 organism case study," *PLoS ONE*, vol. 6, no. 11, Article ID e27587, 2011.

[211] S. Renuse, R. Chaerkady, and A. Pandey, "Proteogenomics," *Proteomics*, vol. 11, no. 4, pp. 620–630, 2011.

[212] J. Cox and M. Mann, "Quantitative, high-resolution proteomics for data-driven systems biology," *Annual Review of Biochemistry*, vol. 80, pp. 273–299, 2011.

Safety and Complications of Medical Thoracoscopy

Shimaa Nour Moursi Ahmed,[1,2] **Hideo Saka,**[1] **Hamdy Ali Mohammadien,**[2]
Ola Alkady,[2] **Masahide Oki,**[1] **Yoshimasa Tanikawa,**[3] **Rie Tsuboi,**[1]
Masahiro Aoyama,[3] **and Keiji Sugiyama**[1]

[1]*Department of Respiratory Medicine, National Hospital Organization Nagoya Medical Center, Nagoya, Aichi 460-0001, Japan*
[2]*Department of Respiratory Medicine, Sohag University Hospital, Nasr City Street, Sohag 82524, Egypt*
[3]*Department of Respiratory Medicine and Clinical Immunology, Toyota Kosei Hospital, 500-1 Ibohara Josuicho, Toyota-Shi 470-0396, Japan*

Correspondence should be addressed to Hideo Saka; saka@med.nagoya-u.ac.jp

Academic Editor: Isamu Sugawara

Objectives. To highlight the possible complications of medical thoracoscopy (MT) and how to avoid them. *Methods.* A retrospective and prospective analysis of 127 patients undergoing MT in Nagoya Medical Center (NMC) and Toyota Kosei Hospital. The data about complications was obtained from the patients, notes on the computer system, and radiographs. *Results.* The median age was 71.0 (range, 33.0–92.0) years and 101 (79.5%) were males. The median time with chest drain after procedure was 7.0 (range, 0.0–47.0) days and cases with talc poudrage were 30 (23.6%). Malignant histology was reported in 69 (54.3%), including primary lung cancer in 35 (27.5), mesothelioma in 18 (14.2), and metastasis in 16 (12.6). 58 (45.7%) revealed benign pleural diseases and TB was diagnosed in 15 (11.8%). 21 (16.5%) patients suffered from complications including lung laceration in 3 (2.4%), fever in 5 (3.9%) (due to hospital acquired infection (HAI) in 2, talc poudrage in 2, and malignancy in 1), HAI in 2 (1.6%), prolonged air-leak in 14 (11.0%), and subcutaneous emphysema in 1 (0.8%). *Conclusions.* MT is generally a safe procedure. Lung laceration is the most serious complication and should be managed well. HAI is of low risk and can be controlled by medical treatment.

1. Introduction

MT is used increasingly by chest physicians and has become, after bronchoscopy, the second most important endoscopic technique in respiratory medicine [1]. It is considered to be one of the main areas of interventional pulmonology and an important part of a specialist pleural disease service [2, 3].

Thoracoscopy is the oldest invasive interventional technique in the recent history of respiratory medicine. It was initially performed in 1910 by an internist from Sweden, Hans-Christian Jacobaeus. Jacobaeus was the first to use the term thoracoscopy that he described as "replacing fluid with air" in order to examine the pleural surfaces of two patients with tuberculous pleurisy. Jacobaeus later developed a therapeutic application for thoracoscopy by using thermocautery to lyse adhesions and create a pneumothorax to treat tuberculosis (Jacobaeus operation) [4].

At the end of the 1990s, semirigid (or flex-rigid) thoracoscope was successfully introduced as a new instrument for thoracoscopy [5]. Pulmonologists who used to work with a flexible bronchoscope found it more familiar. It allows easy lateral vision or even retro visualization of the point of entry, but its main limitations are small biopsies taken through the small working channel and the difficulty to lyse the adhesions [6].

The application of MT is mainly for diagnosing pleural effusion and for performing talc poudrage pleurodesis in malignant pleural effusion and recurrent spontaneous pneumothorax [7]. For the diagnosis of malignant pleural disease, MT has consistently been demonstrated to be superior to fluid cytology and "blind" closed needle biopsy [8–10] with a sensitivity of up to 95% [11]. A recent study comparing MT with CT-guided Abrams needle biopsy demonstrated no significant difference with the two techniques, although the advantage of thoracoscopy remains that pleurodesis can be performed after pleural fluid removal during the procedure [12].

It also plays a crucial role in staging non-small-cell lung cancer and guiding treatment and prognosis, as the documentation of pleural metastasis renders the patient inoperable (stage M1a) [13]. It can be useful as well to provide large biopsies required for the application of molecular techniques, such as the use of molecular markers, for example, epidermal growth factor receptor; these markers participate in the modern staging of malignant diseases and provide possibilities for potential therapies [14]. Other nonroutine and more complex applications of MT are in the treatment of empyema, in lung biopsy with forceps, and in cervical sympathectomy; these procedures are considered advanced, need more experience, and should definitely be performed by experts and highly trained thoracoscopists [15].

MT in the hands of experienced physicians is safe with mortality of 0.35% (95% confidence interval (CI) 0.19–0.54%) and likely to be less if diagnostic procedures alone are performed [16]. This compares favorably with mortality from transbronchial biopsy (0.22–0.6%) [17] and mediastinoscopy (0.17%) [18]. Pain is frequently reported after the procedure and may be more common when using talc poudrage for pneumothorax when compared with malignant effusion [19]. There has been previous concern with respect to the development of acute respiratory distress syndrome (ARDS) following talc poudrage, [20] which was likely to be from the grade of talc utilized [21]. Major complications (empyema, hemorrhage, port site tumor growth, bronchopleural fistula and/or persistent air leak, postoperative pneumothorax, and pneumonia) occur in 1.8% (95% CI 1.4–2.2%) and minor complications (subcutaneous emphysema, minor hemorrhage, operative skin site infection, fever, and atrial fibrillation) occur in 7.3% (95% CI 6.3–8.4%) [16].

The aim of this study is to evaluate the safety of MT and the possible complications that can occur during and after the procedure.

2. Materials and Methods

2.1. Patients. We performed a retrospective and prospective analysis of 127 patients undergoing MT for diagnostic and therapeutic purposes in NMC during the period of 2007 to 2015 and Toyota Kosei Hospital during the period of 2011 to 2015. The retrospective analysis included patients during the period of 2007 to 2013 in NMC and during the period of 2011 to 2013 in Toyota Kosei Hospital and prospective analysis included the patients during 2014 and 2015 for both.

During the period of our study, the total number of patients was 139 but we excluded 10 patients due to defective data required for analysis and the other 2 patients were excluded due to failure to complete MT. The patients' data was obtained from the hospital computerized system. The case notes were examined for any report of complications and radiographs were examined for outcome. The histology and relevant microbiology reports were obtained from the laboratory computerized system.

2.2. MT and Chest Tube Management. MT was performed by experienced physicians using The Olympus semirigid LTF-260 thoracoscopy. The patients were in the lateral position with local anesthesia and conscious sedation using midazolam and fentanyl in NMC and only local anesthesia in Toyota Kosei Hospital, with ECG and pulse oximetry monitoring throughout.

About 5 to 10 biopsies were taken from the parietal pleura depending on the macroscopic findings and 4 g of graded talc (Steritalc®, Novatech, La Ciotat, France) poudrage was used during pleurodesis. All patients had 16 F chest drains after the procedure through the same entry port as the thoracoscopy. Intercostal drains were connected to an underwater seal and negative suction (-10 to $-20\,cm/H_2O$) was used till the drained fluid becomes less than 150 mL/day.

2.3. Prethoracoscopic Investigations. All patients were subjected to pleural fluid analysis, chest X-ray, chest CT, chest ultrasonography (US), ECG, and routine liver and kidney functions.

2.4. Thoracoscopic Technique

Premedication. Midazolam 0.4 mg together with fentanyl 0.2 mg was administered to the patients just before the procedure through intravenous line and sometimes during the procedure if it lasted for long time.

Oxygen via nasal cannula was administered during the entire procedure to maintain SpO_2 >90%.

After premedication, the combined scope and forceps were inserted, under local anesthesia, through a trocar with an outer diameter of 10 mm and without valve, in an intercostal space, with the patient resting on the healthy side. A sterile catheter was introduced through the trocar and the residual effusion was taken under sterile conditions. After the pleural cavity had been emptied, the lung and pleura were examined by way of the thoracoscope and any abnormality like adhesions, fibrin deposition, discoloration of the pleura, hyperemia, tuberculous nodules, formation of tumors, and so forth was observed.

Whenever feasible, biopsies were taken, placed immediately in formalin, and sent for microscopic examination. About 5 to 10 biopsies were taken from each patient from the parietal pleura depending on the macroscopic findings.

2.5. Statistical Analysis. Statistical analyses were processed by statistical software program (PASW Statistics 16; SPSS Inc., Chicago, IL, USA). Data were statistically described in terms of frequencies (number of cases), percentages, median, and range when appropriate.

3. Results

The total number of cases was 127 with median age of 71.0 (range, 33.0–92.0) years and 101 (79.5%) were males; as regards smoking, 36 (28.3%) cases were current smokers. The median duration of drainage by intercostal tube after MT was 7.0 (range, 0.0–47.0) days and cases of talc poudrage

TABLE 1: Characteristics of patients undergoing medical thoracoscopy.

Characteristics	The total number of patients 127
Age, median (range), year	71.0 (33.0–92.0)
Sex, no. (%)	
Male	101 (79.5)
Female	26 (20.5)
Smoking status, number (%)	
Nonsmoker	44 (34.6)
Smoker	36 (28.3)
Ex-smoker	47 (37)
The affected side, number (%)	
Right	69 (54.3)
Left	55 (43.3)
Bilateral	3 (2.4)
Nature of pleural fluid analysis, number (%)	
Exudate	124 (97.6)
Transudate	3 (2.3)
Duration of ICT drainage, median (range), days	7.0 (0.0–47.0)
Talc poudrage, number (%)	30 (23.6)

ICT: intercostals tube.
NB: 10 of the cases of exudate were purulent and one was hemorrhagic fluid.

TABLE 2: Diagnostic outcome of medical thoracoscopy in 127 patients.

Malignant (n = 69; 54.3% of total)	Benign (n = 58; 45.7% of total)
Primary lung cancer 35 (27.5% of total)	Nonspecific pleuritis 27 (21.3% of total)
Metastasis to pleura 16 (12.6% of total)	Tuberculosis 15 (11.8% of total)
Mesothelioma 18 (14.2% of total)	Empyema 10 (7.9% of total)
	Hypoalbuminemia 2 (1.6% of total)
	Uremic pleuritis 2 (1.6% of total)
	Drug induced pleuritis 1 (0.9% of total)
	Ruptured bulla 1 (0.9% of total)

NB: Cases of empyema were diagnosed before doing MT; they were not postprocedure complications.

were 30 (23.6%). The details of patients' characteristics are shown in Table 1.

Benign pleural disease was diagnosed in 58 (45.7%), including tuberculosis in 15 (11.8%), empyema in 10 (7.9%), the nonspecific pleuritis in 27 (21.3%), hypoalbuminemia in 2 (1.6%), uremic pleuritis in 2 (1.6%), drug induced pleuritis in 1 (0.9 %), and ruptured bulla in 1 (0.9 % of total). The details are shown in Table 2.

Malignant histology was reported in 69 (54.3%) including primary lung cancer in 35 (27.5%), metastasis in 16 (12.6%),

TABLE 3: The secondary pleural cancers, differentiation, and origins.

(a) Differentiation of the primary lung cancers (n = 35)

Type	Number	(%) of lung cancer
Adenocarcinoma	29	(82.9)
Squamous cell carcinoma	4	(11.4)
Small-cell lung cancer	2	(5.7)

(b) Primary origin of the metastases (n = 16)

Type	Number	(%) of metastases
Lymphoma	4	(25)
Kidney	2	(12.5)
Prostate	2	(12.5)
Ovary	2	(12.5)
Pancreas	2	(12.5)
Pharynx	1	(6.3)
Colon	1	(6.3)
Bladder	1	(6.3)
Thymus	1	(6.3)

TABLE 4: Thoracoscopic complications.

Total number of patients 127, patients with complications 21 (16.5%)	
Type	N (%) of total
Lung laceration	3 (2.4)
Fever	5 (3.9)
HAI	2 (1.6)
Prolonged air leak	14 (11.0)
Subcutaneous emphysema	1 (0.8)
Bleeding	0
ARDS	0
Mortality due to procedure	0

HAI, hospital acquired infection; ARDS, acute respiratory distress syndrome.

and mesothelioma in 18 (14.2%). The frequency of different histological types of lung cancer was adenocarcinoma in 29 (82.9%), squamous-cell carcinoma in 4 (11.4%), and small-cell carcinoma in 2 (5.7%). The most common source of metastasis was lymphoma in 4 (25%). The details are shown in Tables 2 and 3.

No mortality was related to the procedure of MT. No major bleeding from the biopsy sites or hemoptysis was observed. Complications occurred in 21 (16.5%) cases including lung lacerations in 3 (2.4%), fever in 5 (3.9%) (due to HAI in 2, talc poudrage in 2, and malignancy in 1), HAI in 2 (1.6%), prolonged air leak in 14 (11.0%), and subcutaneous emphysema in 1 (0.8%). The details are shown in Table 4.

MT failed in two cases: the first case was due to extensive adhesions which rendered introducing the MT and the second one was a case of left primary spontaneous haemopneumothorax due to continuous bleeding from the ruptured emphysematous bulla.

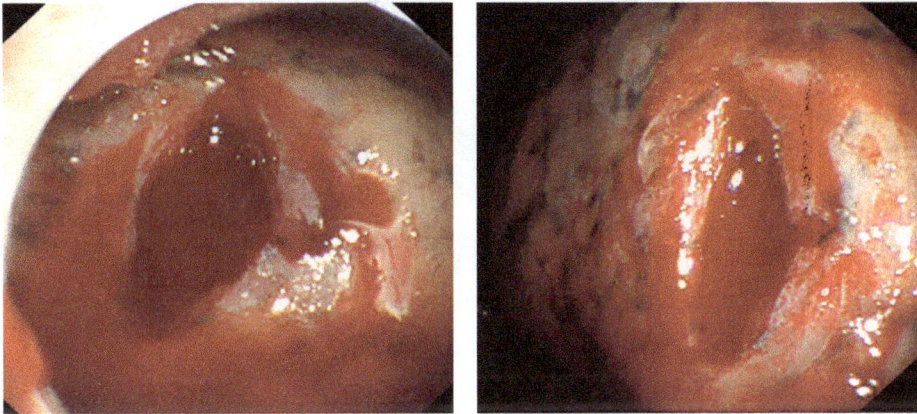

FIGURE 1: Lung laceration in one of the patients following introducing the trocar.

4. Discussion

Although this study was done on a large number of patients (127), the rate of complications was not so severe 16.5% ($n = 21$). The most serious complication was lung laceration which occurred in 3 cases, all of them occurred during introducing the trocar and did not exceed 1.5 cm in length as illustrated in Figure 1. Two of them were managed during performing MT by calling the cardiothoracic surgeon and the application of polyglycolic acid (PGA) mesh and fibrin glue over the site of the laceration under local anesthesia without any complications during and after the procedure but the third case was neglected during the procedure and that resulted in air leak and subcutaneous emphysema after procedure which increased and indicated urgent surgical intervention to close the laceration.

To prevent the occurrence of lung laceration, some authors advocate the creation of pneumothorax a few hours or even the day before the thoracoscopy. However, direct introduction of a blunt trocar into the thoracic wall without prior induction of pneumothorax is safe and effective, especially if there is enough pleural fluid. The trocar should always be inserted perpendicular to the chest wall with a rotating motion. It is safer to locate the tip over the border of the inferior rib at the chosen port of entry, in order to prevent damage to the intercostal vessels and nerves. The introduction of the trocar can be troublesome especially in cases of pleural adhesions. When the physician is not sure about the presence of tight adhesions between the lung and the chest wall at the chosen site of entry, a digital dissection and direct exploration of the port of entry with the telescope may be helpful [22]. Chest US can be also very helpful to identify loculations in the pleural cavity and to locate the best entry site for thoracoscopy [23].

Actually, US was done before MT in the 3 cases complicated with lung lacerations, pneumothorax was created before introducing MT, and there were no extensive adhesions which may play a role in the occurrence of lung laceration, but the main cause was vigorous maneuver during introducing the trocar.

The second and important complication in this study was fever; it occurred in 5 cases due to different causes. Fever was grade 1 in all cases according to Common Terminology Criteria for Adverse Events (CTCAE) version 4.0. Two of them occurred after talc poudrage and lasted only for two days and improved with antipyretics. The third case developed fever due to malignancy; this patient was diagnosed as pleural metastasis from renal cell carcinoma and did not improve with antipyretics or antibiotics. Already the patient presented with fever before performing MT, and it lasted with him until the discharge with exclusion of other causes. The fourth and fifth cases developed HAI in the form of worsening of the already diagnosed empyema after improvement following MT which was done for drainage and adhesiolysis; the fourth patient was of old age (70 years old) with bad general condition and stayed in hospital for one month; he developed fever two days after the procedure and improved after one week with antibiotics. The fifth patient has the same situation like the fourth one (being 76 years old, bad general condition, and long hospital stay for 33 days). He was complicated with septicemia and developed fever three days after the procedure which lasted for 2 days and then the patient died. Prolonged hospital stay with the bad general condition may play important role in the development of HAI.

There were 11 cases of death but not related to MT; the main cause was malignancy and the presence of other comorbidities as hepatic and renal diseases.

The median time for drainage by intercostal tube after procedure was 7.0 (range, 0.0–47.0) days. In this study, long drainage time was due to prolonged air leak and incomplete lung reexpansion especially in neoplastic patients and patients diagnosed as empyema with other comorbidities and bad general condition. Cases complicated with prolonged air leak were 14 (11.0%) including 7 cases with malignancy, 6 cases with empyema, and one case with TB.

With respect to developing postprocedure infections, this represents an area that can potentially be modified by improved patient management immediately after the procedure including active chest physiotherapy and early mobilization to reduce basal atelectasis, all practices that can be learnt

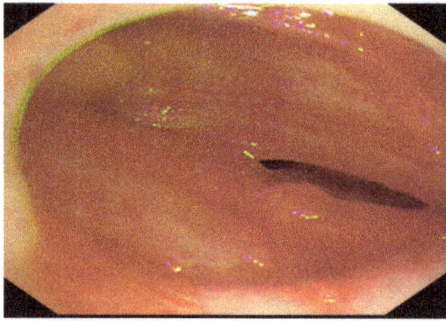

FIGURE 2: Obliteration of the pleural space due to extensive adhesions and pleural thickening.

from our surgical colleagues [23, 24]. The use of a one-off dose of intravenous broad spectrum antibiotic at the time of the procedure may also lead to a reduction of infections following thoracoscopy, although this practice varies among physicians and was not routine practice during the study period. The rates in this study of empyema, pneumonia, and 1-month mortality compare favorably with other large thoracoscopy series [25, 26].

MT failed in two cases: the first case was due to the presence of severe adhesions which rendered introducing MT so we gave up MT for the safety of the patient and thoracotomy was done. Chest US was used to determine the best site for introducing the trocar but the presence of extensive adhesions caused obliteration of the pleural cavity as illustrated in Figure 2. The second was a case of primary left haemopneumothorax due to spontaneous rupture of an emphysematous bulla, which was diagnosed before MT by chest CT. This indicated the presence of large amount of left pleural effusion with a rim of pneumothorax and a large apical emphysematous bulla, and thoracocentesis revealed hemorrhagic pleural effusion. The findings of bloody pleural effusion and normal pleura were observed during the procedure. Active bleeding was not clear but over 2,000 mL of hemorrhagic fluid was drained. A semiurgent video assisted thoracoscopic surgery (VATS) was indicated after the procedure, which was done on the next day for resection of the bulla.

5. Conclusions

In conclusion, medical thoracoscopy is generally a safe procedure. Lung laceration is the most serious complication and should be managed well. HAI is of low risk and can be controlled by medical treatment.

Abbreviations

MT: Medical thoracoscopy
HAI: Hospital acquired infection
ARDS: Acute respiratory distress syndrome
US: Ultrasonography.

Competing Interests

The authors declare no competing interests regarding the publication of this paper.

Acknowledgments

The authors are grateful to Dr. Akiko Kada, MD, Ph.D., from the clinical research center in NMC for helping them in the statistical analysis of the data.

References

[1] R. Loddenkemper, P. N. Mathur, M. Noppen et al., *Medical Thoracoscopy/Pleuroscopy. Manual and Atlas*, Thieme, Stuttgart, Germany, 2011.

[2] L. M. Seijo and D. H. Sterman, "Interventional pulmonology," *New England Journal of Medicine*, vol. 344, no. 10, pp. 740–749, 2001.

[3] C. E. Hooper, Y. C. G. Lee, and N. A. Maskell, "Setting up a specialist pleural disease service," *Respirology*, vol. 15, no. 7, pp. 1028–1036, 2010.

[4] H. C. Jacobaeus, "The cauterization of adhesions in artificial pneumothorax treatment of pulmonary tuberculosis under thoracoscopic control," *Proceedings of the Royal Society of Medicine*, vol. 16, pp. 45–62, 1923.

[5] A. N. McLean, S. R. Bicknell, L. G. McAlpine, and A. J. Peacock, "Investigation of pleural effusion: an evaluation of the new Olympus LTF semiflexible thoracofiberscope and comparison with Abram's needle biopsy," *Chest*, vol. 114, no. 1, pp. 150–153, 1998.

[6] P. Lee and H. G. Colt, "Rigid and semirigid pleuroscopy: the future is bright," *Respirology*, vol. 10, no. 4, pp. 418–425, 2005.

[7] J.-M. Tschopp, R. Rami-Porta, M. Noppen, and P. Astoul, "Management of spontaneous pneumothorax: stae of the art," *European Respiratory Journal*, vol. 28, no. 3, pp. 637–650, 2006.

[8] R. Loddenkemper and C. Boutin, "Thoracoscopy: present diagnostic and therapeutic indications," *European Respiratory Journal*, vol. 6, no. 10, pp. 1544–1555, 1993.

[9] C. Boutin, J. R. Viallat, P. Cargnino, and P. Farisse, "Thoracoscopy in malignant pleural effusions," *American Review of Respiratory Disease*, vol. 124, no. 5, pp. 588–592, 1981.

[10] R. Menzies and M. Charbonneau, "Thoracoscopy for the diagnosis of pleural disease," *Annals of Internal Medicine*, vol. 114, no. 4, pp. 271–276, 1991.

[11] H. E. Davies, J. E. Nicholson, N. M. Rahman, E. M. Wilkinson, R. J. O. Davies, and Y. C. G. Lee, "Outcome of patients with nonspecific pleuritis/fibrosis on thoracoscopic pleural biopsies," *European Journal of Cardio-Thoracic Surgery*, vol. 38, no. 4, pp. 472–477, 2010.

[12] M. Metintas, G. Ak, E. Dundar et al., "Medical thoracoscopy vs CT scan-guided abrams pleural needle biopsy for diagnosis of patients with pleural effusions: a randomized, controlled trial," *Chest*, vol. 137, no. 6, pp. 1362–1368, 2010.

[13] M. E. Froudarakis, "Diagnosis and management of pleural effusion in lung cancer," in *Pleural Diseases*, D. Bouros, Ed., pp. 427–447, Informa, New York, NY, USA, 2nd edition, 2009.

[14] M. E. Froudarakis, "Thoracoscopy one century later: the oldest interventional technique of modern pneumonology, with great future prospects," *Pneumon*, vol. 23, no. 1, pp. 28–33, 2010.

[15] G. F. Tassi, R. J. O. Davies, and M. Noppen, "Advanced techniques in medical thoracoscopy," *European Respiratory Journal*, vol. 28, pp. 1–9, 2006.

[16] N. M. Rahman, N. J. Ali, G. Brown et al., "Local anaesthetic thoracoscopy: British Thoracic Society pleural disease guideline 2010," *Thorax*, vol. 65, supplement 2, pp. ii54–ii60, 2010.

[17] D. C. Zavala, "Pulmonary hemorrhage in fiberoptic transbronchial biopsy," *Chest*, vol. 70, no. 5, pp. 584–588, 1976.

[18] C. P. Wall, E. A. Gaensler, C. B. Carrington, and J. A. Hayes, "Comparison of transbronchial and open biopsies in chronic infiltrative lung diseases," *American Review of Respiratory Disease*, vol. 123, no. 3, pp. 280–285, 1981.

[19] J.-R. Viallat, F. Rey, P. Astoul, and C. Boutin, "Thoracoscopic talc poudrage pleurodesis for malignant effusions: a review of 360 cases," *Chest*, vol. 110, no. 6, pp. 1387–1393, 1996.

[20] D. H. Rehse, R. W. Aye, and M. G. Florence, "Respiratory failure following talc pleurodesis," *American Journal of Surgery*, vol. 177, no. 5, pp. 437–440, 1999.

[21] M. Noppen, "Who's (still) afraid of talc?" *European Respiratory Journal*, vol. 29, no. 4, pp. 619–621, 2007.

[22] F. Rodríguez-Panadero and B. R. Romero, "Complications of thoracoscopy," in *Thoracoscopy for Pulmonologists: A Didactic Approach*, P. Astoul, G. Tassi, and J.-M. Tschopp, Eds., pp. 209–217, Springer, Berlin, Germany, 2014.

[23] A. R. L. Medford, "Additional cost benefits of chest physician-operated thoracic ultrasound (TUS) prior to medical thoracoscopy (MT)," *Respiratory Medicine*, vol. 104, no. 7, pp. 1077–1078, 2010.

[24] J. A. Brooks-Brunn, "Postoperative atelectasis and pneumonia: risk factors," *American Journal of Critical Care*, vol. 4, no. 5, pp. 340–351, 1995.

[25] J. A. Brooks-Brunn, "Postoperative atelectasis and pneumonia," *Heart and Lung*, vol. 24, no. 2, pp. 94–115, 1995.

[26] K. Viskum and B. Enk, "Complications of thoracoscopy," *Poumon et le Coeur*, vol. 37, no. 1, pp. 25–28, 1981.

3

Reconstructive Surgery for Head and Neck Cancer Patients

Matthew M. Hanasono

The University of Texas M.D. Anderson Cancer Center, 1515 Holcombe Boulevard, Unit 443, Houston, TX 77030, USA

Correspondence should be addressed to Matthew M. Hanasono; mhanasono@mdanderson.org

Academic Editor: Andrea Figus

The field of head and neck surgery has gone through numerous changes in the past two decades. Microvascular free flap reconstructions largely replaced other techniques. More importantly, there has been a paradigm shift toward seeking not only to achieve reliable wound closure to protect vital structures, but also to reestablish normal function and appearance. The present paper will present an algorithmic approach to head and neck reconstruction of various subsites, using an evidence-based approach wherever possible.

1. Introduction

The field of head and neck reconstructive surgery is a dynamic one. Advances made in the last decade are mostly secondary to expanded use of microvascular free flaps [1]. Several flaps, including the anterolateral thigh, fibula osteo-cutaneous, and suprafascial radial forearm fasciocutaneous free flaps, have emerged as workhorse flaps for reconstructing a wide variety of defects. As the anatomy of these flaps has become more familiar, their reliability and versatility have increased. Reliable wound closure without exposure of vital structures is no longer the only priority. Preserving function, including speech and swallowing, and restoring appearance are the goals in every reconstruction. Free flap success rates now routinely exceed 95 percent or better at most centers [1–3]. On top of this, minimizing flap donor site morbidity is an important consideration. Because of the high rate of recurrence as well as long-term complications following major head and neck resections and reconstructions, preservation of recipient vessel options and flap donor sites should also be a consideration. In the following paper, an algorithmic approach to mid-facial, mandibular, oral cavity, and pharyngoesophageal reconstruction will be reviewed and expected outcomes discussed.

2. Mid-Facial Reconstruction

Management of mid-facial defects is among the most complicated and controversial areas of head and neck oncologic reconstruction. Options include use of prosthetic obturators, pedicled flaps, and free flaps, sometimes combined with grafts or alloplasts [4]. The popularity of pedicled flaps has declined in recent years due to limited reach and volume. Prosthetic obturators remain a good solution for some patients with limited defects. For extensive defects, obturators may be difficult or impossible to retain, particularly in edentulous patients [5]. Furthermore, obturators are inappropriate for defects that involve resection of the skull base, orbital contents, orbital floor, or soft tissues of the face. Finally, some patients may not like the inconvenience of an obturator, which must be removed and cleaned regularly and periodically adjusted or replaced for fit and/or hygiene.

Mid-facial reconstructions with various bony and soft tissue free flaps have been described, and the best technique remains a subject of debate [6–11]. One of the fundamental problems with reconstructing the mid-face is that the defects created by oncologic resection are highly variable. Such defects usually not only involve the maxillary bones, but also may include a number of adjacent facial and cranial bones, as well as soft tissues of the face, palate, and orbit. Successful outcomes in mid-facial reconstruction involve not only a mastery of a broad range of reconstructive flaps and craniofacial plating techniques, but also an understanding of the requirements for prosthetic rehabilitation, which is used not only in place of reconstruction in some cases, but also often in concert with local and distant tissue transfer procedures.

2.1. Regional Anatomy and Nomenclature. The central structures of the mid-face are the paired maxillary bones, which are fused in the midline to form the upper jaw. The maxillary bones contribute to the roof of the mouth, the floor and lateral wall of the nasal cavity, and the floor and medial walls of the orbit. Each maxilla attaches laterally to the zygomatic bones, which comprise part of the orbital floor and the lateral orbital wall and provide shape to the cheek. In addition to the zygomatic bones, the maxillae also articulate with the frontal and ethmoid bones of the cranium and the nasal, lacrimal, inferior nasal conchal, palatine, and vomer bones of the face.

Many maxillary tumors extend into or arise from the orbit, which is a conical structure that contains the eye, extraocular muscles, and extraocular fat, as well as blood vessels and cranial nerves II, III, IV, V, and VI. The superior margin of the orbit is the frontal bone, the inferior margin is the maxilla, palatine, and zygomatic bones, the medial margin is the frontal, lacrimal, and ethmoid bones, and the lateral margin is the zygomatic and sphenoid bones. The orbit lies below the anterior cranial fossa, above the maxillary sinus, lateral to the nasal cavity, and anterior to the middle cranial fossa (medially) and the temporal fossa (laterally). From the orbital rim, the orbit tapers posteriorly to an apex, the entrance of the optic canal. Two large discontinuities, the superior and inferior orbital fissures, converge upon one another in the back of the orbit just lateral to the apex.

Oncologic resections of maxillary tumors can be quite variable [12]. There is no consensus in the literature on the nomenclature of types of maxillectomy. In many publications the term "partial" and the term "subtotal" have been used interchangeably. Spiro et al. [12] divided maxillectomies into limited, subtotal, and total depending on whether the resection involved predominantly one wall, at least two walls including the palate, or the entire maxilla. Others subclassify partial maxillectomy into infrastructure (where only the upper alveolus and hard palate below the level of nasal floor are removed), medial (where medial wall of maxilla often along with the medial 1/3rd of inferior orbital wall and the medial orbital wall is removed), suprastructure (where all the walls of maxilla, except for hard palate and upper alveolus, are removed), and subtotal (where all the walls of maxilla, except for the orbital floor and the zygomatic buttress, are removed) [13].

Orbital exenteration involves removal of all the orbital contents, in contrast to enucleation, which involves removal of only the globe. This technique is used for many adnexal cancers involving the eyelid with orbital extension. When the eyelid skin and orbicularis muscles are not involved in the cancerous process, such as in some palpebral conjunctival and orbital cancers, the anterior lamella of the eyelid (skin or musculocutaneous layer) can be spared and used for coverage of exenterated orbital defect. As a matter of aesthetic preference, the eyelids are still removed by some surgeons and replaced by skin from the reconstructive flap. In extended orbital exenteration, cancers of the paranasal sinuses, nasal cavity, and periorbital and facial soft tissues extending to the orbit require more radical surgical ablation including one or more orbital bony walls, as well as other structures such as the sinuses and facial skin. Both total maxillectomy and suprastructure maxillectomy may be combined with orbital exenteration, technically making it an extended orbital exenteration but more often referred to as an orbitomaxillectomy by most surgeons.

2.2. Reconstructive Approach. Medial maxillectomy involves resection of the medial wall of the maxilla and inferior turbinate. This surgery is usually indicated for benign or low-grade tumors arising from the lateral nasal wall, formerly performed through a lateral rhinotomy incision, and it is now frequently performed endoscopically. If no other structures are removed, reconstruction is unnecessary. For the remainder of maxillary and orbital resections, reconstruction or rehabilitation must be addressed with flaps, grafts, and/or prosthetics.

In terms of reconstruction, there are several key considerations. The status of the palate is the main determinator of which flap type, if any, is best suited for reconstructing the defect [5]. The amount of hard and soft palate resected as well as the location of the resection and the plans for dental restoration will dictate whether a prosthetic obturator is indicated or a bony or soft tissue flap should be performed. The status of the orbital floor is important if the orbital contents are to be preserved. Accurate reconstruction here, with grafts, implants, or bony flaps, is mandatory for useful eye function. If an extended orbital exenteration or orbitomaxillectomy is performed, a pedicled or free flap may be indicated to separate the orbit from the nasal cavity and sinuses or occasionally the intracranial cavity. A pedicled or free flap may also be needed to serve as lining of the remaining orbit for an orbital prosthetic when one is desired by the patient. A final consideration is whether facial skin and soft tissues, such as the lips, eyelids, or nose, will be included in the resection. Facial skin may be reconstructed with local tissues (e.g., cervicofacial rotation flap) or a pedicled or free flap, while other facial structures are usually addressed separately, most commonly with local tissue techniques (e.g., paramedian forehead flap for nasal reconstruction).

2.2.1. Suprastructure Maxillectomy. Suprastructure maxillectomies result in defects that do not involve the palate. Suprastructure defects that do not violate the bony orbit do not necessarily need reconstruction. An exception is when facial soft tissues are included in the resection and soft tissue cheek reconstruction is needed. Another exception may be when intracranial contents at the skull base have been exposed. In the latter case, a bulky soft tissue free flap that obliterates the maxillary sinus is recommended to isolate the intracranial cavity from the nasal cavity by creating a watertight seal against the dura or brain, thereby preventing cerebrospinal fluid leaks and meningitis, although small defects can sometimes be sealed with local or pedicled flaps, such as the temporoparietal fascia flap.

2.2.2. Unilateral Posterior Palatomaxillectomy. While any number of palatoalveolar defects is possible, Okay et al. [5] have recommended distinguishing defects based on whether function can be satisfactorily restored with an obturator or if a free flap is required. Palatoalveolar defects that spare both canine teeth can often be successfully treated with an obturator. In these cases, cantilever forces resulting in unstable prosthetic retention are minimized because of the favorable root morphology of the canine adjacent to the obturator and the substantial arch length provided by the remaining alveolus. Thus, defects including unilateral posterior palatomaxillectomy defects or anterior defects limited to the premaxilla, which bears the 4 incisor teeth, can be obturated and should be considered separately from those that cannot, including those that involve half the palate and those that involve the entire anterior arch or whole palate.

Based on this information, unilateral palatomaxillectomy defects posterior to the canine tooth can usually be treated with an obturator. However, some patients may still prefer to undergo autologous reconstruction due to inconvenience, hygiene issues, residual instability, mainly in edentulous patients, and long-term costs associated with periodic adjustment and replacement of the prosthesis [13–15]. Additionally, exposure of the intracranial contents, loss of the orbital floor or orbital contents, and resection of the facial soft tissues are indications for free flap reconstruction. Alternately, a temporalis muscle flap can be tunneled into the defect and placed against the skull base, if exposed, and, if large enough, close the palatal defect [16].

Soft tissue free flaps are our first choice for closure posterior palatomaxillary defects [16–18]. The aesthetic challenge is usually to provide adequate volume to the cheek to support the facial soft tissues and avoid a hollow appearance. An analogous situation is present in the mandible, where posterior mandibular reconstruction with soft tissue flaps can often achieve good results with regard to both function and appearance, provided the flap has adequate bulk. Restoration of posterior maxillary dentition, which is not easily visible even when smiling, is not a priority to many patients.

The anterolateral thigh (ALT) or rectus abdominis myocutaneous (RAM) free flaps are usually well suited to provide the appropriate amount of tissue for posterior palatomaxillary reconstruction (Figure 1). These flaps tend to be thicker in Western patients and will partially obliterate the maxillary sinus. Both flaps can be dissected such that their muscular components can be minimized and the flaps can be safely defatted in patients with more subcutaneous adipose tissue than desired. By utilizing distal perforators, the pedicle length is usually satisfactory in both flaps to reach the neck blood vessels without need for interposition vein grafting. Suturing to the palatal mucosa should take place over the bony palatal remnant to avoid an oronasal fistula, or holes can be drilled in the bony palate and a deep layer of sutures can be placed through them for an extra degree of wound closure stability.

For all free flap reconstructions in the mid-face, the facial artery and vein or the superficial temporal artery and vein are the preferred recipient vessels when available. When the facial artery and vein are used as recipient blood vessels, a subcutaneous tunnel is created within the cheek to the neck. Care is taken not to injure the parotid duct during tunnel creation by dissecting anterior to the Stensen's duct orifice. Facial nerve injury is avoided by staying within the subcutaneous plane, as in a facelift.

2.2.3. Unilateral Hemipalatomaxillectomy.

Unlike unilateral posterior palatomaxillectomy defects, those where the resection of the palate and alveolus extends anterior to the canine tooth defects are difficult to obturate because of the greater cantilever forces acting on the prosthesis, which must also rely on less dentition for retention. Free flap selection for these defects is somewhat controversial. Soft tissue free flaps are usually more straightforward surgically [16–18]. However, they do not provide a rigid skeletal framework, which can result in a loss of anterior maxillary projection on the side of the defect and cannot accept osseointegrated implants for dental restoration. To accommodate a conventional dental prosthesis, the soft tissue flap must not protrude excessively into the oral cavity. However, achieving a concave palatal reconstruction with soft tissue flaps can be technically challenging, especially if the lateral portion of the defect includes some or all of the buccal mucosa.

The author favors the use of osteocutaneous free flaps for hemipalatomaxillectomy defects in highly functional patients with a reasonable oncologic prognosis (Figure 3). Besides providing better anterior projection, osteocutaneous free flaps offer the possibility of osseointegrated implants for dental restoration. A caveat is that postoperative radiation therapy may render placement of osseointegrated implants risky, thus defeating one of the main purposes of bony reconstruction. In such cases, options include initial placement of an obturator, if possible, followed by delayed osteocutaneous free flap reconstruction following the conclusion of radiation or proceeding with immediate bony reconstruction and simultaneous osseointegrated implant placement. Some centers do perform delayed osseointegrated implant placement even into irradiated bony free flaps after treatment with hyperbaric oxygen therapy, although the efficacy of this strategy still needs to be established.

In terms of bony free flap selection, many donor sites have been suggested, including the fibula, scapula, radius, rib, and iliac crest [6–11]. The author favors the fibula because of its high quality bone stock that easily accommodates osseointegrated implants and tolerates the multiple osteotomies necessary to shape the bone so that it resembles the mid-facial form [19]. Regardless of which flap is used, osteotomies should be made to simulate the complex shape of the native maxilla as closely as possible. While it is tempting to simply place vascularized bone in a nonanatomic position and shape, our experience is that the soft tissues of the cheek will eventually contract and reveal the shape of the underlying bone, especially when postoperative radiation is administered.

2.2.4. Bilateral Palatomaxillectomy.

Bilateral palatomaxillectomy defects that involve loss of the anterior maxillary alveolar arch, including the canine teeth, need bony reconstruction to maintain mid-facial height, width, and projection. They also require bony reconstruction for dental restoration with osseointegrated implants, which are usually necessary to retain a prosthesis. Bilateral palatomaxillectomy defects can rarely, if ever, be stably obturated [19–21]. Although other

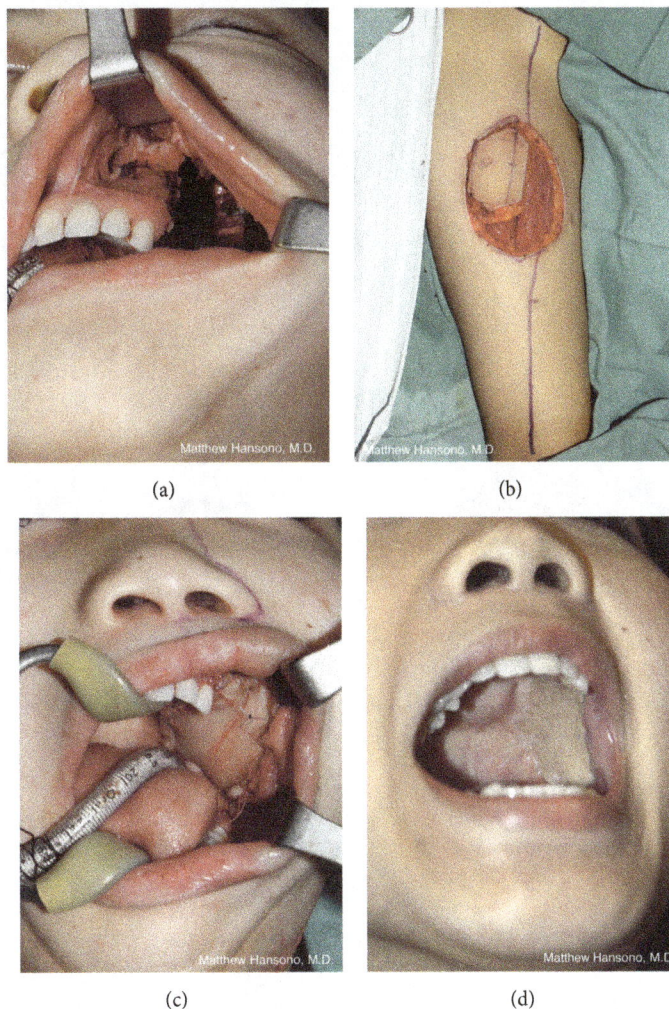

FIGURE 1: Posterior palatomaxillary defect following tumor removal (a). An anterolateral thigh free flap is harvested, measuring approximately 5 × 5 cm (b). Flap inset (c). Postoperative appearance (d).

osteocutaneous free flaps have been advocated, the fibula free flap is our preferred flap for bilateral palatomaxillectomy reconstruction for the same reasons noted above. In addition, for sizable defects involving both maxillary bones, the fibula offers the longest length of bone of the various flap options.

In our experience, 14 to 16 cm of bone length is typically needed to reconstruct a bilateral maxillectomy defect [19]. The lateral surface of the fibula bone is used to restore the vertical maxillary height, measured from the orbital rim to the occlusal plane of the hard palate, by orienting it such that it faces anteriorly on the face. The peroneal vessels, therefore, assume a posterior position facing the maxillary sinus. Some flexor hallucis longus muscle is usually included with the flap in order to obliterate the maxillary sinus cavity and provide adequate soft tissue around the vascular pedicle to prevent its desiccation. The skin paddle of the flap is used to reconstruct the palatal defect and the nasal surface of the flap is left to mucosalize spontaneously in most cases.

When the bony defect extends more laterally or posteriorly on one side than another, that side is usually preferred for the microvascular anastomosis due to closer proximity to the recipient blood vessels. Alternately, the side with better recipient blood vessels, if any, is selected. The leg that is ipsilateral to the side of the planned microvascular anastomosis is chosen as the fibula osteocutaneous free flap donor side so that the skin paddle can be used to restore the palate with tension on the cutaneous perforators. Vein grafts are used when pedicle length is inadequate to reach the recipient vessels. The facial blood vessels are usually preferred as recipients when available, due to their proximity to the defect and their good size match to the peroneal blood vessels.

After the resection is complete, a titanium reconstruction plate is fashioned based on the defect in the approximate shape of the Greek letter "omega" in the transverse plane (Figure 2). The configuration of the reconstruction plate is such that it simulates the width and projection of the native maxilla. The lateral portions of the reconstruction plate must be long enough to allow two or three screw fixations to the remaining zygomatic bones laterally.

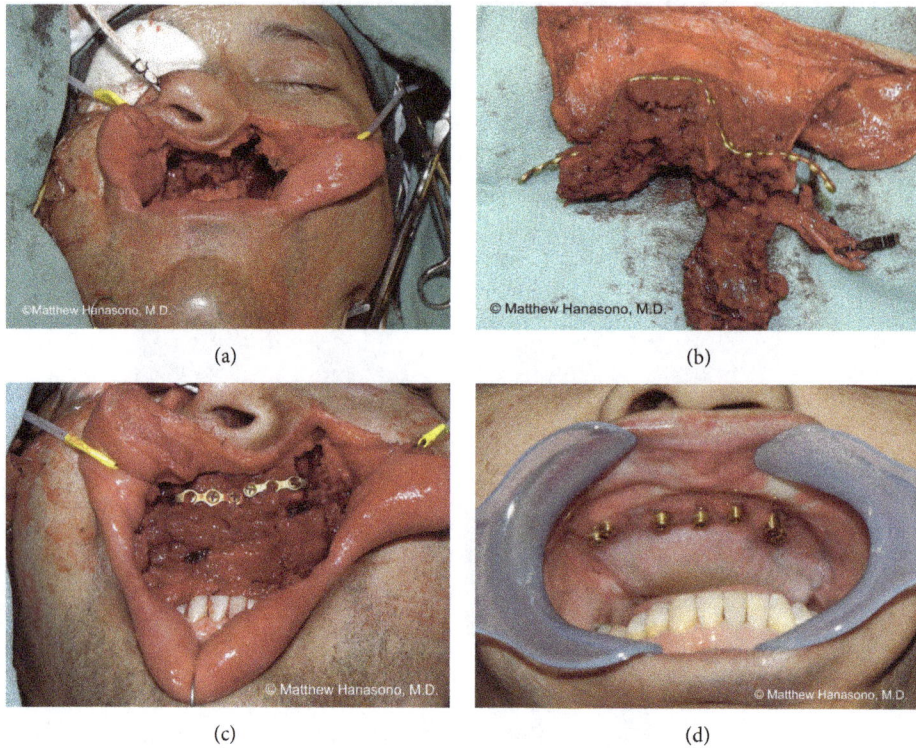

FIGURE 2: Anterior bilateral palatomaxillary defect following tumor removal (a). A fibula osteocutaneous free flap is osteotomized then rigidly fixated to resemble the Greek letter "omega" in the transverse plane (b). Flap inset (c). Postoperative appearance (d). The skin paddle is used to close the palatal defect, while the bone restores mid-facial height, width, and projection. Osseointegrated implants have been placed.

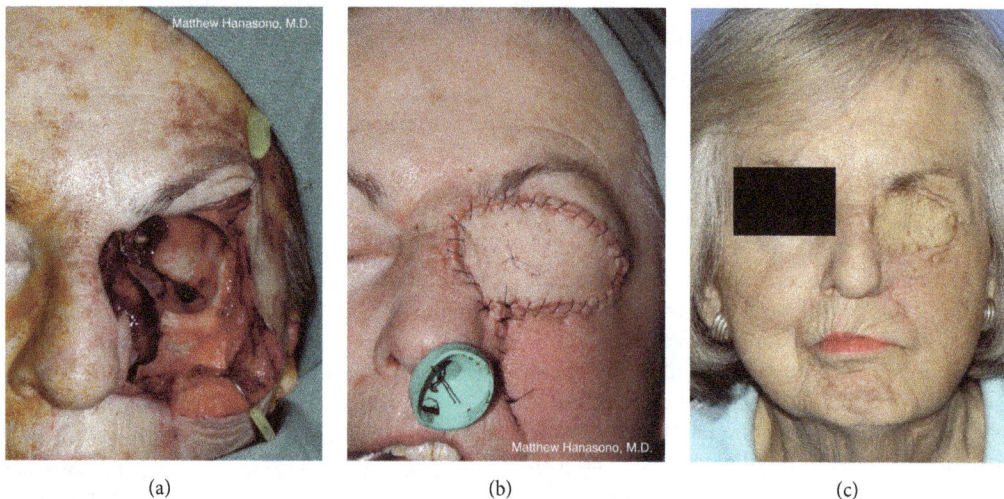

FIGURE 3: Orbitomaxillectomy defect following tumor removal (a). An anterolateral thigh free flap is used to close the defect and isolate the orbital cavity from the sinonasal cavities (b). A soft nasal trumpet is used to stent the nasal cavity open. Postoperative appearance (c).

Closing wedge osteotomies are performed on the fibular bone with a reciprocating saw, taking care not to injure the vascular pedicle. When reconstructing bilateral maxillectomy defects, the lateral portions of the "omega" recreate the malar regions. The central portion of the fibula free flap restores the maxillary alveolus. For unilateral (see *unilateral hemi-palatomaxillectomy*, above) or less than complete bilateral defects, a shorter segment of bone is used and one or more osteotomies can be omitted (i.e., the fibular bone resembles a half or incomplete "omega").

The portion of the fibula free flap that replaces the anterior maxillae is inset at the vertical level of the resected alveolus, rather than at the level of the dentition, to provide room for an implant-retained dental prosthesis. A slight downward angulation (about 20–25 degrees) of the portion of the fibula used to recreate the anterior maxillae is usually desirable to fully restore vertical facial height [22, 23].

Dental restoration with osseointegrated implants is performed three to six months after fibula free flap reconstruction. In patients with significant subcutaneous adipose tissue in their fibula free flap skin paddle, thinning of the fat is usually performed simultaneous with placement of the implants. Partial or total hardware removal is sometimes necessary in order to place the osseointegrated dental implants.

2.3. Orbital Floor Defects. Our experience suggests that, when supported by a soft tissue free flap, the orbital floor can usually be successfully reconstructed with bone grafts or alloplasts, even when postoperative radiation therapy is administered. Many surgeons, however, feel that bone grafts are relatively more resistant to radiation-associated complications than alloplasts are [24]. In a recent review of orbital floor reconstruction for trauma, Kirby et al. [25] found that autologous bone reconstructions were more likely to be complicated by orbital dystopia and enophthalmos compared to titanium mesh and porous polyethylene reconstructions, possibly due to increased difficulty in shaping the reconstructed orbital floor, irregular thickness, and unpredictable resorption. Obviously, alloplastic materials have the advantage of being available in virtually unlimited quantities and carry with them no donor site morbidity.

When using the fibula osteocutaneous free flap for reconstructing hemipalatomaxillectomy and bilateral palatomaxillectomy defects that include resection of the orbital floor, some soleus or flexor hallucis longus muscle can be included with the fibula free flap to support a bone graft or alloplastic orbital floor reconstruction. A double-barreled design to reconstruct both the floor and the hard palate is possible but challenging because of the limited space in the mid-face [26]. Patients who have had a complication following nonvascularized reconstruction can usually be reconstructed secondarily with a bony free flap, such as the fibula, scapula, and serratus anterior with rib, or radial forearm osteocutaneous free flaps.

In patients who have had orbital wall reconstruction, periodic light perception and visual acuity checks are necessary to rule out optic nerve injury or globe compression. Any signs of decreased vision should prompt an immediate ophthalmology consult and potential return to the operating room. Extraocular movements should be assessed as well, and a forced duction test at the conclusion of the surgery should always be performed.

2.4. Orbital Exenteration Defects. The primary goal of reconstruction is to line the orbital cavity with durable tissue as well as to exclude the nasal or sinus cavities when the medial or inferior orbital wall has been removed and protect the brain when the orbital roof has been removed. Additionally, the patient's desire for prosthetic rehabilitation should be considered when planning the reconstruction. A deep orbital cavity facilitates prosthetic fit while a bulky flap that sits flush with the face or bulges outward may not securely hold a prosthesis without osseointegrated implants. A bulky flap may also cause the prosthesis to protrude unnaturally.

Healing by secondary intention and granulation may be the simplest treatment after tumor resection. The entire process can take months and requires daily wound care with wet to dry dressings. When completely healed by secondary intention, the orbital cavity is only slightly shallowed with granulation tissue but allows easy inspection for local tumor recurrence. Wound closure can be accelerated by using a meshed or unmeshed split thickness skin graft to line the orbital cavity. Similar to healing by secondary intention, the split thickness skin grafting of the orbital defect also results in excellent visualization of the orbital cavity. Due to their thinness, skin graft reconstructions usually result in a deep orbital cavity that provides an excellent fit for an orbital prosthesis if one is desired by the patient. When there is no history of prior radiation and no postoperative radiation is planned, secondary intention and skin grafting even on bare orbital bone are usually successful methods for addressing the standard orbital exenteration wound.

If radiation is planned after surgery or if radiation has been given previously, more durable, well-vascularized lining of the orbital cavity with soft tissue rather than just spontaneous epithelialization or skin graft coverage is necessary to avoid chronic bone exposure and osteoradionecrosis. Among local pedicled flaps used, the most common ones are the temporalis muscle flap and temporoparietal fascia flap. The temporalis muscle flap, based on the anterior and posterior deep temporal arteries arising from the internal maxillary artery is thin enough to permit a reasonably secure fit for orbital prostheses, even without osseointegrated implants but results in a depression at the donor site, which may be cosmetically unfavorable in many patients [27]. The temporoparietal fascia flap covered by a split-thickness skin graft may be preferable in that there is no donor site deformity. In both cases, reach of these two flaps may be limited and it may be necessary to remove the lateral orbital wall in order to cover the entire orbital cavity. Large scalp or forehead flaps should be avoided when other reconstructive options are available because of their donor site disfigurement.

In extended orbital exenteration, the size of the cavity usually necessitates soft tissue coverage larger than what local or regional flaps can provide [28]. An exception is the resection of the lateral orbital wall alone, which is usually inconsequential from a reconstructive standpoint. The orbital cavity may still be reconstructed with a skin graft or regional flap. In addition, limited defects of the medial orbital wall can often still be reconstructed with a temporalis muscle flap. For all other defects, reconstruction should be performed with a microvascular free flap. A multitude of soft tissue free flaps are satisfactory for reconstruction of the extended orbital exenteration cavity.

Our preference is to reconstruct the cavity with a radial forearm fasciocutaneous free flap in cases where the bony resection is limited [27]. This flap provides an adequate amount of tissue with relatively little bulk in nonobese patients to accommodate an orbital prosthetic without revision surgery. In cases where the bony resection is more extensive a larger, bulkier flap is preferred. The RAM or the ALT free flaps are good choices in this situation [27]. Both flaps may be designed such that muscle tissue obliterates the sinuses and creates a seal over any exposed dura, preventing infection with sinonasal bacterial flora. Bulkier flaps such as these are required to restore mid-facial volume and preserve cheek contour.

Orbital exenteration performed in concert with a suprastructure maxillectomy (i.e., orbitomaxillectomy) adds another reconstructive priority: closure of the nasal cavity to prevent the escape of air and nasal drainage. Because the formation of a sinonasocutaneous fistula along the suture line between the medial flap (or native cheek skin) and the nose can be difficult to treat, every effort should be made to obtain a secure closure. While thin fasciocutaneous flaps that result in a concave orbital cavity are beneficial for patients with isolated orbital exenteration defects that wish to have an orbital prosthesis, for patients with orbitomaxillectomy defects, bulkier free flaps that obliterate the orbital cavity in order to minimize the chance of a fistula as well as maintain cheek contour are indicated. The rectus abdominis free flap, harvested as a myocutaneous flap or as a muscle-sparing variant (i.e., muscle-sparing rectus abdominis free flap or deep inferior epigastric perforator flap), is suitable and can be tailored to the specifics of the defect in terms of size, volume, and desired pedicle length. The ALT free flap also works well for orbitomaxillectomy reconstruction (Figure 3). A myocutaneous ALT free flap, incorporating some or all of the thickness of the vastus lateralis muscle, can be used when the thigh is thin and has insufficient adipose tissue to restore cheek contour.

Defects involving both an orbital exenteration defect and a palatomaxillectomy defect are best reconstructed with flaps that allow for multiple skin paddles to close the three defects (external orbital skin, nasal lining, and palatal coverage) separately allowing for airtight skin-to-skin and skin-to-mucosa closure. Both the RAM free flap and ALT free flap are usually good choices here as well, again tailoring the flap design to include more or less muscle based on the extent of the defect. In cases where the pedicle of the ALT free flap only gives rise to a single cutaneous perforator, a portion of the skin paddle can be deepithelialized to reconstruct two or more surfaces. It is the author's preference to usually leave a "raw" (noncutaneous) flap surface facing the nasal cavity and allow it to spontaneously remucosalize.

2.5. Complications. In our experience, the success rate of free flaps used in mid-facial reconstruction is as high as free flaps used to reconstruct other head and neck defects [17]. Because of the greater distance from the cervical recipient blood vessels, there is the potential for pedicle length to be inadequate. In such instances, interposition vein grafting is preferable to performing anastomoses under tension. Also, care must be taken to make an adequately large subcutaneous tunnel for the pedicle to reach the neck without compression.

Specific to maxillary and orbital reconstruction is the potential for oronasal (i.e., palatal) fistulae and sinonasocutaneous fistulae, usually near the medial canthus [17]. Closure along palatal and facial suture lines must be multilayered and meticulous. Nasal obstruction should be avoided as air under pressure can cause wound breakdown along lateral rhinotomy incisions and medial orbital incisions. In our experience, late occurring fistulae in irradiated patients rarely heal spontaneously and usually require another free flap for closure.

With regard to orbital reconstruction, there is a potential for graft or implant exposure along the orbital rim when tissues are thin and poorly vascularized, especially when incisions are placed over bony prominences or titanium hardware. In such cases, consideration should be given to placing flap tissue between bone grafts, implants, or hardware and the cheek or eyelid skin or to replacing the skin with a flap skin. Also, accurate positioning of the reconstructed orbital walls is critical to avoiding orbital content entrapment, enthophthalmos or exophthalmos, vertical dystopia (eyes at different levels), or even blindness due to elevated intraocular pressures or impingement of the optic nerve if grafts and implants are placed too far posteriorly in the region of the orbital apex.

3. Mandibular Reconstruction

Reconstruction of the mandible can be quite complex and time-consuming following resection of cancers. Mandibular defects frequently involve composite tissues including oral mucosa and soft tissue structures, mandibular bone, and, in some cases, external skin. Nevertheless, many advances have been made in mandibular reconstruction in the past two decades, including the development of vascularized bone flaps, low profile, high tensile strength reconstruction plates, the ability to restore dentition with osseointegrated implants, and the incorporation of computer-aided design (CAD) and computer-aided manufacturing (CAM) into the surgical planning.

Goals of mandibular reconstruction include reestablishing the shape of the lower third of the face, creating a surface for mastication or dental restoration, preventing deviation of the jaw leading to malocclusion, maintaining free movement of the temporomandibular joint, and providing a stable wound that does not result in an orocutaneous fistula. In addition, mandibular reconstruction should not result in tethering the tongue in a way that affects speech or deglutition or introduce redundant tissue that can obstruct the airway or compromise oral hygiene. The reconstruction must also be reliable and long lasting. Mandibular reconstruction that results in early fracture or extrusion of bone flaps or grafts, as well as reconstruction plates, results in a situation that is frequently even more difficult to treat than the initial defect [29].

3.1. Regional Anatomy. The mandible provides the bony support for the lower third of the face and bears the lower teeth. Each side of the mandible consists of a lateral horizontal portion, called the body, a perpendicular portion, called the ramus, an alveolar process along the upper border of the mandible, which bears the teeth, a condyle, which forms the temporomandibular joint with the temporal bone, and a coronoid process, which is a triangular bony projection, anterior to the condyle. The paired mandibular bones join anteriorly in the midline at the symphysis. The portion of the body just lateral to the symphysis is referred to as the parasymphyseal region. The body and the ramus meet in a region termed the angle of the mandible (also known as the gonial angle). There are two foramina on each side of the mandible: the mandibular foramen on the deep side, which is penetrated by the inferior alveolar nerve, a branch of the mandibular division of the trigeminal (V) nerve, and the mental foramen on the superficial side, from which the mental nerve, a continuation of the interior alveolar nerve, emerges inferior to the second premolar tooth and supplies sensation to the lower lip.

Many muscles attach to the bony mandible. Anteriorly, the paired genioglossus muscles attach to the inner surface of the mandible at the mentum, lateral to the lower part of the symphysis. Immediately inferior to the attachment of the genioglossus muscles is the attachment point of the paired geniohyoid muscles. The mylohyoid, digastric, and the superior pharyngeal constrictor muscles also attach to the inner surface of the mandible along its inferior, inner border. Loss of the anterior mandible, therefore, can have profound effects on swallowing and protection from aspiration due to posterior displacement of the tongue and limited laryngeal elevation, which can also contribute to airway obstruction. Because of this, close airway monitoring and strong consideration for prophylactic (usually temporary) tracheostomy are indicated. Patients need to be counseled regarding potential impairment of swallowing and chronic aspiration following anterior mandibular resection. Speech can also be affected and the tongue will have limited protrusion.

The muscles of mastication insert along the posterior mandible. The temporalis muscle inserts mostly onto the coronoid process, while the masseter muscle inserts broadly along the lateral surface of the mandibular ramus and posterior body. The lateral pterygoid muscles attach to the condylar neck on each side, while the medial pterygoid muscles, which serve to depress the mandible and open the mouth, insert on the medial surface of the angle. Loss of the posterior portion of the mandible, therefore, results in impaired mandibular movement on the affected side. Even with reconstruction, mouth opening and closing will be dependent upon the actions of the contralateral muscles of mastication. Tension from the medial and lateral pterygoid muscles will tend to rotate the mandible toward the side of the resection.

3.2. Reconstructive Approach. Options for treating mandibular defects include performing no reconstruction with primary closure of the oral soft tissues to themselves, reconstruction with metal plates, nonvascularized bone grafts, osteomyocutaneous pedicled flaps, soft tissue pedicled or free flaps, and osseous or osteocutaneous free flaps.

3.3. Mandibular Reconstruction with Reconstruction Plates. Mandibular reconstruction with a reconstruction plate that spans a segmental bony mandibular defect was a more popular technique prior to the development of microvascular free bone flaps. Some centers continue to utilize reconstructive plates when a patient is deemed unsuitable for a prolonged operative procedure involving free tissue transfer or when microvascular expertise is unavailable. However, experience

has shown that such reconstructions are at high risk for complications, including plate fracture, and/or exposure, either intraorally or through the skin of the cheek or chin [30].

To help decrease the rate of exposure, many surgeons have combined reconstruction plates with a pectoralis major muscle or myocutaneous pedicled flap or a soft tissue free flap. However, Wei et al. [29] still reported a complication rate of 69% in patients reconstructed with soft tissue free flaps, primarily the anterolateral thigh fasciocutaneous free flap and a reconstruction plate, in a series of 80 patients. Plate exposure was the most common complication, followed by soft tissue deficiency, deformity of the lateral face, intraoral contracture, trismus, and osteoradionecrosis. Thirty-one percent of the patients with complications ultimately underwent a secondary salvage procedure with a fibula osteocutaneous flap.

Overall, complication rates associated with a reconstructive plate and soft tissue flap are reported to be between 21 and 87 percent [30, 31]. Anterior defects are associated with a higher rate of plate extrusion than lateral defects as are defects in patients undergoing radiation treatment or with a history of prior irradiation. In addition, larger defects result in significantly higher failure rates than smaller defects.

Even when patients are reasonable candidates for a free flap, some surgeons advocate plate or plate and soft tissue flap reconstruction in patients with advanced cancers and a limited life expectancy, since surgery is usually shorter and recovery is usually faster. However, this approach must be carefully considered on a case-by-case basis, because the incidence of plate-related complications is high. In addition, the results are rarely ideal due to persistent contour deformity and malocclusion. Secondary salvage of such complications with vascularized bone flaps can be performed but tends to be much more difficult than if it is performed at the time of the resection due to more challenging dissection of recipient vessels and greater difficulty restoring accurate occlusion secondary to postoperative and radiation therapy-associated scar contracture.

3.4. Nonvascularized Bone Grafts. Autogenous bone grafts can be used for mandibular reconstruction. The bone is revascularized by a process of creeping substitution. Sources of cortical bone graft include iliac crest, split calvarium, and rib. Nonvascularized bone grafts may be used in defects less than about 5 cm long. High failure rates are frequently seen in longer segments and in anterior defects. Preoperative or postoperative radiation therapy is a contraindication due to high rates of extrusion, resorption, and infection, and, therefore, use of nonvascularized bone grafts for mandible reconstruction is usually restricted to patients with benign disease or who require mandibular surgery for orthognathic rather than oncologic indications. Metallic mesh or Dacron trays filled with cancellous bone chips have also been used for limited defects. This technique is associated with a high rate of extrusion and bone graft dissolution, especially in cancer patients, and has generally fallen out of favor.

3.5. Vascularized Bone Flaps. Mandibular reconstruction with vascularized bone flaps transferred by microsurgical anastomosis should be considered the gold standard in oncologic reconstruction [32, 33]. Use of vascularized bone flaps is associated with early bony union, generally within six weeks. Vascularized bone flaps demonstrate very little bony resorption. Unlike nonvascularized bone grafts, bone flaps can be used to reconstruct large segmental bone losses and can tolerate radiation therapy without resorption, fracture, or extrusion. The commonly used bone flaps may be harvested with a cutaneous or muscular component that allows for simultaneous soft tissue reconstruction. Some flaps can be harvested simultaneously with oncologic resection or cervical vessel dissection by a second team to save time. Some vascularized bone flaps can reliably accept osseointegrated implants, which require a minimum of 6 to 7 mm of bone height for stable placement [34].

Pedicled bone flaps, such as the pectoralis major muscle with rib or sternal bone and the trapezius muscle with scapula, have also been described [35]. The pectoralis osteomyocutaneous flap can be used for anterior defects and the trapezius osteomyocutaneous flap for lateral defects. The lack of reliability, particularly of the distal flap that supplies the bone, limited ability to shape and configure both the soft tissue, and the bony flap components to fit the defect, restricted reach, and limited availability of bone make these two flaps secondary options after free bone flaps. Their use is primarily of historic significance.

3.5.1. Fibula Free Flap. The fibula osteocutaneous flap is probably the most frequently used choice for mandibular reconstruction (Figure 4) [32, 33]. The fibula bone is primarily an ankle stabilizer and provides the origin for several muscles of the lower leg but is expendable provided that the distal several centimeters of the bone, including the lateral malleolus, are spared. A 22 to 25 centimeters segment of fibula bone may be harvested in the adult patient, permitting reconstruction of near-total mandibular defects with a single flap.

The vascular supply of the fibula free flap is the peroneal artery and vein. It is important to examine both lower extremities and palpate for dorsalis pedis and posterior tibial pulses preoperatively [36]. In addition to pathologic conditions, it is important to rule out the possibility of peroneal arteria magna, an anatomic variant where the peroneal artery is the dominant arterial inflow to the distal lower extremity and a fibula free flap is contraindicated [37]. A patient with findings consistent with arterial insufficiency or venous stasis may not be a candidate for a fibula free flap. When the pedal arteries are not palpable or the circulation to the lower extremity is questionable, additional studies may be required, such as conventional, magnetic resonance, or computed tomographic angiography of the lower extremities, prior to performing fibula free flap harvest.

The choice of leg is based on the anticipated side of the recipient blood vessels and expected need for extra- or intraoral lining. The author usually prefers to use the leg that is contralateral to the side of the recipient blood vessels when intraoral lining is needed based on the location of the septocutaneous perforators that travel along the posterior-lateral border of the fibula in its native position on the leg.

The flap is oriented so that the pedicle is on the lingual side, to minimize external compression and allow plate placement on the lateral aspect of the fibula and, for posterior defects, is usually placed posteriorly close to the branches of the external carotid artery and the internal jugular vein.

Osteotomies may be completed while the flap is left *in situ* or during the inset of the flap into the mandibular defect. Performing the osteotomies while the pedicle is still attached to the leg has the advantage of minimizing ischemia time. Also, any injuries to the pedicle can be identified well in advance of revascularization, an advantage that is perhaps most important when rigid fixation and skin paddle inset are performed prior to the microvascular anastomosis. Other surgeons prefer to perform osteotomies after the pedicle is divided due to increased freedom of movement, potentially avoiding traction injury to the pedicle blood vessels.

The author prefers to use a locking titanium reconstruction plate to secure the osteotomized fibula to the remaining native mandibular segments. Some surgeons have had success with using smaller, very low profile miniplates. Such plates have the advantage of permitting fine adjustments to the final shape of the reconstructed mandible while locking reconstruction plates are considered to possess superior stability and are able to tolerate higher loads.

In certain cases, a double-barrel approach to mandibular reconstruction is used to increase bony height [38]. In this technique, reconstruction proceeds in the usual manner but the distal portion of the fibula is turned back 180 degrees onto the proximal fibula for additional height of the reconstructed mandible to more closely approximate the height of the normal dentulous mandible. The double barrel technique is best suited for reconstruction anterior mandibular defects, as the normal height of the mandible is greater in this region. Laterally, the width of a single fibular segment closely approximates the height of the native mandible [22]. When a single width of fibula is used, the fibula is aligned with the lower border of the mandible, rather than the alveolus, in order to achieve the best possible external contour.

Malocclusion following mandibular reconstruction may still not occur infrequently. Whenever possible, the mandible is preplated prior to mandibular resection so that the reconstruction can be designed to maintain the spatial orientation of the native mandible. When preplating is not feasible due to an exophytic tumor, pathologic fracture, or prior resection, use of an external fixator can be considered. More recently, use of computer planning and rapid prototype modeling has helped improve outcomes, particularly when preplating is not feasible [39–41].

3.5.2. Iliac Crest Free Flap. The iliac crest free flap provides a generous amount of cortical and cancellous bone for mandibular reconstruction. The deep circumflex iliac vessels comprise the vascular pedicle of the iliac crest free flap and demonstrate consistent anatomy, reasonable length (average of eight to ten centimeters), and appropriate vessel diameter (average of two to three millimeters) for microsurgical application. The blood supply of the iliac crest bone flap is robust, incorporating both nutrient perforators and periosteal vessels allowing the flap to tolerate multiple osteotomies.

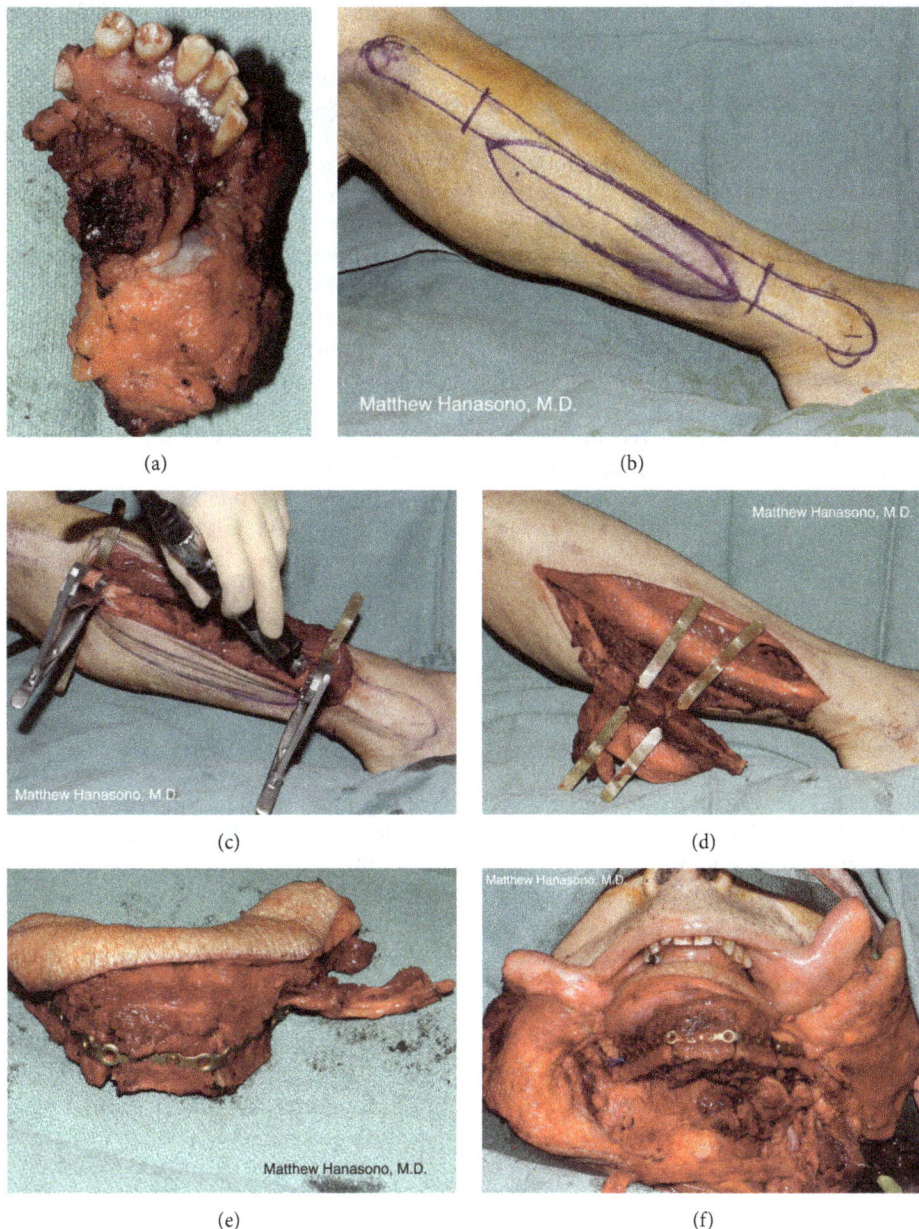

FIGURE 4: Composite anterior mandibular resection for a large invasive floor of mouth cancer (a). Skin markings for a fibula osteocutaneous free flap (b). Approximately 5 to 7 cm of proximal and distal bone are left *in situ* (c). Osteotomies for shaping the fibula can be made prior to or after pedicle division (d). Fibula osteocutaneous free flap after rigid fixation with a titanium reconstruction plate (e). Flap inset (f).

The iliac crest bone may be harvested as a full-thickness bicortical or as a partial-thickness unicortical (inner cortex) bone flap. Unicortical bone flaps are associated with a superior donor site appearance and theoretically less donor site morbidity but less bone stock [42]. The natural curved contour of the bone is often considered ideal for lateral mandibular reconstruction. Reconstruction of anterior defects usually requires an osteotomy. The bone stock, particularly when harvested full-thickness, reliably accommodates osseointegrated dental implants.

The flap may be harvested as a bone-only flap or with an associated skin and/or muscle paddle for reconstruction of composite defects. The skin paddle, which is nourished by several perforators arising from the deep circumflex iliac vessels, may be as wide as 9 to 12 cm and still be closed primarily in most patients. Previously, osteocutaneous iliac crest free flaps included harvesting a cuff of external oblique muscle, internal oblique muscle, and transversalis fascia with the skin paddle, but in recent years perforator dissection has been more commonly performed, resulting in a less bulky soft tissue component [43]. Even when the skin island is dissected as a perforator flap without a muscular component, iliac crest osteocutaneous free flaps may be excessively bulky in some patients and can require substantial primary or later revisionary thinning or use of a second, thinner flap for soft tissue reconstruction. Alternately, a separate internal oblique muscle paddle, based on the ascending branch of the deep circumflex iliac artery, which arises within 1 cm of the anterior superior iliac spine, can also be harvested for reconstruction of composite defects and provide a thin layer of soft tissue coverage.

The donor site, while hidden in clothing, may result in a contour deformity and/or hernia. Gait abnormalities also occur not infrequently. Harvesting the bone flap as a split-cortical flap decreases the morbidity of the flap by preserving hip contour, minimizing gait disturbances, and providing better support for the abdominal viscera resulting in a decreased risk for hernia. Meticulous hemostasis and closed suction drainage of the donor site are recommended as there is significant potential for donor site hematomas and seromas. Obesity is a relative contraindication to performing reconstruction with the iliac crest free flap due to difficulty in flap dissection and increased risk for postoperative donor site hernias.

3.5.3. Scapular Free Flap. Another alternative for mandibular reconstruction is the scapular free flap. The scapula flap has traditionally been based on the circumflex scapular artery. The length of the pedicle can be increased several centimeters by including the more proximal subscapular vessels. The subscapular vessels are also of larger caliber than the circumflex scapular vessels, which may be an advantage in performing the microvascular anastomosis.

The bone may be harvested from either the lateral or the medial edge of the scapula. The lateral scapular bone flap, based on the vertically oriented parascapular branch of the circumflex scapular artery, has a shorter vascular pedicle but is thicker. The medial scapular bone flap, based on the horizontally oriented cutaneous scapular branch of the circumflex scapular artery, is thinner but associated with a longer pedicle and minimal disturbance of the teres major and minor muscles and the glenohumeral joint, resulting in less postoperative shoulder stiffness. Approximately 10 to 14 centimeters of linear bone may be harvested from either the lateral or medial aspect of the scapula.

A skin paddle, based on a cutaneous branch of the circumflex scapular artery, can be harvested with the osseous portion of the flap if needed. For larger defects, a chimeric flap utilizing the subscapular regional blood supply can be harvested to include a scapular or parascapular skin paddle and the latissimus dorsi (with or without an overlying skin paddle) and serratus anterior muscles [44–46]. The serratus anterior can be harvested with a rib to allow for a second bony reconstruction. Furthermore, a thoracodorsal artery perforator skin flap can also be harvested rather than a latissimus dorsi muscle or myocutaneous flap along with other flaps arising from the subscapular axis. The potential configurations are numerous.

Another variation of the scapular osseous flap involves utilizing the angular branch of the thoracodorsal artery [46]. This branch usually arises from the latissimus dorsi branch of the thoracodorsal artery and lies within the submuscular fat pat beneath the superior edge of the latissimus dorsi and teres major muscles. It enters the scapular bone near the inferior angle or tip of the scapula. Basing the scapular flap on this branch allows for a longer pedicle, up to 17 cm if dissected to the axillary artery, and reliably supplies the medial, lateral, and angular portions of the scapular bone. The author has used it in anterior mandibular reconstructions in patients who are not candidates for fibula free flap reconstruction [45]. In this case, the curved shape of the scapular tip nicely restores the shape of the anterior mandible without the need for osteotomies for shaping. However, a major disadvantage of the scapular bone, regardless of its pedicle blood supply, is that it is often quite thin and does not consistently provide enough bone stock for osseointegrated implant placement.

Although a potentially reliable donor site, the scapula flap requires careful planning for positioning the patient during flap harvest, preparation of recipient vessels, microvascular anastomosis, and flap inset. The location of the scapula makes it very difficult to perform a two-teamed approach for harvesting the flap and preparation of the recipient site. Patients may note a degree of shoulder stiffness and limited abduction following the harvest of the scapula flap. Because of this, physiotherapy should routinely be part of the postoperative course.

3.5.4. Radial Forearm Free Flap. For soft tissue reconstruction of the head and neck, the radial forearm fasciocutaneous free flap has a reliable, long (up to 20 centimeters) vascular pedicle. The flap is thin and pliable and can be made sensate by neurorrhaphy of the lateral antebrachial cutaneous nerve to the inferior alveolar nerve. This flap can also be designed as an osteocutaneous flap by inclusion of the anterior (volar) cortex of the radial bone. Up to 14 centimeters of unicortical radius nourished by periosteal branches from the radial artery may be harvested for selected osseous defects. However, the use of the osteocutaneous radial forearm free flap is typically not a first line option due to the limited thickness of the bone that may be harvested without disturbing the structural mechanics of the hand and the risk for radial bone fracture in the forearm after harvest [47].

From a third to a half of the radius may be harvested for limited bony defects. Care must be taken not to detach the flexor pollicis longus muscle attachment to the radius, although a portion of the muscle is included in the flap as a muscle cuff that contains the radial artery perforators nourishing the bone. The distal limit of the bony flap is the insertion of the brachioradialis tendon and the proximal limit is the pronator teres muscle insertion. Osseointegrated implant placement in the radial bone flap has been accomplished but it is generally accepted that these are less reliable than those performed in the other bone flaps.

The donor site morbidity following the harvest of an osteocutaneous radial forearm free flap can be significant. Tendon rupture, carpal tunnel syndrome, and a significant motor weakness have been reported [47]. Radial bone fracture is estimated to occur about 15 percent of the time. Some surgeons suggest prophylactically plating the radius in the same setting as harvesting the flap. Nonetheless, the potential for chronic hand weakness or pain coupled with the thinner donor bone stock of the radial forearm osteocutaneous flap decreases enthusiasm in using this flap as a primary choice in reconstruction of load-bearing segmental mandibular defects, particularly in the anterior mandible.

3.6. Reconstructive Algorithm. Concerning the various types of flap choices for osseous mandibular reconstruction, each flap varies in terms of pedicle length, skin paddle, flap length, ability to accept osseointegrated implants, and patient morbidity. The iliac crest and fibula free flaps most reliably accept osseointegrated implants consistently due to their thickness [48]. The scapular free flap offers numerous soft tissue reconstruction options when harvested as part of a chimeric free flap with other skin and muscle components supplied by the subscapular arterial axis and may provide adequate bone stock for osseointegrated implants in select patients. The skin paddle of the radial forearm free flap is highly reliable and thin, making inset easier. In terms of vascular pedicle length, the radial osteocutaneous free flap has the longest available potential vascular pedicle. This option may be appealing in the patient with an absence of satisfactory local recipient vessels. However, this flap is limited by the very thin bone stock it provides and the risk for radial bone fracture at the donor site, as mentioned. The fibula free flap provides the longest amount of bone, has a good pedicle length and caliber, and, when dissected appropriately, has a reliable skin paddle. Based on its versatility, as well as acceptable donor site morbidity, the fibula free flap is the preferred method of mandibular reconstruction for those defects in which a vascularized bone flap is indicated at most centers, with other free flap choices being secondary and based on soft tissue needs, donor site availability, risk for complications, and patient positioning.

The specific reconstructive technique chosen should also depend on the location of the mandibular defect. Although several defect classification systems have previously been described, the decision-making process can be simplified by considering whether the mandibular defect is anterior, lateral, or posterior. Anterior defects involve the region of the parasymphysis and symphysis, anterior to the first bicuspid. The lateral defects occur posterior to the canine, encompassing some or all of the mandibular body, and extend to the angle of the mandible or the mid-ramus but spare enough of the ramus and condyle to preserve joint movement and allow for titanium plate fixation. Posterior defects are those that involve the condyle and can be limited to the ramus or extend anteriorly to encompass the body up to the parasymphysis. Therefore, the presence of the condyle and upper ramus of the mandible differentiates lateral defects from posterior defects.

3.6.1. Anterior Mandibular Defects. The anterior mandible may be involved with floor of mouth and anterior tongue cancers, as well as occasionally with lower lip cancers by direct extension. As with all cancers invading the mandible, a preoperative computed tomography (CT) scan is requisite, and evidence of cortical invasion will be an indication that a segmental mandibulectomy will be required. Note that tumors that abut the mandible but do not invade the cortex are often treated with a marginal mandibulectomy (removal

of the upper or lingual bony cortex of the mandible) and can usually be covered with a soft tissue pedicled or free flap alone.

Any defect that includes the anterior mandible should be reconstructed with vascularized bone whenever possible (Figure 4). Failure to reconstruct the anterior mandible results in the so-called "Andy Gump" deformity, a condition that is disfiguring and may be functionally problematic in terms of mastication, pooling of saliva, loss of oral competence, and even airway support. It is in this region that the mandible forms a curve and provides projection to the lower face, and, therefore, bony reconstruction is required to maintain facial symmetry.

The linear bone of the fibula will require one or more wedge-shaped osteotomies to restore the curvature of the mandible. Whenever possible, it helps to prebend the titanium reconstruction plate to the native mandible prior to the resection. The reconstruction plate is used as a guide for shaping the fibula free flap (or other bone flap). The simplest technique for planning the osteotomies is by cutting a paper or plastic template, such as a sterile paper ruler, to fit the shape of the titanium plate. More recently, computer-generated cutting guides have become available that facilitate making precise osteotomies at the angles dictated by the preoperative plan created using computer-aided design software (Figure 5).

The mandibular height in the dentulous patient is greater in this region than the lateral mandible, averaging 33.5 mm in males and 31.1 mm in females [22]. By comparison, the width of the lateral surface of the fibula averages 17.9 mm in men and 13.1 mm in women [22]. Hence, a double-barrel configuration may be desirable in the anterior mandible. In such cases, the lower "barrel" of the fibula should ideally project anteriorly several millimeters further than the upper "barrel" to maintain both chin projection and occlusion. If a single-barrel configuration is used, the fibula is inset so that it matches the occlusion of the maxilla. In edentulous patients, the mandible will tend to overrotate and anterior projection can be substantially increased. In such cases, the fibula will need to be set back considerably (1 to 2 cm or more) if there are no plans for dental restoration to limit mandibular excursion and avoid the appearance of a severe prognathia.

3.6.2. Posterior Mandibular Defects. Posterior mandibular resections may result following the surgical treatment of many different types of cancers, including retromolar trigone cancers, tonsillar and lateral pharyngeal wall cancers, and base of tongue cancers. A number of primary bone tumors that develop from impacted third molars can require resection of this part of the mandible as well. In some cases, large buccal, maxillary, and soft palate cancers can extend inferiorly and involve the posterior mandible. Finally, deeply invasive skin cancers, parotid cancers, and temporal bone cancers can require removal of the posterior portion of the mandible, although, in such cases, there will not necessarily be a mucosal defect.

It is established that reconstruction with vascularized bone flaps is preferred for defects that include the anterior mandible to minimize complications and to maximize oral

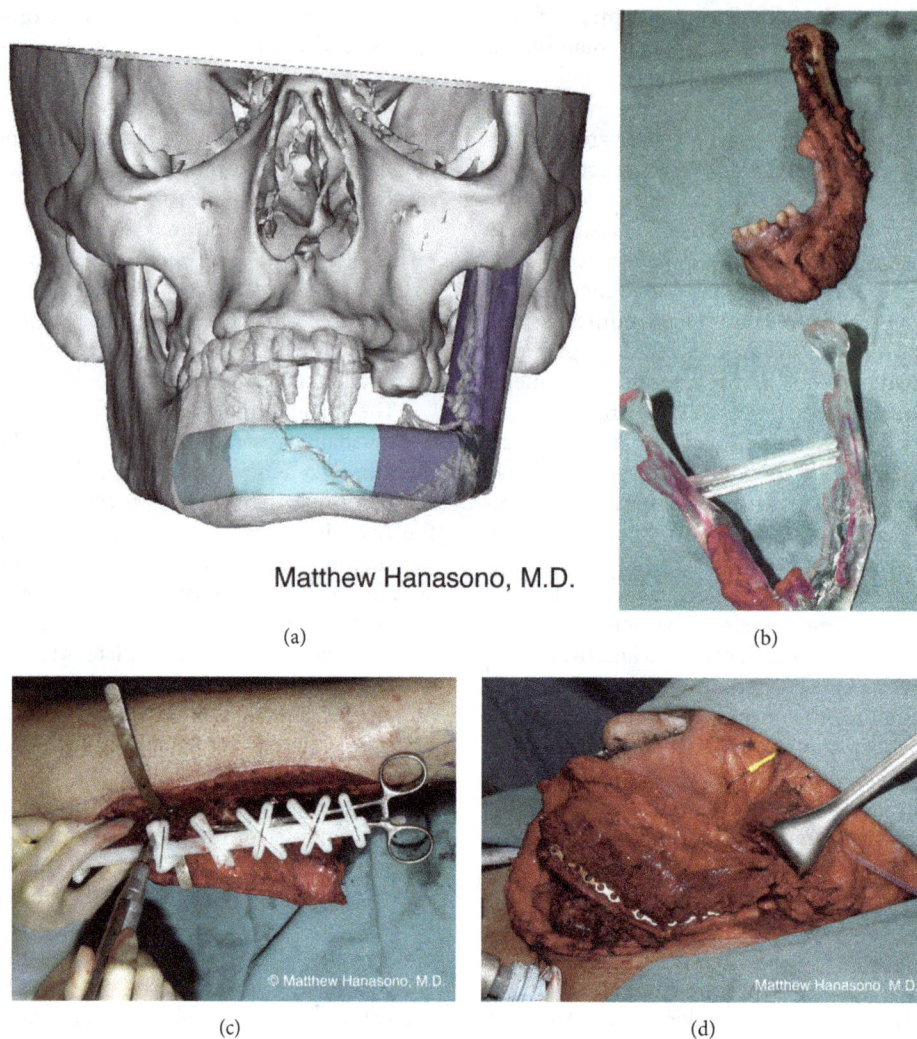

Matthew Hanasono, M.D.

(a)

(b)

(c)

(d)

FIGURE 5: Virtual plan for mandibular reconstruction using computer-assisted design software (figure courtesy of Medical Modeling, Incorporated, Golden, CO) (a). Comparison of mandibular specimen to rapid prototype model (b). Computer-generated slotted cutting guide used to help make osteotomies in a fibula osteocutaneous free flap (c). Flap inset (d).

function. Reconstruction of the posterior mandible, specifically those in which the condyle and sufficient subcondylar ramus to accommodate secure fixation with titanium hardware is lacking, is more controversial. Use of soft tissue alone with reasonable results has been reported [49, 50]. In these reports, soft tissue free flaps such as the anterolateral thigh (ALT) free flap and the rectus abdominis myocutaneous (RAM) free flap were found to allow single flap closure with adequate tissue bulk to replace the missing mandible and associated soft tissues as well as providing a skin paddle to resurface the oral mucosal defect (Figure 6).

Soft tissue reconstruction can result in acceptable cosmetic appearance, speech, and swallowing function [49, 50]. Other advantages include potentially reduced operative time compared to bony flap harvest and shaping, faster recovery, and a low complication rate. Furthermore, in cases where the posterior mandible has been resected, bony reconstruction may not have significant advantages as the ipsilateral

masticatory musculature is generally not reconstructable, nor is there perfect replacement for the condylar joint (see below).

When soft tissue is used, the flap must be adequately bulky to prevent substantial deviation of the mandible toward the resected side. Anticipating soft tissue atrophy, especially when postoperative radiation is administered, some volume overcorrection is desirable. A pectoralis major myocutaneous pedicled flap may also give satisfactory results in posterior mandibular reconstruction. However, the pectoralis major myocutaneous pedicled flap can be limited in reach and arc of rotation for very high or posterior defects. Because late contraction of the pedicle may also cause a descent of the bulk of the flap toward the neck or result in limited neck mobility, the author considers pectoralis major myocutaneous flaps a second choice to a bulky soft tissue free flap. Whether bony or soft tissue reconstruction is utilized, there will be risk for malocclusion due to loss of the condyle and temporomandibular joint disruption. Nonedentulous patients tend to experience

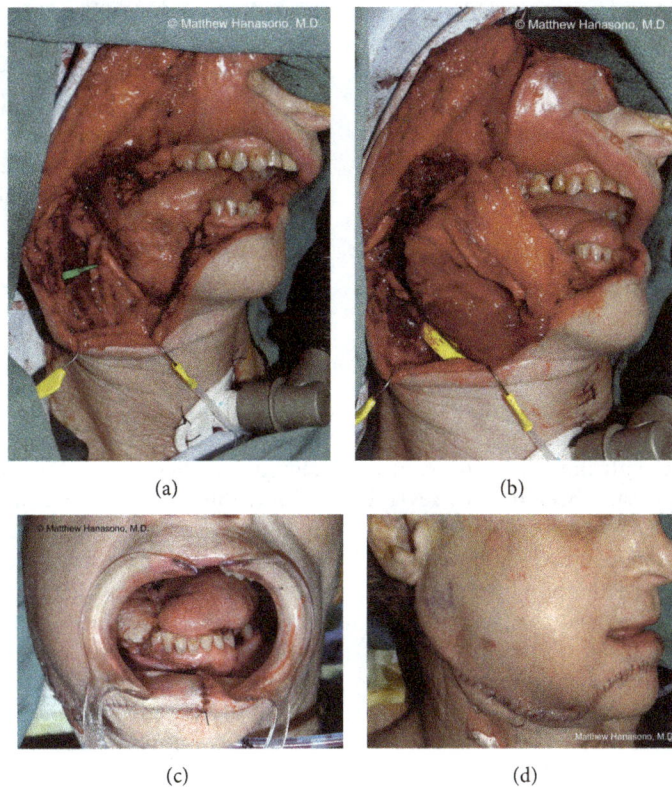

FIGURE 6: Posterior mandibular defect following tumor resection (a). Anterolateral thigh myocutaneous free flap inset (b). Skin paddle to close oral defect (c). External appearance (d).

fewer problems with malocclusion since they can use their remaining teeth to guide their jaws into the proper occlusal relationship.

Although satisfactory functional and cosmetic results for posterior mandible reconstruction with soft tissue free flap reconstruction can be achieved, bony reconstruction is probably still best for highly functional patients who are able to tolerate more extensive operations and bony free flap harvest. In our experience, occlusion is usually, although not always, superior with bony reconstruction [50]. As the defect extends more anteriorly, both the improved occlusion and cosmetic appearance owing to maintaining a better-defined jawline favor bony reconstruction.

3.6.3. Condylar Defects. The temporomandibular joint is a diarthrodial joint in which the condyle of the mandible is separated from the glenoid fossa of the temporal bone by a cartilaginous disc. Derangement of the joint or removal of the disc or condyle can lead to pain, instability, or trismus. Movement of the temporomandibular joint is complex and is comprised of both a rotational and a gliding process. Numerous methods of condylar and temporomandibular joint reconstruction have been described. Because of its complexity, no uniformly satisfactory technique has been found and reconstruction of this region remains a subject of controversy.

Reconstruction of the rest of the mandible is addressed whenever appropriate with osseous or osteocutaneous free

flap reconstruction as described above. Tumors of the superior ramus rarely invade the temporomandibular joint, and if enough of the upper ramus can be spared, the optimal reconstruction would be to fixate the bony free flap to the mandibular remnant. However, the superior cut in posterior segmental mandibulectomies often results in minimal subcondylar bone being left behind, making stable fixation with rigid titanium plates difficult or impossible. In many cases, the condyle is, therefore, completely removed. In addition, all masticatory muscles are detached from the mandible and the ligamentous support of the joint is disrupted.

Reconstruction of the condyle with titanium prostheses has been described. While some success has been noted, complications including infection, plate fracture, extrusion, and erosion into the middle cranial fossa are not uncommon. For this reason, such prostheses, even those with a silicone cap, have largely been abandoned in most centers. This technique should generally be avoided in cancer patients, who are at elevated risk for complications, particularly because of the frequent need for radiation therapy.

Reconstruction with costal cartilage grafts has also been described. The costochondral graft appears to be most useful in isolated condylar defects, providing a soft articulating surface with the glenoid fossa. In larger defects, such as is the case in most oncologic resections, a nonvascularized cartilaginous graft lacks adequate length and stability and is prone to resorption, particularly in cases where postoperative radiation therapy is given.

Temporomandibular joint reconstruction with plating of the native condyle onto a vascularized bone flap as a graft has been described by Hidalgo [51]. In a series of 14 patients who underwent hemimandibular resection, the resected condyle was mounted on a free vascular bone flap as a nonvascularized graft. Some condylar resorption was noted in a few patients but this did not correlate with a decrease in function. It was felt that use of the native condyle aided in accurate free bone flap placement. No recurrences stemming from the transplanted condyle were observed. Wax et al. [52] attempted this technique in 2 patients, one of whom had displacement of the condyle out of the glenoid fossa and the second had poor cosmetic and functional outcomes. Experience with this procedure has not otherwise been described in the literature.

Replacement of the condyle with the fibular head or a contoured, rounded fibular end has also been used by several centers, including our own. A pseudoarthrosis is thought to form. The end of the bony flap can be anchored by a suture that extends from the fibular periosteum or a hole drilled in the bone to the cut end of the pterygoid tendon or a hole drilled into the lip of the glenoid fossa to minimize drift of the bony flap end out of the temporomandibular joint. The end of the fibular bone flap is rounded with a cutting burr and fits into the glenoid fossa.

3.6.4. Lateral Mandibular Defects.

Lateral mandibular defects usually arise from extension of lateral tongue and floor of mouth cancers, buccal cancers, and submandibular gland cancers. Osteoradionecrosis may also be an indication for lateral mandibular resection, since this region of the mandible frequently receives substantial radiation during the treatment of oropharyngeal cancers, while the condyle, ramus, and parasymphyseal regions are relative spared.

Missing lateral segments are usually bridged with bone. Bony reconstruction allows for very accurate results, including restoration of preoperative occlusion. Here too, vascularized bone flaps are usually preferred, but nonvascularized bone grafts may be considered for very small defects in healthy wound beds that have neither been radiated nor are expected to be radiated postoperatively. Some surgeons feel that reconstruction plates can be used to bridge lateral defects, however, because there is a significant risk of plate fracture over time, as mentioned above, this type method should be avoided if at all possible. In general, reconstruction of such defects with bony free flaps is usually straightforward as few, if any, osteotomies are required. Also, the height of the midpoint of the mandibular body averages only 25.7 mm in males and 24.5 mm in females, so double-barreled fibular reconstruction, which is more time-consuming and complicated, is usually unnecessary [22].

In combined lateral and posterior defects (i.e., defects in which the condyle and subcondylar region cannot be spared that also extend anteriorly to involve the mandibular body), as well as in patients who are not good candidates for bony free flap reconstruction, soft tissue reconstruction can be performed. If lateral segments are not reconstructed with bone, the posterior mandibular segment bearing the condyle should be removed to prevent eventual erosion of the bone medially into the oral cavity caused by the continued pull of the pterygoid muscles. In many cases, satisfactory functional and aesthetic results can be achieved with a pedicled or free soft tissue flap for lateral and posterior-lateral defects, just as in purely posterior defects as described above. However, the more anterior the defect extends, the more noticeable a contour deformity will be due to the absence of the lower mandibular bony margin and a visible "step-off" where the native mandible ends. Additionally, the more anterior the defect extends, the greater the potential for malocclusion is as the mandible rotates toward the side of the defect due to the pull of the contralateral pterygoid muscles.

3.7. Massive Defects.

In selected cases, head and neck reconstruction may require a second microvascular free flap or regional pedicled flap for closure of extensive defects to achieve the best functional and aesthetic results [53, 54]. Such reconstructions may be limited by the availability of recipient blood vessels. Strategies such as the use of chimeric flaps (e.g., the scapular bone/latissimus dorsi muscle/serratus anterior muscle flap), vein grafting to more distant recipient vessels, such as the transverse cervical or contralateral neck vessels, and the "piggy backing" technique, where one flap is anastomosed to the pedicle of another flap, may be required [55].

One commonly used combination is the use of a soft tissue skin or myocutaneous flap for intraoral reconstruction, such as when there is a substantial glossectomy defect, and a bony flap such as the fibula to restore the mandible. A thin-pliable flap, such as the radial forearm flap, is recommended for reconstruction of a hemiglossectomy defect, while a bulkier ALT or RAM free flap is recommended for near-total or total glossectomy defects. While the use of a large skin paddle from a single fibula osteocutaneous free flap may close the oral wound, a two-flap procedure is advocated to maintain tongue mobility in patients who can tolerate an extended surgery and have a reasonable oncologic prognosis in order to optimize the functional outcome.

When there is a through and through defect, an osteocutaneous bone flap is usually used with its skin paddle providing the intraoral lining and a soft tissue free flap providing the external coverage (Figure 7). Another option is the use of a chimeric osteocutaneous scapular-latissimus dorsi (or thoracodorsal artery perforator) free flap or 2-skin paddle fibula osteocutaneous free flap (when more than one set of cutaneous perforating blood vessels are present). The pectoralis major myocutaneous pedicled flap may also be used to reconstruct the external cheek defect, although this flap is usually reserved as a "lifeboat" in case of complications such as a flap loss or fistula.

Occasionally, a maxillary and mandibular defect is encountered and may be another indication for a two-free flap reconstruction. In such cases, a myocutaneous ALT or rectus abdominis flap is used for unilateral maxillary and buccal reconstruction and a fibula osteocutaneous free flap is used for mandibular reconstruction. However, limited mandibular defects combined with palatomaxillary defects can often be addressed with a single large ALT or RAM free flap when the mandibular defect does not involve the anterior mandible, such as might arise from a retromolar trigone

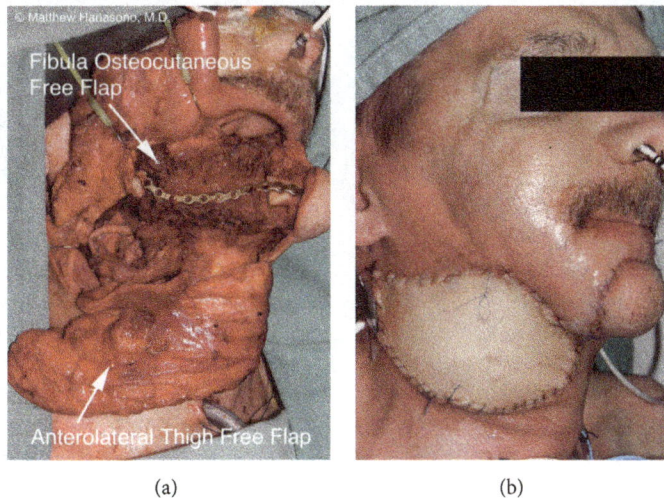

(a)   (b)

FIGURE 7: A fibula osteocutaneous free flap for mandibular and intraoral reconstruction and an anterolateral thigh free flap for external neck skin reconstruction (a). Completed reconstruction (b).

tumor that extends superiorly or a posterior palatal tumor that extends inferiorly.

3.8. Osseointegrated Implants. Dental rehabilitation may be achieved by the use of fixed or removal prostheses that are retained by osseointegrated dental implants. The efficacy of this technique has been demonstrated in the noncancer edentulous population. Use of osseointegrated dental implants requires adequate bone stock and a well-vascularized recipient tissue bed with stable soft tissue coverage. Placement of osseointegrated implants into the remaining edentulous native mandible or free vascularized bone flaps has been very successful in carefully selected patients [56]. Implants must be surrounded by a minimum of 1 mm of healthy bone. The fibula and iliac crest free flaps offer the best bone stock for osseointegration, while the scapula and radial forearm do so less reliably. Implant failure is increased in patients who smoke or have had radiation therapy or poor oral hygiene with dental infections.

The choice of timing for placement of osseointegrated implants, either primarily at the time of microvascular free bone flap reconstruction or secondarily after initial healing, has been completed depending on a number of factors including whether the resected lesion was benign or malignant, status of adjacent skin and soft tissues, plans for postoperative radiation, and patient motivation. Some authors regard radiotherapy to host bone as a contraindication to implant placement. Urken et al. [57] reported a 92-percent success rate of endosteal dental implants in vascularized mandibular reconstructions. The rate of implant success in which implants placed were irradiated postoperatively was 86 percent; implants placed into previously irradiated bone had a 64 percent success rate. Other issues that are debated include whether implants should be placed prior to or after radiation therapy, the maximum radiation dose associated with acceptable risk for implant placement, and the length of time that should elapse after radiation treatment prior to implant placement in delayed cases.

3.9. Complications. Specific to bony free flap mandibular reconstruction, malunions and nonunions are rare. If they occur, they can many times be successfully treated with debridement of the bone edges and rigid fixation, provided the free flap remains viable. Fistulae can occur and should be treated promptly with irrigation and debridement if there is purulent fluid in the vicinity of the pedicle, anastomosis, or cervical recipient vessels to prevent thrombosis or vascular rupture.

We allow patients who undergo fibula free flap reconstruction to ambulate as early as postoperative day 2, even in a splint, with weight bearing as tolerated on the affected limb. While not ambulating, we require the patient to keep the donor limb elevated at all other times, whether in bed or in a chair, to facilitate skin graft healing. Donor site complications occur in about 30 percent of patients, the vast majority of which are managed conservatively [58]. It may take up to 3 months for patients to return to their baseline of ambulatory status following fibula free flap harvest. Long-term complications are relatively uncommon but may include persistent weakness, ankle instability, great toe contracture, and decreased ankle mobility.

4. Oral Cavity and Pharyngoesophageal Reconstruction

The oral cavity is the most common site for squamous cell carcinoma of the head and neck. The tongue and floor of the mouth are the most common sites for primary cancers in the United States whereas buccal cancer is most common in some regions in Asia. The organs in the oral cavity, particularly the tongue, play critical roles in speech and swallowing. The base of the tongue is more important for swallowing function, whereas the oral tongue is more important for speech and food manipulation. Proper reconstruction of these vital organs in the oral cavity is necessary to maintain the airway, avoid fistulae, restore speech and swallowing function, and improve quality of life and self-image.

Pharyngoesophageal defects are most commonly the result of a total laryngopharyngectomy for squamous cell carcinoma in the laryngeal region or hypopharynx. Other etiologies include benign strictures, pharyngocutaneous fistulas, and thyroid cancer by direct extension. Since radiotherapy has become the primary treatment for early stages of squamous cell carcinoma in these regions, many pharyngoesophageal defects are the results of salvage laryngopharyngectomy following chemoradiation failure, making reconstruction more challenging. The goals of reconstruction are to provide alimentary continuity, protection of important structures such as the carotid artery, and restoration of speech and swallowing.

4.1. Regional Anatomy. The oral cavity is bounded by the lips anteriorly and the base of tongue and soft palate posteriorly. Subsites of the oral cavity include the floor of mouth, oral tongue (anterior two-thirds of the tongue, up to the circumvallate papillae), buccal mucosa, hard palate, mandibular and maxillary alveolar ridges, and retromolar trigones. The oral tongue is a critical structure for speech articulation and manipulating food. The hypoglossal (XII) nerve innervates all the muscles of the tongue except for the palatoglossus, which is innervated by the vagus (X) nerve. The facial (VII) nerve, via the chorda tympani, and the lingual (V3) nerve are responsible for taste and sensation of the oral tongue, respectively. Squamous cell carcinomas arising from the mucosa are the most common type of cancer affecting the oral cavity. Salivary gland cancers, arising from the submandibular, sublingual, and minor salivary glands, are the next most common.

The pharynx is divided into the nasopharynx, oropharynx, and hypopharynx. The nasopharynx extends from the skull base to the level of the soft palate. Most cancers of the nasopharynx are treated with combined radiation and chemotherapy and surgical defects in this region are rare. The oropharynx extends from the soft palate to the hyoid bone. The soft palate, tonsils, tonsillar pillars, base of tongue, and the pharyngeal walls at this level are all considered parts of the oropharynx. The soft palate prevents nasal regurgitation while the base of tongue and pharyngeal walls, which contain constrictor muscles, play a critical role in deglutition. The hypopharynx extends from the hyoid bone to the cricopharyngeus muscle, which is the most important component of the upper esophageal sphincter. The piriform sinuses, postcricoid area, and posterior pharyngeal wall comprise the hypopharynx. The hypopharynx may be the site of primary cancers, again most commonly squamous cell carcinomas, or may be involved in laryngeal cancers by direct extension.

4.2. Oral Cavity Defects

4.2.1. Floor of Mouth Defects. If no bone is exposed and there is no communication with the neck, floor of mouth defects can be allowed to mucosalize spontaneously or skin grafted. Partial skin graft loss is common for oral cavity

reconstruction; however, areas of loss usually remucosalize spontaneously.

Small defects of the floor of mouth with bone exposure can be repaired with a facial artery musculomucosal (FAMM) flap (Figure 8). The FAMM flap is based on the facial artery and includes a portion of the buccinator muscle in addition to the buccal mucosa and is usually useful for small defects up to about 2 cm in width that enable primary closure of the donor site [59–61]. The blood supply to the FAMM flap is the facial artery. When elevating a FAMM flap, a small amount of buccinator muscle is included in the flap, along with the buccal mucosa and the facial artery. Venous drainage depends mainly on the buccal venous plexus. The FAMM flap can be superiorly based on the angular artery to repair palatal defects but needs to be inferiorly based on the main facial artery in order to be rotated to the floor of the mouth. Prior to elevation, a handheld Doppler ultrasound is used to trace the course of the facial artery. The width of the flap is limited by the amount of laxity in the buccal mucosa that allows primary closure of the donor site, usually around 2 cm.

The submental flap is another local option that can be harvested with a width of 4 to 6 cm, depending on the redundancy of the submental skin, while allowing primary closure of the donor site. This flap is supplied by the submental branches of the facial artery and vein [62–64]. The anterior belly of the digastric muscle is usually included to ensure adequate perfusion since the small arterial and venous blood supply, which is often not visualized within the submental fat, is deep to the muscle about 70 percent of the time and superficial 30 percent of the time. The pivot point is roughly at the angle of the mandible. Both the submental and FAMM flap may be unavailable as options following neck dissection in which the facial artery is ligated.

The pedicled pectoralis major myocutaneous (PMMC) flap or pectoralis major muscle flap covered by a skin graft can be also used for extensive floor of mouth as well as many other oral cavity reconstructions. These flaps are based on the thoracoacromial artery and can reliably cover most oral cavity defects. The skin paddle of the PMMC flap is reliable when designed to include adequate cutaneous perforators [65]. As mentioned above, disadvantages of the pedicled pectoralis major flap include limited reach, neck contracture due to fibrosis of the proximal muscle, and, if a lot of proximal muscle is included in the flap, an unsightly bulge in the neck. Despite these drawbacks, pectoralis major flaps are still frequently used in patients who are poor free flap candidates, as an additional flap in conjunction with a free flap to reconstruct massive defects or as a secondary option in the event of a free flap failure. In contrast, for patients who are in satisfactory medical condition with a reasonable functional and oncologic prognosis, free flaps are the gold standard.

The radial forearm fasciocutaneous (RFF) free flap is useful for moderate to large floor of mouth defects since it is thin and pliable thus preventing compromised speech or swallowing due to excess bulk or tethering of the tongue. The RFF is based on the radial artery and is rapidly harvested with a long pedicle thereby facilitating head and neck reconstruction. Drawbacks of the RFF flap are decreased circulation to

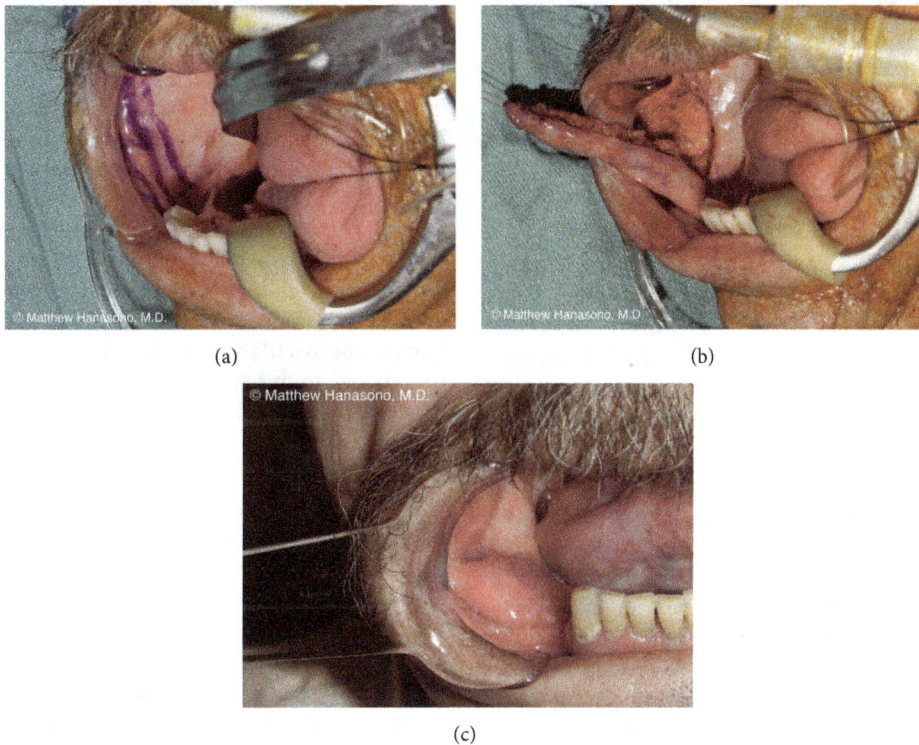

FIGURE 8: Design of a facial artery musculomucosal pedicled flap for a lateral floor of mouth and mandibular gingival defect (a). The flap is elevated and includes a portion of the buccinator muscle and the facial artery, which is deep to the muscle (b). Postoperative appearance (c).

the hand, risk for tendon exposure due to incomplete skin graft take and a relatively unfavorable donor site appearance.

Several steps are taken to minimize donor site morbidity following RFF flap harvest. The author prefers to use the venae comitantes as vein outflow rather than the cephalic vein. In many patients, the cephalic vein is far away from the radial artery. Including the cephalic vein requires a flap design that is more dorsal, resulting in a more noticeable donor site scar. Designing the skin paddle more proximally to avoid the wrist crease when the dimensions of the defect permit also decreases morbidity by not having watches or bracelets rub against the skin graft postoperatively. A suprafascial harvest, in which the fascia investing the forearm muscles and tendons is spared, may decrease donor site morbidity without compromising flap viability [66, 67]. The superficial radial sensory nerve more easily avoided by staying in the suprafascial plane, but, nevertheless needs to be identified and consciously preserved. The venae comitantes are usually no larger than 1.5 mm in diameter before they converge; therefore, the vein is usually taken above the convergence of the venae comitantes, where the diameter is greater than 2.5 mm in most cases.

An alternative to the RFF free flap is the ulnar artery perforator (UAP) flap [68]. The UAP flap relies on discrete perforators that usually arise 8 cm or more proximal to the hamate bone. Tendon exposure following UAP flap is more limited than in the RFF. The donor site is more hidden and small defects can be closed primarily when the arm skin is lax, as in the elderly. Ulnar forearm skin is usually less hairy

than radial forearm skin and just as thin. There are usually one to three true perforators arising from the ulnar artery and its accompanying venae comitantes.

The disadvantage of the UAP flap is that the pedicle is shorter, usually 4 to 5 cm long. However, in most head and neck reconstructions, the recipient vessels are within short reach. Therefore, a long vascular pedicle is not needed. Also, dissection along the ulnar nerve can be tedious and transient paresthesias can be experienced by the patient postoperatively. Because of the potentially lower donor site morbidity, the UAP flap is often selected over the radial forearm flap when a long pedicle is not needed.

The distal border of the flap is usually proximal the wrist crease to avoid tendon exposure. Dissection is usually performed under tourniquet control. Suprafascial dissection is performed until the perforators are seen medially and laterally where the fascia is incised and subfascial dissection is carried out. The perforators are small, and, therefore, meticulous dissection is required. The ulnar nerve is carefully separated from the ulnar artery and vein and retraction of the nerve should be avoided. The medial antebrachial cutaneous nerve is included in the flap for sensory reinnervation.

For floor of mouth resections that result in substantial submandibular dead space, slightly bulkier flaps, such as the ALT free flap, are useful. The ALT free flap is particularly useful in head and neck reconstruction because it can be transferred either as a fasciocutaneous flap or as a myocutaneous flap depending on the reconstructive needs. When harvested as a fasciocutaneous free flap, it is usually intermediate in thickness between the RFF flap and the RAM flap. The RAM flap is based on the deep inferior epigastric vessels and is too bulky in most patients with isolated floor of mouth defects. Although the bulk of the flap can be decreased by harvesting it as a fasciocutaneous flap based on the deep inferior epigastric perforator (DIEP) vessels, even without the rectus abdominis muscle the DIEP flap is usually thicker than the ALT free flap.

4.2.2. Buccal Mucosa Defects. The goal of reconstruction for defects involving the buccal mucosa is to prevent cicatricial trismus. Primary closure can be used for small defects, and split- or full-thickness grafts can be used for moderate ones. For defects involving the majority of the buccal mucosa, a thin, pliable fasciocutaneous free flap such as the RFF or UAP flaps are needed to prevent scar contracture from limiting mouth opening. The ALT flap may also be used in thin patients and may have the advantage of decreased donor site morbidity as compared to forearm flaps. The ALT free flap can also be thinned considerably at the time of surgery, taking care not to injure the perforator blood supply and the subdermal vascular plexus of the flap, as well as reduced secondarily with suction-assisted lipectomy. Buccal mucosa resections that result in through and through cheek defects often require reconstruction with flaps that can either be folded on themselves, deepithelializing a portion of the flap to allow wound closure at the flap margin, or harvested with dual skin paddles. ALT and RAM free flaps can be designed with more than one skin paddle, allowing separate reconstruction of the buccal mucosa and external cheek skin with a single flap. The RFF and UAP flaps can often be safely split when there are multiple branches of the pedicle vessel supplying the proximal and distal skin paddle, but their size usually required them to be used for smaller cheek defects.

4.2.3. Tongue Defects. Partial tongue defects can be closed primarily or with full thickness skin grafts to prevent graft contracture. If primary closure or a graft is likely to result in significant tongue tethering, a flap is usually indicated for closure. In practical terms, flaps are commonly required for defects approaching half the tongue and larger. Additionally, a through and through defect communicating with the dissected neck is usually best addressed with a flap to decrease the risk of fistula.

For hemiglossectomy defects, a thin, pliable flap is needed to preserve tongue mobility, although a small amount of bulk is also needed to obliterate the oral cavity dead space with the mouth closed and not create a funnel for secretions to drain directly into the larynx. The goal is to allow the residual tongue to contact the premaxilla and palate for speech articulation, as well as to be able to sweep and clear the oral cavity, and move food and secretions from anterior to posterior [69–71]. Here again, most surgeons prefer the RFF free flap oriented such that the distal end of the flap is used to reconstruct the anterior portion of the tongue (Figure 9). Adequate flap width is needed to prevent tethering the tip of the tongue to the floor of mouth and to recreate a sulcus. Bulkier free flaps or the PMMC flap can also be used in

more extensive resections; however these options typically have inferior results in terms of speech and swallowing.

In addition to the RFF or UAP free flaps, a regional option for partial and hemiglossectomy reconstruction is the supraclavicular artery island flap (SCAIF), provided the flap is long enough, based on the patient's anatomy, not to result in tethering of the reconstructed tongue [72–77]. The SCAIF is an axial pattern flap based on the supraclavicular artery, which is usually a branch of the transverse cervical artery that originates from the thyrocervical trunk, although on rare occasions it can arise from the suprascapular artery. The supraclavicular artery is a thin diameter vessel that can be reliably found in the supraclavicular triangle, between the clavicle, sternocleidomastoid and trapezius muscles, from which it travels toward the acromion.

On the day of surgery, the pedicle location is confirmed using Doppler ultrasound. A suture can be fixated at the pivot point and the radius of rotation and skin paddle length can be estimated and marked out with a surgical marker. An elliptical skin paddle is then designed according to the defect and also includes an additional 2 to 3 cm of skin medial to the pedicle origin. The skin paddle may be up to 6 to 8 cm wide and still be closed primarily in some patients, depending on the skin laxity of the shoulder area. Lengthwise, the flap can extend up to 3 cm distal to the acromion. The length of the SCAIF skin island can be increased by delaying the flap, elevating it but returning it to its original position without rotation for a period of about 7 days.

The skin incision is carried down through the skin and subcutaneous tissue through the fascia of the anterior deltoid muscle. The SCAIF is then dissected from distal to proximal in a subfascial plane. As the flap is harvested more proximally, the underside of flap is checked with a handheld Doppler to confirm inclusion of the supraclavicular artery. The pedicle can also be visualized in the medial third of the flap by transillumination of the skin. Proximally, a 1 to 2 cm cuff of subcutaneous fat surrounding the pedicle is preserved to avoid injury to the source vessel. Several sensory nerves are encountered during the dissection and can be divided to increase the arc of flap rotation. Once the flap dissection is completed lateral to the pedicle, the remaining medial skin incisions are performed to complete the skin island paddle.

The strategy for reconstruction following near total and total glossectomy is different than for hemiglossectomy [78–81]. A bulkier flap is required to reconstruct the greater volume of resection and flaps such as the RAM or ALT are commonly used. Swallowing and speech outcomes are better when the flap can be made convex into the oral cavity. To do so, it is helpful to design the flap to be somewhat wider than the oral defect, at least 8 to 9 cm in most cases, anticipating some atrophy of the flap with time, particularly if postoperative radiation will be administered. Additionally, many surgeons believe that laryngeal suspension using permanent sutures between the hyoid bone and mandible helps to prevent prolapse of the flap and also improves functional results by elevating the larynx. Laryngeal suspension from the mandible is performed with permanent circumhyoid sutures placed through drill holes on both sides of the mentum.

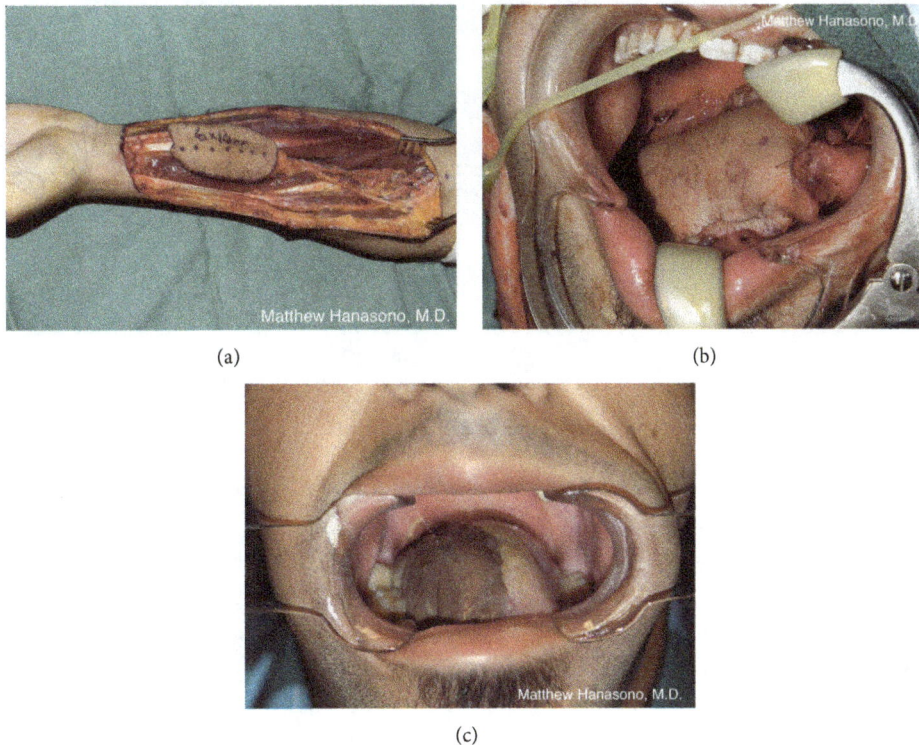

(a)

(b)

(c)

FIGURE 9: Radial forearm free flap harvest for a right hemiglossectomy reconstruction (a). Flap inset (b). Postoperative appearance (c).

If at all possible, concave reconstructions creating a trough-like area should be avoided since pooling of secretions in the oral cavity can result in aspiration. Regardless, the patient should be counseled preoperatively about the possibility of unintelligible speech, inability to swallow, and chronic aspiration. The possibility of long-term tube-feeding and tracheostomy dependency following a total or subtotal glossectomy should always be discussed.

Although the complex motor function of the tongue cannot be restored with current reconstructive techniques, sensory reinnervation of free flaps is well documented [82, 83]. The RFF free flap can be made potentially sensate by coapting the lateral antebrachial cutaneous nerve to the stump of the lingual nerve using standard techniques. Similarly, the ALT and RAM free flaps can be made sensate by anastomosis of the lateral circumflex femoral and intercostal nerves, respectively, to the lingual nerve. Sensory recovery is variable. Thin free flaps, such as the RFF, have been shown to recover some sensation spontaneously even if nerve repair is not performed [84]. It remains unclear, however, whether the amount of sensibility typically recovered secondary to nerve repair actually translates into improved speech or swallowing [85].

Following hemiglossectomy reconstruction with the techniques described above, more than 90% of patients are able to resume an oral diet without the need for tube feeding, and most patients can tolerate a regular or soft diet, depending on their dental status. Tumor recurrence, a bulky flap, and aspiration can result in an inability to resume an oral diet. Aspiration occurs frequently in patients when the surgical resection extends to the epiglottis. With proper training by

speech pathologists, most motivated patients can relearn how to swallow. Nearly all patients who have undergone a hemiglossectomy and reconstruction should be able to have their feeding tubes removed and speak intelligibly. Functional outcomes after total or subtotal glossectomy reconstruction remain disappointing. Overall, approximately half of the patients require partial or complete tube feeding.

4.3. Pharyngeal Defects. Many oropharyngeal cancers are more radiosensitive than oral cancers and radiotherapy is increasingly used as primary treatment in an effort to decrease morbidity secondary to surgical resection. Nevertheless, surgical resection is still indicated for extensive tumors, such as those that involve both the oral cavity and the oropharynx, and for recurrent cancers. The goals of reconstruction for the oropharynx include restoring continuity to the aerodigestive tract and replacing the volume of the tongue base in order to maintain swallowing function without aspiration.

Defects of the tonsillar fossa and pharyngeal walls can be reconstructed with a skin graft or allowed to heal by secondary intention when they are small and superficial. Deep wounds, such as those that result in communication with the neck contents, require a flap for closure. These defects are typically closed with thin flaps such as the RFF or ALT (in nonobese patients) to avoid obstructing the airway or interfere with swallowing (Figure 10) [86]. Isolated base of tongue defects can sometimes be closed primarily. Partial defects, including those occurring in continuity with a tonsillar or retromolar trigone resection, are best reconstructed

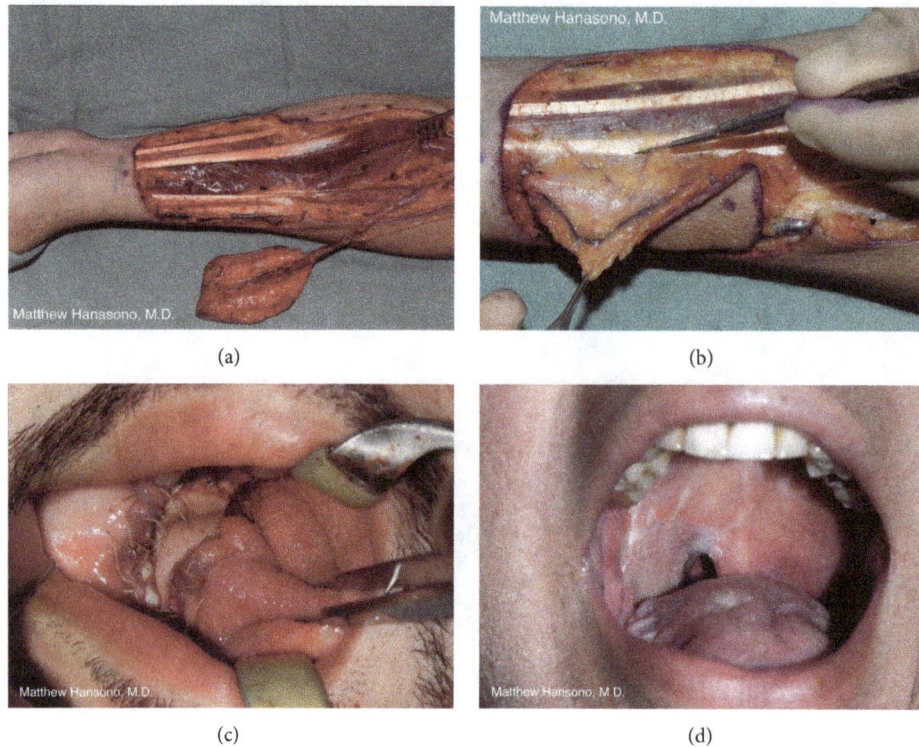

FIGURE 10: Radial forearm free flap harvest for a right oropharyngeal defect (a). To minimize donor site morbidity, a suprafascial harvest technique is used (b). Flap inset (c). Postoperative appearance demonstrating excellent mouth opening (d).

with a thin to moderate thickness fasciocutaneous free flap. Reconstruction of tongue base defects occurring as part of a near-total or total glossectomy requires bulkier flaps as discussed above.

Most tumors involving the hypopharynx, including both primary hypopharyngeal tumors and extensive laryngeal tumors, are malignant and are treated by laryngopharyngectomy. In such cases, reconstruction involves restoring a part or the entire circumference of the hypopharynx, sometimes extending to the cervical esophagus, thus restoring the continuity between the oral cavity and the distal esophagus for swallowing. Flaps are indicated for circumferential defects or for partial defects when primary closure results in a narrowed pharynx that will cause dysphagia or obstruction. Microvascular free flaps have replaced regional pedicled flaps, such as the PMMC flap, due to their lower fistula rates [87]. Free flap options include the jejunal free flap and fasciocutaneous free flaps, such as the ALT and the RFF free flaps.

The jejunal free flap is supplied by vascular arcades arising from the superior mesenteric artery and vein. A suitable segment located 20 to 30 cm from the ligament of Treitz is selected and the flap is isolated on a single arcade. The length of the jejunal segment required for the reconstruction is based on the pharyngeal defect, usually around 10 to 15 cm [88–91]. The flap can be split along the antimesenteric border to increase the diameter so that it is of suitable diameter to match that of the oropharynx and is inset into the defect in an isoperistaltic manner. Care must be taken to avoid redundancy as this may result in regurgitation and dysphagia.

Warm ischemia time should be limited to less than 2 hours to avoid ischemia reperfusion injury. Intestinal continuity is restored in the abdomen and the wound is closed in a standard fashion after a feeding jejunostomy tube and a gastrostomy tube are inserted.

The ALT free flap is another option for hypopharyngeal reconstruction [92–97]. To create a 3 cm diameter lumen, a 9.4 cm wide flap is required, based on the formula, circumference = $\pi \times$ diameter. Compared to the RAM free flap, the ALT free flap is usually thinner in most patients and thus more suitable for creation of a neopharyngeal conduit. The RFF free flap is also useful for hypopharyngeal reconstruction, particularly in partial circumference defects or in obese patients with excessive thigh thickness (Figure 11) [98, 99]. Some hypopharyngeal resections may spare a significant amount of the pharynx, and, occasionally, small or benign tumors can be resected with preservation of the larynx. In such cases, small fasciocutaneous flaps, such as the RFF free flap, are best suited to restoring pharyngeal continuity as a patch.

An advantage of the jejunal free flap is the avoidance of an additional suture line when reconstructing circumferential defects. The primary disadvantage of the jejunal free flap is the need for a laparotomy, which may result in postoperative ileus as well as the risks of anastomotic leakage of the repaired small intestine and potential late bowel obstruction due to adhesion formation. The ALT free flap is associated with minimal donor site morbidity but may be excessively thick in obese patients, although it usually tolerates aggressive thinning down to a thickness of around 0.5 cm, as long as

(a)

(b)

(c)

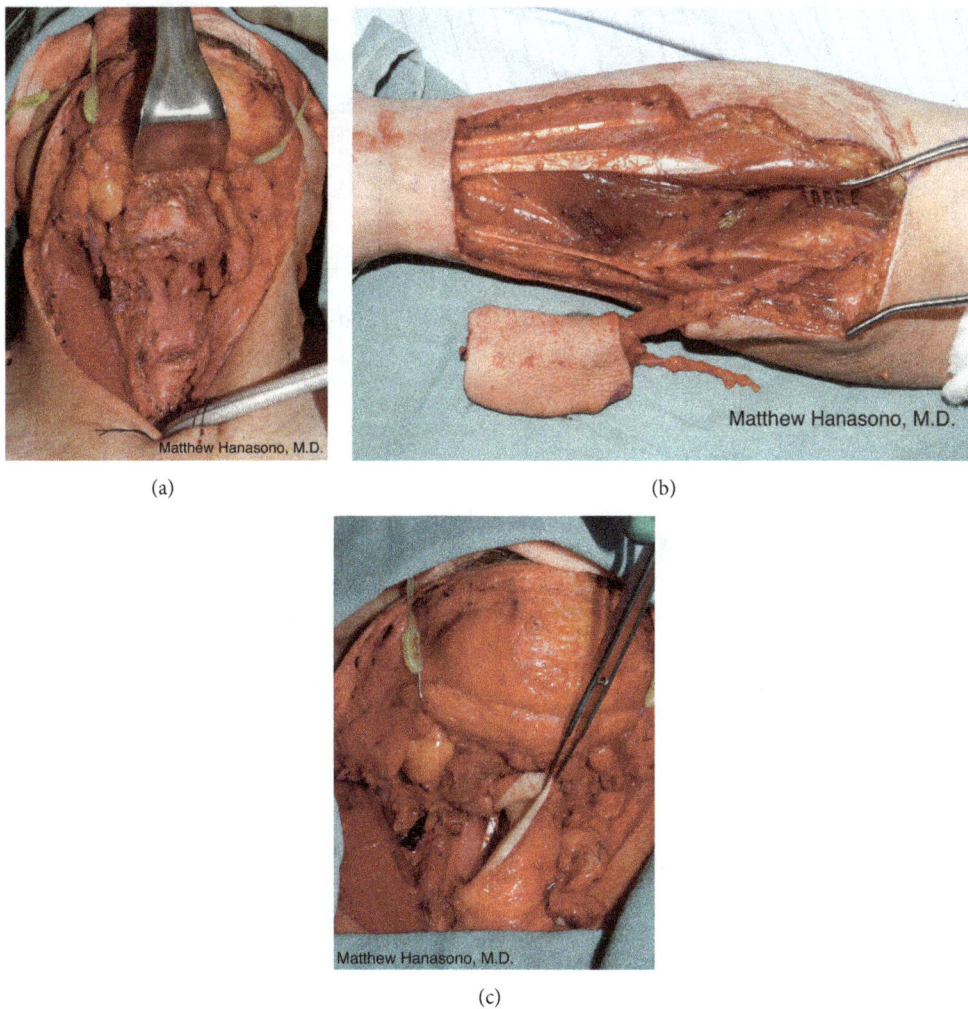

FIGURE 11: A partial circumference pharyngeal defect following a laryngopharyngectomy for recurrent laryngeal cancer (a). A radial forearm free flap was harvested for reconstruction (b). Flap inset over a nasogastric feeding tube (c).

the perforator and a cuff of subcutaneous tissue around it are carefully preserved. Both flaps are reliable with low rates of postoperative pharyngocutaneous fistula formation.

Radiation and chemotherapy are now used as primary therapy for laryngeal cancers in most centers. Thus surgical resections tend to most commonly be performed for cancer salvage, increasing the difficulty of reconstruction and the risk of wound healing complications, such as fistula [100]. In addition, previously irradiated neck skin tends to contract after skin flap elevation and may be at high-risk necrosis and wound dehiscence if closed under tension. In addition to potential exposure of the carotid artery and jugular vein, a wound dehiscence in the region of the tracheal stoma or pharyngeal closure could result in infection or fistula.

Reconstruction of the anterior neck skin often requires a second flap, either another free flap or a pedicled flap. The PMMC flap or pectoralis major muscle flap covered by a skin graft is frequently used to reconstruct the anterior neck skin (Figure 12). An elegant solution is to use a single flap to reconstruct both the pharynx and the anterior neck

skin. The ALT free flap can often be designed with 2 skin paddles based on independent cutaneous perforating blood vessels that join together proximally within the main vascular pedicle, thus requiring only a single set of arterial and venous anastomoses to complete the reconstruction [101]. When more than one perforator is not available, the vastus lateralis muscle can be included with the ALT free flap and skin grafted to reconstruct the neck skin defect. Alternatively, the ALT free flap or other fasciocutaneous free flaps can be partially deepithelialized and a portion of the skin paddle can be used to reconstruct the neck skin defect.

An additional advantage of utilizing a second skin paddle from an ALT free flap for neck reconstruction is that it allows easy monitoring for microvascular anastomotic patency. When there is no external skin paddle, many surgeons utilize an internal Doppler (Cook-Schwartz Doppler) to monitor the buried free flap used for pharyngoesophageal reconstruction [102]. A third alternative is to design the ALT flap with two skin paddles, when there is more than one perforator, and temporarily leave the second skin paddle exteriorized

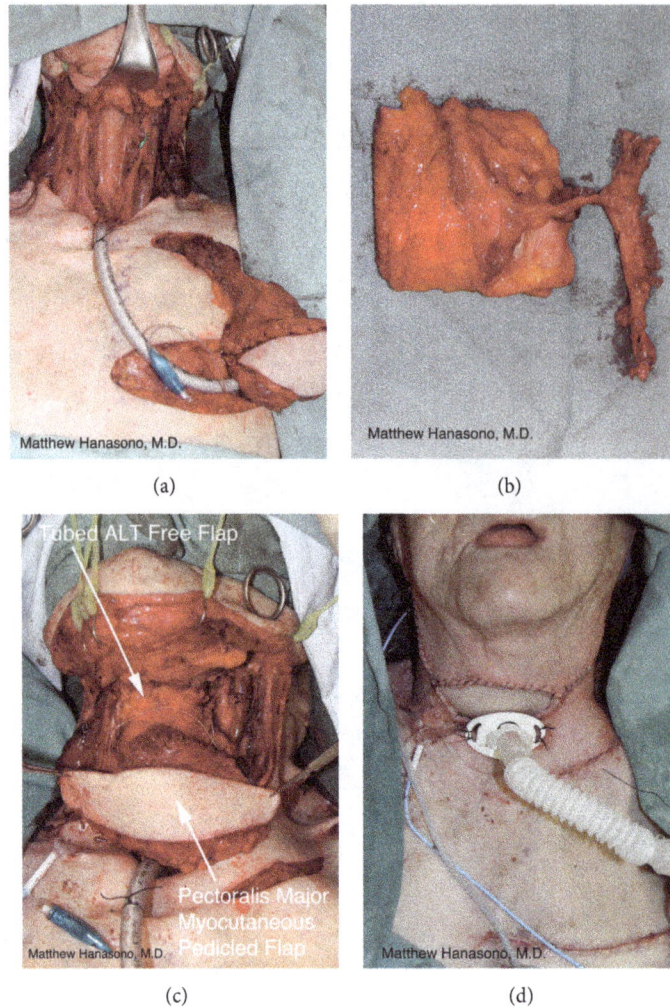

(a)   (b)

(c)   (d)

FIGURE 12: A total circumference pharyngeal defect following a laryngopharyngectomy for recurrent laryngeal cancer (a). A pectoralis major myocutaneous pedicled flap is dissected for neck skin coverage. The anterolateral thigh flap was dissected as a perforator flap and subsequently tubed (b). Inset of flaps (c). Postoperative appearance (d).

through the neck incision, attached by its perforating blood vessel and a small amount of septal fascia [103]. This "monitoring" skin paddle is excised at the bedside prior to hospital discharge by ligating the perforator and amputating the skin paddle at the level of the neck skin. The small cutaneous defect can be left to heal secondarily or closed with one or two sutures under local anesthesia. The jejunal free flap is also often harvested longer than needed and a portion of the distal jejunum is exteriorized through the neck incision as a monitoring segment.

Vocal rehabilitation following laryngopharyngectomy can be accomplished by a number of methods, including use of an electrolarynx or a tracheoesophageal puncture (TEP) prosthesis. The TEP prosthesis is inserted into a surgically created hole between the posterior trachea and the cervical esophagus. If necessary, the hole can be placed through the reconstructive flap. The creation of the TEP can be performed at the time of reconstruction or in delayed manner, following flap healing. A one-way valve is part of the TEP prosthesis and

allows shunting of air from the trachea to the pharynx and mouth for phonation when the tracheal stoma is occluded.

4.3.1. Outcomes. In our group's early experience with 114 consecutive anterolateral thigh flaps used for pharyngoesophageal reconstruction, mean intensive care unit stay was 1.9 ± 2.2 days, and mean hospital stay was 9.0 ± 4.7 days [95]. Pharyngocutaneous fistulae and strictures occurred in 9% and 6% of patients, respectively. Ninety-one percent of patients tolerated an oral diet without the need for tube feeding. By comparison, in the jejunal flap reconstruction, the average hospital stay was 13 days and average intensive care unit stay was 3 days. The incidence of ileus and bowel obstruction was 9%, abdominal hernia, 6%, and anastomotic stricture, 19%. Overall, 65% of patients tolerated an oral diet without supplemental tube feeding, and 23% were partially tube-feed dependent, and 12% were totally tube-feed dependent. Fluent tracheoesophageal speech was achieved in 22% of patients who received a TEP. The quality of tracheoesophageal speech following jejunal flap reconstruction is usually characterized as "wet" or "cavernous" compared with that following a fasciocutaneous flap reconstruction or a total laryngectomy with primary pharyngeal repair.

4.4. Complications. Neck wound infection is the result of prolonged wound exposure and oral contamination during surgery. Many patients with oral cancer have poor oral hygiene because of pain. Prior chemoradiation and radiation therapy can also increase the risk of infection. Copious irrigation and obliteration of dead spaces are important for preventing postoperative wound infection. Once infection occurs, early drainage and thorough debridement and irrigation may enable primary wound closure over a drain; otherwise, the wound should be left open to allow further drainage. Serial operative irrigation and drainage procedures may be helpful in the worst cases. If there is dead space or vascular exposure occurs following debridement, pectoralis major muscle flap reconstruction of the neck may be indicated to protect the carotid artery, especially in patients who have had prior radiation therapy.

Wound dehiscences and fistulae can result from technical suturing errors, compromised tissue quality, most commonly due to prior irradiation and/or surgery, or wound infection. In our experience, pharyngocutaneous fistulas occur in about 9% of patients with ALT flap pharyngoesophageal reconstructions [97]. Fistula rates are similar in partial and circumferential reconstructions. There is the theoretical concern that the longitudinal seam of a tubed fasciocutaneous flap or two longitudinal suture lines in a partial defect might result in a higher incidence of fistula formation than the jejunal flap, which is a natural tube and only requires proximal and distal suture lines. However, in our group's experience, the fistula rate with the ALT flap is not significantly higher than with the jejunal flap. Fistulae usually develop between one and four weeks after surgery and manifest as leakage of saliva or liquids or, in some patients, as a purulent neck infection.

Once a fistula is identified, oral intake is withheld and local wound care is initiated. Small fistulas, in the absence of tumor recurrence or distal obstruction, usually heal spontaneously with conservative management. Therefore, a modified barium swallow (MBS) study is repeated about two weeks later to determine if the leakage has stopped. Larger fistulas or those with infection should be evaluated with CT to rule out abscess. The location of the fistula relative to the carotid artery and internal jugular vein is also evaluated. Any abscess around the carotid artery, especially in patients who have undergone previous radiation therapy should be drained and irrigated and consideration should be given to using a pectoralis major muscle flap to protect the carotid artery. Early intervention may achieve rapid healing and prevent life-threatening complications. With aggressive intervention, persistent fistulas are rare, therefore, if a fistula does persist, the patient should be evaluated for possible tumor recurrence and distal obstruction/stricture.

Anastomotic strictures usually occur at the distal anastomosis several months or years following reconstruction. Spatulation of the esophagus at the time of flap inset may reduce the risk of stricture formation. If a patient develops dysphagia after reconstruction, anastomotic strictures should be suspected and an MBS study was performed to confirm the diagnosis. Endoscopic balloon dilatation is our preferred initial treatment. Repeated dilatations may be required in some patients. In refractory cases, surgical enlargement of the strictured area may require an additional flap, such as the RFF free flap.

5. Conclusions

The 1990s saw a proliferation of free flap reconstruction for head and neck defects as they were demonstrated to be more reliable and result in superior functional and aesthetic outcomes compared to most prior techniques. In the past decade, algorithms were developed for flap selection based on evidence and experience, further improving outcomes and decreasing complications. Flaps are selected to minimize donor site morbidity, including perforator-based flaps, such as the anterolateral thigh free flap. Currently, advances in head and neck reconstruction are focused in further refinement, such as use of computer-assisted design and rapid prototype modeling to plan surgery. The future will undoubtedly bring further breakthroughs in reconstructive surgery in an effort to restore normalcy and allow for more complete oncologic resection with the goal of improving cancer cure rates and quality of life.

Conflict of Interests

The author declares that there is no conflict of interests regarding the publication of this paper.

References

[1] M. M. Hanasono, M. T. Friel, C. Klem et al., "Impact of reconstructive microsurgery in patients with advanced oral cavity cancers," *Head and Neck*, vol. 31, no. 10, pp. 1289–1296, 2009.

[2] D. A. Hidalgo, J. J. Disa, P. G. Cordeiro, and Q.-Y. Hu, "A review of 716 consecutive free flaps for oncologic surgical defects: refinement in donor-site selection and technique," *Plastic and Reconstructive Surgery*, vol. 102, no. 3, pp. 722–732, 1998.

[3] K. E. Blackwell, "Unsurpassed reliability of free flaps for head and neck reconstruction," *Archives of Otolaryngology: Head and Neck Surgery*, vol. 125, no. 3, pp. 295–299, 1999.

[4] S. Archibald, S. Jackson, and A. Thoma, "Paranasal sinus and midfacial reconstruction," *Clinics in Plastic Surgery*, vol. 32, no. 3, pp. 309–325, 2005.

[5] D. J. Okay, E. Genden, D. Buchbinder, and M. Urken, "Prosthodontic guidelines for surgical reconstruction of the maxilla: a classification system of defects," *The Journal of Prosthetic Dentistry*, vol. 86, no. 4, pp. 352–363, 2001.

[6] Y.-M. Chang, O. K. Coskunfirat, F.-C. Wei, C.-Y. Tsai, and H.-N. Lin, "Maxillary reconstruction with a fibula osteoseptocutaneous free flap and simultaneous insertion of osseointegrated dental implants," *Plastic and Reconstructive Surgery*, vol. 113, no. 4, pp. 1140–1145, 2004.

[7] X. Peng, C. Mao, G.-Y. Yu, C.-B. Guo, M.-X. Huang, and Y. Zhang, "Maxillary reconstruction with the free fibula flap,"

Plastic and Reconstructive Surgery, vol. 115, no. 6, pp. 1562–1569, 2005.

[8] S. Yazar, M.-H. Cheng, F.-C. Wei, S.-P. Hao, and K.-P. Chang, "Osteomyocutaneous peroneal artery perforator flap for reconstruction of composite maxillary defects," *Head and Neck*, vol. 28, no. 4, pp. 297–304, 2006.

[9] J. R. Clark, M. Vesely, and R. Gilbert, "Scapular angle osteomyogenous flap in postmaxillectomy reconstruction: defect, reconstruction, shoulder function, and harvest technique," *Head and Neck*, vol. 30, no. 1, pp. 10–20, 2008.

[10] E. M. Genden, D. Wallace, D. Buchbinder, D. Okay, and M. L. Urken, "Iliac crest internal oblique osteomusculocutaneous free flap reconstruction of the postablative palatomaxillary defect," *Archives of Otolaryngology—Head and Neck Surgery*, vol. 127, no. 7, pp. 854–861, 2001.

[11] J. S. Brown, D. C. Jones, A. Summerwill et al., "Vascularized iliac crest with internal oblique muscle for immediate reconstruction after maxillectomy," *British Journal of Oral and Maxillofacial Surgery*, vol. 40, no. 3, pp. 183–190, 2002.

[12] R. H. Spiro, E. W. Strong, and J. P. Shah, "Maxillectomy and its classification," *Head and Neck*, vol. 19, no. 4, pp. 309–314, 1997.

[13] M. A. Moreno, R. J. Skoracki, E. Y. Hanna, and M. M. Hanasono, "Microvascular free flap reconstruction versus palatal obturation for maxillectomy defects," *Head and Neck*, vol. 32, no. 7, pp. 860–868, 2010.

[14] E. M. Genden, D. Okay, M. T. Stepp et al., "Comparison of functional and quality-of-life outcomes in patients with and without palatomaxillary reconstruction: a preliminary report," *Archives of Otolaryngology—Head and Neck Surgery*, vol. 129, no. 7, pp. 775–780, 2003.

[15] S. N. Rogers, D. Lowe, D. McNally, J. S. Brown, and E. D. Vaughan, "Health-related quality of life after maxillectomy: a comparison between prosthetic obturation and free flap," *Journal of Oral and Maxillofacial Surgery*, vol. 61, no. 2, pp. 174–181, 2003.

[16] P. G. Cordeiro and E. Santamaria, "A classification system and algorithm for reconstruction of maxillectomy and midfacial defects," *Plastic and Reconstructive Surgery*, vol. 105, no. 7, pp. 2331–2346, 2000.

[17] M. M. Hanasono, A. K. Silva, P. Yu, and R. J. Skoracki, "A comprehensive algorithm for oncologic maxillary reconstruction," *Plastic and Reconstructive Surgery*, vol. 131, no. 1, pp. 47–60, 2013.

[18] P. G. Cordeiro and C. M. Chen, "A 15-year review of mid-face reconstruction after total and subtotal maxillectomy: part I. Algorithm and outcomes," *Plastic and Reconstructive Surgery*, vol. 129, no. 1, pp. 124–136, 2012.

[19] M. M. Hanasono and R. J. Skoracki, "The omega-shaped fibula osteocutaneous free flap for reconstruction of extensive midfacial defects," *Plastic and Reconstructive Surgery*, vol. 125, no. 4, pp. 160e–162e, 2010.

[20] J. S. Brown, S. N. Rogers, D. N. McNally, and M. Boyle, "A modified classification for the maxillectomy defect," *Head & Neck*, vol. 22, pp. 17–26, 2000.

[21] J. S. Brown and R. J. Shaw, "Reconstruction of the maxilla and midface: introducing a new classification," *The Lancet Oncology*, vol. 11, no. 10, pp. 1001–1008, 2010.

[22] E. I. Chang, M. W. Clemens, P. B. Garvey, R. J. Skoracki, and M. M. Hanasono, "Cephalometric analysis for microvascular head and neck reconstruction," *Head and Neck*, vol. 34, no. 11, pp. 1607–1614, 2012.

[23] M. M. Hanasono, R. F. Jacob, L. Bidaut, G. L. Robb, and R. J. Skoracki, "Midfacial reconstruction using virtual planning, rapid prototype modeling, and stereotactic navigation," *Plastic and Reconstructive Surgery*, vol. 126, no. 6, pp. 2002–2006, 2010.

[24] P. G. Cordeiro and C. M. Chen, "A 15-year review of midface reconstruction after total and subtotal maxillectomy: part II. Technical modifications to maximize aesthetic and functional outcomes," *Plastic and Reconstructive Surgery*, vol. 129, no. 1, pp. 139–147, 2012.

[25] E. J. Kirby, J. B. Turner, D. L. Davenport, and H. C. Vasconez, "Orbital floor fractures: outcomes of reconstruction," *Annals of Plastic Surgery*, vol. 66, no. 5, pp. 508–512, 2011.

[26] E. D. Rodriguez, M. Martin, R. Bluebond-Langner, M. Khalifeh, N. Singh, and P. N. Manson, "Microsurgical reconstruction of posttraumatic high-energy maxillary defects: establishing the effectiveness of early reconstruction," *Plastic and Reconstructive Surgery*, vol. 120, no. 7, 2007.

[27] M. M. Hanasono, J. C. Lee, J. S. Yang, R. J. Skoracki, G. P. Reece, and B. Esmaeli, "An algorithmic approach to reconstructive surgery and prosthetic rehabilitation after orbital exenteration," *Plastic and Reconstructive Surgery*, vol. 123, no. 1, pp. 98–105, 2009.

[28] M. M. Hanasono, D. S. Utley, and R. L. Goode, "The temporalis muscle flap for reconstruction after head and neck oncologic surgery," *The Laryngoscope*, vol. 111, no. 10, pp. 1719–1725, 2001.

[29] F.-C. Wei, N. Celik, W.-G. Yang, I.-H. Chen, Y.-M. Chang, and H.-C. Chen, "Complications after reconstruction by plate and soft-tissue free flap in composite mandibular defects and secondary salvage reconstruction with osteocutaneous flap," *Plastic and Reconstructive Surgery*, vol. 112, no. 1, pp. 37–42, 2003.

[30] P. B. Mariani, L. P. Kowalski, and J. Magrin, "Reconstruction of large defects postmandibulectomy for oral cancer using plates and myocutaneous flaps: a long-term follow-up," *International Journal of Oral and Maxillofacial Surgery*, vol. 35, no. 5, pp. 427–432, 2006.

[31] T. Shpitzer, P. J. Gullane, P. C. Neligan et al., "The free vascularized flap and the flap plate options: comparative results of reconstruction of lateral mandibular defects," *Laryngoscope*, vol. 110, no. 12, pp. 2056–2060, 2000.

[32] D. A. Hidalgo, "Fibular free flap: a new method of mandible reconstruction," *Plastic and Reconstructive Surgery*, vol. 84, no. 1, pp. 71–79, 1989.

[33] P. G. Cordeiro, J. J. Disa, D. A. Hidalgo, and Q. Y. Hu, "Reconstruction of the mandible with osseous free flaps: a 10-year experience with 150 consecutive patients," *Plastic and Reconstructive Surgery*, vol. 104, no. 5, pp. 1314–1320, 1999.

[34] H. Seikaly, J. Chau, F. Li et al., "Bone that best matches the properties of the mandible," *Journal of Otolaryngology*, vol. 32, no. 4, pp. 262–265, 2003.

[35] G. A. Robertson, "A comparison between sternum and rib in osteomyocutaneous reconstruction of major mandibular defects," *Annals of Plastic Surgery*, vol. 17, no. 5, pp. 421–423, 1986.

[36] B. S. Lutz, F. C. Wei, S. H. Ng, I. H. Chen, and S. H. T. Chen, "Routine donor leg angiography before vascularized free fibula transplantation is not necessary: a prospective study in 120 clinical cases," *Plastic and Reconstructive Surgery*, vol. 103, no. 1, pp. 121–127, 1999.

[37] Y.-M. Chang, C. G. Wallace, C.-Y. Tsai, Y.-F. Shen, Y.-M. Hsu, and F.-C. Wei, "Dental implant outcome after primary

implantation into double-barreled fibula osteoseptocutaneous free flap-reconstructed mandible," *Plastic and Reconstructive Surgery*, vol. 128, no. 6, pp. 1220–1228, 2011.

[38] B. S. Lutz, F.-C. Wei, S.-H. Ng, I.-H. Chen, and S. H. T. Chen, "Routine donor leg angiography before vascularized free fibula transplantation is not necessary: a prospective study in 120 clinical cases," *Plastic and Reconstructive Surgery*, vol. 103, no. 1, pp. 121–127, 1999.

[39] M. M. Hanasono and R. J. Skoracki, "Computer-assisted design and rapid prototype modeling in microvascular mandible reconstruction," *Laryngoscope*, vol. 123, no. 3, pp. 597–604, 2013.

[40] J. P. Levine, A. Patel, P. B. Saadeh, and D. L. Hirsch, "Computer-aided design and manufacturing in craniomaxillofacial surgery: the new state of the art," *Journal of Craniofacial Surgery*, vol. 23, no. 1, pp. 288–293, 2012.

[41] A. K. Antony, W. F. Chen, A. Kolokythas, K. A. Weimer, and M. N. Cohen, "Use of virtual surgery and stereolithography-guided osteotomy for mandibular reconstruction with the free fibula," *Plastic and Reconstructive Surgery*, vol. 128, no. 5, pp. 1080–1084, 2011.

[42] S. M. Shenaq and M. J. A. Klebuc, "Refinements in the iliac crest microsurgical free flap for oromandibular reconstruction," *Microsurgery*, vol. 15, no. 12, pp. 825–830, 1994.

[43] T. Şafak, M. J. A. Klebuc, E. Mavili, and S. M. Shenaq, "A new design of the iliac crest microsurgical free flap without including the "obligatory" muscle cuff," *Plastic and Reconstructive Surgery*, vol. 100, no. 7, pp. 1703–1709, 1997.

[44] A. J. Wagner and S. W. Bayles, "The angular branch: maximizing the scapular pedicle in head and neck reconstruction," *Archives of Otolaryngology—Head and Neck Surgery*, vol. 134, no. 11, pp. 1214–1217, 2008.

[45] M. M. Hanasono and R. J. Skoracki, "The scapular tip osseous free flap as an alternative for anterior mandibular reconstruction," *Plastic and Reconstructive Surgery*, vol. 125, no. 4, pp. 164e–166e, 2010.

[46] S. Seneviratne, C. Duong, and G. I. Taylor, "The angular branch of the thoracodorsal artery and its blood supply to the inferior angle of the scapula: an anatomical study," *Plastic and Reconstructive Surgery*, vol. 104, no. 1, pp. 85–88, 1999.

[47] A. Thoma, R. Khadaroo, O. Grigenas et al., "Oromandibular reconstruction with the radial-forearm osteocutaneous flap: experience with 60 consecutive cases," *Plastic and Reconstructive Surgery*, vol. 104, no. 2, pp. 368–378, 1999.

[48] J. J. Disa, D. A. Hidalgo, P. G. Cordeiro, R. M. Winters, and H. Thaler, "Evaluation of bone height in osseous free flap mandible reconstruction: an indirect measure of bone mass," *Plastic and Reconstructive Surgery*, vol. 103, no. 5, pp. 1371–1377, 1999.

[49] A. Mosahebi, A. Chaudhry, C. M. McCarthy et al., "Reconstruction of extensive composite posterolateral mandibular defects using nonosseous free tissue transfer," *Plastic and Reconstructive Surgery*, vol. 124, no. 5, pp. 1571–1577, 2009.

[50] M. M. Hanasono, J. P. Zevallos, R. J. Skoracki, and P. Yu, "A prospective analysis of bony versus soft-tissue reconstruction for posterior mandibular defects," *Plastic and Reconstructive Surgery*, vol. 125, no. 5, pp. 1413–1421, 2010.

[51] D. A. Hidalgo, "Condyle transplantation in free flap mandible reconstruction," *Plastic and Reconstructive Surgery*, vol. 93, no. 4, pp. 770–783, 1994.

[52] M. K. Wax, C. P. Winslow, J. Hansen et al., "A retrospective analysis of temporomandibular joint reconstruction with free fibula microvascular flap," *Laryngoscope*, vol. 110, no. 6, pp. 977–981, 2000.

[53] F.-C. Wei, F. Demirkan, H.-C. Chen, and I.-H. Chen, "Double free flaps in reconstruction of extensive composite mandibular defects in head and neck cancer," *Plastic and Reconstructive Surgery*, vol. 103, no. 1, pp. 39–47, 1999.

[54] M. M. Hanasono, Y. E. Weinstock, and P. Yu, "Reconstruction of extensive head and neck defects with multiple simultaneous free flaps," *Plastic and Reconstructive Surgery*, vol. 122, no. 6, pp. 1739–1746, 2008.

[55] M. M. Hanasono, Y. Barnea, and R. J. Skoracki, "Microvascular surgery in the previously operated and irradiated neck," *Microsurgery*, vol. 29, no. 1, pp. 1–7, 2009.

[56] Y.-M. Chang, E. Santamaria, F.-C. Wei et al., "Primary insertion of osseointegrated dental implants into fibula osteoseptocutaneous free flap for mandible reconstruction," *Plastic and Reconstructive Surgery*, vol. 102, no. 3, pp. 680–688, 1998.

[57] M. L. Urken, D. Buchbinder, H. Weinberg, C. Vickery, A. Sheiner, and H. F. Biller, "Primary placement of osseointegrated implants in microvascular mandibular reconstruction," *Otolaryngology: Head and Neck Surgery*, vol. 101, no. 1, pp. 56–73, 1989.

[58] A. O. Momoh, P. Yu, R. J. Skoracki, S. Liu, L. Feng, and M. M. Hanasono, "A prospective cohort study of fibula free flap donor-site morbidity in 157 consecutive patients," *Plastic and Reconstructive Surgery*, vol. 128, no. 3, pp. 714–720, 2011.

[59] J. Pribaz, W. Stephens, L. Crespo, and G. Gifford, "A new intraoral flap: Facial artery musculomucosal (FAMM) flap," *Plastic and Reconstructive Surgery*, vol. 90, no. 3, pp. 421–429, 1992.

[60] J. J. Pribaz, J. G. Meara, S. Wright, J. D. Smith, W. Stephens, and K. H. Breuing, "Lip and vermilion reconstruction with the facial artery musculomucosal flap," *Plastic and Reconstructive Surgery*, vol. 105, no. 3, pp. 864–872, 2000.

[61] L. Dupoirieux, L. Plane, C. Gard, and M. Penneau, "Anatomical basis and results of the facial artery musculomucosal flap for oral reconstruction," *British Journal of Oral and Maxillofacial Surgery*, vol. 37, no. 1, pp. 25–28, 1999.

[62] D. Martin, J. F. Pascal, J. Baudet et al., "The submental island flap: a new donor site. Anatomy and clinical applications as a free or pedicled flap," *Plastic and Reconstructive Surgery*, vol. 92, no. 5, pp. 867–873, 1993.

[63] S. B. Uppin, Q. G. Ahmad, P. Yadav, and K. Shetty, "Use of the submental island flap in orofacial reconstruction—a review of 20 cases," *Journal of Plastic, Reconstructive and Aesthetic Surgery*, vol. 62, no. 4, pp. 514–519, 2009.

[64] O. Magden, M. Edizer, V. Tayfur, and A. Atabey, "Anatomic study of the vasculature of the submental artery flap," *Plastic and Reconstructive Surgery*, vol. 114, no. 7, pp. 1719–1723, 2004.

[65] H. Rikimaru, K. Kiyokawa, Y. Inoue, and Y. Tai, "Three-dimensional anatomical vascular distribution in the pectoralis major myocutaneous flap," *Plastic and Reconstructive Surgery*, vol. 115, no. 5, pp. 1342–1352, 2005.

[66] B. S. Lutz, F.-C. Wei, S. C. N. Chang, K.-H. Yang, and I. Chen, "Donor site morbidity after suprafascial elevation of the radial forearm flap: a prospective study in 95 consecutive cases," *Plastic and Reconstructive Surgery*, vol. 103, no. 1, pp. 132–137, 1999.

[67] S. C. Chang, G. Miller, C. F. Halbert, K. H. Yang, W. C. Chao, and F. C. Wei, "Limiting donor site morbidity by suprafascial dissection of the radial forearm flap," *Microsurgery*, vol. 17, no. 3, pp. 136–140, 1996.

[68] B. H. Haughey, "Tongue reconstruction: concepts and practice," *Laryngoscope*, vol. 103, no. 10, pp. 1132–1141, 1993.

[69] M. L. Urken, J. F. Moscoso, W. Lawson, and H. F. Biller, "A systematic approach to functional reconstruction of the oral cavity following partial and total glossectomy," *Archives of Otolaryngology—Head and Neck Surgery*, vol. 120, no. 6, pp. 589–601, 1994.

[70] D. B. Chepeha, T. N. Teknos, J. Shargorodsky et al., "Rectangle tongue template for reconstruction of the hemiglossectomy defect," *Archives of Otolaryngology—Head and Neck Surgery*, vol. 134, no. 9, pp. 993–998, 2008.

[71] P. Yu, E. I. Chang, J. C. Selber, and M. M. Hanasono, "Perforator patterns of the ulnar artery perforator flap," *Plastic and Reconstructive Surgery*, vol. 129, no. 1, pp. 213–220, 2012.

[72] V. Q. Vinh, T. Van Anh, R. Ogawa, and H. Hyakusoku, "Anatomical and clinical studies of the supraclavicular flap: analysis of 103 flaps used to reconstruct neck scar contractures," *Plastic and Reconstructive Surgery*, vol. 123, no. 5, pp. 1471–1480, 2009.

[73] P. H. Liu and E. S. Chiu, "Supraclavicular artery flap: a new option for pharyngeal reconstruction," *Annals of Plastic Surgery*, vol. 62, no. 5, pp. 497–501, 2009.

[74] E. S. Chiu, P. H. Liu, and P. L. Friedlander, "Supraclavicular artery island flap for head and neck oncologic reconstruction: Indications, complications, and outcomes," *Plastic and Reconstructive Surgery*, vol. 124, no. 1, pp. 115–123, 2009.

[75] E. S. Chiu, P. H. Liu, R. Baratelli, M. Y. Lee, A. E. Chaffin, and P. L. Friedlander, "Circumferential pharyngoesophageal reconstruction with a supraclavicular artery Island flap," *Plastic and Reconstructive Surgery*, vol. 125, no. 1, pp. 161–166, 2010.

[76] A. G. Anand, E. J. Tran, C. P. Hasney, P. L. Friedlander, and E. S. Chiu, "Oropharyngeal reconstruction using the supraclavicular artery island flap: a new flap alternative," *Plastic and Reconstructive Surgery*, vol. 129, no. 2, pp. 438–441, 2012.

[77] T. T. Sands, J. B. Martin, E. Simms, M. M. Henderson, P. L. Friedlander, and E. S. Chiu, "Supraclavicular artery island flap innervation: anatomical studies and clinical implications," *Journal of Plastic, Reconstructive & Aesthetic Surgery*, vol. 65, no. 1, pp. 68–71, 2012.

[78] A. T. Lyos, G. R. D. Evans, D. Perez, and M. A. Schusterman, "Tongue reconstruction: outcomes with the rectus abdominis flap," *Plastic and Reconstructive Surgery*, vol. 103, no. 2, pp. 442–447, 1999.

[79] Y. Kimata, M. Sakuraba, S. Hishinuma et al., "Analysis of the relations between the shape of the reconstructed tongue and postoperative functions after subtotal or total glossectomy," *Laryngoscope*, vol. 113, no. 5, pp. 905–909, 2003.

[80] Y. Yamamoto, T. Sugihara, Y. Furuta, and S. Fukuda, "Functional reconstruction of the tongue and deglutition muscles following extensive resection of tongue cancer," *Plastic and Reconstructive Surgery*, vol. 102, no. 4, pp. 993–998, 1998.

[81] P. Yu, "Reinnervated anterolateral thigh flap for tongue reconstruction," *Head and Neck*, vol. 26, no. 12, pp. 1038–1044, 2004.

[82] E. Santamaria, F. C. Wei, I. H. Chen, and D. C. C. Chuang, "Sensation recovery on innervated radial forearm flap for hemiglossectomy reconstruction by using different recipient nerves," *Plastic and Reconstructive Surgery*, vol. 103, no. 2, pp. 450–457, 1999.

[83] M. L. Shindo, U. K. Sinha, and D. H. Rice, "Sensory recovery in noninnervated free flaps for head and neck reconstruction," *Laryngoscope*, vol. 105, no. 12, pp. 1290–1293, 1995.

[84] J. P. M. Vriens, R. Acosta, D. S. Soutar, and M. H. C. Webster, "Recovery of sensation in the radial forearm free flap in oral reconstruction," *Plastic and Reconstructive Surgery*, vol. 98, no. 4, pp. 649–656, 1996.

[85] Y. Kimata, K. Uchiyama, S. Ebihara et al., "Comparison of innervated and noninnervated free flaps in oral reconstruction," *Plastic and Reconstructive Surgery*, vol. 104, no. 5, pp. 1307–1313, 1999.

[86] M. E. Zafereo, R. S. Weber, J. S. Lewin, D. B. Roberts, and M. M. Hanasono, "Complications and functional outcomes following complex oropharyngeal reconstruction," *Head and Neck*, vol. 32, no. 8, pp. 1003–1011, 2010.

[87] J. J. Disa, A. L. Pusic, D. A. Hidalgo, and P. G. Cordeiro, "Microvascular reconstruction of the hypopharynx: defect classification, treatment algorithm, and functional outcome based on 165 consecutive cases," *Plastic and Reconstructive Surgery*, vol. 111, no. 2, pp. 652–660, 2003.

[88] J. J. Coleman, J. M. Searles, T. R. Hester et al., "Ten years experience with the free jejunal autograft," *The American Journal of Surgery*, vol. 154, no. 4, pp. 389–393, 1987.

[89] J. J. Coleman III, K.-C. Tan, J. M. Searles, T. R. Hester, and F. Nahai, "Jejunal free autograft: analysis of complications and their resolution," *Plastic and Reconstructive Surgery*, vol. 84, no. 4, pp. 589–595, 1989.

[90] M. A. Schusterman, K. Shestak, E. J. de Vries et al., "Reconstruction of the cervical esophagus: free jejunal transfer versus gastric pull-up," *Plastic and Reconstructive Surgery*, vol. 85, no. 1, pp. 16–21, 1990.

[91] G. P. Reece, M. A. Schusterman, M. J. Miller et al., "Morbidity and functional outcome of free jejunal transfer reconstruction for circumferential defects of the pharynx and cervical esophagus," *Plastic and Reconstructive Surgery*, vol. 96, no. 6, pp. 1307–1316, 1995.

[92] P. Yu, "Characteristics of the anterolateral thigh flap in a western population and its application in head and neck reconstruction," *Head and Neck*, vol. 26, no. 9, pp. 759–769, 2004.

[93] P. Yu and G. L. Robb, "Pharyngoesophageal reconstruction with the anterolateral thigh flap: a clinical and functional outcomes study," *Plastic and Reconstructive Surgery*, vol. 116, no. 7, pp. 1845–1855, 2005.

[94] E. M. Genden and A. S. Jacobson, "The role of the anterolateral thigh flap for pharyngoesophageal reconstruction," *Archives of Otolaryngology—Head & Neck Surgery*, vol. 131, no. 9, pp. 796–799, 2005.

[95] P. Yu, J. S. Lewin, G. P. Reece, and G. L. Robb, "Comparison of clinical and functional outcomes and hospital costs following pharyngoesophageal reconstruction with the anterolateral thigh free flap versus the jejunal flap," *Plastic and Reconstructive Surgery*, vol. 117, no. 3, pp. 968–974, 2006.

[96] D. J. Murray, R. W. Gilbert, M. J. J. Vesely et al., "Functional outcomes and donor site morbidity following circumferential pharyngoesophageal reconstruction using an anterolateral thigh flap and salivary bypass tube," *Head and Neck*, vol. 29, no. 2, pp. 147–154, 2007.

[97] P. Yu, M. M. Hanasono, R. J. Skoracki et al., "Pharyngoesophageal reconstruction with the anterolateral thigh flap after total laryngopharyngectomy," *Cancer*, vol. 116, no. 7, pp. 1718–1724, 2010.

[98] B. Azizzadeh, S. Yafai, J. D. Rawnsley et al., "Radial forearm free flap pharyngoesophageal reconstruction," *Laryngoscope*, vol. 111, no. 5, pp. 807–810, 2001.

[99] J. Scharpf and R. M. Esclamado, "Reconstruction with radial forearm flaps after ablative surgery for hypopharyngeal cancer," *Head and Neck*, vol. 25, no. 4, pp. 261–266, 2003.

[100] D. W. Chang, C. Hussussian, J. S. Lewin, A. A. Youssef, G. L. Robb, and G. P. Reece, "Analysis of pharyngocutaneous fistula following free jejunal transfer for total laryngopharyngectomy," *Plastic and Reconstructive Surgery*, vol. 109, no. 5, pp. 1522–1527, 2002.

[101] P. Yu, "One-stage reconstruction of complex pharyngoesophageal, tracheal, and anterior neck defects," *Plastic and Reconstructive Surgery*, vol. 116, no. 4, pp. 949–956, 2005.

[102] M. K. Wax, "The role of the implantable Doppler probe in free flap surgery," *The Laryngoscope*, vol. 124, supplement 1, pp. S1–S12, 2014.

[103] R. E. H. Ferguson and P. Yu, "Techniques of monitoring buried fasciocutaneous free flaps," *Plastic and Reconstructive Surgery*, vol. 123, no. 2, pp. 525–532, 2009.

4

The Biological Metallic versus Metallic Solution in Treating Periprosthetic Femoral Fractures: Outcome Assessment

Serafino Carta, Mattia Fortina, Alberto Riva, Luigi Meccariello, Enrico Manzi, Antonio Di Giovanni, and Paolo Ferrata

Department of Medical and Surgical Sciences and Neuroscience, Section of Orthopedics and Traumatology, University of Siena, University Hospital "Santa Maria alle Scotte", Siena, Italy

Correspondence should be addressed to Luigi Meccariello; drlordmec@gmail.com

Academic Editor: Jacek Cezary Szepietowski

Introduction. The periprosthetic fracture of the femur is, in order of frequency, the fourth leading cause (5.9%) of surgical revision. Our study aims to demonstrate how the grafting of bone splint betters the outcomes. *Materials.* We treated 15 periprosthetic femoral fractures divided into two groups: PS composed of 8 patients treated with plates and splints and PSS involving 7 patients treated only with plates. The evaluation criteria for the two groups during the clinical and radiological follow-up were the quality of life measured by the Short Form (36) Health Survey (SF-36), Harris Hip Score (HHS), Modified Cincinnati Rating System Questionnaire (MCRSQ), bone healing measured by the Radiographic Union Score (RUS), postoperative complications, and mortality. The evaluation endpoint was set at 24 months for both groups ($p < 0.05$). *Results.* The surgery lasted an average of 124.5 minutes for the PS group and 112.6 minutes for the PSS. At 24 months all clinical and radiographic scores were $p < 0.05$ for the PS group. During follow-up 4 patients (2 in each group) died of causes not related to surgery. *Conclusions.* The use of the metal plate as opposed to cortical allogenic splint should be taken into consideration as a noteworthy point for periprosthetic femoral fractures.

1. Introduction

Fractures around the hip joints are commonly defined as periprosthetic fractures in opposition to specific fractures of the prosthetic components whose treatment requires the total or partial removal of the implants and their replacement. The number of orthopedic hip and knee implants is progressively increasing, due to the aging of the population. The highest number of complications in total arthroprosthesis is represented by the loosening and osteolysis. The degree of osteolysis increases over the time for the stress exercised on the implants and the progressive age-related structural changes of the bone leading to fractures [1, 2]. From a Mayo Clinic study in the US we may see that the incidence of supracondylar fractures after total knee replacement is 0.6–2.5%. Such fractures may occur more than 10 years after the first implant. However the incidence of periprosthetic hip fractures after the first implant was 1.1% and increased to 4% after the complete

revision [2]. The implant may impair healing of the fracture due to endosteal ischemia [3]. Percentages of nonunion for proximal supracondylar fractures of total knee prosthesis are higher than those for fractures. The surgeon must restore the biomechanical integrity of the bone. This requires the restoration of a biological environment in which the bone can heal completely and resume its stability and support functions [4–9]. The treatment must include the soft tissue preservation in order to preserve the periosteal and/or endosteal blood supply. The surgeon should minimize the periosteal damage and consider the possibility of using bone grafts if the biological environment is compromised [4–9]. The patient's condition should be optimized. The goals of treatment are early functional recovery, in order to prevent pulmonary complications, bedsores, osteoporosis from disuse, and all the other complications of a prolonged bed rest, and the restoration of the axial alignment to help prevent the eccentric stress on the prosthesis and promote stabilization and early mobilization of the limb and prevent stiffness and muscle atrophy. The goals of treatment must be [4–9]

(1) restoring the best possible anatomical axis;

(2) obtaining the stability of both the prosthetic implant and the fracture;

(3) obtaining early patient mobilization;

(4) possibly guarantying a return to the quality of life before the trauma.

Modern conservation of cancellous or cortical bone matrix technologies allow in orthopedic surgery the use, as an aid, of biological materials of bone grafts to recreate a successful recovery of the medial wall and then bring the femoral structure to bear, once again, preinjury mechanical loads. Moreover, many authors and biomechanical studies on cadavers have shown that the medial splint is an indispensable counterfort to the medial plate in the osteosynthesis of periprosthetic hip and knee fractures. The purpose of our study is to demonstrate how the grafting of bone splint associated with the best metal plate improves fracture consolidation, functional recovery, and quality of life, compared to internal fixation with a simple plate [10–12].

2. Materials and Methods

From January 2010 to December 2014, at the UOC Orthopedics and Traumatology University of the AOUS Policlinico Santa Maria alle Scotte of Siena, we treated 15 diaphyseal periprosthetic femur, hip, and knee fractures. We divided the patients into two groups.

All patients were informed in a clear and comprehensive way of the two types of treatment and other possible surgical and conservative alternatives. Patients were treated according to the ethical standards of the Helsinki Declaration and were invited to read, understand, and sign the informed consent form.

The two patient groups were formed based on the patient's choice to undergo such treatment. Exclusion criteria included fractures caused by hematological or oncological pathologies, the age being less than 65, and patients who did not adhere to a minimum follow-up of 24 months.

The first group (PS) was represented by 8 patients treated with plate, ring, screws, and bone splint and bone grafts for the hip or knee periprosthetic fracture. The population of the PS group at the time of the trauma had a mean age of 77.8 years (range 70–89); the relation between the sexes (m : f) was 0.6 (3 : 5). The fractures were classified according to the Vancouver classification for the periprosthetic fracture of the hip and that of Rorabeck for the knee and they were so divided: Vancouver B2: 2; Vancouver C: 3; Rorabeck Type 2: 2; Rorabeck Type 3: 1 (Table 1). All patients underwent presurgery anesthetic visit. The preoperative risk for the most part was based on the ASA physical status classification system: III in 6 cases; 5 (62.5%) patients required a place in the intensive care unit for a postoperative recovery (Table 1). The most frequent comorbidities were the cardiovascular diseases which affected 75% (6 patients) of PS population and 62.5% (5 patients) of the patients had three or more comorbidities

at the time of the trauma (for a more detailed description see Table 2). 50% of the patients ($n = 4$) were undergoing pharmacological treatment for osteoporosis at the time of the trauma. The average years of follow-up were 2.3 (range 1–4). All patients in the PS group were treated with bone from cadaveric bank that was implanted only after routine procedures according to protocol. In the immediate postoperative period, all patients followed a personalized physiotherapy program, according to their medical conditions.

The second group (PSS) was represented by 7 patients suffering from periprosthetic hip fractures treated exclusively with plate and screws while the knee (fractures) was treated with plate or revision prosthesis. The PS group population at the time of the trauma had an average age of 75.3 years (range 67–81); the ratio between sexes (m : f) was of 0.75 (3 : 4). Even in this group the fractures were classified according to the Vancouver classification for the periprosthetic fractures of the hip and that of Rorabeck for those of the knee and they were so divided: Vancouver B2: 2; Vancouver C: 3; Rorabeck Type 2: 2; Rorabeck Type 3: 1 (Table 1). All patients underwent presurgery anesthetic visit. The preoperative risk for the most part was based on the ASA physical status classification system: III in 4 cases; 5 (71.42%) patients required a place in the intensive care unit for a postoperative recovery (Table 1).

The most frequent comorbidity was the Diabetes Mellitus involving 85.71% (6 patients) of PS population and 71.42% (5 patients) of the patients had three or more comorbidities at the time of the trauma (for a more detailed description see Table 2). 85.71% of the patients ($n = 6$) were undergoing pharmacological treatment for osteoporosis at the time of the trauma. The average years of follow-up were 2.3 (range 1–5). The chosen criteria to evaluate the two groups during the clinical and radiological follow-up were the quality of life measured by the Short Form (36) Health Survey's (SF-36) overall score [13], the hip function and quality of life related to it, measured by the Harris Hip Score (HHS) [14], the knee function and quality of life related to it, measured by the Modified Cincinnati Rating System Questionnaire (MCRSQ) [15], the bone healing measured by Radiographic Union Score (RUS) [16], and postoperative complications.

The evaluation endpoint was set at 24 months for both groups.

3. Statistical Analysis

Descriptive statistics were used to summarize the characteristics of the study group and subgroups, including means and standard deviations of all continuous variables. The t-test was used to compare continuous outcomes. The Fisher's exact test (groups are smaller than 10 patients) was used to compare categorical variables. The statistical significance was defined as $p < 0.05$. We used Pearson correlation coefficient (r) to compare the predictive score of outcomes and quality of life. Statistical analyses were performed with SPSS v.15.0 (SPSS Inc., an IBM Company, Chicago, IL, USA). Mean ages (and their standard deviations) of the patients were rounded at the closest year. The predictive score of outcomes and quality of life and their standard deviations were approximated at

TABLE 1: Description of population.

	PS	PSS
Number of patients	8	7
Average of age in years	77.8	75.3
Range of patients age in years	70–89	67–81
Gender ratio (m : f)	0.6 (3 : 5)	0.75 (3 : 4)
Fractures type according to Vancouver and Rorabeck classification	Vancouver B2: 2 Vancouver C: 3 Rorabeck 2: 2 Rorabeck 3: 1	Vancouver B2: 2 Vancouver C: 3 Rorabeck 2: 1 Rorabeck 3: 1
ASA physical status classification system	ASA I: 0 ASA II: 2 ASA III: 6 ASA IV: 0	ASA I: 0 ASA II: 3 ASA III: 4 ASA IV: 0
Number of patients that needed a place in intensive care	5 (62.5%)	5 (71.42%)
Patients treated for osteoporosis	4 (50%)	6 (85.71%)
Average years of follow-up after periprosthetic fracture	2.3	2.3
Range of years of follow-up after periprosthetic fracture	1–4	1–5

TABLE 2: Patients' comorbidity.

	PS (%)	PSS number (%)
Comorbidity		
Cardiovascular diseases	6 (75%)	5 (71.42%)
Stroke	4 (50%)	1 (14.29%)
Respiratory diseases	5 (62.5%)	6 (85.71%)
Nefro-urologic diseases	5 (62.5%)	2 (28.57%)
Diabetes mellitus	4 (50%)	6 (85.71%)
Rheumatic diseases	4 (50%)	7 (100%)
Parkinson's disease	1 (12.5%)	2 (28.57%)
Smokers	1 (12.5%)	3 (42.86%)
Use of steroids	7 (87.5%)	7 (100%)
Number of comorbidities for patient		
1	1 (12.5%)	1 (14.29%)
2	2 (25%)	1 (14.29%)
≥3	5 (62.5%)	5 (71.42%)

the first decimal while Pearson correlation coefficient (r) was approximated at the second decimal.

4. Results

The surgery lasted an average of 124.5 minutes (92–186) for the PS group and 112.6 minutes in the PSS group (79 min–192 min).

The quality of life before the trauma SF-36, for the PS group, was about 72.3 (range 62.3–86.4) points while that of the PSS group was 74.2 (range 64.3–88.5) points; there was no statistically significant difference between the two groups ($p > 0.5$). In the sixth month the SF-36 score was 57.8 (range 43.6–74.3) for the PS group, while that of PSS was 54.3 (range 41.6–74.5); there was a statistically significant difference ($p < 0.05$) in favor of the PS group. For a more detailed description see Figure 1.

HHS before the trauma, for the PS group, was about 86.3 (range 78.2–96.8) points while that of the PSS group was 85.9 (range 77.2–96.4) points. There was no statistically significant difference between the two groups ($p > 0.5$). In the sixth month, the HHS score was 73.5 (range 66.7–82.1) for the PS group while that of PSS was 70.4 (range 62.7–80.2); there was a statistically significant difference ($p < 0.05$) in favor of the group PS. For a more detailed description see Figure 2.

MCRSQ before the trauma, for the PS group, was about 86.5 (range 74.2–98.8) points while that of the PSS group was 86.2 (range 74.2–98.8) points. There was no statistically significant difference between the two groups ($p > 0.5$). At the twelfth month, the HHS score was 84.3 (range 74.3–94.6) for the PS group while that of PSS was 78.3 (range 68.3–88.3). There was a statistically significant difference ($p < 0.05$) in favor of the PS group. For a more detailed description see Figure 3.

Regarding the trend of bone healing on a 1-year follow-up measured by RUS, in the twelfth month, there was a statistically significant difference ($p < 0.05$) in favor of the PS group (Figure 4). Bone healing occurred in the PS group on average of 9.6 months after surgery while in the PSS group bone healing occurred 12.4 months postoperatively (Figure 4).

The patients had an indication to the progressive load on average 50.6 days after surgery.

We have not lost any patients from the two groups of up to 24 months of follow-up.

In the PS group, there were 6 complications; the two most frequent were cardiac decompensation (25%, $n = 2$) and myocardial infarction (25%, $n = 2$); after a 2-year follow-up there were 2 deaths, 25% of the total population (Table 3).

In the PSS group there were 12 complications, the most frequent was cardiac decompensation (42.86%, $n = 3$); after a 2-year follow-up there were 2 deaths, 28.57% of the total population (Table 3).

Time from the trauma	Average SF-36 PS	Average SF-36 PSS
Before the trauma	72.3 (range 62.3–86.4)	74.2 (range 64.3–88.5)
0	23.5 (range 15.6–44.8)	26.3 (range 16.8–47.2)
I month from the trauma	32.5 (range 23.9–52.3)	33.8 (range 24.2–53.1)
III months from the trauma	46.3 (range 32.8–58.7)	45.6 (range 32.8–58.6)
VI months from the trauma	57.8 (range 43.6–74.3)	54.3 (range 41.6–74.5)
XII months from the trauma	69.8 (range 52.3–84.8)	63.7 (range 50.3–82.7)
XXIV months from the trauma	76.3 (range 54.4–89.3)	64.5 (range 50.3–82.7)

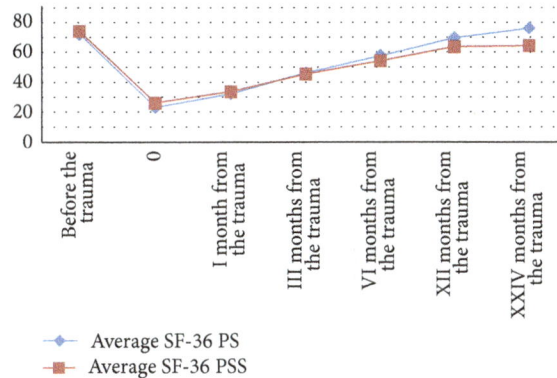

— Average SF-36 PS
— Average SF-36 PSS

FIGURE 1: Trend of the follow-up to two years of quality of life measured by the Short Form (36) Health Survey (SF-36). At the sixth month of follow-up there was already a statistically significant difference ($p < 0.05$) in favor of the PS Group.

TABLE 3: Postoperative complications during all the follow-up.

	PS (%)	PSS (%)
Respiratory infections	1 (12.5%)	1 (14.29%)
Cardiac failure	2 (25%)	3 (42.86%)
DVE (Deep Venous Thrombosis)	0 (0%)	0 (0%)
Urinary infection	0 (0%)	2 (28.57%)
Gastrointestinal bleeding	0 (0%)	2 (28.57%)
Myocardial infarction	2 (25%)	2 (28.57%)
Ictus/tia	1 (12.5%)	2 (28.57%)
Number of complications for patient:		
1	1 (12.5%)	1 (14.29%)
2	1 (12.5%)	2 (28.57%)
≥3	1 (12.5%)	2 (28.57%)
Numbers of deaths		
After two years of follow-up	2 (25%)	2 (28.57%)

There was no statistically significant difference between the two groups ($p > 0.5$) for postoperative mortality.

5. Discussion

More than 80,000 hip replacement operations are performed in Italy every year: a procedure that represents one of the major achievements of modern orthopedic surgery. The complexity of the factors influencing the success of the operations in clinical terms does not facilitate the use of outcome indicators [17]. Current expectations of success have thus made it possible to extend the range to pathologies and age groups initially considered at high risk. Many prospective studies report as future projections an increase of periprosthetic femur and knee fractures. Gathering information on the patients' quality of life in clinical trials of high methodological level is the basis of progress in prosthetic hip and knee surgery. It is known, however, that the most recent and sophisticated clinical trial methodologies emphasize the need for an assessment of a rigorous and standardized outcome [18]. Clinical research in prosthetic hip and knee surgery has focused, in recent years, on the analysis of the results, in order to reveal common features of the various methods in terms of benefits and complications, but also the differences of specific centers and institutions [19]. Similar analysis conducted in different geographical areas (USA, France) has shown how a measuring index of the great diffusion as the Harris Hip Score (HHS), until now considered an undisputed standard and only recently statistically validated [20], actually provides a partial evaluation of the patient's perspective on the pathology and the surgical procedure: only a share of the major causes of the patient's complaints and disability are examined by the questionnaire, while it ignores other complaints (night pain, sexual activity, sleep disorders, etc.) which have a high subjective meaning [13]. In applying a similar procedure to the prosthetic hip and knee surgery, many authors agree to use a combined generic questionnaire (SF-36) [14, 15] for the correct determination to evaluate the quality of life of patients subject to revision of prosthetic implants. In the evaluation of the prosthetic hip surgery a significant problem is the presence of "comorbidity," that is, the role played by the associated pathologies, especially in the elderly. If we consider that the majority of implants has high survival rates (above 90%)

Time from the trauma	Average HHS PS	Average HHS PSS
Before the trauma	86.3 (range 78.2–96.8)	85.9 (range 77.2–96.4)
0	15.6 (range 9.3–24.6)	17.7 (range 10.4–25.1)
I month from the trauma	32.6 (range 22.8–52.8)	35.4 (range 23.2–54.8)
III months from the trauma	56.9 (range 49.6–68.8)	54.3 (range 47.1–66.4)
VI months from the trauma	73.5 (range 66.7–82.1)	70.4 (range 62.7–80.2)
XII months from the trauma	77.3 (range 70.8–92.1)	72.5 (range 68.3–86.4)
XXIV months from the trauma	82.6 (range 72.4–94.3)	74.6 (range 70.2–87.5)

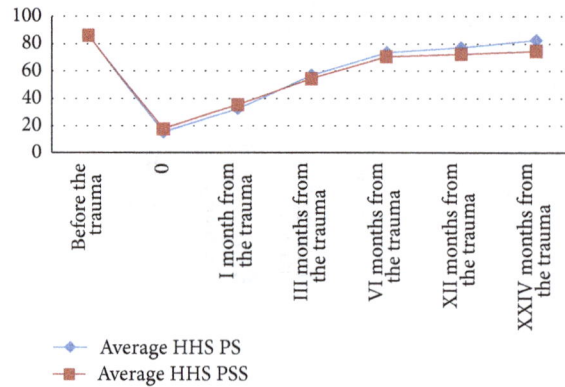

FIGURE 2: Trend hip function and quality of life related to it for 2-year follow-up measured by Harris Hip Score (HHS). At six months there was a statistically significant difference ($p < 0.05$) in favor of the PS group.

Time from the trauma	Average MCRSQ PS	Media MCRSQ average PSS
Before the trauma	86.5 (range 74.2–98.8)	86.2 (range 74.2–98.8)
0	25.3 (range 18.2–34.8)	26.8 (range 18.2–34.8)
I month from the trauma	46.3 (range 34.8–56.3)	46.2 (range 34.6–56.3)
III months from the trauma	64.2 (range 60.1–74.1)	64.6 (range 60.3–74.3)
VI months from the trauma	76.3 (range 68.3–88.3)	76.3 (range 68.3–88.3)
XII months from the trauma	84.3 (range 74.3–94.6)	78.3 (range 68.3–88.3)
XXIV months from the trauma	90.7 (range 80.4–98.3)	80.3 (range 70.3–88.3)

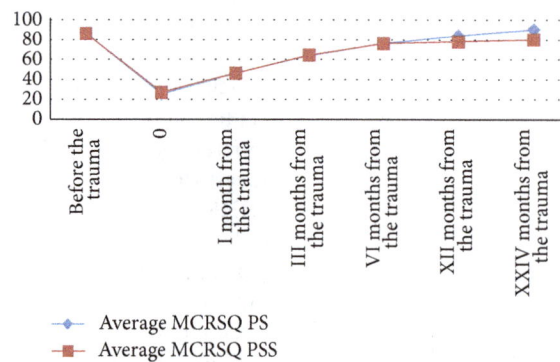

FIGURE 3: Trend of knee function and quality of life related to it for two-year follow-up measured by the Modified Cincinnati Rating System Questionnaire (MCRSQ). At twelve months there was a statistically significant difference ($p < 0.05$) in favor of the PS group.

10 years after surgery and that, to date, in Italy the average age of a patient undergoing this type of operation is of about 70 years, we can easily imagine how associated musculoskeletal, but also cardiovascular, respiratory, and neurological, pathologies produce a continuous decay of functional indexes, which affect the result regardless of the hip or knee prosthesis [16]. This "problem" influences the general measures, as the femoral periprosthesic fractures, as recently documented by Ritter and Albohm [21]. The collection of a comorbidity index may facilitate, in the analysis phase,

XR UNION	Average RUS PS	Average RUS PSS
I month from the trauma	1.5 (range 1-2)	1.4 (range 1-2)
III months from the trauma	2.5 (range 2-3)	2.4 (range 2-3)
VI months from the trauma	3.1 (range 3-4)	3 (range 3-3)
XII months from the trauma	3.8 (range 3-4)	3.1 (range 3-4)
XXIV months from the trauma	4	3.1 (range 3-4)

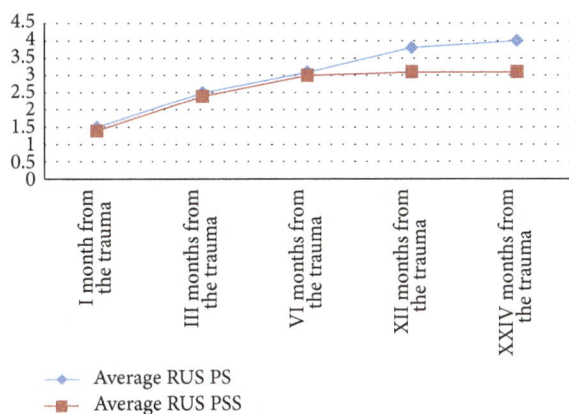

FIGURE 4: Trend of bone healing in two-year follow-up measured by Radiographic Union Score (RUS). At the twelfth month there was a statistically significant difference ($p < 0.05$) in favor of the PS group.

the stratification of patients and has been highly recommended by several authors. Not surprisingly it was Sir John Charnley, father of the modern prosthetic hip surgery and careful scholar of the results of the method he perfected, that designed a simple system to differentiate patients with monoarticular (class A), bilateral (class B) disease or suffering from other chronic diseases (class C), which proves to be still very useful in longitudinal studies [22]. From the surgical point of view in the majority of cases of type B Vancouver fracture (60–75%) [23], the stem may appear mobilized (B2). A surgical alternative to the methods presented by us in these cases is to replace the femoral stem using long stem uncemented prosthesis which is able to exceed the fracture, twice the cortical diameter [24], so as to obtain a good stability, similar to that obtained with an intramedullary nail. Many authors recommend the use of uncemented long stems with a distal porous coating because the use of cement in the fracture can lead to nonhealing and, for the interposition in the fracture, also general risks such as air embolism and vascular problems due to the exothermic reaction during polymerization [25].

In the Vancouver C type fractures (fracture distal to the femoral stem) [26], the femoral stem is generally stable and therefore these injuries can be treated by applying the general concepts of reduction and osteosynthesis, typical for common femoral fracture. It is important to obtain a good anatomic axis reduction and ensure a good stability. To achieve these results, in our opinion, it is preferable to reduce the fracture with ORIF "open" technique and stabilize it with a plate that allows the simultaneous use of screws and/or cerclage. In situations where the subprosthetic fracture is very distal to the stem, to affect the pars metaphyseal distal femur,

we can consider a "closed" reduction and stabilization with an intramedullary retrograde nail [26]. The same principle of retrograde nailing in Type 2 or Type 3 Rorabeck is considered by many authors to be a simple, safe, and minimally invasive treatment of femoral periprosthetic knee fractures [26], with high success rates related to the ability of the system to ensure a good axial, angular, and rotational stability which allows early mobilization of the prosthetic knee. Retrograde nailing is not recommended in the presence of very distal and comminuted femur fractures in which the space for the insertion of the distal locking screws may be insufficient. The nailing is also not recommended in the presence of ipsilateral hip replacement since it creates a less resistant area between the stems of the two implants such as causing a fracture in the free interposed zone. The osteosynthesis with plate is primarily recommended in comminuted fractures of the more distal portion of the femur on stable implants (Type 2 Rorabeck), where the construct with multiple converging screws with angular stability provides mechanical stability to the axial and torsional forces acting on bones often osteoporotic [27]. The development of plates with polyaxial screws also allows insertion of screws around any prosthetic implant. Many authors consider useful, especially in highly comminuted fractures, the use of such plates with angular stability with bridge fittings, bypassing the fracture, as long as a correct axial alignment is guaranteed [27]. When possible, the use of LISS plate (Less Invasive Stabilization System) with minimally invasive MIPO technique (Minimally Invasive Plate Osteosynthesis) allows a minimal dissection of the soft tissue and periosteum, reduced blood loss, and reduced risk of infection [27]. The plate osteosynthesis is especially useful in the presence of an implant in the proximal femur (prosthetic rod or pertrochanteric nail) being equipped with monocortical stability screws that permit overlap pin of the distal portion of the implant, so as to avoid an increase of stress between two implants. Ultimately a stable internal fixation with a reduced damage to soft tissues allows an early functional recovery [27]. The use of the plate and the graft of allogenic femoral cortical splint in the treatment of periprosthetic femoral fractures is not a new technique and it has been extensively described by many authors [28]. J.-W. Wang and C.-J. Wang [29] in 2002 recommended the use of a compression plate opposed to cortical splint. Wang's group reported a fracture consolidation rate of 100%, but they also reported a case of osteomyelitis and one malunion after a maximum follow-up of 68 months [29]. From 1996 to 2007, Font-Vizcarra et al. [11] in their study reported a retrospective review of 21 patients who had periprosthetic femoral fractures and were treated with plate and screws instead of allogenic frozen cortical stick. The group was made up of 16 women and 5 men with an average age 80.3 years at time of surgery. Three patients were not available at follow-up and four died within a few weeks after discharge. The remaining 14 patients were evaluated clinically and radiologically with a mean follow-up of 3.2 years. The consolidation of the fracture was observed in 13 patients, and the integration of the transplant occurred in 12 patients. One of the 14 patients developed a deep infection with staphylococcus coagulase-negative, with a satisfying result after surgical debridement and antibiotic therapy. There were no cases of nonunion or implant failure. At final evaluation, the mean EQ-5D VAS score was 64 (ranging from 40 to 90 points) and the EQ-5D mean health index adapted to the Spanish population was 0.57. We used the SF-36's overall score to measure the patients quality of life because we want to understand: evaluating individual patients health status; researching the cost-effectiveness of a treatment; monitoring and comparing disease burden. We are also aware that it has the following limitations: the survey does not take into consideration a sleep variable; the survey has a low response rate in the >65 population.

The mean Oxford hip score was 31.2. The results described by Font-Vizcarra et al. [11] support the use of cortical allograft for these fractures to increase the chance of fracture healing and improve bone biomechanics. The same authors believed that the cortical splint opposed to plate and screws is particularly suitable for the B1 and C fractures in which decreased bone density is present [11].

From the qualitative point of view of the hip function and the quality of life, the patients were given two questionnaires: the HHS and the SF-12 (the simplified form of SF-36). As shown in the new study by Dettoni et al. [30], the validations to adaptation of the Italian population to the HHS, HHS, and SF-12 are correlated with each other. The same correlation can be taken between SF-36 and MCRSQ [31]. All scientific literature agrees that the simple fracture of the proximal femur in an elderly patient with many comorbidities can result, one year after the trauma, in death, entrapment, significant reduction in quality of life, and loss of autonomy in normal activities of normal life [32]. The literature has demonstrated that both morbidity and mortality in the patients suffering from periprosthetic fracture are similar to those of the geriatric hip fracture population. As such, the early restoration of function and ambulation is critical in patients with these injuries, and effective surgical strategies to achieve these goals are essential [32].

The treatment of periprosthetic fractures is very complex and the results are very variable. The treatment for each case must be individualized. Custom-made prosthesis may be used in places where the prosthesis is well fixed in the femur. The goal is to obtain stable fracture fixation and a secure and well-fixed femoral component in proper alignment which allows for early mobilization of the patient to prevent any complications associated with prolonged recumbency in old age [33].

In 2003, Peters et al. [12] in a cadaveric study compared the stability of the periprosthetic femur fracture using the single metal plate of cortical bone splint opposed to a metal plate and the use of two cortical slats with rings. The cadaveric studies were carried out by loading the weight on one leg and climbing the stairs with a force of 2250 Newtons. Stability and optimum implant resistance by loading on one lower limb were achieved in the group of two cortical bone slats and rings. In climbing stairs the most performing implant was the one with cortical bone splint opposed to the metal plate and screws. The authors concluded that the plate alone was not enough to achieve good biomechanical outcomes for this type of fractures.

When comparing the total femoral allograft with osteosynthesis using plate and screws the use of a cortical graft (splint) and a plate is more rigid than the plate itself but it is not as rigid as using two plates positioned orthogonally [34]. The modulus of elasticity is similar between the cortical allograft and host bone but the allogeneic bone splint reduces stress shielding [34]. The use of allogenic cortical splint has the potential to add stem cells, cancellous bone, and bone matrix [35] and is therefore particularly useful for patients who are known to be commonly affected by osteoporosis [35]. Rates of 89–100% of the consolidation of fractures have been reported by using cortical allografts with or without contraposition of plate for periprosthetic femoral fractures [29], and the addition of allograft cancellous bone may increase the rate of fracture healing [35]. In fact Kim et al. [36] revealed that the 16-year rate of survival of the components was 91% with bone allograft strut and the mean Harris Hip Score was 39 ± 10 points before revision and improved to 86 ± 14 points at 16-year follow-up ($p = 0.02$) and the mean preoperative WOMAC score was 62 ± 29 (41–91) points and improved to 22 ± 19 (11–51) points at 16-year follow-up ($p = 0.003$). Fractures treated with plate fixation are more rigid and do not form the same robust callus as those treated with intramedullary nails [37]. Furthermore, the presence of the plate with or without the bone allograft strut obscures the evaluation of the lateral cortex, and many reviewers commented on the difficulty in its scoring. This difficulty is reported in experimental work, where the intraclass correlation coefficient (between RUST and modified RUST) values of individual cortices that demonstrated the lowest agreement for the lateral cortex in plate fixation are seen. The goal of the modified RUST or RUS score described in many articles is to gain a greater range of scores during the crucial time of healing when callus was bridging [37].

The cortical allografts allow personalized fixation without the expense of having a custom-made implant. The use of the slats makes prosthetic revision surgery longer than using the plate alone. The increasing complexity of the most extensive surgery for dissection of the soft tissue and periosteal detachment [38] may explain a high rate of complications; the authors show a 17% of complications [38] and the deep infection has a rate of 4–13% [38]. The great mass of dead bone can increase the rate of deep infection the same way a devitalized bone produces the growth of bacteria leading to infection. The transmission of infectious diseases is possible with the use of allogeneic transplant, but the protocols in use in bone banks have reduced this risk [38].

Complete resorption of the cortical bone splint has rarely been reported in practice; however, the stages that precede this resorption have been observed [38]. In our case history the most recent X-ray examination has shown the melting, but not the reabsorption, and this indicates a cortical graft revascularization [38], which was especially evident in the revisions of knee periprosthetic fractures [38].

6. Conclusions

From the data available in the literature and from our experience we can say that the use of the metal plate opposed to the cortical allogenic splint should be considered as a noteworthy point for periprosthetic femur fractures in the hip and knee arthroplasty, where there is bone loss and/or a potential mechanical instability. We have shown that the potential benefit from the association of a metal plate with cortical allogenic splint increases bone quality, reduces stress shielding, increases the percentage of probability of fracture consolidation, makes the system more stable, reduces complications, and improves patient quality of life due to a shorter functional recovery. However the customization of the transplant must be considered against the potential disadvantages of the lengthening of surgical time and the complexity of the surgery, the risk of infections, the nonunion, mortality, and transmission of infectious diseases.

Competing Interests

All authors disclose no financial and personal relationships with other people or organizations that could inappropriately influence (bias) their work. Examples of potential competing interests include employment, consultancies, stock ownership, honoraria, paid expert testimony, patent applications/registrations, and grants or other funding.

References

[1] S. Della Corte, V. Crispino, M. Iavarone et al., "The Periprosthetic fractures, Epidemiology and treatment: our experience," *AITOG OGGI*, vol. 2, pp. 26–31, 2013.

[2] D. J. Berry, "Epidemiology of periprosthetic fractures after major joint replacement: hip and knee," *Orthopedic Clinics of North America*, vol. 30, pp. 183–190, 1999.

[3] B. A. Masri, R. M. D. Meek, and C. P. Duncan, "Periprosthetic fractures evaluation and treatment," *Clinical Orthopaedics and Related Research*, vol. 420, pp. 80–95, 2004.

[4] M. Ehlinger, F. Bonnomet, and P. Adam, "Periprosthetic femoral fractures: the minimally invasive fixation option," *Orthopaedics & Traumatology: Surgery & Research*, vol. 96, no. 3, pp. 304–309, 2010.

[5] P. J. Dougherty, D.-G. Kim, S. Meisterling, C. Wybo, and Y. Yeni, "Biomechanical comparison of bicortical versus unicortical screw placement of proximal tibia locking plates: a cadaveric model," *Journal of Orthopaedic Trauma*, vol. 22, no. 6, pp. 399–403, 2008.

[6] D. A. Herrera, P. J. Kregor, P. A. Cole, B. A. Levy, A. Jönsson, and M. Zlowodzki, "Treatment of acute distal femur fractures above a total knee arthroplasty: systematic review of 415 cases (1981–2006)," *Acta Orthopaedica*, vol. 79, no. 1, pp. 22–27, 2008.

[7] H.-S. Han, K.-W. Oh, and S.-B. Kang, "Retrograde intramedullary nailing for periprosthetic supracondylar fractures of the femur after total knee arthroplasty," *Clinics in Orthopedic Surgery*, vol. 1, no. 4, pp. 201–206, 2009.

[8] E. Tsiridis, S. Krikler, and P. V. Giannoudis, "Periprosthetic femoral fractures: current aspects of management," *Injury*, vol. 38, no. 6, pp. 649–650, 2007.

[9] M. Ehlinger, J. M. Cognet, and P. Simon, "Traitement des fractures fémorales sur matériel par voie mini-invasive et remise en charge immédiate : apport des plaques à vis bloquées (LCP). Série préliminaire," *Revue de Chirurgie Orthopédique et Réparatrice de l'Appareil Moteur*, vol. 94, no. 1, pp. 26–36, 2008.

[10] G. J. Macpherson, T. Gotterbarm, P. R. Aldinger, H. Mau, and S. J. Breusch, "Long-term fate of femoral allograft for periprosthetic fracture around a revision knee arthroplasty: a case report and review of the literature," *Hard Tissue*, vol. 2, no. 3, article 25, 2013.

[11] L. Font-Vizcarra, J. A. Fernández-Valencia, X. Gallart, J. M. Segur, S. Prat, and J. Riba, "Cortical strut allograft as an adjunct to plate fixation for periprosthetic fractures of the femur," *HIP International*, vol. 20, no. 1, pp. 43–49, 2010.

[12] C. L. Peters, K. N. Bachus, and J. S. Davitt, "Fixation of periprosthetic femur fractures: a biomechanical analysis comparing cortical strut allograft plates and conventional metal plates," *Orthopedics*, vol. 26, no. 7, pp. 695–699, 2003.

[13] J. M. Fielden, P. H. Gander, J. G. Horne, B. M. F. Lewer, R. M. Green, and P. A. Devane, "An assessment of sleep disturbance in patients before and after total hip arthroplasty," *Journal of Arthroplasty*, vol. 18, no. 3, pp. 371–376, 2003.

[14] J. E. Ware and C. D. Sherbourne, "The MOS 36-item short-form health survey (Sf-36). I. conceptual framework and item selection," *Medical Care*, vol. 30, no. 6, pp. 473–483, 1992.

[15] J. E. Ware Jr. and B. Gandek, "Overview of the SF-36 Health Survey and the International Quality of Life Assessment (IQOLA) Project," *Journal of Clinical Epidemiology*, vol. 51, no. 11, pp. 903–912, 1998.

[16] E. Romanini, R. Padua, G. Zanoli, L. Massari, A. Soccetti, and M. Tartarone, "Rapporto costi benefici nelle scelte terapeutiche nel paziente anziano: quali benefici e come misurarli?" *Giornale Italiano di Ortopedia e Traumatologia*, vol. 26, no. 1, pp. S440–S446, 2000.

[17] W. J. Hozack, R. H. Rothman, T. J. Albert, R. A. Balderston, and K. Eng, "Relationship of total hip arthroplasty outcomes to other orthopaedic procedures," *Clinical Orthopaedics and Related Research*, no. 344, pp. 88–93, 1997.

[18] M. E. Kantz, W. J. Harris, K. Levitsky, J. E. Ware Jr., and A. R. Davies, "Methods for assessing conditionspecific and generic functional status outcomes after total knee replacement," *Medical Care*, vol. 30, no. 5, supplement, pp. MS240–MS252, 1992.

[19] C. Villani, E. Romanini, M. C. Giordano, P. Persiani, and F. Casella, "Artroprotesi totale d'anca non cementata: valutazione patient-oriented a medio termine," *Giornale Italiano di Ortopedia e Traumatologia*, vol. 26, no. 2, pp. 67–73, 2000.

[20] P. Soderman and H. Malchau, "Is the Harris hip score system useful to study the outcome of total hip replacement?" *Clinical Orthopaedics and Related Research*, no. 384, pp. 189–197, 2001.

[21] M. A. Ritter and M. J. Albohm, "Overview: maintaining outcomes for total hip arthroplasty. The past, present, and future," *Clinical Orthopaedics and Related Research*, vol. 344, pp. 81–87, 1997.

[22] J. Charnley, "The long-term results of low-friction arthroplasty of the hip performed as a primary intervention," *Journal of Bone and Joint Surgery—Series B*, vol. 54, no. 1, pp. 61–76, 1972.

[23] C. P. Duncan and B. A. Masri, "Fractures of the femur after hip replacement," in *Istructional Course Lectures*, D. W. Jackson, Ed., pp. 293–304, AAOS, Rosemont, Ill, USA, 1995.

[24] D. S. Garbuz, B. A. Masri, and C. P. Duncan, "Periprosthetic fractures of the femur: principles of prevention and management," in *Instructional Course Lectures*, W. D. Cannon, Ed., vol. 47, pp. 237–242, A.A.O.S., Rosemont, Ill, USA, 1998.

[25] S. J. Incavo, D. M. Beard, F. Pupparo, M. Ries, and J. Wiedel, "One-stage revision of periprosthetic fractures around loose cemented total hip arthroplasty," *American Journal of Orthopedics*, vol. 27, no. 1, pp. 35–41, 1998.

[26] M. H. Gonzalez, R. Barmada, D. Fabiano, and W. Meltzer, "Femoral shaft fracture after hip arthroplasty: a system for classification and treatment," *Journal of the Southern Orthopaedic Association*, vol. 8, no. 4, pp. 240–251, 1999.

[27] A. Hagel, H. Siekmann, and K.-S. Delank, "Periprosthetic femoral fracture—an interdisciplinary challenge," *Deutsches Arzteblatt International*, vol. 111, no. 39, pp. 658–664, 2014.

[28] S. Otte, J. Fitzek, C. Wedemeyer, F. Löer, M. von Knoch, and G. Saxler, "Reinforcement of deficient femur with inlay strut grafts in revision hip arthroplasty: a small series," *Archives of Orthopaedic and Trauma Surgery*, vol. 126, no. 10, pp. 649–653, 2006.

[29] J.-W. Wang and C.-J. Wang, "Supracondylar fractures of the femur above total knee arthroplasties with cortical allograft struts," *Journal of Arthroplasty*, vol. 17, no. 3, pp. 365–372, 2002.

[30] F. Dettoni, P. Pellegrino, M. R. La Russa et al., "Validation and cross cultural adaptation of the Italian version of the harris hip score," *HIP International*, vol. 25, no. 1, pp. 91–97, 2015.

[31] N. J. Greco, A. F. Anderson, B. J. Mann et al., "Responsiveness of the international knee documentation committee subjective knee form in comparison to the western ontario and mcmaster universities osteoarthritis index, modified cincinnati knee rating system, and short form 36 in patients with focal articular cartilage defects," *American Journal of Sports Medicine*, vol. 38, no. 5, pp. 891–902, 2010.

[32] A. Nauth, M. T. Nousiainen, R. Jenkinson, and J. Hall, "The treatment of periprosthetic fractures," *Instructional Course Lectures*, vol. 64, pp. 161–173, 2015.

[33] C. P. Pal, P. Singh, D. Kumar, and A. Singh, "Periprosthetic femoral fracture with broken implant insitu:—a treatment prospect," *Journal of Orthopaedic Case Reports*, vol. 4, no. 3, pp. 12–15, 2014.

[34] J. K. Choi, T. R. Gardner, E. Yoon, T. A. Morrison, W. B. Macaulay, and J. A. Geller, "The effect of fixation technique on the stiffness of comminuted Vancouver B1 periprosthetic femur fractures," *Journal of Arthroplasty*, vol. 25, supplement 6, pp. 124–128, 2010.

[35] F. S. Haddad and C. P. Duncan, "Cortical onlay allograft struts in the treatment of periprosthetic femoral fractures," *Instructional Course Lectures*, vol. 52, pp. 291–300, 2003.

[36] Y.-H. Kim, J.-W. Park, J.-S. Kim, and D. Rastogi, "High survivorship with cementless stems and cortical strut allografts for large femoral bone defects in revision THA," *Clinical Orthopaedics and Related Research*, vol. 473, no. 9, pp. 2990–3000, 2015.

[37] J. Litrenta, P. Tornetta, S. Mehta et al., "Determination of radiographic healing: an assessment of consistency using RUST and modified RUST in metadiaphyseal fractures," *Journal of Orthopaedic Trauma*, vol. 29, no. 11, pp. 516–520, 2015.

[38] J. Tomás Hernández and K. Holck, "Periprosthetic femoral fractures: when I use strut grafts and why?" *Injury*, vol. 46, supplement 5, pp. S43–S46, 2015.

5

The Protective Effects of Alpha-Lipoic Acid and Coenzyme Q$_{10}$ Combination on Ovarian Ischemia-Reperfusion Injury

Ahmet Ali Tuncer,[1] Mehmet Fatih Bozkurt,[2] Tulay Koken,[3] Nurhan Dogan,[4] Mine Kanat Pektaş,[5] and Didem Baskin Embleton[1]

[1]*Department of Pediatric Surgery, Afyon Kocatepe University Hospital, 03000 Afyonkarahisar, Turkey*
[2]*Department of Pathology, Faculty of Veterinary Medicine, Afyon Kocatepe University, 03000 Afyonkarahisar, Turkey*
[3]*Department of Biochemistry, Afyon Kocatepe University Medical Faculty, 03000 Afyonkarahisar, Turkey*
[4]*Department of Biostatistics, Afyon Kocatepe University Medical Faculty, 03000 Afyonkarahisar, Turkey*
[5]*Department of Obstetrics & Gynecology, Afyon Kocatepe University Hospital, 03000 Afyonkarahisar, Turkey*

Correspondence should be addressed to Ahmet Ali Tuncer; drtaali@yahoo.com

Academic Editor: João Quevedo

Objective. This study aims to evaluate whether alpha-lipoic acid and/or coenzyme Q$_{10}$ can protect the prepubertal ovarian tissue from ischemia-reperfusion injury in an experimental rat model of ovarian torsion. *Materials and Methods.* Forty-two female preadolescent Wistar-Albino rats were divided into 6 equal groups randomly. The sham group had laparotomy without torsion; the other groups had torsion/detorsion procedure. After undergoing torsion, group 2 received saline, group 3 received olive oil, group 4 received alpha-lipoic acid, group 5 received coenzyme Q$_{10}$, and group 6 received both alpha-lipoic acid and coenzyme Q$_{10}$ orally. The oxidant-antioxidant statuses of these groups were compared using biochemical measurement of oxidized/reduced glutathione, glutathione peroxidase and malondialdehyde, pathological evaluation of damage and apoptosis within the ovarian tissue, and immunohistochemical assessment of nitric oxide synthase. *Results.* The left ovaries of the alpha-lipoic acid + coenzyme Q$_{10}$ group had significantly lower apoptosis scores and significantly higher nitric oxide synthase content than the left ovaries of the control groups. The alpha-lipoic acid + coenzyme Q$_{10}$ group had significantly higher glutathione peroxidase levels and serum malondialdehyde concentrations than the sham group. *Conclusions.* The combination of alpha-lipoic acid and coenzyme Q$_{10}$ has beneficial effects on oxidative stress induced by ischemia-reperfusion injury related to ovarian torsion.

1. Introduction

Ovarian torsion is defined as the total or partial rotation of the ovary, the fallopian tube, or both, around its vascular axis. This clinical situation is an emergency of pediatric surgery and gynecology as it causes abdominal pain which requires surgery. Therefore, detorsion of the ovary is surgically performed to maintain its proper circulation [1, 2].

Ovarian torsion and detorsion (T/D) induce ischemia-reperfusion injury which leads to the occurrence of morphological, histological, and biochemical alterations within the ovarian tissue. This is due to a pathological process, which is named ischemia-reperfusion injury. As the ischemic tissue receives an excessive supply of molecular oxygen during reperfusion, acute ischemic injury is worsened by the products of oxidative stress including free radicals and oxygen reactive species. These products cause lipid peroxidation which impairs the permeability of cell membranes and disrupts the integrity of cells [3–6].

Alpha-lipoic acid (ALA) is found naturally within the mitochondria. It is an essential cofactor for pyruvate dehydrogenase and alpha-ketoglutarate dehydrogenase. The coupling of ALA and its reduced form (dihydrolipoic acid) is described as the "ideal," "unique," and "universal antioxidant" [7]. It has been demonstrated that ALA protects various membrane systems from oxidative injury including neuronal membranes, erythrocyte membranes, and mitochondrial membranes [8–10]. The efficiency of ALA has been shown in diabetes mellitus, atherosclerosis, ischemia-reperfusion diseases, multiple sclerosis, cognitive losses, and senile dementia [11].

Coenzyme Q_{10} (CoQ_{10}) is a strong antioxidant which provides stabilization of cell membranes by participating in the mitochondrial electron transport chain. This molecule also acts as a cofactor in the synthesis of adenosine triphosphate (ATP) by oxidative phosphorylation. It has been shown that CoQ_{10} inhibits lipid peroxidation, scavenges free oxygen radicals, and increases the utilization of oxygen in energy production [12–14].

Free radicals which occur as a result of ischemia-reperfusion and oxidative stress affect the phospholipids on the cell membrane and they create phosphoryl choline and ceramide on the scale of neutral sphingomyelinase (n-SMase). Ceramide leads to caspase activation and activates apoptosis. CoQ_{10} decreases apoptosis by affecting both the creation of free radicals and n-SMase step. Likewise, alpha-lipoic acid prevents apoptosis both by sweeping free oxygen radicals as an antioxidant and by affecting the caspase system [15, 16].

The present study aims to evaluate whether ALA, CoQ_{10}, or the combination of both can be used to protect prepubertal ovarian tissue from ischemia-reperfusion injury in an experimental rat model of ovarian torsion.

2. Materials and Methods

This study was approved by the Ethical Committee of Afyon Kocatepe University for Animal Experiments (number: 59269667/281, date: 15.02.2013). The experiments in this study were performed in accordance with the guidelines for animal research.

2.1. Study Design. The rats that were included in the experiment had intact circadian rhythm and ad libitum feeding within their natural environment. Forty-two female preadolescent Wistar-Albino rats (mean age: 4 weeks, weight range: 40–45 g) were divided into 6 equal groups randomly.

All surgical operations were performed under intramuscular 50 mg/kg ketamine (Ketasol 10%, Richter Pharma AG, Wels, Austria) and 10 mg/kg xylazine (Alfazyne 2%, Alfasan International BV, Woerden, Netherlands) anesthesia. Rats were placed in the dorsal recumbent position. A 1.5 cm midline laparotomy incision was made under sterile conditions so that the abdomen was opened and the large intestines were separated gently. In order to visualize the left ovary, large intestines are placed on the left side of the rat's abdomen. After the left ovary was found, it was made to undergo torsion of 720 degrees clockwise and then fixated to the anterior abdominal wall with a single 5/0 prolene suture. Afterwards, the abdominal incision was repaired with continuous sutures. Rats were covered with gauze to be protected from hypothermia and they recovered from the effects of anesthesia in approximately 30 minutes. Medication was given orally with gavage after an hour postoperatively; detorsion was

performed at the 3rd hour and bilateral oophorectomy and blood samples were taken at the 9th hour postoperatively. The reason for choosing postoperative 9th hour for biochemical, histopathological, and immunohistochemical evaluation is based on pharmacokinetic properties of the molecules. When ALA is taken orally, it is rapidly absorbed and reaches plasma peak levels in 30 minutes to 1 hour [17]. In contrast, coenzyme Q_{10} reaches peak plasma levels in about 4–6 hours after its oral administration [18].

Group 1 (sham group) included 7 rats that had laparotomy without torsion. Group 2 (saline group) consisted of 7 rats that underwent T/D and received saline orally (Polifleks 0.9% NaCl, Eczacıbaşı-Baxter, Istanbul, Turkey). Group 3 (olive oil group) included 7 rats that had T/D and received olive oil orally (Taris, Izmir, Turkey). Group 4 (ALA group) consisted of 7 rats that underwent T/D and received ALA orally (100 μM/kg/day, ≥99% titration in olive oil, Sigma-Aldrich Chemie GmbH, Steinheim, Germany). Group 5 (CoQ_{10} group) included 7 rats that had T/D and received CoQ_{10} orally (10 mg/kg/day, ≥98% titration in olive oil, Sigma-Aldrich Chemie GmbH, Steinheim, Germany). Group 6 (ALA + CoQ_{10}) included 7 rats that underwent T/D and received both ALA and CoQ_{10} orally. As both ALA and CoQ_{10} were administered in olive oil solutions in the treatment groups, an olive oil group was included to rule out whether olive oil itself would exert antioxidant effects.

2.2. Biochemical Analysis for Oxidant-Antioxidant Status. Blood samples were collected into heparinized tubes and were examined in the biochemistry laboratory of the study center. Serum levels of oxidized/reduced glutathione (GSH) and malondialdehyde (MDA) concentrations were determined by high-performance liquid chromatograph (HPLC) in the isocratic phase in the Agilent 1100 series instrument with fluorescent detection (Ex:515, Em:553 nm for MDA; Ex:385, Em:515 for GSH) using a kit from Chromsystems Chemicals GmbH (glutathione kits, Chromsystems Chemicals, Munich, Germany; malondialdehyde kits, Chromsystems Chemicals, Munich, Germany). The results were evaluated as μmol/g hemoglobin for GSH and μmol/L hemoglobin for MDA.

Serum levels of glutathione peroxidase were determined using glutathione peroxidase kits (glutathione peroxidase assay kits, Cayman Chemicals, Ann Arbor, USA). ELISA microanalyzer was used for absorbance assays (ChemWell 2910, Awareness Technology Inc., Palm City, USA). The results were evaluated as U/g hemoglobin for glutathione peroxidase.

2.3. Histopathological Evaluation. Since the study was carried out on ovarian tissues of preadolescent rats, the pathologist was unable to evaluate the ovarian reserve based on the counts of primordial, preantral, and antral follicles. In order to specify the ovarian damage histopathologically, at least five microscopic sections were examined and semiquantitative scores were obtained. The presence of follicular cell degeneration, hyperemia, hemorrhage, and inflammation were used as the criteria for ovarian injury. Each specimen was scored using a scale ranging from 0 to 3 (0: none; 1: mild; 2: moderate;

3: severe) [19]. The ovarian sections were analyzed by the same pathologist who was blinded to experiment groups.

2.4. TUNEL Assay for Apoptosis. Paraffin blocks were prepared for histopathological examination and 5 μm sections from these blocks were transferred to positive charged slides for TUNEL assay. Nuclease-free proteinase K (0.6 units/mL, pH 8.0) incubation was applied (in 37°C oven, for 10 minutes) for antigen retrieval. After washing with PBS, 10-minute 3% hydrogen peroxide application was made at room temperature for blocking of endogenous peroxidase activities. Sections were transferred into humidity chamber and a commercial apoptosis kit (In Situ Cell Death Detection Kit, POD (cat. number 1 684 817), Roche Diagnostics GmbH, Mannheim, Germany) was applied according to the manufacturer's procedure: slides are incubated in TUNEL mixture for 1 hour at 37°C and then they are incubated for 30 minutes in converter pod at 37°C. All slides were stained with AEC chromogen. For counterstain, Mayer's hematoxylin staining was performed. After each step, sections were washed with PBS. The immunoreactivity for apoptosis was graded from 0 to 4 with a light microscope in terms of density and distribution of staining: (0) no positivity on stroma and follicles, (1) mild positivity only in follicles, (2) moderate positivity in follicles and slight positivity in stroma, (3) moderate positivity in follicles and stroma, and (4) severe positivity in follicles and stroma.

2.5. Immunohistochemical Assay for Nitric Oxide Synthase (NOS). Streptavidin-biotin-peroxidase complex (VECTAS-TAIN Elite ABC Kit PK-6101, Vector Laboratories, Peterborough, UK) method was used. Briefly, 5 μm tissue sections were mounted on positive charged slides from paraffin blocks. Deparaffinized and rehydrated sections were transferred into 3% hydrogen peroxide for blocking endogenous peroxides and then antigen retrieving processes were carried out. Nonspecific immunoglobulins were blocked with nonimmune sera. Antibodies against NOS (C-terminal-polyclonal 1/40 dilution (ab15203), Abcam, Cambridge, UK) were applied to the sections. Then, biotinylated secondary antibody and streptavidin-peroxidase were dropped on the tissue sections. After this process, sections were visualized with 3-amino-9-ethylcarbazole chromogen (AEC substrate kit (code number 00-2007), Invitrogen, Basel, Switzerland). The immunoreactivity for NOS was graded from 0 to 4 with a light microscope in terms of density and distribution of staining: (0) no positivity in stroma and follicles, (1) mild positivity in follicles, (2) moderate positivity in follicles and slight positivity in stroma, (3) moderate positivity in follicles and stroma, and (4) severe positivity in follicles and stroma.

2.6. Statistical Analysis. Collected data were analyzed by MedCalc (version 12.7.5.0, Ghent, Belgium). Continuous variables were expressed as mean $\pm$ standard deviation (range: minimum–maximum) whereas categorical variables were denoted as mean rank. Kruskal-Wallis test and Mann-Whitney U test were used for the comparisons. Conover-Inman post hoc test was used to determine the groups

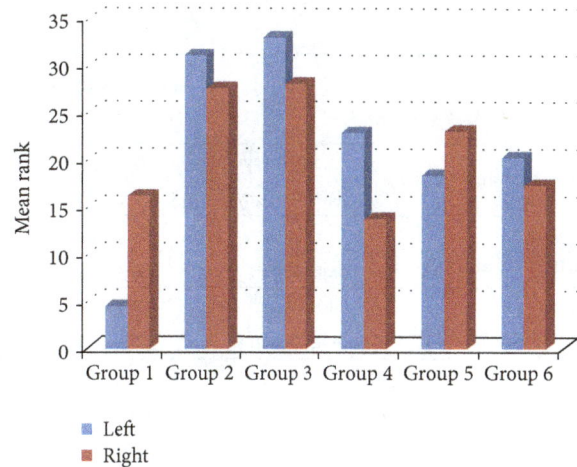

FIGURE 1: Mean rank of apoptosis.

between which statistical significance exists. Two-tailed P values less than 0.05 were accepted to be statistically significant.

3. Results

Table 1 compares the pathological scoring of the sham, control, and study groups (Table 1). When compared to the right ovaries, the left ovaries had significantly higher apoptosis scores in the saline, olive oil, ALA, CoQ$_{10}$, and ALA + CoQ$_{10}$ groups ($P = 0.003$, $P = 0.002$, $P = 0.001$, $P = 0.002$, and $P = 0.008$, resp.). The right ovaries of the sham, control, and study groups were statistically similar in aspect of apoptosis scores ($P = 0.07$). The left ovaries of the ALA + CoQ$_{10}$ group had significantly lower apoptosis scores than the left ovaries of the saline and olive oil groups ($P = 0.001$ for both) (Figures 1 and 2). The ALA, CoQ$_{10}$, and ALA + CoQ$_{10}$ groups had statistically similar apoptosis scores ($P_{4-5} = 0.430$, $P_{4-6} = 0.556$, and $P_{5-6} = 0.612$).

The right and left ovaries had statistically similar NOS level in the sham, control, and study groups ($P = 0.530$, $P = 0.644$, $P = 0.367$, $P = 0.709$, $P = 0.947$, and $P = 0.578$, resp.). The right ovaries of the ALA + CoQ$_{10}$ group had significantly higher NOS content than the right ovaries of the saline and olive oil groups ($P = 0.001$ for both). The left ovaries of the ALA + CoQ$_{10}$ group had significantly higher NOS content than the left ovaries of the saline and olive oil groups ($P = 0.001$ for both) (Figures 3 and 4). The ALA, CoQ$_{10}$, and ALA + CoQ$_{10}$ groups had statistically similar NOS content but NOS content of the ALA + CoQ$_{10}$ group tended to be higher than those of the ALA and CoQ$_{10}$ groups ($P_{4-5} = 0.126$, $P_{4-6} = 0.248$, and $P_{5-6} = 0.378$).

When compared with the left ovaries of the saline and olive oil groups, the left ovaries of the ALA, CoQ$_{10}$, and ALA + CoQ$_{10}$ groups had significantly lower ovarian damage scores ($P = 0.03$). However, there were no statistically significant differences among the study groups ($P_{4-5} = 0.1$, $P_{4-6} = 1.00$, and $P_{5-6} = 0.1$) (Figure 5). The right and left ovaries of the sham group were statistically similar whereas the left

TABLE 1: Pathological scoring of all groups.

		Apoptosis score Mean ± std. deviation	P	Nitric oxide synthase Mean ± std. deviation	P	Histopathological evaluation Mean ± std. deviation	P
Group 1 (sham) ($n = 7$)	Left ovary	1.0 ± 0.0	0.259	0.2 ± 0.1	0.530	0.0 ± 0.0	1.00
	Right ovary	0.7 ± 0.2		0.3 ± 0.1		0.0 ± 0.0	
Group 2 Control (saline) ($n = 7$)	Left ovary	3.8 ± 0.9	0.003*	1.3 ± 0.6	0.644	2.7 ± 0.48	0.001*
	Right ovary	3.6 ± 0.7		1.7 ± 0.8		0.71 ± 0.48	
Group 3 Control (olive oil) ($n = 7$)	Left ovary	3.7 ± 0.5	0.002*	1.7 ± 0.5	0.367	2.8 ± 0.37	0.001*
	Right ovary	3.6 ± 0.7		2.0 ± 0.6		0.85 ± 0.69	
Group 4 (ALA) ($n = 7$)	Left ovary	2.7 ± 1.1	0.001*	2.3 ± 1.1	0.709	1.7 ± 0.48	0.005*
	Right ovary	0.6 ± 0.1		2.4 ± 1.3		0.57 ± 0.53	
Group 5 (CoQ_{10}) ($n = 7$)	Left ovary	2.6 ± 1.4	0.002*	2.4 ± 1.2	0.947	1.7 ± 0.75	0.015*
	Right ovary	1.1 ± 0.3		2.1 ± 0.9		0.7 ± 0.48	
Group 6 (ALA + CoQ_{10}) ($n = 7$)	Left ovary	2.5 ± 1.3	0.008*	2.6 ± 1.4	0.578	1.7 ± 0.48	0.014*
	Right ovary	0.9 ± 0.1		2.6 ± 1.5		0.57 ± 0.78	

*$P < 0.05$ was accepted to be statistically significant.

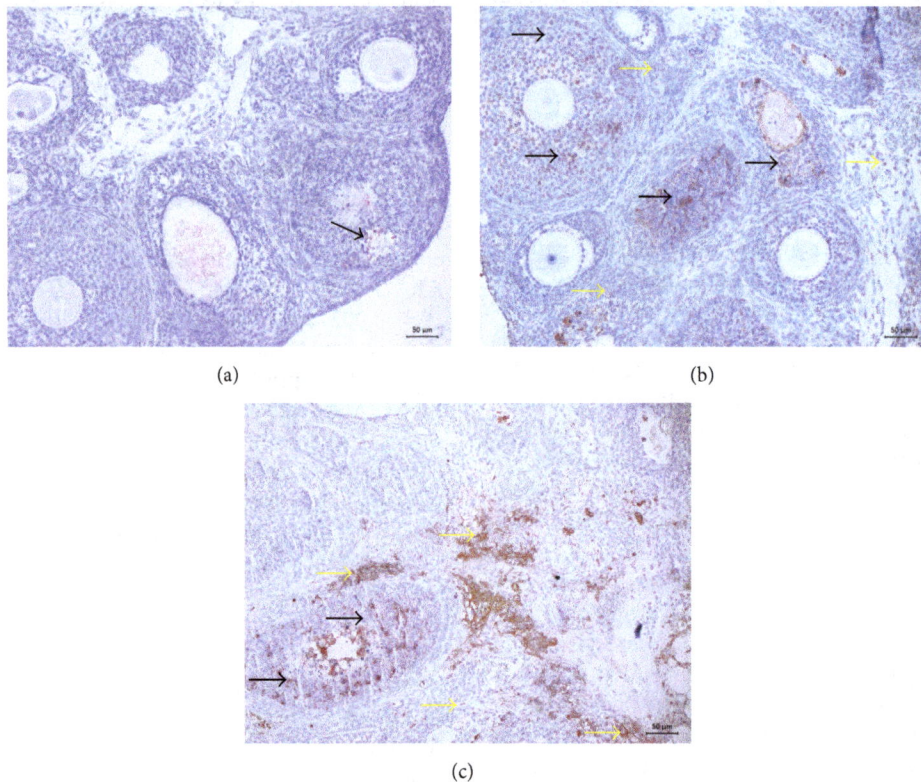

(a)

(b)

(c)

FIGURE 2: Slight TUNEL positivity in follicular cells (arrow) in group 1 (a). Moderate TUNEL positivity in follicular cells (arrows) and slight positivity in stroma (yellow arrows) in group 6 (b). Severe TUNEL positivity in follicular cells (arrows) and stroma (yellow arrows) in group 2 (c). ×50. TUNEL method. AEC chromogen. Gill's (I) Hematoxylin.

ovaries of the remaining groups had significantly higher tissue damage scores than those of the contralateral ovaries (P values are enlisted in Table 1).

The biochemical assessments of the oxidant-antioxidant statuses of the sham, control, and study groups were compared (Figure 6). All six groups were statistically similar with respect to serum glutathione concentrations ($P = 0.069$). When compared with the sham group, the ALA + CoQ_{10} group had significantly higher glutathione peroxidase levels and serum malondialdehyde concentrations ($P = 0.007$ and $P = 0.027$, resp.). There were no statistically significant differences between the glutathione peroxidase levels of the control

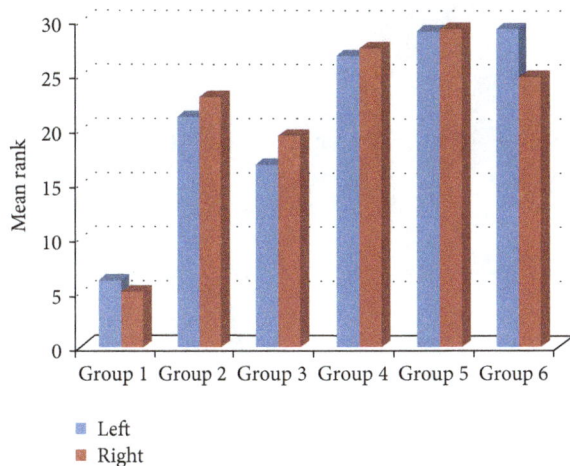

FIGURE 3: Mean rank of NOS immunoreactivity.

groups (groups 2 and 3) and the ALA, CoQ_{10}, and ALA + CoQ_{10} groups ($P_{2-4} = 0.687$, $P_{2-5} = 0.360$, $P_{2-6} = 0.117$, $P_{3-4} = 0.402$, $P_{3-5} = 0.576$, and $P_{3-6} = 0.802$; $P_{4-5} = 0.609$, $P_{4-6} = 0.276$, and $P_{5-6} = 0.564$). There were no statistically significant differences between serum malondialdehyde concentrations of the control groups (groups 2 and 3) and the ALA, CoQ_{10}, and ALA + CoQ_{10} groups but malondialdehyde levels of the ALA + CoQ_{10} group tended to be lower than those of the ALA and CoQ_{10} groups ($P_{2-4} = 0.446$, $P_{2-5} = 0.420$, $P_{2-6} = 0.067$, $P_{3-4} = 0.372$, $P_{3-5} = 0.349$, and $P_{3-6} = 0.050$; $P_{4-5} = 0.965$, $P_{4-6} = 0.286$, and $P_{5-6} = 0.306$). When compared with the control group, the ALA + CoQ10 group had lower serum malondialdehyde concentrations ($P = 0.05$).

4. Discussion

Ischemia refers to the decrease in blood supply of an organ which results in the breakdown of ATP and lipid peroxides so that the generation of lactic acid and hypoxanthine is enhanced. As blood supply normalizes during reperfusion, xanthine oxidase converts hypoxanthine to uric and superoxide radicals. These radicals consist of hydrogen peroxide, hydroxyl radicals, and superoxide anions. Superoxide radicals cause lipid peroxidation, which impairs the permeability of cell membranes, disrupt cellular integrity, and, thus, lead to cell damage. The production of nitric oxide and peroxynitrite is also accelerated in case of reperfusion followed by ischemia [20–23]. In this study, the apoptosis scores of the left ovaries were significantly lower than those of the right ovaries in the saline, olive oil, ALA, CoQ_{10}, and ALA + CoQ_{10} groups. This finding indicates that a model of ischemia-reperfusion has been established successfully in all of the control and study groups.

ALA has been addressed as an efficient glutathione substitute which can increase cellular glutathione content and improve the antioxidant status of the myocardium [24]. It has been also reported that ALA protects against hepatic ischemia-reperfusion injury in rats [25]. The administration of ALA before the torsion of spermatic cord exerted significant protective effects against ischemia-reperfusion

injury [26]. These protective effects may be attributed to the reduction of lipid peroxidation and the reinforcement of antioxidant defense mechanisms including glutathione and glutathione peroxidase [24–26].

A number of studies have focused on the utilization of CoQ_{10} for the prevention and treatment of ischemia-reperfusion injury in many organs. Kalayci et al. made up a model of brain ischemia-reperfusion injury and found that malondialdehyde levels were significantly reduced in rats that received a single dose of 10 mg/kg CoQ_{10} intraperitoneally [14]. Erol et al. concluded that CoQ_{10} treatment was able to decrease malondialdehyde levels in an experimental model of testicular ischemia-reperfusion injury [13]. Similarly, Ozler et al. reported that an intraperitoneal injection of CoQ_{10} could decrease oxidative stress markers significantly in a rat model of ovarian ischemia-reperfusion injury [19].

As for the present study, the administration of ALA or CoQ_{10} via oral route resulted in a decrease in apoptosis scores and an increase in NOS content of the ovaries that underwent torsion and subsequent detorsion. The NOS make up a group of enzymes that catalyze the production of nitric oxide from L-arginine. Nitric oxide is an important cellular signaling molecule that modulates the protection against oxidative damage. The increase in NOS content of the ovaries treated with ALA + CoQ_{10} indicates the antioxidant activity of the aforementioned molecules [27, 28].

In addition, ALA treatment caused an increase in serum glutathione peroxidase levels and a decrease in serum malondialdehyde concentrations. However, these alterations were not statistically significant. Such discrepancy may be the result of relatively smaller cohort size, oral route of administration for antioxidant molecules, relatively shorter follow-up period after surgery, and relatively insufficient dose of ALA administration. Oral route was preferred for the administration of antioxidant molecules because the availability and utility of these agents in clinical settings were a concern of this study. The other power-limiting factors were the inability to measure the tissue concentrations of oxidant and antioxidant molecules and the failure in specifying ovarian contents of endothelial and inducible NOS separately. These failures might be attributed to the relatively small size of prepubertal ovarian tissues.

The findings of the present study indicate a cumulative increase in NOS and a cumulative decrease in malondialdehyde levels for the combination of ALA and CoQ_{10}. Yet, these alterations have been regarded as statistically insignificant. These findings imply that the combination of ALA and CoQ_{10} could improve ATP synthesis and reverse some of the cell damage caused by the reduction of energy availability. Moreover, this combination would extinguish the hazardous effects of oxidative stress which are primarily induced by the impairment of respiratory chain. An underlying factor for this synergetic effect might be that the combination treatment could diminish one or more of the final common pathways of mitochondrial dysfunction so that mitochondrial ATP production is improved [29, 30]. Another explanation may be the fact that the combination of two antioxidant agents would be more effective than an individual antioxidant agent because different antioxidants complement each other. Thus,

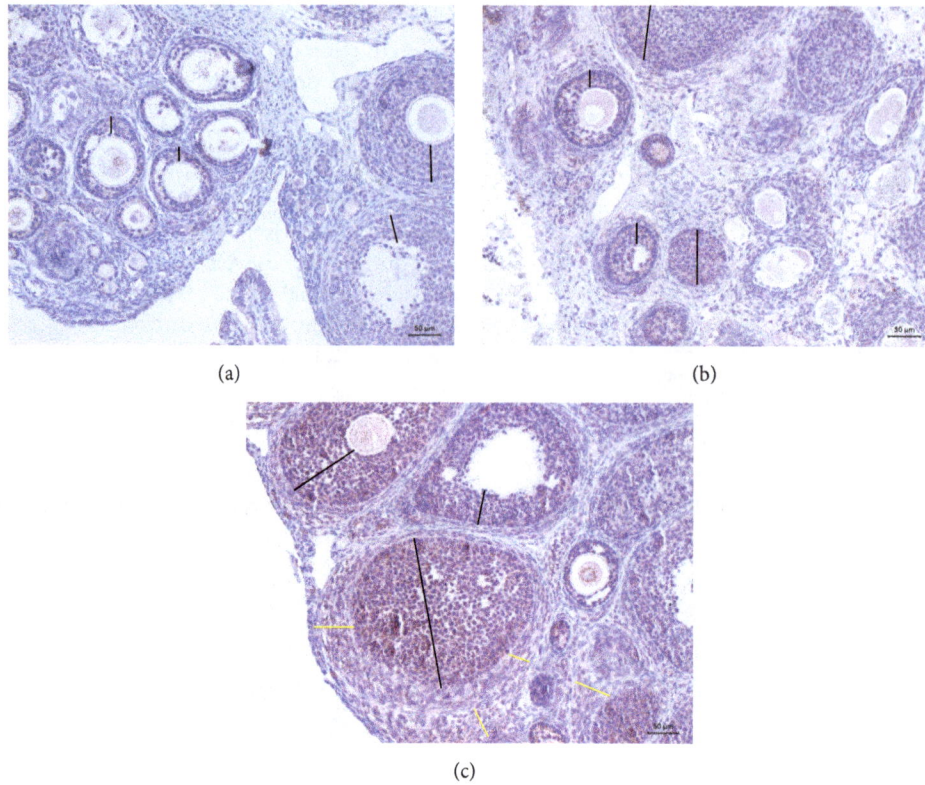

FIGURE 4: Slight NOS positivity in follicular cells (lines) (a). Moderate NOS positivity in follicular cells in group 3 (lines) (b). Severe NOS positivity in follicular cells (lines) and stroma (yellow lines) in group 6 (c). ×50. ABC peroxidase. AEC chromogen. Gill's (I) Hematoxylin.

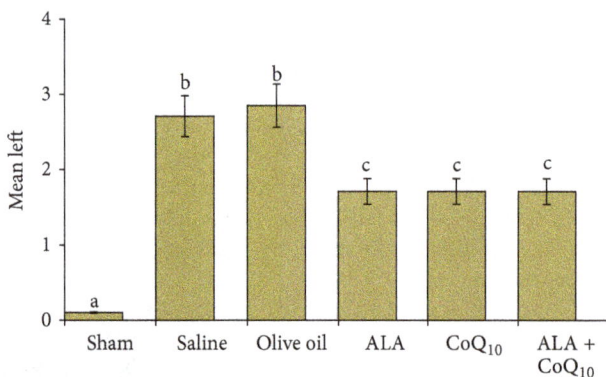

FIGURE 5: When compared with the left ovaries of the saline and olive oil groups, the left ovaries of the alpha-lipoic acid, coenzyme Q_{10}, and alpha-lipoic acid + coenzyme Q_{10} groups had significantly lower ovarian damage scores ($P = 0.03$). The same letters indicated that the difference was statistically insignificant but different letters showed that there was statistical significance between the groups.

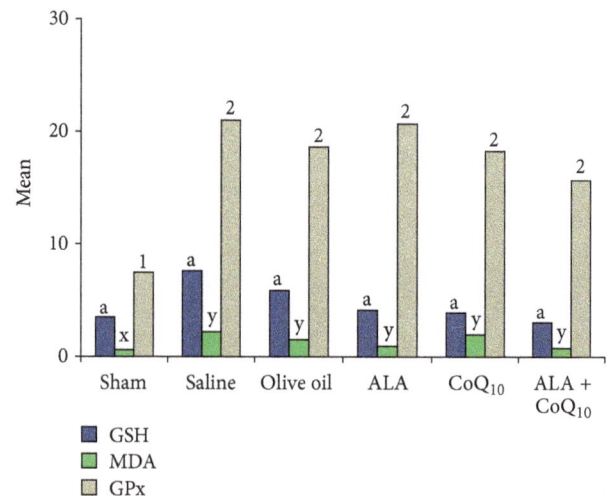

FIGURE 6: When compared with the sham group, the alpha-lipoic acid + coenzyme Q_{10} group had significantly higher glutathione peroxidase levels and serum malondialdehyde concentrations ($P = 0.007$ and $P = 0.027$, resp.). When compared with the control group, the alpha-lipoic acid + coenzyme Q_{10} group had lower serum malondialdehyde concentrations ($P = 0.05$). The same letters indicated that the difference was statistically insignificant but different letters showed that there was statistical significance between groups ("a" for glutathione; "1, 2" for malondialdehyde; and "x, y" for glutathione peroxidase).

there would be an increase in the total antioxidant capacity that is required to respond to the outburst of free radicals and reactive oxygen species [31].

Although the left ovaries have undergone torsion and subsequent detorsion in this study, the NOS content of the right ovary in the ALA + CoQ_{10} group has been found to be significantly higher. This finding can be explained by the reduction in blood supply of the right ovary. This reduction is caused by the vasoconstriction which is induced by the increase in the sympathetic activity after the torsion/detorsion procedure. On the other hand, no significant differences could be detected among the study groups in aspect of apoptosis. This failure could be due to the relatively small cohort size and the differences in the pathological examination techniques [32].

5. Conclusion

The findings of this study imply that the combination of ALA and CoQ_{10} has beneficial effects on oxidative stress induced by ischemia-reperfusion injury in an experimental model of ovarian torsion. These beneficial effects appear to be more pronounced within the ovarian tissue but less prominent in peripheral circulation. This finding may be due to the relatively shorter follow-up period after the administration of ALA or CoQ_{10}.

Further research is warranted to clarify the effects of ALA and CoQ_{10} on the prepubertal ovarian tissues which have been exposed to ischemia-reperfusion injury.

Competing Interests

The authors report no competing interests.

Acknowledgments

The authors declare that this study has received financial support from the Scientific Research Project Coordination Unit of Afyon Kocatepe University (12.TUS.03).

References

[1] A. S. Laganà, V. Sofo, F. M. Salmeri et al., "Oxidative stress during ovarian torsion in pediatric and adolescent patients: changing the perspective of the disease," *International Journal of Fertility and Sterility*, vol. 9, no. 4, pp. 416–423, 2015.

[2] C. Rey-Bellet Gasser, M. Gehri, J.-M. Joseph, and J.-Y. Pauchard, "Is it ovarian torsion? A systematic literature review and evaluation of prediction signs," *Pediatric Emergency Care*, vol. 32, pp. 256–261, 2016.

[3] S. Yaman Tunc, E. Agacayak, N. Y. Goruk et al., "Protective effects of honokiol on ischemia/reperfusion injury of rat ovary: An Experimental Study," *Drug Design, Development and Therapy*, vol. 10, pp. 1077–1083, 2016.

[4] I. Sayar, S. Bicer, C. Gursul, M. Gürbüzel, K. Peker, and A. Işik, "Protective effects of ellagic acid and ozone on rat ovaries with an ischemia/reperfusion injury," *Journal of Obstetrics and Gynaecology Research*, vol. 42, no. 1, pp. 52–58, 2016.

[5] M. S. Bostanci, M. Bakacak, F. Inanc et al., "The protective effect of G-CSF on experimental ischemia/reperfusion injury in rat ovary," *Archives of Gynecology and Obstetrics*, vol. 293, no. 4, pp. 789–795, 2016.

[6] Ü. M. Ural, Y. B. Tekin, I. Sehitoglu, Y. Kalkan, and M. C. Cüre, "Biochemical, histopathological and immunohistochemical evaluation of the protective and therapeutic effects of thymoquinone against ischemia and ischemia/reperfusion injury in the rat ovary," *Gynecologic and Obstetric Investigation*, vol. 81, no. 1, pp. 47–53, 2016.

[7] S. Ghibu, B. Lauzier, S. Delemasure et al., "Antioxidant properties of alpha-lipoic acid: effects on red blood membrane permeability and adaptation of isolated rat heart to reversible ischemia," *Molecular and Cellular Biochemistry*, vol. 320, no. 1-2, pp. 141–148, 2009.

[8] T. Yang, Z. Xu, W. Liu, B. Xu, and Y. Deng, "Protective effects of alpha-lipoic acid on MeHg-induced oxidative damage and intracellular Ca^{2+} dyshomeostasis in primary cultured neurons," *Free Radical Research*, vol. 50, no. 5, pp. 542–556, 2016.

[9] S. Hwang, J. W. Byun, J. S. Yoon, and E. J. Lee, "Inhibitory effects of α-lipoic acid on oxidative stress-induced adipogenesis in orbital fibroblasts from patients with graves ophthalmopathy," *Medicine*, vol. 95, no. 2, Article ID e2497, 2016.

[10] S. Zavareh, I. Karimi, M. Salehnia, and A. Rahnama, "Effect of in vitro maturation technique and alpha lipoic acid supplementation on oocyte maturation rate: focus on oxidative status of oocytes," *International Journal of Fertility and Sterility*, vol. 9, no. 4, pp. 442–451, 2015.

[11] J. M. May, Z.-C. Qu, and S. Mendiratta, "Protection and recycling of α-tocopherol in human erythrocytes by intracellular ascorbic acid," *Archives of Biochemistry and Biophysics*, vol. 349, no. 2, pp. 281–289, 1998.

[12] G. Lenaz, R. Fato, G. Formiggini, and M. L. Genova, "The role of Coenzyme Q in mitochondrial electron transport," *Mitochondrion*, vol. 7, pp. S8–S33, 2007.

[13] B. Erol, M. Bozlu, V. Hanci, H. Tokgoz, S. Bektas, and G. Mungan, "Coenzyme Q10 treatment reduces lipid peroxidation, inducible and endothelial nitric oxide synthases, and germ cell-specific apoptosis in a rat model of testicular ischemia/reperfusion injury," *Fertility and Sterility*, vol. 93, no. 1, pp. 280–282, 2010.

[14] M. Kalayci, M. M. Unal, S. Gul et al., "Effect of coenzyme Q10 on ischemia and neuronal damage in an experimental traumatic brain-injury model in rats," *BMC Neuroscience*, vol. 12, article 75, 2011.

[15] P. Navas, J. M. Villalba, and R. Cabo, "The importance of plasma membrane coenzyme Q in aging and stress responses," *Mitochondrion*, vol. 7, pp. 34–40, 2007.

[16] J. Moungjaroen, U. Nimmannit, P. S. Callery et al., "Reactive oxygen species mediate caspase activation and apoptosis induced by lipoic acid in human lung epithelial cancer cells through Bcl-2 down-regulation," *Journal of Pharmacology and Experimental Therapeutics*, vol. 319, no. 3, pp. 1062–1069, 2006.

[17] R. Hermann, J. Mungo, P. J. Cnota, and D. Ziegler, "Enantiomer-selective pharmacokinetics, oral bioavailability, and sex effects of various alpha-lipoic acid dosage forms," *Clinical Pharmacology: Advances and Applications*, vol. 6, pp. 195–204, 2014.

[18] J. Garrido-Maraver, M. D. Cordero, M. Oropesa-Ávila et al., "Coenzyme Q10 therapy," *Molecular Syndromology*, vol. 5, no. 3-4, pp. 187–197, 2014.

[19] A. Ozler, A. Turgut, N. Y. Görük, U. Alabalik, M. K. Basarali, and F. Akdemir, "Evaluation of the protective effects of CoQ_{10} on ovarian I/R injury: an experimental study," *Gynecologic and Obstetric Investigation*, vol. 76, no. 2, pp. 100–106, 2013.

[20] S. Somuncu, M. Cakmak, G. Dikmen, H. Akman, and M. Kaya, "Ischemia-reperfusion injury of rabbit ovary and protective effect of trapidil: an experimental study," *Pediatric Surgery International*, vol. 24, no. 3, pp. 315–318, 2008.

[21] Y. Ergun, A. Koc, K. Dolapcioglu et al., "The protective effect of erythropoietin and dimethylsulfoxide on ischemia-reperfusion injury in rat ovary," *European Journal of Obstetrics Gynecology and Reproductive Biology*, vol. 152, no. 2, pp. 186–190, 2010.

[22] A. Oral, F. Odabasoglu, Z. Halici et al., "Protective effects of montelukast on ischemia-reperfusion injury in rat ovaries subjected to torsion and detorsion: biochemical and histopathologic evaluation," *Fertility and Sterility*, vol. 95, no. 4, pp. 1360–1366, 2011.

[23] M. A. Osmanağaoğlu, M. Kesim, E. Yuluğ, A. Menteşe, and S. C. Karahan, "Ovarian-protective effects of clotrimazole on ovarian Ischemia/reperfusion injury in a rat ovarian-torsion model," *Gynecologic and Obstetric Investigation*, vol. 74, no. 2, pp. 125–130, 2012.

[24] S. Ghibu, C. Richard, C. Vergely, M. Zeller, Y. Cottin, and L. Rochette, "Antioxidant properties of an endogenous thiol: alpha-lipoic acid, useful in the prevention of cardiovascular diseases," *Journal of Cardiovascular Pharmacology*, vol. 54, no. 5, pp. 391–398, 2009.

[25] E. Dulundu, Y. Ozel, U. Topaloglu et al., "Alpha-lipoic acid protects against hepatic ischemia-reperfusion injury in rats," *Pharmacology*, vol. 79, no. 3, pp. 163–170, 2007.

[26] S. B. Guimarães, J. M. V. Santos, A. A. Aragão, O. de Sandes Kimura, P. H. U. Barbosa, and P. R. L. de Vasconcelos, "Protective effect of α-lipoic acid in experimental spermatic cord torsion," *Nutrition*, vol. 23, no. 1, pp. 76–80, 2007.

[27] K. L. Chan, "Role of nitric oxide in ischemia and reperfusion injury," *Current Medicinal Chemistry—Anti-Inflammatory & Anti Allergy Agents*, vol. 1, no. 1, pp. 1–13, 2002.

[28] R. Schulz, M. Kelm, and G. Heusch, "Nitric oxide in myocardial ischemia/reperfusion injury," *Cardiovascular Research*, vol. 61, no. 3, pp. 402–413, 2004.

[29] M. C. Rodriguez, J. R. MacDonald, D. J. Mahoney, G. Parise, M. F. Beal, and M. A. Tarnopolsky, "Beneficial effects of creatine, CoQ10, and lipoic acid in mitochondrial disorders," *Muscle and Nerve*, vol. 35, no. 2, pp. 235–242, 2007.

[30] S. K. Jain and G. Lim, "Lipoic acid decreases lipid peroxidation and protein glycosylation and increases ($Na^+ + K^+$)- and Ca^{++}-ATPase activities in high glucose-treated human erythrocytes," *Free Radical Biology and Medicine*, vol. 29, no. 11, pp. 1122–1128, 2000.

[31] M. Valko, C. J. Rhodes, J. Moncol, M. Izakovic, and M. Mazur, "Free radicals, metals and antioxidants in oxidative stress-induced cancer," *Chemico-Biological Interactions*, vol. 160, no. 1, pp. 1–40, 2006.

[32] M. Cakmak, M. Kaya, M. Barlas et al., "Histologic and ultrastructural changes in the contralateral ovary in unilateral ovarian torsion: an experimental study in rabbits," *Tokai Journal of Experimental and Clinical Medicine*, vol. 18, no. 3–6, pp. 167–178, 1993.

6

Percutaneous Septal Ablation in Hypertrophic Obstructive Cardiomyopathy: From Experiment to Standard of Care

Lothar Faber

Department of Cardiology, Heart and Diabetes Center North Rhine-Westphalia, University Hospital of the Ruhr University Bochum, Georgstraße 11, 32545 Bad Oeynhausen, Germany

Correspondence should be addressed to Lothar Faber; lfaber@hdz-nrw.de

Academic Editor: Jesus Peteiro

Hypertrophic cardiomyopathy (HCM) is one of the more common hereditary cardiac conditions. According to presence or absence of outflow obstruction at rest or with provocation, a more common (about 60–70%) obstructive type of the disease (HOCM) has to be distinguished from the less common (30–40%) nonobstructive phenotype (HNCM). Symptoms include exercise limitation due to dyspnea, angina pectoris, palpitations, or dizziness; occasionally syncope or sudden cardiac death occurs. Correct diagnosis and risk stratification with respect to prophylactic ICD implantation are essential in HCM patient management. Drug therapy in symptomatic patients can be characterized as treatment of heart failure with preserved ejection fraction (HFpEF) in HNCM, while symptoms and the obstructive gradient in HOCM can be addressed with beta-blockers, disopyramide, or verapamil. After a short overview on etiology, natural history, and diagnostics in hypertrophic cardiomyopathy, this paper reviews the current treatment options for HOCM with a special focus on percutaneous septal ablation. Literature data and the own series of about 600 cases are discussed, suggesting a largely comparable outcome with respect to procedural mortality, clinical efficacy, and long-term outcome.

1. Etiology, Pathogenesis, and Pathophysiology of HCM

Hypertrophic cardiomyopathy (HCM [1–70]) is a cardiac condition morphologically characterized by unexplained myocardial hypertrophy. Extent and distribution of wall thickening are highly variable; the interventricular septum is most often involved, while the right ventricle is rarely affected. The prevalence of the disease is considered to be around 0.2%; in >50% of patients HCM has a familiar background [3, 6–8]. Inheritance shows an autosomal-dominant pattern, with an incomplete and highly variable penetrance. Mutations have been found in >2 dozens of genes coding for sarcomeric proteins or those involved in myocardial energy metabolism; the condition therefore has been characterized as a "sarcomeric disease" [42–48]. Histologically, the prominent findings in HCM are myocardial disarray, hypertrophy, and fibrosis [49–59]. Not only the myocardial walls but also the coronary vasculature walls are often thickened which may decrease coronary reserve and lead to myocardial ischemia in the absence of occlusive atherosclerosis. In addition, myocardial bridging is a rather frequent finding, and mitral valve leaflets may be elongated [13–15].

Left ventricular systolic function as expressed by the ejection fraction is normal in the vast majority of patients, although modern imaging techniques frequently show impaired longitudinal systolic deformation of the affected myocardium. In addition, fibrosis and hypertrophy lead to increased myocardial stiffness and impairment of diastolic left ventricular function early in the disease process [5, 6, 8, 31, 32, 54–57]. Elevated filling pressures and a reduced stroke volume with stress may thus be present as in other entities characterized as "heart failure with preserved ejection fraction" (HfpEF), and left atrial dilatation is a typical morphological finding in HCM patients. A late stage of the disease with a dilated left ventricle and reduced ejection fraction may be observed in up to 5% of cases.

Independent from the functional limitation, a wide spectrum of supraventricular and ventricular arrhythmias may occur at every stage during the disease course. Again, fibrosis and disarray play an important role as the arrhythmogenic substrate; myocardial ischemia due to hypertrophy and thickened vessel walls may be an additional trigger [6, 8, 51, 58, 59]. Sudden cardiac death is a feared complication of the disease and sometimes its first manifestation. Among young (<35 years) athletes dying suddenly, HCM (usually the nonobstructive phenotype) is considered to be responsible for about 30%. The dissociation between morphology, functional status, and arrhythmogenic risk is a major problem of HCM management. Sudden cardiac death, often occurring during or after strenuous exercise, is more common in younger and previously asymptomatic patients. Stroke and heart failure related death seems to prevail in elderly cohorts.

An important distinction in HCM is between the nonobstructive (hypertrophic nonobstructive cardiomyopathy: HNCM) and the obstructive (HOCM) phenotype of the disease (Figure 1). Dependent on the distribution of hypertrophy within the left ventricle, the septal curvature, the size and configuration of the mitral valve, and left ventricular loading conditions, about 60–70% of HCM patients develop a dynamic obstruction between a "high-pressure" and a "low-pressure" compartment of the left ventricle [2–6, 8, 9, 19, 33–35]. Typically this obstruction is located between the subaortic septum and parts of the mitral valve ("SAM" phenomenon: systolic anterior movement) and is associated with mitral regurgitation. SAM-associated mitral regurgitation shows a typical posterolateral jet direction that can be used for differentiation towards primary mitral regurgitation (Figure 2). In a minority of cases outflow obstruction may be located in the midcavity region, in the apex, or occasionally in the right ventricular outflow tract. The hemodynamic significance of obstruction seems to depend on the size of the LV compartment that is working against increased afterload; apical gradients are considered to be less significant. A substantial degree of variability has been described regarding gradient severity, and provocation (by physical exercise, preload reduction, inotropic agents, or postextrasystolic augmentation) is essential to distinguish between HNCM and HOCM both during echocardiographic and invasive hemodynamic studies [6, 8, 19].

2. Symptoms, Clinical Workup, and Natural History in HCM

Typical symptoms in HCM patients are dyspnea, angina, or dizziness on exertion. A marked day-to-day variability is typical for the disease. Palpitations or syncope occurring both with and without exercise are reported by 20–30% of patients. Recurrent syncope and a family history of sudden cardiac death (at <45 years) have to be actively asked for because these features are considered risk factors [20] for sudden arrhythmogenic death. On the other hand, a severe HCM phenotype on imaging studies does not necessarily preclude normal exercise capacity or even athletic performance.

Cardiac auscultation is usually normal in patients with HNCM. The characteristic auscultatory finding in HOCM is the variable systolic murmur which accentuates with preload

reduction (e.g., with a Valsalva maneuver) and which diminishes with increase of afterload (e.g., with squatting). All types of ECG changes may be present; the typical ECG changes in HNCM are "giant negative T waves" and "pseudoinfarction Q waves" in HOCM. ECG changes may precede the phenotype on imaging studies by decades. Holter monitoring should be performed for risk stratification in every HCM patient since the finding of nonsustained VT's is another risk marker. Stress testing is useful to objectively measure the degree of functional limitation and to check the blood pressure response to exercise which is considered another risk factor for sudden cardiac death (see below).

The diagnosis of HCM can usually be made by noninvasive imaging techniques (echocardiography with its different modalities, cardiac magnetic resonance imaging, and multislice computed tomography). A multimodal approach is useful in many patients since the full extent of wall thickening is sometimes missed by 2-dimensional echocardiography, and cardiac magnetic resonance imaging with contrast enhancement allows for additional assessment of fibrosis. The degree and the distribution of hypertrophy are highly variable, ranging from isolated thickening of individual myocardial segments that merely exceed the normal LV wall thickness of <12 mm up to diffuse and massive hypertrophy of >50 mm. A wall thickness of >30 mm has to be actively looked for since this is the fifth risk factor for sudden cardiac death [6, 8, 17, 20].

Invasive studies are needed to exclude coexistent coronary artery disease, to visualize the anatomy of the septal perforator arteries if septal ablation is considered, and to perform endomyocardial biopsy if a myocardial storage disease is suspected. The level of suspicion for such a storage disease should be high in presence of a low-voltage ECG. A prevalence of storage diseases of up to 10% has been reported in "HCM" series [6, 8]. Diastolic LV performance and the outflow gradients can also be assessed invasively. The role of invasive electrophysiology studies for risk stratification is uncertain.

Natural history in HCM is highly variable [5, 6, 8, 28, 37–41]. In most cases the diagnosis is made during adolescence until early adulthood, and symptoms are slowly progressive. Disease manifestation in childhood is considered prognostically ominous. Late manifestation, however, is typical in carriers of the myosin-binding protein C mutation. Prognosis is determined by arrhythmic events in younger patients, typically independent of symptoms in this group, and by cardiac failure and stroke in elderly patients. In nonselected cohorts, the annual mortality rate is reported to be around 1%/year; in high-risk group this figure rises up to 5-6% [6, 8, 19].

3. Therapeutic Considerations for HOCM: Risk Management, Medical Therapy, Pacemakers, and Surgery

Whether or not obstruction or symptoms are present, HCM patients should not engage in competitive sports [6, 8, 71]. A limitation with respect to moderate physical activities

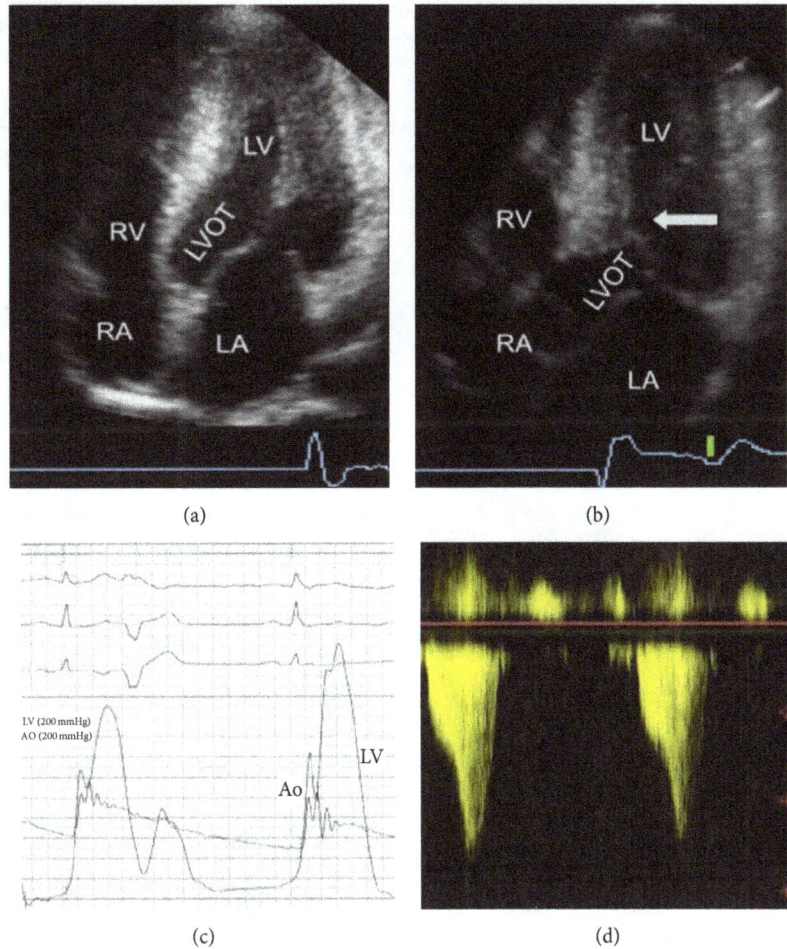

FIGURE 1: 2D-echocardiographic findings in hypertrophic nonobstructed cardiomyopathy (HNCM, (a)) with predominant thickening of the apical segments and a wide open, unobstructed outflow tract (LVOT) and in hypertrophic obstructive cardiomyopathy (HOCM, (b)) with a protruding subaortic septum making systolic contact with the mitral valve (SAM-phenomenon, arrow). (c) shows simultaneous pressure tracing from the LV and the aorta demonstrating the outflow gradient and the Brockenbrough sign. The corresponding Doppler profiles are shown in (d). The gradient increases from 40 to 140 mm Hg. The typical CW-Doppler flow profile of left ventricular outflow obstruction in HOCM has a late-peaking signal indicating dynamic obstruction involving contracting muscle as opposed to the more symmetrical signal of fixed valvular stenosis. The peak pressure gradient equals $4 \times (\text{peak velocity})^2$. LA: left atrium; RA: right atrium; LV: left ventricle; Ao: aorta; and IVS: interventricular septum.

in asymptomatic patients, however, does not seem to be justified. Outflow obstruction may exacerbate with alcohol intake, and the turbulent flow in the LVOT together with the obstruction-associated mitral regurgitation includes an increased risk for infective endocarditis [72, 73]. HCM patients in atrial fibrillation are endangered by thromboembolic stroke; oral anticoagulation is thus mandatory in these cases [6, 8]. All HCM patients should be risk-stratified [6, 8, 20, 74–82] since the implantation of an ICD reliably reduces arrhythmogenic cardiac events.

Risk stratification in HCM is based on the presence versus absence of five major risk factors, each one with a relatively low positive individual predictive value. However, combining them their significance considerably increases. These risk markers are (see above) as follows:

(i) a "malignant" family history (of sudden cardiac death at <45 years),

(ii) recurrent unexplained syncope,

(iii) nonsustained ventricular tachycardia on Holter monitoring,

(iv) inadequate blood pressure rise with exercise (i.e., failure to rise by >20 mm Hg or a fall of >20 mm Hg after an initial rise),

(v) excessive LVH (>30 mm) in any region.

Patients without any of the listed risk markers seem to have a favorable prognosis, although cases of SCD have been reported with a completely negative list of risk factors. Other aspects that suggest a benign disease course are a normal or near-normal ECG, advanced age >65 years at diagnosis, and a preserved exercise tolerance on cardiopulmonary stress testing. On the other hand, in individuals carrying two or more of these risk markers, ICD implantation should be strongly considered. Whether just one risk factor is sufficient

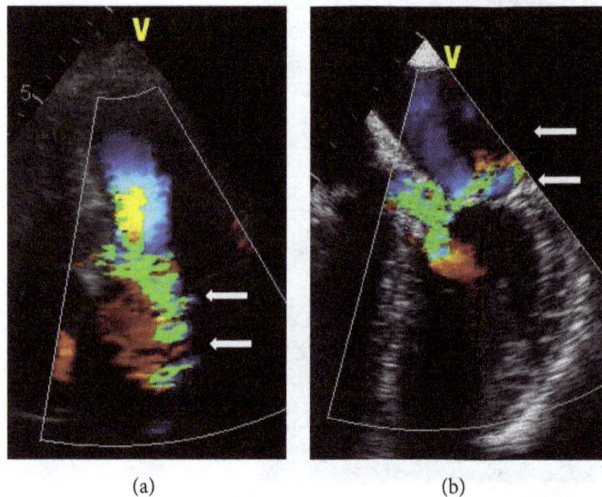

(a)   (b)

FIGURE 2: Typical mitral regurgitation associated with SAM and subaortic LVOT obstruction with a posterolateral jet orientation (arrows) in a transthoracic (a) and transesophageal view (b). LA: left atrium; RA: right atrium; LV: left ventricle; Ao: aorta; and IVS: interventricular septum.

for primary ICD prophylaxis is controversially discussed. In our practice a malignant family history is a strong argument for an ICD even if this is the only risk marker.

Recently, the documentation of areas of marked late gadolinium enhancement/fibrosis on cardiac MRI has been linked to an increased risk [8, 21–23, 53, 57, 67]. In addition, very early onset of the disease, the presence of an apical aneurysm and of myocardial bridging, objective signs of myocardial ischemia, marked left atrial dilatation, and supraventricular tachyarrhythmias have been linked to future adverse events, although in smaller patient cohorts. Patients with a late dilated stage of the disease seem to be a high-risk category of its own with a very unfavorable prognosis.

Medical therapy with negatively inotropic drugs (beta-blockers, calcium antagonists of the verapamil type, and disopyramide) is the first line of treatment in order to reduce symptoms and improve quality of life [83–86] in patients with HOCM. Additional antifibrillatory effects may be present for beta-blockers, while verapamil is supposed to have a positive effect on diastolic LV function. Beta-blocker dosage for symptom control should be uptitrated to a resting heart rate of 50–60 beats/min. The effect of disopyramide on obstruction seems to exceed that of the two other drugs; however, disopyramide is no longer available in central Europe.

The antiarrhythmic properties of the different drugs are welcomed in many patients. On the other hand, latent conduction abnormalities may exacerbate in individual cases. Furthermore, about 5–10% of patients may have a paradoxical hemodynamic response to verapamil. The initiation of treatment with verapamil and disopyramide therefore should be monitored closely. Overall, in many patients, the effect of drug treatment vanishes over the years, and none of these strategies are really "evidence-based." Drugs that lead to a marked pre- or afterload reduction or those with

positive inotropic effects are contraindicated in HOCM since they may produce drastic exacerbation of obstruction and hemodynamic collapse.

Medical therapy in HCM without obstruction, either in "deobstructed" HOCM after a septal reduction intervention or in primary HNCM, may be understood as HFpEF treatment. In order to optimize left ventricular filling time, heart rate should be tightly controlled using beta-blockers or verapamil-type calcium antagonists. Diuretics and ACE inhibitors/AT receptor antagonists may be used for signs of congestion or concomitant hypertension. Occasionally, an outflow tract obstruction may be produced in initially nonobstructive patients by vigorous afterload reduction; thus we again recommend echo-Doppler monitoring of the initial phase of therapy. Animal experiments and a recently published study in human HNCM [86] suggest inhibition or even reversal of fibrosis with AT receptor antagonist treatment.

Atrial fibrillation with loss of active ventricular filling-in is often associated with a considerable drop in exercise tolerance and an increased risk of embolic events. Anticoagulants should be promptly administered, and Amiodarone can prevent recurrence of atrial fibrillation. Ablation therapy of atrial fibrillation is an additional option; however, outcomes are less favorable as compared to patients without structural heart disease. End-stage disease should be treated as severe heart failure of other etiologies, including modern assist device strategies and heart transplantation.

Surgical myectomy, developed in the late fifth and the sixth decade of the 20th century, traditionally has been the treatment of choice for HCM patients with drug-refractory symptoms and significant outflow obstruction [87–97]. The procedure aims at removing a part of the protruding septal myocardium (Figure 3) via a transaortic approach and leaves a clearly visible septal trough on imaging studies (Figure 4) and usually a left bundle-branch block on the surface ECG in >50% of the patients treated (Figure 6). The depth and extent of septal resection can be tailored to the individual anatomy, thus also addressing midcavity obstruction or papillary muscle abnormalities if present. Furthermore, valvular correction/replacement or coronary bypass grafting can be combined with the reduction of septal myocardium if necessary. Perioperative monitoring by transesophageal echocardiography has become a routine procedure. The rate of pacemaker dependency is reported to be ≤5%.

Reports on >2000 patients undergoing (isolated) myectomy consistently demonstrated clinical and hemodynamic success rates of >90% together with operative mortality rates that finally were reduced to <1-2% in experienced centers. A favorable effect on the hypertrophic process and a positive prognostic influence [94] are suspected from long-term observations of postmyectomy patients; however, a randomized study against medical treatment does not exist. Favorable results of myectomy were also reported in specific subsets including pediatric patients as well as cases with atypical or midcavity obstruction. Taking all this together, myectomy has set the standard of safety and efficacy of treatment for symptomatic obstructive HCM; and all alternatives should be measured against this standard.

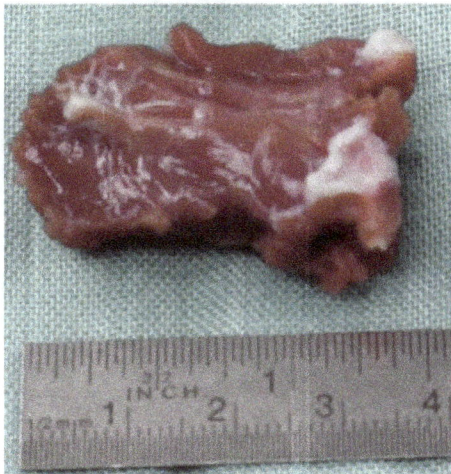

FIGURE 3: Septal myocardium removed during a myectomy procedure. According to septal thickness and location of the obstruction, a block of myocardium of $4.0 \times 1.5 \times 0.8$ cm was removed from the subaortic septum.

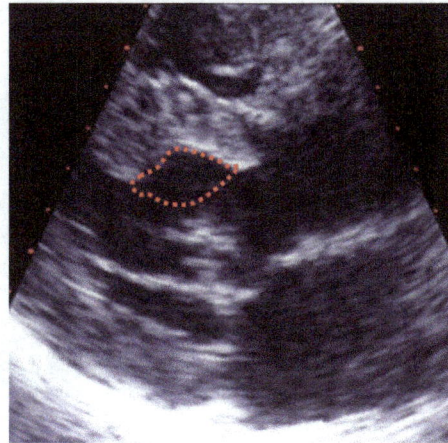

FIGURE 4: Echocardiographic visualization of the septal trough (dotted line) produced by a myectomy procedure.

After some observations concerning LVOT gradient reduction with pacing, dual-chamber pacemaker implantation was introduced as a less invasive alternative to myectomy in the ninth decade of the 20th century. Pacing from the RV apex with a short AV-delay may be understood as a combination of a global negative inotropic effect and some outflow tract opening due to delayed activation of the basal septum. A gradient reduction of 50–90% has been reported. Enthusiasm for this approach, however, was tempered since a considerable placebo effect became obvious in several randomized trials [98]. At present, we consider AV sequential pacing a "niche indication" for

(1) patients with left bundle-branch block (and thus a very high risk for complete AV block during septal ablation (see below)),

(2) patients who need an ICD for risk reduction anyway,

(3) selected patients with isolated midcavity obstruction.

4. Septal Ablation: From Experiment to Standard of Care

From 1995 onwards, therapeutic options for HOCM dramatically changed by the introduction of percutaneous septal ablation [99–140]. In 1994, after obtaining ethical approval for a limited series of cases to undergo this new procedure, Sigwart performed the first three septal ablations in elderly, highly symptomatic HOCM patients who were unable to tolerate surgical myectomy. The positive results of these first cases were published in 1995 [99], followed by a widespread adoption of the new technique.

The septal ablation procedure produces a circumscript necrosis by injection of 96% ethanol (or other toxic agents; see below) into a septal perforator artery supplying the septal bulge involved in outflow obstruction (Figure 5). Several components of the procedure had earlier been tested or used clinically and in other scenarios. In the early 1980 years, the group of Sigwart reported on the effect of temporary balloon occlusion within a coronary vessel on myocardial function and thickening [100]. Brugada and coworkers, among others, used the injection of absolute ethanol into coronary arteries to eliminate arrhythmogenic foci [101]. The group of Kuhn and coworkers [102, 103] reported on temporary gradient reduction in HOCM following temporary balloon occlusion of septal perforator arteries. Even the use of intraprocedural contrast echocardiography had been outlined in a research proposal as early as 1989 [104]. Several acronyms have been introduced for the technique (in alphabetical order and probably incomplete): alcohol/ethanol septal ablation (ASA/ESA), nonsurgical myocardial reduction (NSMR), percutaneous transluminal septal myocardial ablation (PTSMA), or transcoronary ablation of septal hypertrophy (TASH), reflecting slightly different procedural strategies and/or operator preference.

The septal lesion produced by the procedure often closely resembles a myectomy trough (Figures 5 and 6), and it also reproduces the hemodynamic effect of a surgical myectomy with reduction/elimination of the outflow gradient, SAM, and the SAM-associated mitral regurgitation. After the procedure, about 50–60% of the patients show a right bundle-branch block pattern on surface ECG and have transient complete heart block during the procedure. Across all reported series including the learning curve of the individual investigator groups, periprocedural mortality of septal ablation was 1–4%, at present 1-2%. This holds true both for several single-center series and for multicenter registries [115, 116, 127]. The injected ethanol doses gradually decreased over the years (from >5 to 1–3 mL), leading to smaller infarctions and less AV conduction problems. However, the rate of pacemaker implantation still varies considerably (between <5 and up to 20%, in patients with preexisting left bundle-branch block: >60%; see above). Following a local remodeling process, the morphologic and hemodynamic treatment result should be judged no earlier than after 3–6 months. At that time point, gradients usually are reduced by 80–90%, associated with an

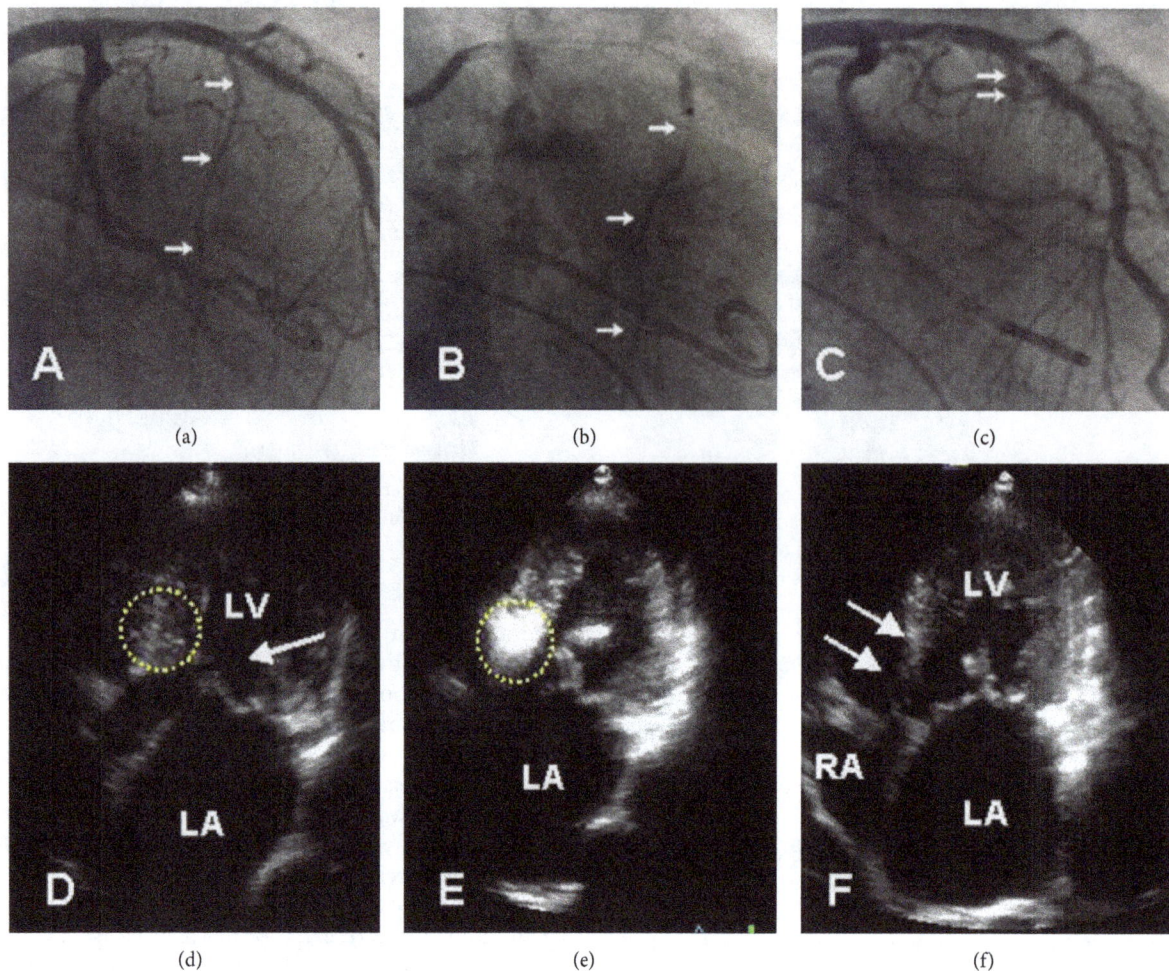

FIGURE 5: Angiographic ((a)–(c)) and echocardiographic ((d)–(f)) aspect of an echotargeted septal ablation procedure (in our practice denominated as PTSMA). A guidewire is advanced into the target vessel (arrows in (a)). Subsequently, an over-the-wire balloon is introduced. The correct position and fit of the balloon are verified by contrast injection (arrows in (b)) through the central catheter lumen. The vessel stump after alcohol injection and removal of the balloon is shown in (c) (arrows). In (d), the dotted circle marks the septal target area including the SAM-septal contact zone. Contrast injection into the target vessel (e) precisely highlights this area. After 3–6 months, akinesia and thinning of the subaortic septum are clearly visible, comparable to a myectomy trough.

increase in exercise capacity by 20% and an improvement of diastolic LV function markers. During the past two decades septal ablation has gained wide acceptance as the nonsurgical alternative of choice for patients with hypertrophic cardiomyopathy, significant outflow obstruction, and symptoms refractory to medical treatment.

4.1. Septal Ablation Procedure. A detailed description of the technique has been repeatedly published by our and other groups, differing in several technical aspects [99, 106, 108, 109, 112–116]. In general, two phases of technical development can be described. From roughly 1995 to 1998, during a phase of initial deployment of the new technique, relatively high doses (in some cases >10 mL) of ethanol were injected almost always into the first septal perforator artery, not guided by any imaging techniques. This era, including the early learning curve in most groups, resulted in relatively good clinical efficacy, with reductions in gradient and improvement in

symptoms, but with rather high complication rates, including complete heart block requiring pacemaker implantation in an unacceptable large proportion of patients undergoing the procedure and also probably underreported, distant myocardial infarction or death from inadvertent spillage of ethanol.

During the next phase, roughly between 1999 and 2009, the incorporation of myocardial contrast echo as a guide in order to select the correct septal perforator substantially increased procedural safety. Furthermore, careful follow-up of postablation patients demonstrated that it was not necessary to completely eliminate obstruction during the ablation session, leading to a substantial reduction of the injected amount of alcohol (currently to roughly 2 mL or 1 mL per cm of myocardial thickness in the target region). The pacemaker implantation rate was brought down by scoring systems to estimate the risk of procedure-related persisting or recurrent conduction problems.

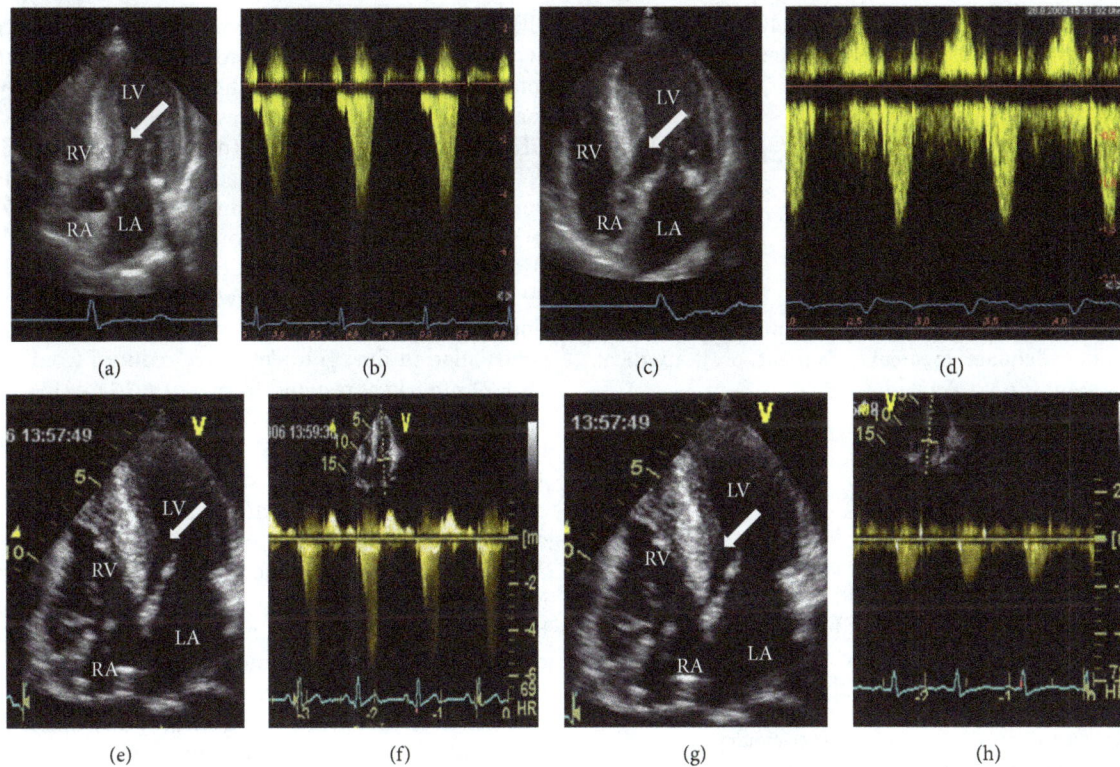

FIGURE 6: Echocardiographic aspect of HOCM before/after a myectomy ((a)–(d)) and after a percutaneous septal ablation ((e)–(h)). Both cases show marked thickening of the midcavity and subaortic septum (arrows in (a) and (e)) at baseline together with a substantial outflow acceleration to >5 m/s corresponding to an outflow gradient of 100 mm Hg at rest ((b) and (f)). After the respective intervention there is thinning of the subaortic septum (arrows in (c) and (g)) and normalisation of LV outflow to <2 m/s, that is, absence of a resting gradient. The different ECG patterns of QRS widening with a LBBB pattern in C/D after myectomy and a RBBB pattern after septal ablation are also visible. LA: left atrium; RA: right atrium; RV: right ventricle; and LV: left ventricle.

There is still consensus that a temporary pacemaker lead should be routinely inserted in all patients. The outflow gradient may be monitored using simultaneous pressure recordings from the left ventricular apex and the ascending aorta. A standard short (10–12 mm) over-the-wire balloon catheter is introduced into the target septal branch presumed to be responsible for the blood supply to the septal area involved in obstruction. The balloon is inflated, and the effect on obstruction is measured.

In contrast to other techniques that strongly rely on this effect, in our practice as well as in most other centers the correct vessel selection is assured by injecting 1-2 mL of a nontoxic echocardiographic contrast agent through the central lumen of the balloon catheter under simultaneous transthoracic echocardiographic monitoring. This approach exactly shows the septal area that will be attacked, that is, the future area of necrosis (Figure 4). Opacification of any other cardiac structures has to be securely excluded [109]. Currently, in about 15% a target vessel change is necessary based on echocardiographic findings (usually contrast in areas distant from the septal target region) or for the same reason the procedure has to be stopped [120, 130]. Only if the target region is correctly marked, 1–3 mL of 96% alcohol (i.e., 1 mL per 1 cm of septal thickness) is slowly injected through

the central lumen of the balloon catheter under analgesic medication (5–10 mg of morphine) and continuous fluoroscopic control. Ten minutes after the last alcohol injection the balloon is deflated and removed, ensuring that no alcohol backwash occurs into the left anterior descending artery. A final angiogram excludes LAD damage and verifies septal branch occlusion, and a final hemodynamic measurement is performed. The duration of postinterventional monitoring is controversially discussed. Since an artificial myocardial necrosis has been created, we suggest a monitoring duration of at least 48 hours (coronary or intensive care unit), with enzyme and ECG controls every 4 hours. Transvenous and transcutaneous pacing equipment should be readily available.

Absolute ethanol is not necessarily the only agent to induce the iatrogenic septal necrosis. Glue septal ablation using cyanoacrylate has been suggested to be a safe and effective approach to reduce septal thickness in patients with septal collateral vessels to the right coronary artery. The authors suggested that immediate glue polymerization prevents its transit through collateral vessels. Significant reductions in LVOT obstruction were observed, but long-term durability of this technique has not yet been demonstrated. Other cytotoxic agents that may be used are microcoils or contour emboli, and a small series with less favorable results reported on the use of radiofrequency energy [139, 140] applied either from the right ventricular septum or directly to the left ventricular septum.

4.2. Patient Selection for Septal Ablation.

Criteria for patient selection largely follow those established for septal myectomy. Septal ablation may be considered an alternative to septal myectomy in [6, 8]:

(1) patients with symptoms limiting daily activities (functional class > II, exercise-induced syncope) despite adequate medical treatment or if medical treatment is not tolerated;

(2) patients with a substantial degree of outflow obstruction (pressure drop > 50–60 mm Hg with provocation by a Valsalva maneuver, bicycle stress, or postextrasystolic augmentation);

(3) patients with a suitable left ventricular and coronary morphology, that is, those with a "classical," subaortic obstruction produced by the protruding septum and the "SAM" of the mitral valve and one or more septal perforator arteries that go to this septal area.

Patients with coexisting, significant coronary artery disease in one vessel only may be treated percutaneously first; ablation should be delayed until documentation of a good long-term result of PCI. In cases with multiple (>1) vessel disease, we prefer a surgical approach. In atypical obstruction or midcavity obstruction, the decision must be individualized; ablation is possible [120, 130] but results are less favorable in this subgroup as compared to subaortic obstruction. At present, with respect to the very limited long-term experience with septal ablation and the favorable results of myectomy also in this age group, we are reluctant with ablation in the pediatric population with HOCM.

4.3. Current Results of Septal Ablation.

As stated above, periprocedural mortality figures from experienced centers at present range between 0 and 2%. However, the rate of procedure-related pacemaker implantations still varies considerably, that is, between <5 and up to >20%. With respect to the morphologic and hemodynamic treatment result, across all reported series gradients usually are reduced by 80–90%, associated with an increase in exercise capacity, an improvement of diastolic LV function markers [132], and a reduction of left atrial size. A systematic review found a 30-day mortality of septal ablation around 1.5%, comparable to current survival rates after surgical myectomy. The most frequent complications of septal ablation were dissections of the LAD, cardiac tamponade, fatal bradyarrhythmias, ventricular fibrillation, cardiogenic shock, and pulmonary embolism. Agarwal and colleagues published a meta-analysis of twelve studies [122] comparing the short-term outcome of septal ablation and myectomy. They found no significant differences in short-term mortality (risk difference (RD): 0.01; 95% confidence interval (CI): −0.01 to 0.03).

Our own series now includes 603 patients (selected from a total of 1637 patients evaluated and treated in our HCM clinic). Out of these, 543 patients (90%) received an average dose of 2.4 ± 1.0 mL of ethanol. In 60 patients the intervention was aborted without ethanol injection, mostly for safety reasons/due to contrast echocardiographic findings. CK peak was 507 ± 246 U/L (normal value: <80). Transient AV conduction problems occurred in 245 patients (45%); permanent AV sequential pacing was required in 49 patients (9%). Peri-interventional mortality was 0.9% (5 deaths). After 3 months, self-reported exercise capacity improved in 493 patients (91%), with an average NYHA functional class improvement from 2.9 ± 0.4 to 1.6 ± 0.6; $P < 0.01$. Left ventricular outflow gradients were reduced from 62 ± 34 to 13 ± 21 mm Hg at rest and from 120 ± 36 to 41 ± 39 mm Hg with provocation ($P < 0.0001$). Septal thickness (from 20 ± 4 to 16 ± 4 mm; $P < 0.01$) and left atrial diameter (from 48 ± 7 to 45 ± 7 mm; $P < 0.01$) were also reduced. LV dilatation exceeding the individual normal value, or a global deterioration of systolic LV function, was not observed.

In addition to the comparable in-hospital mortality figures, the limited number of nonrandomized comparisons between septal ablation and (isolated) myectomy shows comparable clinical and hemodynamic results, with a slightly more pronounced improvement with respect to obstruction and exercise capacity following surgery and different surface ECG patterns (after septal ablation: RBBB; after myectomy: LBBB) after intervention [118, 121, 122, 124]. Whether these differences are clinically important or not is unknown. A difference that may be important is the fact that relief from obstruction is usually rapid after myectomy, whereas LV "unloading" after ablation may take several months.

The available publications on long-term effects of septal ablation showed that reduction of septal thickness and outflow gradient seems to continue over a 12-month period, presumably due to ongoing fibrosis and shrinking of the ethanol-induced septal lesion [110, 125–128, 131, 133, 134, 137]. Progressive LV dilatation was not observed; thus the remodeling process seems to remain limited to the region of intervention. Not only septal hypertrophy decreased as a consequence of the therapeutic infarction but also left ventricular posterior wall thickness due to relief of the pressure overload, which in turn indicates that the hypertrophic process in HOCM may not be completely independent of LV afterload. Overall 10-year survival was 90%; the event-free survival in NYHA class II or lower 76% figures again comparable to the reported postsurgical results [110, 131].

Concerns that septal scar induced by alcohol ablation might produce a new arrhythmogenic substrate have thus far not been validated. The long-term survival curves after surgical myectomy and septal ablation seem to be congruent [131, 134]. In one study that reported higher mortality and arrhythmogenic event [137] rates patients had received higher doses of ethanol than currently used. The question whether a successful septal alcohol ablation carries a prognostic benefit besides its symptomatic effect remains unanswered. Recent own data showed that survival in postablation HOCM patients was similar to that in an age-matched background population [131]. The number of risk factors, including the prevalence of nonsustained ventricular tachycardia, was reduced after ablation, and the incidence of sudden cardiac death was low. However, these findings must be confirmed by further investigations; currently we do not support a "prophylactic" intervention that addresses outflow gradients in asymptomatic patients. A meta-analysis comparing myectomy with septal ablation demonstrated absence of differences between the two procedures concerning the incidence of ventricular tachyarrhythmias.

5. Conclusion

Currently, for many patients with symptomatic HOCM, surgical myectomy and septal ablation can both be judged as reasonable options. Both procedures require extensive assessment and careful patient selection, should be performed by experienced operators in the context of a comprehensive program for HCM patients offering all other options (medical treatment, pacemaker and ICD implantation), result in a significant and long-standing clinical and hemodynamic benefit, and have a very acceptable safety profile. Consequently, the 2011 ACCF/AHA Guidelines for the Diagnosis and Management of HCM [8] advocate for septal ablation as a good alternative to surgery in those with significant comorbidity or advanced age and allow the procedure for those at lower surgical risk after a balanced discussion.

This discussion should refer to the individual anatomy, the likelihood of obtaining the desired result with a near-zero gradient, the comorbidities present, the available local expertise, and patient preference. Furthermore, both patient and operator should face the possibility that the ablation session might be ended without ethanol injection in case of lack of an appropriate septal target vessel. In our opinion ablation should be preferentially offered to older patients and to individuals with specific comorbidities and frailties in order to avoid the possible complications of open heart surgery. A preexisting left bundle-branch block increases the risk for pacemaker dependence after septal ablation to nearly 100%. Therefore, these patients preferably should undergo elective pacemaker implantation before ablation.

On the other hand, patients with extreme ventricular thickness (>30 mm) who more often also demonstrate marked myocardial fibrosis will probably have a less favorable outcome with alcohol ablation, and surgery remains a better choice. Surgery may also preferentially be offered in cases in which immediate relief from obstruction is an issue since the full effect of ablation may take several months. Furthermore, patients with concomitant multivessel coronary artery disease, mitral or aortic valve disease, or with anomalous papillary muscle insertion are candidates for operation.

Nearly twenty years after the first experimental cases, it thus appears reasonable to conclude that septal ablation and myectomy should no longer be seen as adversaries, but as partners in order to attain maximum patient benefit. A randomized trial comparing the two procedures has been and remains a major challenge for the future.

Conflict of Interests

The author declares that there is no conflict of interests regarding the publication of this paper.

References

[1] D. Teare, "Asymmetrical hypertrophy of the heart in young adults," *British Heart Journal*, vol. 20, no. 1, pp. 1–8, 1958.

[2] E. Braunwald, C. T. Lambrew, S. D. Rockoff, J. Ross Jr., and A. G. Morrow, "Idiopathic hypertrophic subaortic stenosis, I: a description of the disease based upon an analysis of 64 patients," *Circulation*, vol. 30, pp. 3–119, 1964.

[3] B. J. Maron, "Hypertrophic cardiomyopathy: a systematic review," *Journal of the American Medical Association*, vol. 287, no. 10, pp. 1308–1320, 2002.

[4] P. Spirito, C. E. Seidman, W. J. McKenna, and B. J. Maron, "The management of hypertrophic cardiomyopathy," *The New England Journal of Medicine*, vol. 336, no. 11, pp. 775–785, 1997.

[5] E. D. Wigle, H. Rakowski, B. P. Kimball, and W. G. Williams, "Hypertrophic cardiomyopathy: clinical spectrum and treatment," *Circulation*, vol. 92, no. 7, pp. 1680–1692, 1995.

[6] B. J. Maron, W. J. McKenna, G. K. Danielson et al., "American College of Cardiology/European Society of Cardiology clinical expert consensus document on hypertrophic cardiomyopathy," *Journal of the American College of Cardiology*, vol. 42, pp. 1687–1713, 2003.

[7] B. J. Maron, I. Olivotto, P. Spirito et al., "Epidemiology of hypertrophic cardiomyopathy-related death: revisited in a large non-referral-based patient population," *Circulation*, vol. 102, no. 8, pp. 858–864, 2000.

[8] B. J. Gersh, B. J. Maron, R. O. Bonow et al., "2011 ACCF/AHA guideline for the diagnosis and treatment of hypertrophic cardiomyopathy: executive summary: a report of the American College of cardiology foundation/American heart association task force on practice guidelines," *Circulation*, vol. 124, no. 24, pp. 2761–2796, 2011.

[9] C. Prinz, M. Farr, D. Hering, D. Horstkotte, and L. Faber, "The diagnosis and treatment of hypertrophic cardiomyopathy," *Deutsches Ärzteblatt International*, vol. 108, no. 13, pp. 209–215, 2011.

[10] C. Rapezzi, E. Arbustini, A. L. Caforio et al., "Diagnostic work-up in cardiomyopathies: bridging the gap between clinical phenotypes and final diagnosis: a position statement from the ESC Working Group on myocardial and Pericardial Diseases," *European Heart Journal*, vol. 34, pp. 1448–1458, 2013.

[11] H. G. Klues, A. Schiffers, and B. J. Maron, "Phenotypic spectrum and patterns of left ventricular hypertrophy in hypertrophic cardiomyopathy: morphologic observations and significance as assessed by two-dimensional echocardiography in 600 patients," *Journal of the American College of Cardiology*, vol. 26, no. 7, pp. 1699–1708, 1995.

[12] K. M. Harris, P. Spirito, M. S. Maron et al., "Prevalence, clinical profile, and significance of left ventricular remodeling in the end-stage phase of hypertrophic cardiomyopathy," *Journal of the American College of Cardiology*, vol. 54, no. 3, pp. 191–200, 2009.

[13] H. G. Klues, B. J. Maron, A. L. Dollar, and W. C. Roberts, "Diversity of structural mitral valve alterations in hypertrophic cardiomyopathy," *Circulation*, vol. 85, no. 5, pp. 1651–1660, 1992.

[14] M. S. Maron, I. Olivotto, C. Harrigan et al., "Mitral valve abnormalities identified by cardiovascular magnetic resonance represent a primary phenotypic expression of hypertrophic cardiomyopathy," *Circulation*, vol. 124, no. 1, pp. 40–47, 2011.

[15] E. Schwammenthal, S. Nakatani, S. He et al., "Mechanism of mitral regurgitation in hypertrophic cardiomyopathy: mismatch of posterior to anterior leaflet length and mobility," *Circulation*, vol. 98, no. 9, pp. 856–865, 1998.

[16] M. S. Maron, A. G. Zenovich, S. A. Casey et al., "Significance and relation between magnitude of left ventricular hypertrophy and heart failure symptoms in hypertrophic cardiomyopathy," *American Journal of Cardiology*, vol. 95, no. 11, pp. 1329–1333, 2005.

[17] P. Spirito, P. Bellone, K. M. Harris, P. Bernabò, P. Bruzzi, and B. J. Maron, "Magnitude of left ventricular hypertrophy and risk of sudden death in hypertrophic cardiomyopathy," *The New England Journal of Medicine*, vol. 342, no. 24, pp. 1778–1785, 2000.

[18] I. Olivotto, M. S. Maron, C. Autore et al., "Assessment and significance of left ventricular mass by cardiovascular magnetic resonance in hypertrophic cardiomyopathy," *Journal of the American College of Cardiology*, vol. 52, no. 7, pp. 559–566, 2008.

[19] M. S. Maron, I. Olivotto, A. G. Zenovich et al., "Hypertrophic cardiomyopathy is predominantly a disease of left ventricular outflow tract obstruction," *Circulation*, vol. 114, no. 21, pp. 2232–2239, 2006.

[20] P. M. Elliott, J. Poloniecki, S. Dickie et al., "Sudden death in hypertrophic cardiomyopathy: identification of high risk patients," *Journal of the American College of Cardiology*, vol. 36, no. 7, pp. 2212–2218, 2000.

[21] B. J. Maron, "Contemporary insights and strategies for risk stratification and prevention of sudden death in hypertrophic cardiomyopathy," *Circulation*, vol. 121, no. 3, pp. 445–456, 2010.

[22] M. S. Maron, B. J. Maron, C. Harrigan et al., "Hypertrophic cardiomyopathy phenotype revisited after 50 years with cardiovascular magnetic resonance," *Journal of the American College of Cardiology*, vol. 54, no. 3, pp. 220–228, 2009.

[23] C. Rickers, N. M. Wilke, M. Jerosch-Herold et al., "Utility of cardiac magnetic resonance imaging in the diagnosis of hypertrophic cardiomyopathy," *Circulation*, vol. 112, no. 6, pp. 855–861, 2005.

[24] J. C. C. Moon, N. G. Fisher, W. J. McKenna, and D. J. Pennell, "Detection of apical hypertrophic cardiomyopathy by cardiovascular magnetic resonance in patients with non-diagnostic echocardiography," *Heart*, vol. 90, no. 6, pp. 645–649, 2004.

[25] P. M. Elliott, J. R. Gimeno Blanes, N. G. Mahon, J. D. Poloniecki, and W. J. McKenna, "Relation between severity of left-ventricular hypertrophy and prognosis in patients with hypertrophic cardiomyopathy," *The Lancet*, vol. 357, no. 9254, pp. 420–424, 2001.

[26] B. J. Maron, K. P. Carney, H. M. Lever et al., "Relationship of race to sudden cardiac death in competitive athletes with hypertrophic cardiomyopathy," *Journal of the American College of Cardiology*, vol. 41, no. 6, pp. 974–980, 2003.

[27] D. Corrado, C. Basso, M. Schiavon, and G. Thiene, "Screening for hypertrophic cardiomyopathy in young athletes," *The New England Journal of Medicine*, vol. 339, no. 6, pp. 364–369, 1998.

[28] M. S. Maron, J. J. Finley, J. M. Bos et al., "Prevalence, clinical significance, and natural history of left ventricular apical aneurysms in hypertrophic cardiomyopathy," *Circulation*, vol. 118, no. 15, pp. 1541–1549, 2008.

[29] M. S. Maron, J. R. Lesser, and B. J. Maron, "Management implications of massive left ventricular hypertrophy in hypertrophic cardiomyopathy significantly underestimated by echocardiography but identified by cardiovascular magnetic resonance," *American Journal of Cardiology*, vol. 105, no. 12, pp. 1842–1843, 2010.

[30] I. Olivotto, B. J. Maron, E. Appelbaum et al., "Spectrum and clinical significance of systolic function and myocardial fibrosis assessed by cardiovascular magnetic resonance in hypertrophic cardiomyopathy," *American Journal of Cardiology*, vol. 106, no. 2, pp. 261–267, 2010.

[31] J. B. Geske, P. Sorajja, R. A. Nishimura, and S. R. Ommen, "Evaluation of left ventricular filling pressures by Doppler echocardiography in patients with hypertrophic cardiomyopathy: correlation with direct left atrial pressure measurement at cardiac catheterization," *Circulation*, vol. 116, no. 23, pp. 2702–2708, 2007.

[32] B. J. Maron, P. Spirito, K. J. Green, Y. E. Wesley, R. O. Bonow, and J. Arce, "Noninvasive assessment of left ventricular diastolic function by pulsed Doppler echocardiography in patients with hypertrophic cardiomyopathy," *Journal of the American College of Cardiology*, vol. 10, no. 4, pp. 733–742, 1987.

[33] C. Autore, P. Bernabò, C. S. Barillà, P. Bruzzi, and P. Spirito, "The prognostic importance of left ventricular outflow obstruction in hypertrophic cardiomyopathy varies in relation to the severity of symptoms," *Journal of the American College of Cardiology*, vol. 45, no. 7, pp. 1076–1080, 2005.

[34] P. Elliott, J. Gimeno, M. Tomé, and W. McKenna, "Left ventricular outflow tract obstruction and sudden death in hypertrophic cardiomyopathy," *European Heart Journal*, vol. 27, no. 24, p. 3073, 2006.

[35] M. S. Maron, I. Olivotto, S. Betocchi et al., "Effect of left ventricular outflow tract obstruction on clinical outcome in hypertrophic cardiomyopathy," *The New England Journal of Medicine*, vol. 348, no. 4, pp. 295–303, 2003.

[36] W. J. McKenna and J. E. Deanfield, "Hypertrophic cardiomyopathy: an important cause of sudden death," *Archives of Disease in Childhood*, vol. 59, no. 10, pp. 971–975, 1984.

[37] I. Olivotto, F. Cecchi, S. A. Casey, A. Dolara, J. H. Traverse, and B. J. Maron, "Impact of atrial fibrillation on the clinical course of hypertrophic cardiomyopathy," *Circulation*, vol. 104, no. 21, pp. 2517–2524, 2001.

[38] B. J. Maron, I. Olivotto, P. Bellone et al., "Clinical profile of stroke in 900 patients with hypertrophic cardiomyopathy," *Journal of the American College of Cardiology*, vol. 39, no. 2, pp. 301–307, 2002.

[39] B. J. Maron, S. A. Casey, R. G. Hauser, and D. M. Aeppli, "Clinical course of hypertrophic cardiomyopathy with survival to advanced age," *Journal of the American College of Cardiology*, vol. 42, no. 5, pp. 882–888, 2003.

[40] B. J. Maron, S. A. Casey, T. S. Haas, C. L. Kitner, R. F. Garberich, and J. R. Lesser, "Hypertrophic cardiomyopathy with longevity to 90 years or older," *American Journal of Cardiology*, vol. 109, no. 9, pp. 1341–1347, 2012.

[41] C. J. McLeod, M. J. Ackerman, R. A. Nishimura, A. J. Tajik, B. J. Gersh, and S. R. Ommen, "Outcome of patients with hypertrophic cardiomyopathy and a normal electrocardiogram," *Journal of the American College of Cardiology*, vol. 54, no. 3, pp. 229–233, 2009.

[42] R. Alcalai, J. G. Seidman, and C. E. Seidman, "Genetic basis of hypertrophic cardiomyopathy: from bench to the clinics," *Journal of Cardiovascular Electrophysiology*, vol. 19, no. 1, pp. 104–110, 2008.

[43] A. P. Landstrom and M. J. Ackerman, "Mutation type is not clinically useful in predicting prognosis in hypertrophic cardiomyopathy," *Circulation*, vol. 122, no. 23, pp. 2441–2449, 2010.

[44] P. Richard, P. Charron, L. Carrier et al., "Hypertrophic cardiomyopathy: distribution of disease genes, spectrum of mutations, and implications for a molecular diagnosis strategy," *Circulation*, vol. 107, pp. 2227–2232, 2003.

[45] J. G. Seidman and C. Seidman, "The genetic basis for cardiomyopathy: from mutation identification to mechanistic paradigms," *Cell*, vol. 104, no. 4, pp. 557–567, 2001.

[46] B. J. Maron, J. G. Seidman, and C. E. Seidman, "Proposal for contemporary screening strategies in families with hypertrophic cardiomyopathy," *Journal of the American College of Cardiology*, vol. 44, no. 11, pp. 2125–2132, 2004.

[47] H. Watkins, A. Rosenzweig, D.-S. Hwang et al., "Characteristics and prognostic implications of myosin missense mutations in familial hypertrophic cardiomyopathy," *The New England Journal of Medicine*, vol. 326, no. 17, pp. 1108–1114, 1992.

[48] J. M. Bos, J. A. Towbin, and M. J. Ackerman, "Diagnostic, prognostic, and therapeutic implications of genetic testing for hypertrophic cardiomyopathy," *Journal of the American College of Cardiology*, vol. 54, no. 3, pp. 201–209, 2009.

[49] B. J. Maron and W. C. Roberts, "Quantitative analysis of cardiac muscle cell disorganization in the ventricular septum of patients with hypertrophic cardiomyopathy," *Circulation*, vol. 59, no. 4, pp. 689–706, 1979.

[50] C. Y. Ho, B. López, O. R. Coelho-Filho et al., "Myocardial fibrosis as an early manifestation of hypertrophic cardiomyopathy," *The New England Journal of Medicine*, vol. 363, no. 6, pp. 552–563, 2010.

[51] B. J. Maron, J. K. Wolfson, S. E. Epstein, and W. C. Roberts, "Intramural ('small vessel') coronary artery disease in hypertrophic cardiomyopathy," *Journal of the American College of Cardiology*, vol. 8, no. 3, pp. 545–557, 1986.

[52] J. Shirani, R. Pick, W. C. Roberts, and B. J. Maron, "Morphology and significance of the left ventricular collagen network in young patients with hypertrophic cardiomyopathy and sudden cardiac death," *Journal of the American College of Cardiology*, vol. 35, no. 1, pp. 36–44, 2000.

[53] C. Prinz, M. Schwarz, I. Ilic et al., "Myocardial fibrosis severity on cardiac magnetic resonance imaging predicts sustained Arrhythmic events in hypertrophic cardiomyopathy," *Canadian Journal of Cardiology*, vol. 29, no. 3, pp. 358–363, 2013.

[54] C. Prinz, F. van Buuren, L. Faber et al., "In patients with hypertrophic cardiomyopathy myocardial fibrosis is associated with both left ventricular and left atrial dysfunction," *Acta Cardiologica*, vol. 67, no. 2, pp. 187–193, 2012.

[55] C. Prinz, F. van Buuren, L. Faber et al., "Myocardial fibrosis is associated with biventricular dysfunction in patients with hypertrophic cardiomyopathy," *Echocardiography*, vol. 29, no. 4, pp. 438–444, 2012.

[56] C. Prinz, D. Hering, T. Bitter, D. Horstkotte, and L. Faber, "Left atrial size and left ventricular hypertrophy correlate with myocardial fibrosis in patients with hypertrophic cardiomyopathy," *Acta Cardiologica*, vol. 66, no. 2, pp. 153–157, 2011.

[57] C. Prinz, M. Farr, K. T. Laser et al., "Determining the role of fibrosis in hypertrophic cardiomyopathy," *Expert Review of Cardiovascular Therapy*, vol. 11, no. 4, pp. 495–504, 2013.

[58] F. Cecchi, I. Olivotto, R. Gistri, R. Lorenzoni, G. Chiriatti, and P. G. Camici, "Coronary microvascular dysfunction and prognosis in hypertrophic cardiomyopathy," *The New England Journal of Medicine*, vol. 349, no. 11, pp. 1027–1035, 2003.

[59] C. Basso, G. Thiene, D. Corrado, G. Buja, P. Melacini, and A. Nava, "Hypertrophic cardiomyopathy and sudden death in the young: pathologic evidence of myocardial ischemia," *Human Pathology*, vol. 31, no. 8, pp. 988–998, 2000.

[60] C. Prinz, L. Faber, D. Horstkotte et al., "Evaluation of left ventricular torsion in children with hypertrophic cardiomyopathy," *Cardiology in the Young*, vol. 6, pp. 1–8, 2013.

[61] B. J. Maron and A. Pelliccia, "The heart of trained athletes: cardiac remodeling and the risks of sports, including sudden death," *Circulation*, vol. 114, no. 15, pp. 1633–1644, 2006.

[62] D. Corrado, C. Basso, A. Pavei, P. Michieli, M. Schiavon, and G. Thiene, "Trends in sudden cardiovascular death in young competitive athletes after implementation of a preparticipation screening program," *Journal of the American Medical Association*, vol. 296, no. 13, pp. 1593–1601, 2006.

[63] B. J. Maron, "The electrocardiogram as a diagnostic tool for hypertrophic cardiomyopathy: revisited," *Annals of Noninvasive Electrocardiology*, vol. 6, no. 4, pp. 277–279, 2001.

[64] J. A. Decker, J. W. Rossano, E. O. Smith et al., "Risk factors and mode of death in isolated hypertrophic cardiomyopathy in children," *Journal of the American College of Cardiology*, vol. 54, no. 3, pp. 250–254, 2009.

[65] T. Germans, A. A. M. Wilde, P. A. Dijkmans et al., "Structural abnormalities of the inferoseptal left ventricular wall detected by cardiac magnetic resonance imaging in carriers of hypertrophic cardiomyopathy mutations," *Journal of the American College of Cardiology*, vol. 48, no. 12, pp. 2518–2523, 2006.

[66] T. Butz, F. van Buuren, K. P. Mellwig et al., "Two-dimensional strain analysis of the global and regional myocardial function for the differentiation of pathologic and physiologic left ventricular hypertrophy: a study in athletes and in patients with hypertrophic cardiomyopathy," *International Journal of Cardiovascular Imaging*, vol. 27, no. 1, pp. 91–100, 2011.

[67] R. Chan, B. J. Maron, I. Olivotto, G. Assienza, S. Hong, and J. Lesser, "Prognostic utility of contrast-enhanced cardiovascular magnetic resonance in hypertrophic cardiomyopathy: an international multicenter study," *Journal of the American College of Cardiology*, vol. 59, no. 13, p. E1570, 2012.

[68] L. Faber, C. Prinz, D. Welge et al., "Peak systolic longitudinal strain of the lateral left ventricular wall improves after septal ablation for symptomatic hypertrophic obstructive cardiomyopathy: a follow-up study using speckle tracking echocardiography," *International Journal of Cardiovascular Imaging*, vol. 27, no. 3, pp. 325–333, 2011.

[69] W. Mazur, S. F. Nagueh, N. M. Lakkis et al., "Regression of left ventricular hypertrophy after nonsurgical septal reduction therapy for hypertrophic obstructive cardiomyopathy," *Circulation*, vol. 103, no. 11, pp. 1492–1496, 2001.

[70] Z. Dimitriadis, F. van Buuren, N. Bogunovic, D. Horstkotte, and L. Faber, "Marked regression of left ventricular hypertrophy after outflow desobliteration in HOCM," *Case Reports in Medicine*, vol. 2012, Article ID 546942, 2 pages, 2012.

[71] A. Pelliccia, R. Fagard, H. H. Bjørnstad et al., "Recommendations for competitive sports participation in athletes with cardiovascular disease: a consensus document from the Study Group of Sports Cardiology of the Working Group of Cardiac Rehabilitation and Exercise Physiology and the Working Group of Myocardial and Pericardial Diseases of the European Society of Cardiology," *European Heart Journal*, vol. 26, no. 14, pp. 1422–1445, 2005.

[72] R. Paz, R. Jortner, P. A. Tunick et al., "The effect of the ingestion of ethanol on obstruction of the left ventricular outflow tract in hypertrophic cardiomyopathy," *The New England Journal of Medicine*, vol. 335, no. 13, pp. 938–941, 1996.

[73] P. Spirito, C. Rapezzi, P. Bellone et al., "Infective endocarditis in hypertrophic cardiomyopathy: prevalence, incidence, and indications for antibiotic prophylaxis," *Circulation*, vol. 99, no. 16, pp. 2132–2137, 1999.

[74] B. J. Maron, W.-K. Shen, M. S. Link et al., "Efficacy of implantable cardioverter-defibrillators for the prevention of sudden death in patients with hypertrophic cardiomyopathy," *The New England Journal of Medicine*, vol. 342, no. 6, pp. 365–373, 2000.

[75] B. J. Maron, P. Spirito, W.-K. Shen et al., "Implantable cardioverter-defibrillators and prevention of sudden cardiac death in hypertrophic cardiomyopathy," *Journal of the American Medical Association*, vol. 298, no. 4, pp. 405–412, 2007.

[76] B. J. Maron, M. S. Maron, J. R. Lesser et al., "Sudden cardiac arrest in hypertrophic cardiomyopathy in the absence of conventional criteria for high risk status," *American Journal of Cardiology*, vol. 101, no. 4, pp. 544–547, 2008.

[77] B. J. Maron, C. Semsarian, W.-K. Shen et al., "Circadian patterns in the occurrence of malignant ventricular tachyarrhythmias triggering defibrillator interventions in patients with hypertrophic cardiomyopathy," *Heart Rhythm*, vol. 6, no. 5, pp. 599–602, 2009.

[78] P. Spirito, C. Autore, C. Rapezzi et al., "Syncope and risk of sudden death in hypertrophic cardiomyopathy," *Circulation*, vol. 119, no. 13, pp. 1703–1710, 2009.

[79] B. J. Maron, T. S. Haas, K. M. Shannon, A. K. Almquist, and J. S. Hodges, "Long-term survival after cardiac arrest in hypertrophic cardiomyopathy," *Heart Rhythm*, vol. 6, no. 7, pp. 993–997, 2009.

[80] B. J. Maron and P. Spirito, "Implantable defibrillators and prevention of sudden death in hypertrophic cardiomyopathy," *Journal of Cardiovascular Electrophysiology*, vol. 19, no. 10, pp. 1118–1126, 2008.

[81] L. Monserrat, P. M. Elliott, J. R. Gimeno, S. Sharma, M. Penas-Lado, and W. J. McKenna, "Non-sustained ventricular tachycardia in hypertrophic cardiomyopathy: an independent marker of sudden death risk in young patients," *Journal of the American College of Cardiology*, vol. 42, no. 5, pp. 873–879, 2003.

[82] A. S. Adabag, B. J. Maron, E. Appelbaum et al., "Occurrence and frequency of arrhythmias in hypertrophic cardiomyopathy in relation to delayed enhancement on cardiovascular magnetic resonance," *Journal of the American College of Cardiology*, vol. 51, no. 14, pp. 1369–1374, 2008.

[83] P. Melacini, B. J. Maron, F. Bobbo et al., "Evidence that pharmacological strategies lack efficacy for the prevention of sudden death in hypertrophic cardiomyopathy," *Heart*, vol. 93, no. 6, pp. 708–710, 2007.

[84] M. V. Sherrid, I. Barac, W. J. McKenna et al., "Multicenter study of the efficacy and safety of disopyramide in obstructive hypertrophic cardiomyopathy," *Journal of the American College of Cardiology*, vol. 45, no. 8, pp. 1251–1258, 2005.

[85] S. Nistri, I. Olivotto, M. S. Maron et al., "β blockers for prevention of exercise-induced left ventricular outflow tract obstruction in patients with hypertrophic cardiomyopathy," *American Journal of Cardiology*, vol. 110, no. 5, pp. 715–719, 2012.

[86] Y. J. Shimada, J. J. Passeri, A. L. Baggish et al., "Effects of losartan on left ventricular hypertrophy and fibrosis in patients with nonobstructive hypertrophic cardiomyopathy," *Journal of the American College of Cardiology: Heart Failure*, vol. 1, pp. 480–487, 2013.

[87] B. Heric, B. W. Lytle, D. P. Miller et al., "Surgical management of hypertrophic obstructive cardiomyopathy: early and late results," *Journal of Thoracic and Cardiovascular Surgery*, vol. 110, no. 1, pp. 195–208, 1995.

[88] R. C. Robbins, E. B. Stinson, and P. O. Daily, "Long-term results of left ventricular myotomy and myectomy for obstructive hypertrophic cardiomyopathy," *Journal of Thoracic and Cardiovascular Surgery*, vol. 111, no. 3, pp. 586–594, 1996.

[89] H. D. Schulte, H. Gramsch-Zabel, and B. Schwartzkopff, "Hypertrophische obstruktive Kardiomyopathie: chirurgische Behandlung," *Schweizerische Medizinische Wochenschrift*, vol. 125, pp. 1940–1949, 1995.

[90] H. D. Schulte, W. Bircks, and B. Lösse, "Techniques and complications of transaortic subvalvular myectomy in patients with hypertrophic obstructive cardiomyopathy (HOCM)," *Zeitschrift fur Kardiologie*, vol. 76, no. 3, pp. 145–151, 1987.

[91] A. G. Morrow, B. A. Reitz, S. E. Epstein et al., "Operative treatment in hypertrophic subaortic stenosis. Techniques, and the results of pre and postoperative assessments in 83 patients," *Circulation*, vol. 52, no. 1, pp. 88–102, 1975.

[92] R. B. McCully, R. A. Nishimura, A. J. Tajik, H. V. Schaff, and G. K. Danielson, "Extent of clinical improvement after surgical treatment of hypertrophic obstructive cardiomyopathy," *Circulation*, vol. 94, no. 3, pp. 467–471, 1996.

[93] N. G. Smedira, B. W. Lytle, H. M. Lever et al., "Current effectiveness and risks of isolated septal myectomy for hypertrophic obstructive cardiomyopathy," *Annals of Thoracic Surgery*, vol. 85, no. 1, pp. 127–133, 2008.

[94] S. R. Ommen, B. J. Maron, I. Olivotto et al., "Long-term effects of surgical septal myectomy on survival in patients with obstructive hypertrophic cardiomyopathy," *Journal of the American College of Cardiology*, vol. 46, no. 3, pp. 470–476, 2005.

[95] A. G. Morrow and E. C. Brockenbrough, "Surgical treatment of idiopathic hypertrophic subaortic stenosis: technic and hemodynamic results of subaortic ventriculomyotomy," *Annals of Surgery*, vol. 154, pp. 181–189, 1961.

[96] A. Woo, W. G. Williams, R. Choi et al., "Clinical and echocardiographic determinants of long-term survival after surgical myectomy in obstructive hypertrophic cardiomyopathy," *Circulation*, vol. 111, no. 16, pp. 2033–2041, 2005.

[97] W. Ball, J. Ivanov, H. Rakowski et al., "Long-term survival in patients with resting obstructive hypertrophic cardiomyopathy: comparison of conservative versus invasive treatment," *Journal of the American College of Cardiology*, vol. 58, no. 22, pp. 2313–2321, 2011.

[98] B. J. Maron, R. A. Nishimura, W. J. McKenna, H. Rakowski, M. E. Josephson, and R. S. Kieval, "Assessment of permanent dual-chamber pacing as a treatment for drug-refractory symptomatic patients with obstructive hypertrophic cardiomyopathy: a randomized, double-blind, crossover study (M-PATHY)," *Circulation*, vol. 99, no. 22, pp. 2927–2933, 1999.

[99] U. Sigwart, "Non-surgical myocardial reduction for hypertrophic obstructive cardiomyopathy," *The Lancet*, vol. 346, no. 8969, pp. 211–214, 1995.

[100] U. Sigwart, M. Grbic, J. J. Goy et al., "Left ventricular function after revascularization for coronary occlusion lasting 1-2 hours," *Schweizerische Medizinische Wochenschrift*, vol. 113, no. 45, pp. 1661–1664, 1983.

[101] P. Brugada, H. De Swart, J. L. R. M. Smeets, and H. J. J. Wellens, "Transcoronary chemical ablation of ventricular tachycardia," *Circulation*, vol. 79, no. 3, pp. 475–82, 1989.

[102] F. Gietzen, C. Leuner, T. Gerenkamp, and H. Kuhn, "Relief of obstruction in hypertrophic cardiomyopathy by transient

occlusion of the first septal branch of the left coronary artery," *European Heart Journal*, vol. 15, pp. 125–126, 1994.

[103] H. Kuhn, F. Gietzen, C. Leuner, and T. Gerenkamp, "Induction of subaortic septal ischaemia to reduce obstruction in hypertrophic obstructive cardiomyopathy," *European Heart Journal*, vol. 18, no. 5, pp. 846–851, 1997.

[104] G. Berghöfer, Einfluß der Septumperfusion auf die Obstruktion der linksventrikulären Ausflußbahn bei HOCM (personal communication in 1998), 1989.

[105] E. Braunwald, "Induced septal infarction: a new therapeutic strategy for hypertrophic obstructive cardiomyopathy," *Circulation*, vol. 95, no. 8, pp. 1981–1982, 1997.

[106] P. Boekstegers, P. Steinbigler, A. Molnar et al., "Pressure-guided nonsurgical myocardial reduction induced by small septal infarctions in hypertrophic obstructive cardiomyopathy," *Journal of the American College of Cardiology*, vol. 38, no. 3, pp. 846–853, 2001.

[107] S. M. Chang, N. M. Lakkis, J. Franklin, W. H. Spencer III, and S. F. Nagueh, "Predictors of outcome after alcohol septal ablation therapy in patients with hypertrophic obstructive cardiomyopathy," *Circulation*, vol. 109, no. 7, pp. 824–827, 2004.

[108] L. Faber, H. Seggewiss, and U. Gleichmann, "Percutaneous transluminal septal myocardial ablation in hypertrophic obstructive cardiomyopathy: results with respect to intraprocedural myocardial contrast echocardiography," *Circulation*, vol. 98, no. 22, pp. 2415–2421, 1998.

[109] L. Faber, P. Ziemssen, and H. Seggewiss, "Targeting percutaneous transluminal septal ablation for hypertrophic obstructive cardiomyopathy by intraprocedural echocardiographic monitoring," *Journal of the American Society of Echocardiography*, vol. 13, no. 12, pp. 1074–1079, 2000.

[110] L. Faber, A. Meissner, P. Ziemssen, and H. Seggewiss, "Percutaneous transluminal septal myocardial ablation for hypertrophic obstructive cardiomyopathy: long term follow up of the first series of 25 patients," *Heart*, vol. 83, no. 3, pp. 326–331, 2000.

[111] R. Flores-Ramirez, N. M. Lakkis, K. J. Middleton, D. Killip, W. H. Spencer III, and S. F. Nagueh, "Echocardiographic insights into the mechanisms of relief of left ventricular outflow tract obstruction after nonsurgical septal reduction therapy in patients with hypertrophic obstructive cardiomyopathy," *Journal of the American College of Cardiology*, vol. 37, no. 1, pp. 208–214, 2001.

[112] F. H. Gietzen, C. J. Leuner, U. Raute-Kreinsen et al., "Acute and long-term results after transcoronary ablation of septal hypertrophy (TASH)," *European Heart Journal*, vol. 20, no. 18, pp. 1342–1354, 1999.

[113] C. Knight, A. S. Kurbaan, H. Seggewiss et al., "Nonsurgical septal reduction for hypertrophic obstructive cardiomyopathy: outcome in the first series of patients," *Circulation*, vol. 95, no. 8, pp. 2075–2081, 1997.

[114] H. Kuhn, H. Seggewiss, F. H. Gietzen, P. Boekstegers, L. Neuhaus, and L. Seipel, "Catheter-based therapy for hypertrophic obstructive cardiomyopathy: first in-hospital outcome analysis of the German TASH Registry," *Zeitschrift fur Kardiologie*, vol. 93, no. 1, pp. 23–31, 2004.

[115] L. Faber, H. Seggewiss, F. H. Gietzen et al., "Catheter-based septalablation for symptomatic hypertrophic obstructive cardiomyopathy: follow-up results of the TASH-registry of the German Cardiac Society," *Zeitschrift fur Kardiologie*, vol. 94, no. 8, pp. 516–523, 2005.

[116] N. M. Lakkis, S. F. Nagueh, N. S. Kleiman et al., "Echocardiography-guided ethanol septal reduction for hypertrophic obstructive cardiomyopathy," *Circulation*, vol. 98, no. 17, pp. 1750–1755, 1998.

[117] J. X. Qin, T. Shiota, H. M. Lever et al., "Conduction system abnormalities in patients with obstructive hypertrophic cardiomyopathy following septal reduction interventions," *American Journal of Cardiology*, vol. 93, no. 2, pp. 171–175, 2004.

[118] J. Xin, T. Shiota, H. M. Lever et al., "Outcome of patients with hypertrophic obstructive cardiomyopathy after percutaneous transluminal septal myocardial ablation and septal myectomy surgery," *Journal of the American College of Cardiology*, vol. 38, no. 7, pp. 1994–2000, 2001.

[119] H. Seggewiss, U. Gleichmann, L. Faber, D. Fassbender, H. K. Schmidt, and S. Strick, "Percutaneous transluminal septal myocardial ablation in hypertrophic obstructive cardiomyopathy: acute results and 3-month follow-up in 25 patients," *Journal of the American College of Cardiology*, vol. 31, no. 2, pp. 252–258, 1998.

[120] H. Seggewiss, "Current status of alcohol septal ablation for patients with hypertrophic cardiomyopathy," *Current Cardiology Reports*, vol. 3, no. 2, pp. 160–166, 2001.

[121] U. S. Valeti, R. A. Nishimura, D. R. Holmes et al., "Comparison of surgical septal myectomy and alcohol septal ablation with cardiac magnetic resonance imaging in patients with hypertrophic obstructive cardiomyopathy," *Journal of the American College of Cardiology*, vol. 49, no. 3, pp. 350–357, 2007.

[122] S. Agarwal, E. M. Tuzcu, M. Y. Desai et al., "Updated meta-analysis of septal alcohol ablation versus myectomy for hypertrophic cardiomyopathy," *Journal of the American College of Cardiology*, vol. 55, no. 8, pp. 823–834, 2010.

[123] P. A. Noseworthy, M. A. Rosenberg, M. A. Fifer et al., "Ventricular arrhythmia following alcohol septal ablation for obstructive hypertrophic cardiomyopathy," *American Journal of Cardiology*, vol. 104, no. 1, pp. 128–132, 2009.

[124] S. Firoozi, P. M. Elliott, S. Sharma et al., "Septal myotomy-myectomy and transcoronary septal alcohol ablation in hypertrophic obstructive cardiomyopathy: a comparison of clinical, haemodynamic and exercise outcomes," *European Heart Journal*, vol. 23, no. 20, pp. 1617–1624, 2002.

[125] P. Sorajja, U. Valeti, R. A. Nishimura et al., "Outcome of alcohol septal ablation for obstructive hypertrophic cardiomyopathy," *Circulation*, vol. 118, no. 2, pp. 131–139, 2008.

[126] F. A. Cuoco, W. H. Spencer III, V. L. Fernandes et al., "Implantable cardioverter-defibrillator therapy for primary prevention of sudden death after alcohol septal ablation of hypertrophic cardiomyopathy," *Journal of the American College of Cardiology*, vol. 52, no. 21, pp. 1718–1723, 2008.

[127] S. F. Nagueh, B. M. Groves, L. Schwartz et al., "Alcohol septal ablation for the treatment of hypertrophic obstructive cardiomyopathy: a multicenter north american registry," *Journal of the American College of Cardiology*, vol. 58, no. 22, pp. 2322–2328, 2011.

[128] C. Prinz, J. Vogt, B. G. Muntean, D. Hering, D. Horstkotte, and L. Faber, "Incidence of adequate ICD interventions in patients with hypertrophic cardiomyopathy supposed to be at high risk for sudden cardiac death," *Acta Cardiologica*, vol. 65, no. 5, pp. 521–525, 2010.

[129] L. Faber, D. Welge, D. Hering et al., "Percutaneous septal ablation after unsuccessful surgical myectomy for patients with hypertrophic obstructive cardiomyopathy," *Clinical Research in Cardiology*, vol. 97, no. 12, pp. 899–905, 2008.

[130] L. Faber, D. Welge, D. Fassbender, H. K. Schmidt, D. Horstkotte, and H. Seggewiss, "One-year follow-up of percutaneous septal

ablation for symptomatic hypertrophic obstructive cardiomyopathy in 312 patients: predictors of hemodynamic and clinical response," *Clinical Research in Cardiology*, vol. 96, no. 12, pp. 864–873, 2007.

[131] M. K. Jensen, C. Prinz, D. Horstkotte et al., "Alcohol septal ablation in patients with hypertrophic obstructive cardiomyopathy: low incidence of sudden cardiac death and reduced risk profile," *Heart*, vol. 99, pp. 1012–1017, 2013.

[132] M. Alam, H. Dokainish, and N. Lakkis, "Alcohol septal ablation for hypertrophic obstructive cardiomyopathy: a systematic review of published studies," *Journal of Interventional Cardiology*, vol. 19, no. 4, pp. 319–327, 2006.

[133] V. L. Fernandes, C. Nielsen, S. F. Nagueh et al., "Follow-Up of Alcohol Septal Ablation for Symptomatic Hypertrophic Obstructive Cardiomyopathy. The Baylor and Medical University of South Carolina Experience 1996 to 2007," *JACC: Cardiovascular Interventions*, vol. 1, no. 5, pp. 561–570, 2008.

[134] P. Sorajja, S. R. Ommen, D. R. Holmes Jr et al., "Survival after alcohol septal ablation for obstructive hypertrophic cardiomyopathy," *Circulation*, vol. 126, pp. 2374–2380, 2012.

[135] A. A. Chen, I. F. Palacios, T. Mela et al., "Acute predictors of subacute complete heart block after alcohol septal ablation for obstructive hypertrophic cardiomyopathy," *American Journal of Cardiology*, vol. 97, no. 2, pp. 264–269, 2006.

[136] T. Lawrenz, F. Lieder, M. Bartelsmeier et al., "Predictors of complete heart block after transcoronary ablation of septal hypertrophy: results of a prospective electrophysiological investigation in 172 patients with hypertrophic obstructive cardiomyopathy," *Journal of the American College of Cardiology*, vol. 49, no. 24, pp. 2356–2363, 2007.

[137] F. J. Ten Cate, O. I. I. Soliman, M. Michels et al., "Long-term outcome of alcohol septal ablation in patients with obstructive hypertrophic cardiomyopathy: a word of caution," *Circulation: Heart Failure*, vol. 3, no. 3, pp. 362–369, 2010.

[138] M. A. Fifer, "Most fully informed patients choose septal ablation over septal myectomy," *Circulation*, vol. 116, no. 2, pp. 207–216, 2007.

[139] T. Lawrenz, B. Borchert, C. Leuner et al., "Endocardial radiofrequency ablation for hypertrophic obstructive cardiomyopathy: acute results and 6 months' follow-up in 19 patients," *Journal of the American College of Cardiology*, vol. 57, no. 5, pp. 572–576, 2011.

[140] A. Oto, K. Aytemir, S. Okutucu et al., "Cyanoacrylate for septal ablation in hypertrophic cardiomyopathy," *Journal of Interventional Cardiology*, vol. 24, no. 1, pp. 77–84, 2011.

7

Control of Pedicle Screw Placement with an Electrical Conductivity Measurement Device: Initial Evaluation in the Thoracic and Lumbar Spine

Olaf Suess[1,2] **and Markus Schomacher**[2,3]

[1]*DRK Kliniken Berlin Westend, Zentrum für Wirbelsäulenchirurgie und Neurotraumatologie, Berlin, Germany*
[2]*Department of Neurosurgery, Charité University Hospital, Berlin, Germany*
[3]*Vivantes Klinikum am Friedrichshain, Neurochirurgische Klinik, Berlin, Germany*

Correspondence should be addressed to Olaf Suess; o.suess@drk-kliniken-berlin.de

Academic Editor: Hassan Serhan

Aim. Transpedicular screw fixation is widely used in spinal surgery. But the insertion of pedicle screws can sometimes be challenging because of the variability in pedicle size and the proximity of nerve roots. *Methods.* We detected intraoperatively the sensitivity for iatrogenic pedicel perforation with a hand-held electronic conductivity measurement device (ECD) that measures electrical conductivity of tissue-medium surrounding the instrument tip. ECD was used to guide the placement of 84 pedicle screws in 15 patients undergoing surgery for tumor or degenerative spinal disease at various spinal levels from T8 to L5. Additionally a CT-scan controlled screw positioning postoperatively. *Results.* The placement was "correct" (no mediocaudal pedicle wall penetration) for 78 of 84 (92,8%) screws, "suboptimal but acceptable" (0–2 mm penetration) for 4 of 84 (4,8%) screws, and "misplaced" (penetration > 2 mm) for 2 of 84 (2,4%) screws. *Conclusion.* Although this study was not designed to compare electronic conductivity technique to other guidance methods, such as fluoroscopy or navigation, a convincing "proof of concept" for ECD use in spinal instrumentation could be demonstrated. Advantages include easy handling without time-consuming setup and reduced X-ray exposure. However, further investigations are necessary to evaluate i.a. the economic aspects for this single-use developed instrument.

1. Introduction

Transpedicular screw placement in the vertebra during posterior operations to stabilize the spine is currently the most widely used and successful technique to treat pathological changes of the spine caused by trauma, tumor, scoliosis, or degenerative diseases [1–5]. But correctly placing the pedicle screw in this operative technique can sometimes be challenging for the surgeon, due to variation in pedicle size and thickness at the various spinal levels and also due to the proximity to the nerve roots [6, 7]. Misplacement of the pedicle screws can cause damage to the dural sac or the exiting nerve roots if the pedicle wall is broken mediocaudally [8–11] (Figure 1).

Currently, various methods are used to attain the most correct pedicle screw placement possible. Among the mechanical aids, there is the possibility of probing the pedicle canal and inserting the pedicle screw by means of a guidewire [7, 12]. Among the imaging techniques, there is the controlled insertion of the pedicle screw during fluoroscopy or the use of computer tomography (CT) or other computer-supported navigation procedures [13–17]. But the use of intraoperative fluoroscopy can expose both the patient and the OR personnel to excessive radiation. Computer-supported navigation requires additional preoperative CT imaging, longer planning time, and more experience of the surgeon in the usage of navigation software and navigation-supported instrumentation [16]. Electrophysiological monitoring techniques, such as measuring motor evoked potentials (MEP) or electromyographic potentials (EMG), can be used to detect affections of the spinal nerves after insertion of the pedicle screw [18–21]. But sometimes, damage due to a misplaced

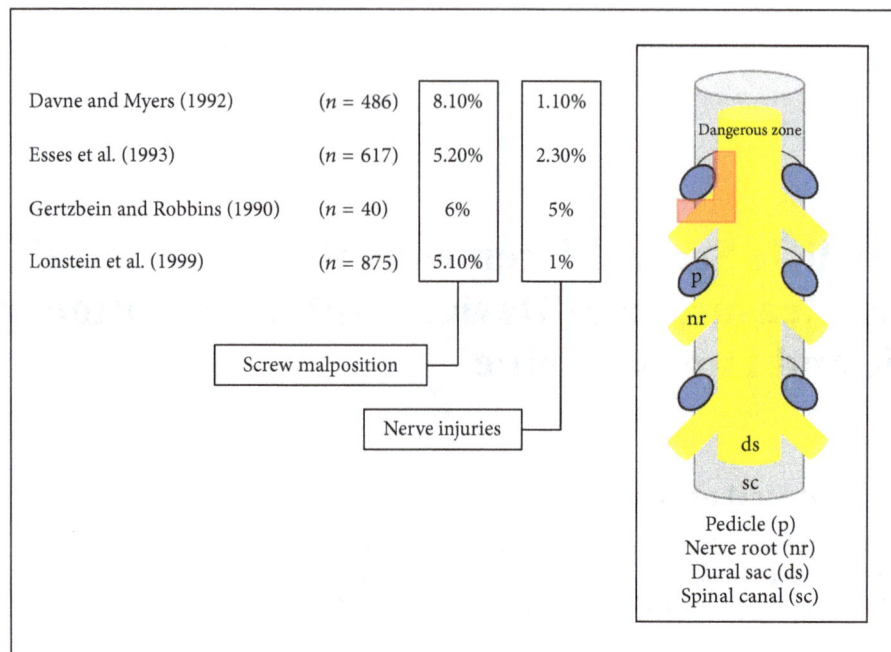

Davne and Myers (1992)	($n = 486$)	8.10%	1.10%
Esses et al. (1993)	($n = 617$)	5.20%	2.30%
Gertzbein and Robbins (1990)	($n = 40$)	6%	5%
Lonstein et al. (1999)	($n = 875$)	5.10%	1%

Screw malposition

Nerve injuries

Dangerous zone

p

nr

ds

sc

Pedicle (p)
Nerve root (nr)
Dural sac (ds)
Spinal canal (sc)

FIGURE 1: Illustration of the proximity of nerve root and dural sac to the pedicle. Misplacement of pedicle screws can cause damage to the dural sac or the exiting nerve roots if the pedicle wall is broken mediocaudally (dangerous zone). Modified figure published in PediGuard™ booklet (SpineVision, Paris, France).

pedicle screw can only be detected after dural or nerve root damage already occurred [22]. Also, they require additional qualified personnel [20].

Currently, an electrical impedance and conductivity measurement device was developed to improve the accuracy of pedicle screw placement. The probe-shaped tool can be used as a mechanical tool for the preparation of a lead canal for the insertion of the pedicle screw. It furthermore measures the electrical conductivity in the surrounding tissue, which changes depending on the tissue type, as shown in earlier animal and clinical feasibility studies [23–26]. These changes in conductivity are then communicated to the surgeon by light and sound signals, enabling the user to better understand the patient's spinal anatomy and to detect iatrogenic pedicle perforations prior to inserting the screw. In initial reports, this implement has demonstrated a high sensitivity (98%) and specificity (99%) for recognizing perforations of the cortex during pedicle screw placement [23–25]. On the other hand, it can be used for intraoperative electromyographic (EMG) monitoring through induction of a small electrical current on the surrounding tissue and nerve, during the localization and evaluation of spinal nerves and nerve roots.

This paper reports on our initial experience with this device in severe degenerative disease and spinal tumor surgery.

2. Methods

2.1. Device. The electrical conductivity device PediGuard (ECD) (SpineVision, Paris, France) comes in three sizes (diameter × length in mm): 2.5 × 40, 3.2 × 45, and 4.0 × 44

(Figure 2), all of which can be used depending on the patient anatomy and level of segment. It is designed as a free-hand pedicle probe. The instrument tip serves as a bipolar electrode, which detects every 0.5 sec the changes of impedance/electrical conductivity in the surrounding tissue, due to changes of the electromagnetic field (Figure 3). These electromagnetic changes are transformed into audio and visual signals via an electronic switching circuit that is housed in the handle. For signaling there is both a speaker housed in the handle for indicating low or high frequency tones in various rhythms and also a two-color LED (green and yellow). A middle tone pitch and medium light frequency of the green LED are produced during the positioning of the instrument tip in the bone. During contact of the instrument tip with the cortex, a drop of the tone pitch and a decrease of the light frequency of the green LED occur, letting the surgeon know that the instrument tip is still in contact with bone tissue. If the cortex is broken through and the tip enters into surrounding soft tissue, a high pitch tone occurs and the green LED reaches a high light frequency, as a warning signal for the surgeon. Illumination of the yellow LED signals a malfunctioning in the measurement system.

2.2. Patients. The ECD was used to place a total of 84 polyaxial screws into 15 patients. The procedures were performed between October 2008 and October 2011. There were 6 male and 9 female patients with a mean age of 61 years (41–83 y). Patients with cardiac pacemakers and severe osteoporosis were excluded from participation according to the manufacturer's recommendations. In 8/15 patients a degenerative disease with DDD, spinal canal stenosis, and

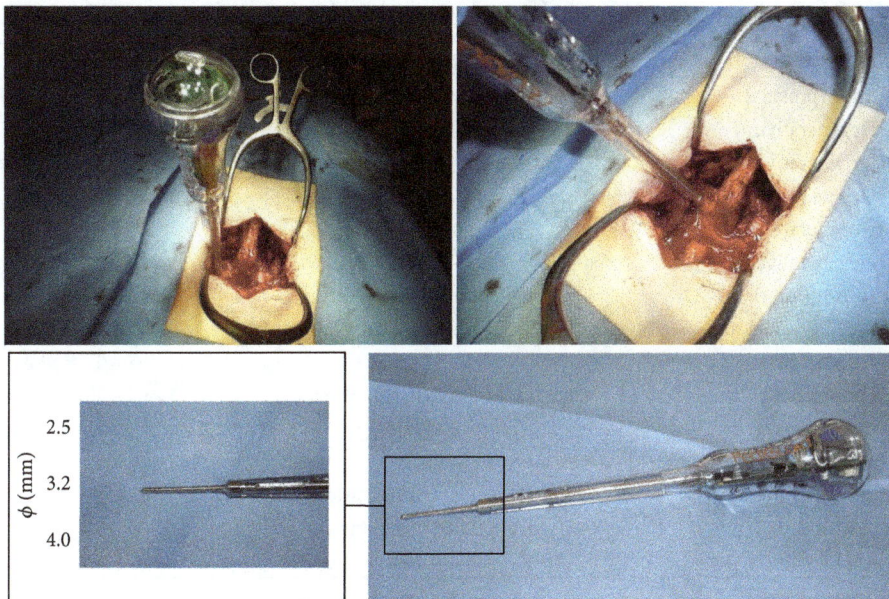

FIGURE 2: Pictures of intraoperative application in a case of lumbar spine surgery of the electrical conductivity device PediGuard (ECD) (SpineVision, Paris, France). The tip of the device comes in three sizes (diameter × length in mm): 2.5 × 40, 3.2 × 45, and 4.0 × 44.

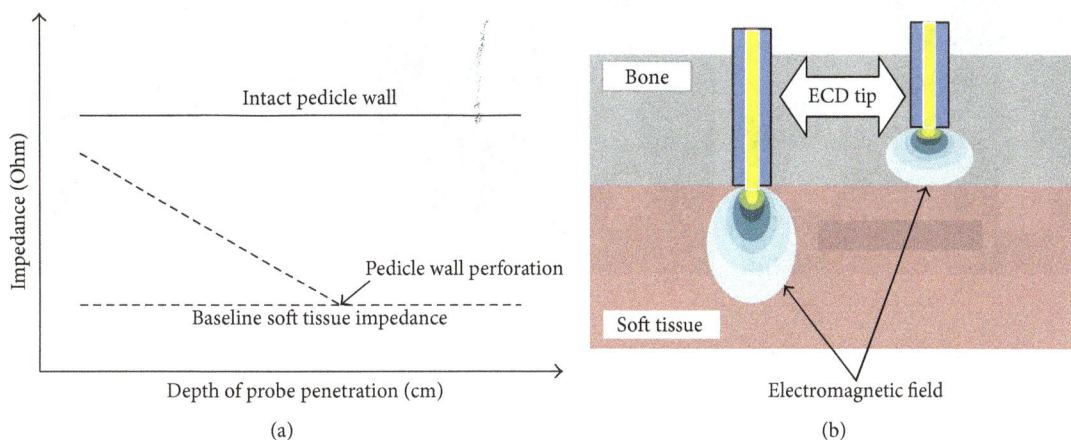

FIGURE 3: (a) Characteristics of the course of probe tip impedance values versus depth of pedicle penetration in an intact pedicle and one with pedicle wall perforation. The impedance values in the intact pedicle remain still above the soft tissue impedance while in perforated pedicle values drop down under the baseline of soft tissue impedance. Modified figure from published version in [22]. (b) Illustration of the electromagnetic field in two media with different electrical conductivity. In bone structure with low electrical conductivity the electromagnetic field is concentrated around the probe tip, whereas in soft tissue with higher electrical conductivity the electromagnetic field around the probe tip is spread out. Modified figure published in PediGuard booklet (SpineVision, Paris, France).

spondylolisthesis was the indication for dorsal instrumentation with a screw/rod system. In the other 7/15 cases a metastatic tumor of the spine (3x adenocarcinoma of the lung, 2x mamma carcinoma, 1x prostate carcinoma, and 1x hypopharynx carcinoma) was operated on. There were 7 single-level and 8 multilevel procedures (Table 1).

2.3. Surgical Procedure. The instrument set was used for dorsal transpedicular stabilization operations on the thoracic and lumbar spine. The access to the vertebrae was in all cases via a dorsal midline access. The facet joints were prepared and an insertion canal was made with the ECD. Polyaxial

screws (XIA, Stryker, USA, and Legacy, Medtronic, USA) with a diameter of 5.5 mm (thoracic) or 6.5 mm (lumbar) and a length of 30–50 mm were placed into the vertebral bodies according to the trajectory given by the ECD. Postoperatively, CT imaging of the spine (1 mm reconstructed slices, 0.7 mm increment, Kernel H70) was used to evaluate the positioning of the pedicle screw (Figure 4).

2.4. Data Evaluation. The placement of the pedicle screws on postoperative CT was evaluated by an independent radiologist and graded into three levels: (a) correct, (b) suboptimal (but acceptable), or (c) misplaced (Figure 4). The position of

TABLE 1: Indication for surgery, surgical procedure, number of screws, and segments operated on.

#	Indication	Procedure	Screws	Segments
1	Tumor (prostate)	Dorsal instrumentation	8	T8–L1
2	Degenerative	PLIF	4	L3-L4
3	Degenerative	PLIF	4	L4-L5
4	Degenerative	PLIF	6	L3–L5
5	Degenerative	PLIF	4	L4-L5
6	Degenerative	PLIF	4	L3-L4
7	Tumor (lung)	Dorsal instrumentation	4	T11–L1
8	Tumor (hypopharynx)	Dorsal instrumentation	8	T11–L4
9	Degenerative	TLIF	6	L2–L4
10	Tumor (lung)	Dorsal instrumentation	8	T8–T12
11	Degenerative	TLIF	4	L4-L5
12	Degenerative	PLIF	6	L3–L5
13	Tumor (mamma)	Dorsal instrumentation	8	T10–L2
14	Tumor (lung)	Dorsal instrumentation	6	T11–L2
15	Tumor (mamma)	Dorsal instrumentation	4	T8-T9

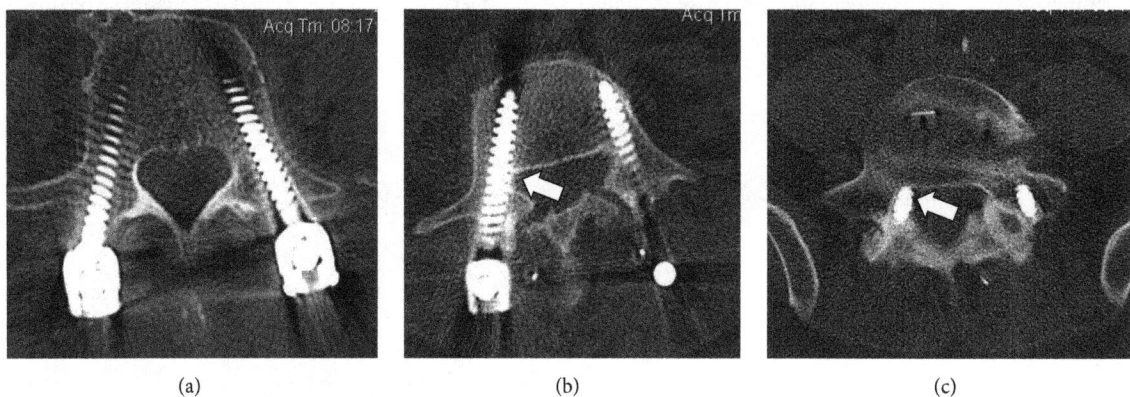

(a) (b) (c)

FIGURE 4: Examples of pedicle screw placement on postoperative CT imaging: (a) "correct" (no mediocaudal pedicle wall penetration), (b) "suboptimal but acceptable" (0–2 mm penetration), and (c) "misplaced" (penetration > 2 mm).

the pedicle screw was rated as "correct" when no screwthread penetration through the mediocaudal pedicle wall could be seen on the postoperative CT (1 mm slice thickness). The position was "suboptimal" (but acceptable) when the screwthread penetrated the pedicle wall less than 2 mm. The position was rated "misplaced" when the pedicle wall was penetrated 2 mm or more by the screwthread [7, 12].

3. Results

Thirty-eight screws (38/84; 45,2%) were placed during posterior instrumented fusion (PLIF) for spondylolisthesis, while the other 46/84 (54,8%) were placed during dorsal instrumentation for spinal tumor (Table 1).

The signal remained constant, while the ECD was advanced forward through the pedicle into the vertebral body in 72/84 (85.7%) pedicle sites. In the other 12/84 (14.3%) sites, sound and LED signals warned for variation in the measured conductivity as a sign for possible pedicle wall penetration.

In these cases, the ECD was slightly moved backwards and redirected in another trajectory through the pedicle until no further warning signal occurred.

The screw placement was graded as "correct" for 78 of 84 (92,8%) screws and "suboptimal" for 4 of 84 screws (4,8%). Hence, 97,6% of the screws were satisfactorily placed, whereas 2 of 84 (2,4%) screws had to be graded "misplaced" (Table 2). In levels T8–T12 5.5 mm polyaxial screws were placed. For these cases the ECD with the 3.2 mm tip was used. Three out of the 32 thoracic screws were suboptimally placed with medial wall penetration of 1 mm and another T9 screw showed 2.5 mm misplacement. In levels L1–L5 6.5 mm polyaxial screws were placed. For these cases the ECD with the 4.0 mm tip was used. Two out of 52 lumbar screws were either suboptimally placed (1x at L4, Figure 4(b)) or misplaced (1x at L5, Figure 4(c)). The "misplaced" screw had a 2.5 mm breakthrough at the medial L5 pedicle wall without direct contact to the transversing nerve root. There was no clinical sign of radiculopathy immediately after surgery or on the 6- and 12-month follow-up examinations. No revision

TABLE 2: Screw placements.

Level	Correct	Suboptimal	Misplaced	Total
T8	5	1		6
T9	4	1	1	6
T10	1	1		2
T11	10			10
T12	8			8
L1	6			6
L2	6			6
L3	12			12
L4	17	1		18
L5	9		1	10
Total	78	4	2	84

surgery was necessary. There were no mechanical failures of the ECD itself during these 15 operations.

4. Discussion

The use of transpedicular screw systems during spinal surgery has become widespread [2, 4, 5, 27], yet the insertion of pedicle screws can sometimes be a challenge for the surgeon because of the variability of size, height, and position of the pedicle in the various pathologies of the spine and also because of the immediate vicinity to exiting nerves and vessels [4, 5, 28]. With the increasing use of this procedure, there is also a rise of the complications associated with transpedicular screw fixation [29]. The operating surgeon must be experienced, in order to avoid risks, lasting deficits, or even reoperation for the patient [8, 9, 30].

In this study, there was a high rate of correct placement of screws with the ECD (92,8%) and a low rate of misplaced screws (2,4%). This is consistent with previously published reports [23–25], as well as gray literature from conferences [26]. Although this is an entirely respectable rate of accuracy, it is only marginally better than the rates previously reported in level-one studies on other methods of pedicle screw placement. The definitive benchmark is a recent meta-analysis on over 37,000 pedicle screws from 130 different studies [31]. That meta-analysis reported that 91.3% of all pedicle screws were accurately placed, and a subgroup analysis of the navigation-assisted in vivo pedicle screws had an accuracy rate of 95.2%. Similarly, an even more recent but narrower meta-analysis on about 7500 screws reported an overall accurate insertion rate of 89.2% and CT-navigation-based accurate insertion rate of 90.8% [32]. Since these recent meta-analyses, a new study evaluated the placement of 150 pedicle screws at T1–T3 using 3D-image guidance; they reported rates of 93.3% correctly placed screws and 6.7% as breaching the pedicle wall by 0–2 mm [33]. A very recent study on 424 lumbosacral pedicle screws placed with conventional open technique and intraoperative fluoroscopy reported correct screw placement for 93.2% of screws, questionable cortical encroachment for 2.8%, penetration ≤ 2 mm for 0.6%, and penetration > 2 mm for 1.6%. They concluded that "the conventional technique [of pedicle screw placement] still remains a practical, safe,

and effective surgical method for lumbosacral fixation" [34]. Given our small sample size and the possible margin of errors, it cannot be concluded that ECD leads to a higher rate of accurate screw placement than conventional techniques, and indeed navigation-based screw placement appears to be slightly more accurate than ECD.

The present study has several important limitations that must be kept in mind. First, the study has no control group using other methods (such as fluoroscopy, navigation, or pure free-hand placement) as a basis for direct comparison. So we cannot draw any conclusions regarding improvement over conventional techniques. Thus, this study can only be regarded as a proof of concept for the electronic conductivity technique in spinal instrumentation. Second, the sample size is too small to serve as a conclusive evaluation, even if it had been designed as a randomized double-blind comparative study. Regrettably, it was not possible for us to enlarge the sample further. Third, the data were all from a single site; the rate of accuracy may be somewhat better or worse in the hands of other surgeons. Clinically, our initial experience was positive enough to warrant further investigation in carefully monitored research settings. We reemphasize the thought that this system has not yet undergone sufficient scientific evaluation for adoption into routine clinical practice (to our knowledge, randomized controlled multicenter studies are said to be initiated by the manufacturer but yet not published). Such RCTs have to prove that the ECD technology really improves patient safety in direct comparison to other conventional methods of pedicle screw placement.

Finally, we must comment on the cost of this device and associated design factors. The device cannot be reused for more than one operation—the outer casing of the device is made of a plastic, which makes it impossible to sterilize the instrument for reuse. The sound and light signals of the device are driven by a built-in internal battery that only lasts about 24 hours before dying out. In order to initially activate the battery, a paper-like tab on the side of the device must be pulled off. Once this paper-like tab is removed, the battery is active and running. There is no way to pause the battery from discharging. If the paper tab is accidentally removed before any operation is scheduled, the battery will die out anyway and the device would be useless. Furthermore, there is no way to open the device and replace the battery. Opening it up would require permanently breaking the plastic outer shell of the device, thus rendering it unusable. Moreover, the plastic shell has small airholes, so the user can hear the beeping tones from the speaker that is inside the handle. But consequently, blood or other patient fluids potentially carrying viruses can get inside the device through these sound-holes, thus contaminating the device so it cannot be safely reused on a second patient while the battery is still running. In the current era of dwindling healthcare budgets and limited resources for single-use instruments (e.g., in the DRG reimbursement system) one has to critically take this fact into consideration when deciding for such an "extra" tool. Even if this device later demonstrates a clinical benefit for patient health and safety (and not merely an increase in surrogate radiographic endpoints), rigorous health economic analyses are needed to determine whether it also has sufficient cost-benefit advantages. Potential ethnography endpoints for cost saving studies could include i.a. anesthetic case time and/or improved efficiency through lower instrument passes, leading to reduced overall operating time.

5. Conclusions

The general engineering concept of measuring electrical conductivity to improve the accuracy of pedicle screw placement appears, in our small initial clinical experience, to be a potentially useful method. The ECD safely allowed detection of changes in the electromagnetic field around the instrument tip as a warning signal for tissue with different consistency to bone. With careful handling, it even allows detection of cortical breaches before full penetration has occurred, giving the surgeon the chance to redirect the trajectory. Further advantages of this technique include easy handling without a time-consuming setup and no additional X-ray exposure. However, further studies should evaluate the advantages of the system in cost-comparison and clinical benefit, because in our viewpoint the economic inefficiency of a single-use product, which is otherwise quite promising, may limit the use in routine spinal surgery.

List of Abbreviations

CT: Computed tomography
DDD: Degenerative disc disease
DRG: Diagnosis related groups
ECD: Electronic conductivity device
EMG: Electromyography
LED: Light-emitting diode
$L(x)$: Lumbar spine level (x)
MEP: Motor evoked potential
mm: Millimeters
MRI: Magnetic resonance imaging
PLIF: Posterior lumbar interbody fusion
RCT: Randomized controlled trial
sec: Seconds
$T(x)$: Thoracic spine level (x).

Competing Interests

The authors declare that they have no competing interests.

Acknowledgments

The authors would like to thank Michael Hanna, PhD (Mercury Medical Research & Writing) for contributing to the revision and writing of the manuscript.

References

[1] L. Hackenberg, T. M. Link, and U. Liljenqvist, "Axial and tangential fixation strength of pedicle screws versus hooks in the thoracic spine in relation to bone mineral density," *Spine*, vol. 27, no. 9, pp. 937–942, 2002.

[2] P. X. Montesano, R. F. McLain, and D. R. Benson, "Spinal instrumentation in the management of vertebral column tumors," *Seminars in Orthopaedics*, vol. 6, no. 4, pp. 237–246, 1991.

[3] M. M. Panjabi, T. Oda, and J.-L. Wang, "The effects of pedicle screw adjustments on neural spaces in burst fracture surgery," *Spine*, vol. 25, no. 13, pp. 1637–1643, 2000.

[4] M. M. Panjabi, K. Takata, V. Goel et al., "Thoracic human vertebrae quantitative three-dimensional anatomy," *Spine*, vol. 16, no. 8, pp. 888–901, 1991.

[5] R. Xu, N. A. Ebraheim, Y. Ou, and R. A. Yeasting, "Anatomic considerations of pedicle screw placement in the thoracic spine: roy-camille technique versus open-lamina technique," *Spine*, vol. 23, no. 9, pp. 1065–1068, 1998.

[6] R. A. Hart, B. L. Hansen, M. Shea, F. Hsu, and G. J. Anderson, "Pedicle screw placement in the thoracic spine: a comparison of image-guided and manual techniques in cadavers," *Spine*, vol. 30, no. 12, pp. E326–331, 2005.

[7] L. Weise, O. Suess, T. Picht, and T. Kombos, "Transpedicular screw fixation in the thoracic and lumbar spine with a novel cannulated polyaxial screw system," *Medical Devices: Evidence and Research*, vol. 1, no. 1, pp. 33–39, 2008.

[8] S. H. Davne and D. L. Myers, "Complications of lumbar spinal fusion with transpedicular instrumentation," *Spine*, vol. 17, no. 6, pp. 184–189, 1992.

[9] S. I. Esses, B. L. Sachs, and V. Dreyzin, "Complications associated with the technique of pedicle screw fixation. A selected survey of ABS members," *Spine*, vol. 18, no. 15, pp. 2231–2239, 1993.

[10] S. D. Gertzbein and S. E. Robbins, "Accuracy of pedicular screw placement in vivo," *Spine*, vol. 15, no. 1, pp. 11–14, 1990.

[11] J. E. Lonstein, F. Denis, J. H. Perra, M. R. Pinto, M. D. Smith, and R. B. Winter, "Complications associated with pedicle screws," *The Journal of Bone & Joint Surgery—American Volume*, vol. 81, no. 11, pp. 1519–1528, 1999.

[12] P. A. Grützner, T. Beutler, K. Wendl, J. von Recum, A. Wentzensen, and L. Nolte, "Navigation an der Brust- und Lendenwirbelsäule mit dem 3D-Bildwandler," *Der Chirurg*, vol. 75, no. 10, pp. 967–975, 2004.

[13] J. D. Witt and S. Kamineni, "The posterior interosseous nerve and the posterolateral approach to the proximal radius," *The Journal of Bone & Joint Surgery*, vol. 80, pp. 240–242, 1998.

[14] C. Bolger and C. Wigfield, "Image-guided surgery: applications to the cervical and thoracic spine and a review of the first 120 procedures," *Journal of Neurosurgery*, vol. 92, no. 2, pp. 175–180, 2000.

[15] T. Laine, T. Lund, M. Ylikoski, J. Lohikoski, and D. Schlenzka, "Accuracy of pedicle screw insertion with and without computer assistance: a randomised controlled clinical study in 100 consecutive patients," *European Spine Journal*, vol. 9, no. 3, pp. 235–240, 2000.

[16] N. D. Glossop, R. W. Hu, and J. A. Randle, "Computer-aided pedicle screw placement using frameless stereotaxis," *Spine*, vol. 21, no. 17, pp. 2026–2034, 1996.

[17] K. T. Foley and M. M. Smith, "Image-guided spine surgery," *Neurosurgery Clinics of North America*, vol. 7, no. 2, pp. 171–186, 1996.

[18] R. M. Beatty, P. McGuire, J. M. Moroney, and F. P. Holladay, "Continuous intraoperative electromyographic recording during spinal surgery," *Journal of Neurosurgery*, vol. 82, no. 3, pp. 401–405, 1995.

[19] B. V. Darden II, K. E. Wood, M. K. Hatley, J. H. Owen, and J. Kostuik, "Evaluation of pedicle screw insertion monitored by intraoperative evoked electromyography," *Journal of Spinal Disorders*, vol. 9, no. 1, pp. 8–16, 1996.

[20] M. Gundanna, M. Eskenazi, J. Bendo, J. Spivak, and R. Moskovich, "Somatosensory evoked potential monitoring of lumbar pedicle screw placement for in situ posterior spinal fusion," *The Spine Journal*, vol. 3, no. 5, pp. 370–376, 2003.

[21] J. P. Lubicky, J. A. Spadaro, H. A. Yuan, B. E. Fredrickson, and N. Henderson, "Variability of somatosensory cortical evoked potential monitoring during spinal surgery," *Spine*, vol. 14, no. 8, pp. 790–798, 1989.

[22] B. S. Myers, C. C. Hasty, D. R. Fioberg, R. D. Hoffman, B. J. Leone, and W. J. Richardson, "Measurement of vertebral cortical integrity during pedicle exploration for intrapedicular fixation," *Spine*, vol. 20, no. 2, pp. 144–148, 1995.

[23] C. Bolger, C. Carozzo, T. Roger et al., "A preliminary study of reliability of impedance measurement to detect iatrogenic initial pedicle perforation (in the porcine model)," *European Spine Journal*, vol. 15, no. 3, pp. 316–320, 2006.

[24] C. Bolger, M. O. Kelleher, L. McEvoy et al., "Electrical conductivity measurement: a new technique to detect iatrogenic initial pedicle perforation," *European Spine Journal*, vol. 16, no. 11, pp. 1919–1924, 2007.

[25] H. Koller, W. Hitzl, F. Acosta et al., "In vitro study of accuracy of cervical pedicle screw insertion using an electronic conductivity device (ATPS part III)," *European Spine Journal*, vol. 18, no. 9, pp. 1300–1313, 2009.

[26] A. Lubansu, J. Brotchi, and Dewitte O, "Evaluation of a hand-held pedicle drilling tool for help in the posterior pedicle screw placement," in *Proceedings of the Belgian Society of Neurosurgery Annual Meeting*, Leuven, Belgium, March 2006.

[27] U. R. Liljenqvist, H. F. H. Halm, and T. M. Link, "Pedicle screw instrumentation of the thoracic spine in idiopathic scoliosis," *Spine*, vol. 22, no. 19, pp. 2239–2245, 1997.

[28] J. L. Berry, J. M. Moran, W. S. Berg, and A. D. Steffee, "A morphometric study of human lumbar and selected thoracic vertebrae," *Spine*, vol. 12, no. 4, pp. 362–367, 1987.

[29] Y. Nohara, H. Taneichi, K. Ueyama et al., "Nationwide survey on complications of spine surgery in Japan," *Journal of Orthopaedic Science*, vol. 9, no. 5, pp. 424–433, 2004.

[30] S. C. Acikbas, F. Y. Arslan, and M. R. Turner, "The effect of transarticular screw misplacement on late spinal stability," *Acta Neurochirurgica*, vol. 145, no. 11, pp. 949–954, 2003.

[31] V. Kosmopoulos and C. Schizas, "Pedicle screw placement accuracy: a meta-analysis," *Spine*, vol. 32, no. 3, pp. E111–E120, 2007.

[32] N.-F. Tian and H.-Z. Xu, "Image-guided pedicle screw insertion accuracy: a meta-analysis," *International Orthopaedics*, vol. 33, no. 4, pp. 895–903, 2009.

[33] J. M. Bledsoe, D. Fenton, J. L. Fogelson, and E. W. Nottmeier, "Accuracy of upper thoracic pedicle screw placement using three-dimensional image guidance," *Spine Journal*, vol. 9, no. 10, pp. 817–821, 2009.

[34] V. Amato, L. Giannachi, C. Irace, and C. Corona, "Accuracy of pedicle screw placement in the lumbosacral spine using conventional technique: computed tomography postoperative assessment in 102 consecutive patients," *Journal of Neurosurgery: Spine*, vol. 12, no. 3, pp. 306–313, 2010.

8

Evaluating the Reproducibility of Motion Analysis Scanning of the Spine during Walking

Aaron Gipsman, Lisa Rauschert, Michael Daneshvar, and Patrick Knott

Chicago Medical School, Rosalind Franklin University of Medicine and Science, 3333 Green Bay Road, North Chicago, IL 60064, USA

Correspondence should be addressed to Aaron Gipsman; aaron.gipsman@my.rfums.org

Academic Editor: Panagiotis Korovessis

The Formetric 4D dynamic system (Diers International GmbH, Schlangenbad, Germany) is a rasterstereography based imaging system designed to evaluate spinal deformity, providing radiation-free imaging of the position, rotation, and shape of the spine during the gait cycle. *Purpose.* This study was designed to evaluate whether repeated measurements with the Formetric 4D dynamic system would be reproducible with a standard deviation of less than +/− 3 degrees. This study looked at real-time segmental motion, measuring kyphosis, lordosis, trunk length, pelvic, and T4 and L1 vertebral body rotation. *Methods.* Twenty healthy volunteers each underwent 3 consecutive scans. Measurements for kyphosis, lordosis, trunk length, and rotations of T4, L1, and the pelvis were recorded for each trial. *Results.* The average standard deviations of same-day repeat measurements were within +/− 3 degrees with a range of 0.51 degrees to 2.3 degrees. *Conclusions.* The surface topography system calculated reproducible measurements with error ranges comparable to the current gold standard in dynamic spinal motion analysis. Therefore, this technique should be considered of high clinical value for reliably evaluating segmental motion and spinal curvatures and should further be evaluated in the setting of adolescent idiopathic scoliosis.

1. Introduction

Adolescent idiopathic scoliosis (AIS) is a common condition affecting between 2 and 4 percent, or an estimated 6 million adolescents, in the United States [1]. Frequent assessment and monitoring of this patient population are necessary to determine an individual's progression of spinal deformity. Healthcare providers most often use spinal radiographs as the standard-of-care for evaluation. X-rays currently offer the most reliable way to quantify the magnitude of the curve but have the disadvantages of exposing patients to harmful radiation. Nash et al. reported that over a three-year period, a group of teenage girls with AIS underwent an average of 22 radiographs [2]. Ronckers et al. found cancer mortality to be 8 percent higher than expected in patients with repeated radiographs for scoliosis, as well as a four times greater relative risk of breast cancer in female patients with spinal disorders [3].

Surface topography is the study of the three-dimensional shape of the surface of the back. Measurement systems using surface topography do not involve exposure to ionizing radiation and are therefore completely safe [4]. According to a study by Knott et al., if surface topography can deliver reliable results, then it should replace radiographs in a certain number of follow-up clinical visits when curve surveillance is necessary and exposure to radiation can be avoided [5]. Other than the Formetric 4D machines, many surface topographical devices have been developed and tested for the purpose of screening for scoliosis [6–20].

The development of the Formetric 3D/4D device by DIERS biomedical technologies has provided a new option for static imaging of the spine. This radiation-free technology uses surface topography of the trunk to analyze surface asymmetry and identify bony landmarks thereby aiding in the evaluation of spinal deformities. As with other surface topography systems, it projects parallel stripes of light onto the back of a standing patient. The distortion of the raster lines provides the basis for calculating the surface topography. A map of 10,000 individual points is obtained and a surface is applied to these points. A large database of CT scans was used to create a mathematical model linking surface topography to spine position. The computer software contains this mathematical model and uses it to predict spinal position whenever exposed to a new topography scan. The Formetric system uses this complex algorithm to produce a three-dimensional computerized representation of the patient's spine [21]. Previous studies have indicated that patient evaluation using the Formetric 3D/4D for static measurements of spinal curvature is comparable to radiographs in terms of its test-retest reproducibility and seems to be a reliable way to monitor AIS patients [21]. According to a study performed using the static Formetric 4D machine, the trunk measurements were extremely reliable, with standard deviations consistent with those of standing radiographs. Measurements were reproducible, with standard deviations of only a few degrees for angular measurements and only a few millimeters for distance measurements [5].

Up until now, the technique of surface topography had only been applied to static imaging. However, physicians often need to analyze patients' movements to diagnose pathological or abnormal changes. Static images may underestimate the magnitude of scoliosis or general spinal curvature deformity. It would be valuable to be able to three-dimensionally analyze the spine under dynamic conditions to better understand the spinal motion in deformities such as scoliosis. Gait analysis is an option for measuring dynamic changes in spinal curvature and position; however it requires a large laboratory with expensive equipment and relies on the eye of the observer.

An alternative to gait analysis is the new version of the Formetric 3D/4D, the Formetric 4D dynamic model. Also developed by DIERS, this device uses similar surface topography techniques as the previous model to enable radiation and contact free analysis of the spine under dynamic conditions. The Formetric 4D dynamic captures images of the patient's back at a rate of 50 frames per second during simple motion (such as walking on a treadmill) for a duration of 5 seconds. Therefore, approximately 250 static images are collected and quickly converted into three-dimensional representations of the patient's spine. The combination of images results in a real-time three-dimensional representation of the shape of the spine in motion during the gait cycle. Objective values from the spine, pelvis, and scapula can be calculated, which may provide benefits in diagnosis and monitoring AIS patients and patients with deficits in postural control.

The goal of this study was to measure the reproducibility of the Formetric 4D dynamic system via analyzing the trunk length, kyphotic angle, lordotic angle, the rotation of the T4 vertebra relative to the pelvis, the rotation of the L1 vertebra relative to the pelvis, and the rotation of the pelvis during the normal gait cycle. Reproducible measurements would support the reliability of this imaging technique, which is the first step towards determining whether it should be further utilized as an effective method for screening, monitoring, and treating scoliosis, as well as other conditions affecting posture. Repeat measurements in subjects with a normal spinal curvature should be the first step in evaluating the technique's accuracy.

Measurements were considered reproducible if the average standard deviations were within +/− 3 degrees, which is the error seen with segmental orientation tracking with

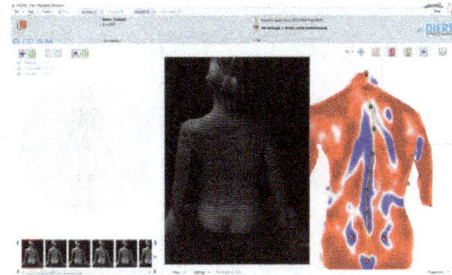

FIGURE 1: Static mode mean curvature screen: the middle image is raster line projection; the far right image is a representation of spinal curvature based surface topography.

the VICON optical motion measurement system, the current gold standard in spinal motion analysis [22]. The VICON system uses cameras to capture real-time complex human motion by recording marker position throughout the range of motion [22]. This optical tracking system is mainly restricted to the gait laboratory setting due to the high cost and volume of equipment, but it is currently the most prevalently used method for dynamic human motion analysis [22, 23]. Thus, it is the best comparison for the reliability of this novel technique of dynamic surface topography measurement.

2. Significance

The justification for this research is, if an accurate nonradiographic method for measuring spinal curvature and motion can be found, clinicians may be able to reduce or eliminate the need to expose young patients to ionizing radiation during their treatment for AIS. This machine may also eliminate the need for a more formal gait laboratory analysis. Gait analysis can be expensive, time consuming, and physically tolling on patients. The goal of this study was to determine whether dynamic surface topography motion analysis can produce reliable measurements. Testing the reproducibility of this system using subjects without any known spinal deformity should be the first step in evaluating the utility of dynamic surface topography as an effective tool for clinical spinal motion analysis.

3. Materials and Methods

The newest version of the Formetric 4D (dynamic feature) was acquired by the Illinois Bone and Joint Institute in 2011 and the principal investigator learned to use the machine according to the manufacturer's basic recommendations. After obtaining approval from the institutional review board, all volunteers were verbally recruited from the Illinois Bone and Joint Institute and Rosalind Franklin University of Medicine and Science by the principal investigator. The main prerequisite was the ability to walk on a treadmill. Inclusion was not based on sex, race, religion, insurance, or socioeconomic status. Participants who did not understand the informed consent or did not wish to participate in the study were excluded. The study included 20 healthy volunteers (7 male and 13 female) between the ages of 20 and 27.

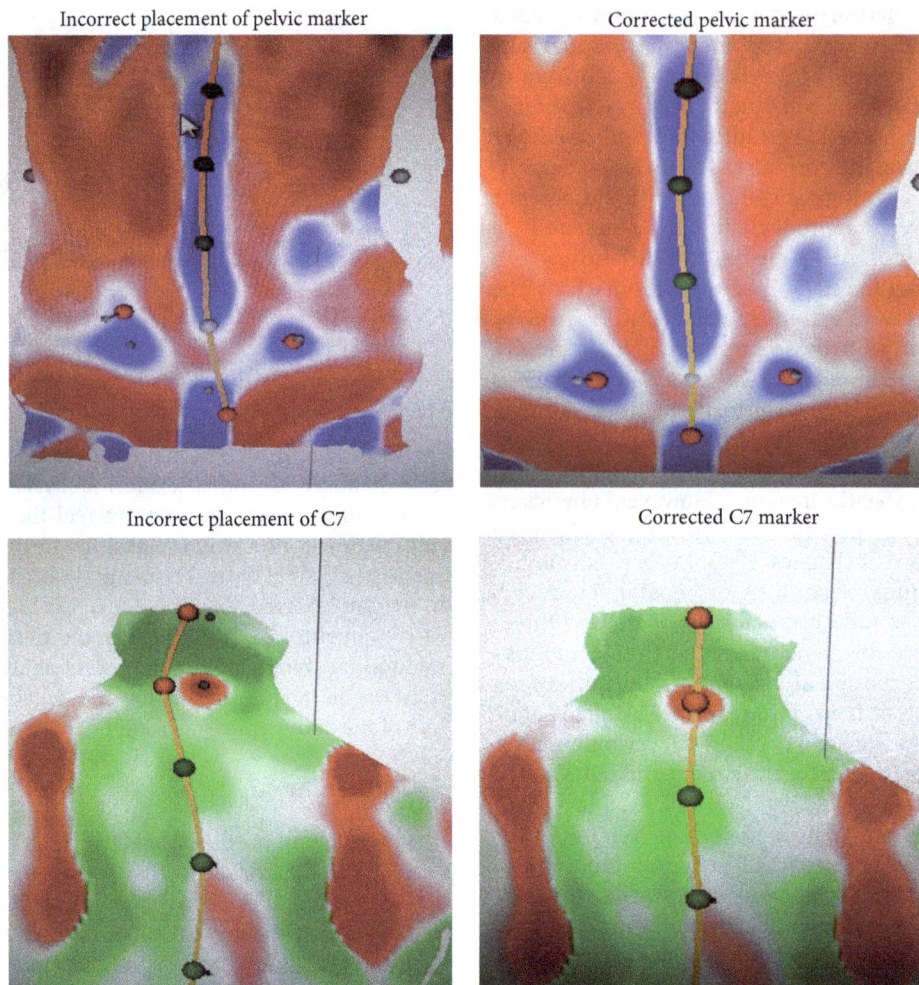

Incorrect placement of pelvic marker | Corrected pelvic marker

Incorrect placement of C7 | Corrected C7 marker

FIGURE 2: Adjustment of markers.

Initially, a pilot study was conducted in order for the investigators to learn how to use the machine better and to identify any potential problems with scanning subjects and obtaining measurements. Based on observations from this pilot study and the general protocol described by the manufacturers, a standardized procedure was developed to minimize any variability introduced by the operator. The protocol is described below.

3.1. Procedure. Subjects were provided with standard disposable exam shorts with elastic waistbands. The investigators ensured that shorts were positioned low enough on the hips so that the upper gluteal cleft was visible. Female subjects were provided with adhesive paper drapes to wear over their breasts. Drapes were adjusted so that they were not visible from the back. Volunteers with long hair were provided with hair clips and the investigators made sure that hair was positioned securely out of the way and completely off of the neck. All necklaces, watches, and so forth, which might have been visible in the frame of view, were removed.

3.1.1. Marker Placement. The primary examiner placed 3 reflective stickers on the subject's back, one on the spinous

process of C7 and one on each of the posterior superior iliac spines (PSIS) in the sacral region. These markers help the machine find these points quickly allowing faster and more accurate data processing. The examiner palpated each location before placing the sticker. Proper marker placement was confirmed with static imaging as follows. After the stickers were placed, subjects were instructed to stand at a marked position on the floor in their normal relaxed position with arms at their side and back to the Formetric 4D camera. With the machine in static mode, the mean curvature screen was selected (Figure 1). The investigators confirmed that the stickers were correctly located in the center of the PSIS depressions (blue dimples) and C7 (red protuberance). The primary examiner adjusted the stickers as necessary according to the surface topography images as shown in Figure 2. Results from a previous study comparing automatic detection of anatomic landmarks using the Formetric 4D versus manual detection by the clinician showed that automatic detection using surface topography was more reliable [24]. Once the reflective stickers were properly placed, they remained there until all measurements were completed.

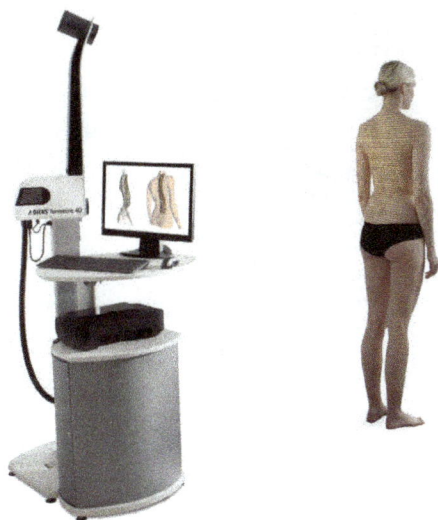

FIGURE 3: Formetric 4D device with raster line projection.

Next, the subject was directed to the treadmill and stood even with the tape marks indicating the 2-meter mark from the Formetric stereo imager.

3.1.2. Camera Positioning and Setup.
The camera column was adjusted based on the subject's height so that the spine was in center view and the green crosshairs were just below the scapula. Any lights/reflective portions of the treadmill were covered and ensured to be out of camera view. Investigators were cautious to make sure subjects' hair was still out of the way, shorts were low enough for visualization of the spine and hips, and frontal drapes for female patients were still out of camera view in this position.

The investigator then clicked the "project stripes" button to turn on the lights. The subject's position on the treadmill was checked to make sure that the stripes of light were sharp and in focus. An example of the Formetric 4D system projecting raster lines onto a representative subject's back is shown in Figure 3.

3.1.3. Lighting Conditions.
Lighting in the exam room was dimmed appropriately so that raster lines projected onto the subject's back were easily visible. Best results were possible with the lights above the patient turned off and the ceiling light on the other side of the room turned on. These conditions were kept consistent for all subjects.

3.1.4. Measurements.
The treadmill was set to 1.8 mph and the subject began walking at a steady, comfortable pace. Investigators closely observed to make sure they were walking at the proper distance from the camera so that the stripes remained in focus and the subject was instructed to walk evenly with the 2 meter tape marks on the treadmill. After 30 seconds of walking, the examiner clicked "start recording" to begin the measurement. Once the 5-second motion image capture was complete, the lights turned off automatically. The examiner stopped the treadmill and the subject rested for 2 minutes, while the Formetric software processed the data. For each subject, these steps were repeated two more times for a total of 3 trials.

3.1.5. Data.
For each trial, the 5-second motion imaging capture recorded at least 3 steps of the gait cycle. Multiple measurements are recorded by the Formetric system with each trial. For this reproducibility study, the investigators looked specifically at the measurements for the maximum and minimum values of kyphosis, lordosis, the rotation of the T4 vertebra, the rotation of L1 vertebra, the rotation of the pelvis, and the trunk length. These parameters were chosen based on clinical significance and ease of obtaining measurements from the computer report. Sample screenshots showing examples of data reporting are shown in Figures 4, 5, and 6.

The investigators averaged the vertebral and pelvic rotations over the 3 steps by recording the 3 peak rotations and the 3 minimum rotations. The averages of each of these parameters from each trial were calculated. In addition, the average values of all three trials for each parameter were calculated. This was then used to calculate the standard deviation for each parameter. For each parameter, the standard deviation was taken from the three trials performed on each subject. These 20 standard deviations (one for each parameter from each subject) were then averaged to determine the average standard deviations for that parameter.

For example, the subject underwent trial number one. Two of the many parameters measured and recorded were the maximum and minimum kyphotic angle. The average kyphotic angle for trial one was then calculated and recorded using the maximum and minimum values. The subject then underwent trials two and three, and the same measurements and calculations were performed. Thus, 3 maximum, 3 minimum, and 3 average values for the kyphotic angle were measured. The 3 values of the same parameter, for example, the three maximum kyphotic angle values (one from each trial), were then averaged in order to obtain an overall average maximum kyphotic angle value for the subject. This overall average for each parameter was used to calculate the standard deviation of the three trials for that specific parameter (such as the maximum kyphotic angle). This was done for each of the parameters mentioned previously. An example of this data collection for a single subject is shown in Table 1.

4. Results

The average standard deviations, the standard errors of the mean, and the ranges from all 12 parameters are listed below in Table 2. When evaluating same-day repeat scans, standard deviations ranged from 0.51 to 2.3 degrees and standard error of the means from 0.14 to 0.51 degrees.

5. Discussion

Surface topography has been used by a number of devices for the surveillance of spinal curve progression in patients with AIS. Previous studies have already shown that the static surface topography measurement with the Formetric 4D

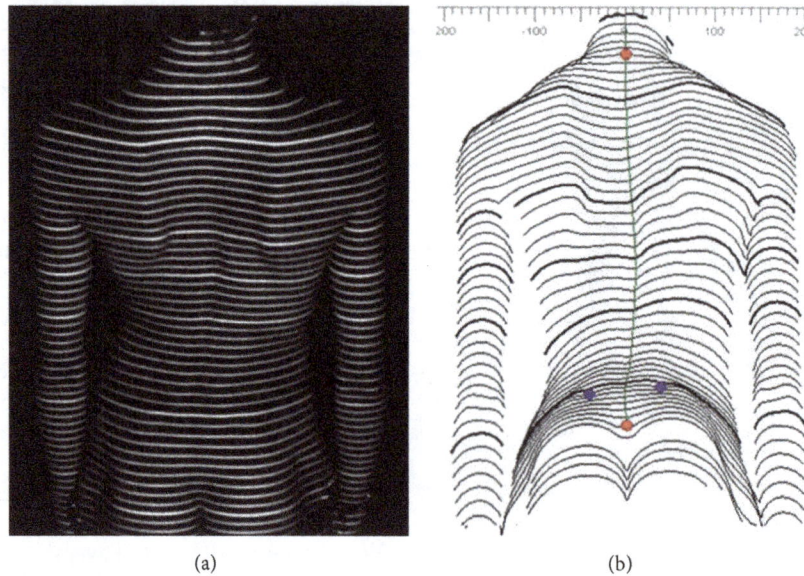

(a)   (b)

FIGURE 4: Raster lines projected onto the surface of subject's back (a) and reproduced computerized surface topography map (b).

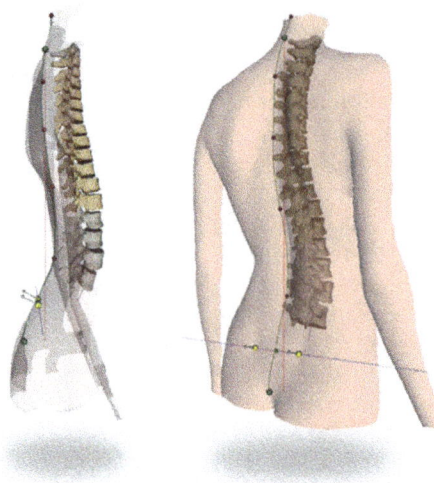

FIGURE 5: Three-dimensional computerized representation of the subject's underlying spine based on surface topography.

is comparable to radiographs in estimating the position of the spine as reported by Frerich et al. [21]. Therefore this technique of dynamic surface topography, which combines multiple static images over a period of time, should be equally capable of predicting the position of the spine under the skin during a dynamic gait cycle. The advantage of the dynamic surface topography feature is that it allows for measurement of additional parameters including degree of vertebral rotations and changes in the spinal curvature throughout the gait cycle, which would be useful in certain clinical situations. This study represents the first step in determining whether dynamic surface topography scanning is a reliable tool for clinical evaluation of patients with spinal deformity.

Limitations of this study include a small sample size ($n = 20$) and the subjects being close in age, skin color, and body habitus. The standard deviation is not as relevant in small sample sizes as it is with large sample sizes. Small sample sizes also make determination of the actual mean more difficult. It is possible that out of three measurements, the middle value of the three is not the one that is most correct. However, it was the variability in the measurements that was the most relevant to the study.

Regarding the limitations of body habitus, the measurements using surface topography were shown to still be reliable when creating an accurate spinal model up to a BMI of 29 [25]. Additionally, Weiss and Seibel's article titled "*Can surface topography replace radiography in the management of patients with scoliosis?*" states "although the correlation between X-ray and surface measurements was comparable with that published before, we cannot conclude that the device can be reliably used in the surveillance of patients

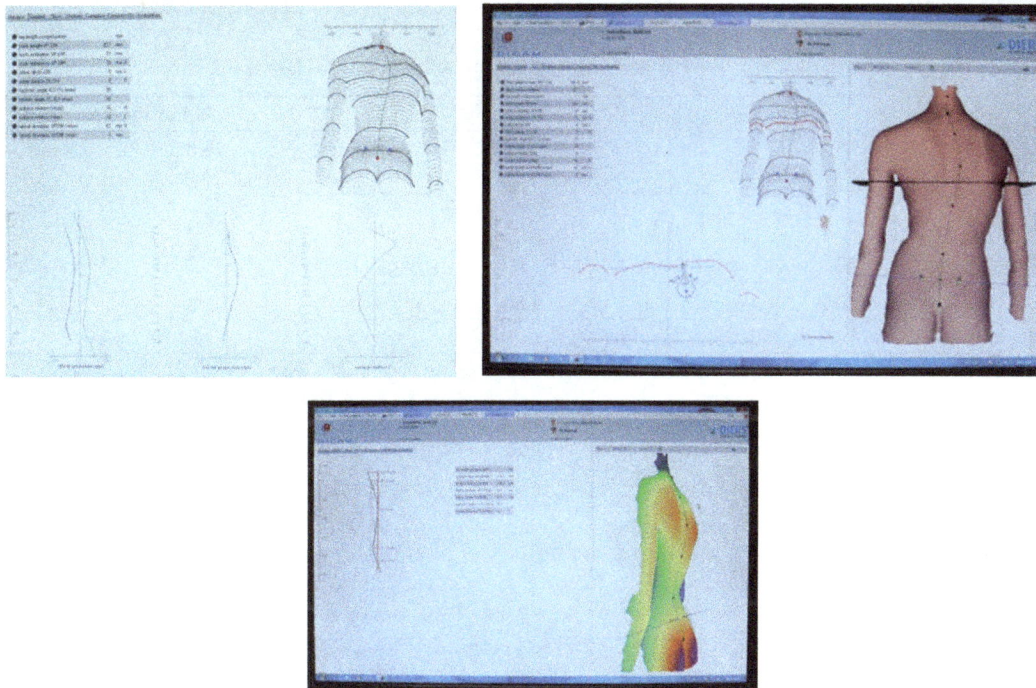

FIGURE 6: Diers Formetric sample data collection screens.

with AIS, as the differences in one case were as high as 38°" [26]. There is a learning curve in using the Formetric scanner, and during training of the examiner the results of the scans may not be as accurate. Additionally, there seem to be a few specific types of deformity that do not lend themselves to topographical scanning well. Extreme thoracic hypokyphosis is one of these, and for a very thin female scoliosis patient with a very flat thoracic curve, the Formetric algorithm may not be able to produce accurate results. This may have been the case with the one patient in Weiss and Seibel's study that had a 38-degree difference between the X-ray and the topographic scan.

The results showed statistically reproducible measurements for healthy subjects undergoing 3 consecutive motion scans. The measurements collected were well within +/− 3 degrees, which is also seen with segmental orientation tracking with the VICON optical motion measurement system (the current gold standard for spinal motion analysis) [23]. Therefore, the technique presented in this study should be considered clinically reproducible. The VICON system is the closest form of motion analysis tracking that is currently used in clinical practice and thus the best measure of success for this study.

6. Conclusion

This study was designed to evaluate the reproducibility of the technique of dynamic surface topography, in association with spinal measurements, in order to determine whether this method can be further utilized in the clinical setting. In the process of conducting the study, standardization protocols were created based on previous findings of a pilot study which evaluated variables such as lighting conditions, height and angle of camera, background materials within camera view, and positioning of clothing and long hair. The results showed a standard deviation of less than +/− 3 degrees and a range of 0.51 degrees to 2.3 degrees with SEM's less than 1 degree for all parameters studied. Thus, this technique of surface topography motion analysis was able to measure clinically relevant, reproducible, and spinal posture data during walking. It is clear that this technique provides reliable measurements for healthy subjects with same-day repeat measurements. Future studies will be aimed at determining the reproducibility of this technique among subjects with spinal deformities such as AIS, as well as evaluating the session to session reproducibility over time. This reproducibility study should potentially serve as a step in the process of the evaluation of other potential applications of this technique, such as spinal motion analysis in patients with spinal fusions, pre- and postoperatively, and the evaluation of the effectiveness of chiropractic medicine pre- and post-manipulation.

Disclosure

Aaron Gipsman, Lisa Rauschert, Patrick Knott, and Michael Daneshvar are coauthors.

Conflict of Interests

The authors have no conflicts of interest to disclose.

TABLE 1: Raw data collected from one subject for all 3 trials.

		Kyphosis				Lordosis		
Trial 1	max 1	65.4	min 1	54.3	max 1	44.8	min 1	40.5
Trial 2	max 2	61.9	min 2	55	max 2	45.5	min 2	40.9
Trial 3	max 3	62.8	min 3	57.7	max 3	45.4	min 3	39.3
	Average max	**63.4**	Average min	**55.7**	Average max	**45.2**	Average min	**40.2**
	SD	1.82	SD	1.80	SD	0.38	SD	0.83
		L1 rotation				T4 rotation		
Trial 1	max 1	2.5	min 1	−0.2	max 1	5	min 1	1
	max 2	3.2	min 2	−0.4	max 2	6	min 2	0
	max 3	4.2	min 3	0.2	max 3	6	min 3	0
	Avg. max	**3.3**	Avg. min	**−0.1**	Avg. max	**5.7**	Avg. min	**0.3**
	SD	0.9	SD	0.3	SD	0.6	SD	0.6
Trial 2	max 1	3.1	min 1	0.5	max 1	7	min 1	1
	max 2	4.9	min 2	−2.4	max 2	9	min 2	−1
	max 3	3.7	min 3	−0.7	max 3	9	min 3	0
	Avg. max	**3.9**	Avg. min	**−0.9**	Avg. max	**8.3**	Avg. min	**0**
	SD	0.9	SD	1.5	SD	1.2	SD	1
Trial 3	max 1	3.8	min 1	−0.9	max 1	6	min 1	−1
	max 2	3.4	min 2	−1	max 2	7	min 2	−2
	max 3	3.4	min 3	−1	max 3	7	min 3	−2
	Avg. max	**3.5**	Avg. min	**−1.0**	Avg. max	**6.7**	Avg. min	**−1.7**
	SD	0.2	SD	0.1	SD	0.6	SD	0.6
		Pelvis rotation						
Trial 1	max 1	1.2	min 1	−2.1				
	max 2	3	min 2	−4.2				
	max 3	4.1	min 3	−3.7				
	Avg max	**2.8**	Avg min	**−3.3**				
	SD	1.5	SD	1.1				
Trial 2	max 1	3.4	min 1	−4.2				
	max 2	1.4	min 2	−5				
	max 3	2.2	min 3	−4.1				
	Avg max	**2.3**	Avg min	**−4.4**				
	SD	1.0	SD	0.5				
Trial 3	max 1	3.4	min 1	−4.5				
	max 2	2.4	min 2	−6.7				
	max 3	2.2	min 3	−3.9				
	Avg max	**2.7**	Avg min	**−5.0**				
	SD	0.6	SD	1.5				
		Trunk Length						
Trial 1	max	463.2	min	459				
Trial 2	max	463.4	min	457.3				
Trial 3	max	462.7	min	455				
	Avg max	**463.1**	Avg min	**457.1**				
	SD	0.4	SD	2.0				

TABLE 2: Average standard deviations, standard error of the mean, and range for spinal parameters studied.

Parameter	Average SD in degrees	SEM in degrees ($n = 20$)	Range of SD (in degrees)
Kyphosis maximum	2.3	0.51	0.23–6.37
Kyphosis minimum	2	0.45	0.47–6.44
Lordosis maximum	1.2	0.27	0.29–4.24
Lordosis minimum	1.2	0.27	0.1–3.07
L1 Rotation maximum	0.51	0.11	0.1–2.3
L1 Rotation minimum	0.58	0.13	0.1–2.8
T4 Rotation maximum	0.68	0.15	0–2.6
T4 Rotation minimum	0.9	0.20	0–3.6
Pelvis rotation maximum	0.62	0.14	0.1–2.7
Pelvis rotation minimum	0.63	0.14	0–3.1
Trunk length maximum	1.53	0.34	0.3–6.1
Trunk length minimum	1.3	0.29	0.4–6.0

Acknowledgments

No funds were received for the performance of this research, although the Formetric 4D machine was loaned to the Illinois Bone and Joint Institute for this evaluation. No funding has been received from or by the manufacturer for this research.

References

[1] B. Reamy and J. B. Slakey, "Adolescent idiopathic scoliosis: review and current concepts," *American Family Physician*, vol. 64, p. 111, 2001.

[2] C. L. Nash Jr., E. C. Gregg, R. H. Brown, and K. Pillai, "Risks of exposure to X-rays in patients undergoing long-term treatment for scoliosis," *The Journal of Bone and Joint Surgery*, vol. 61, no. 3, pp. 371–374, 1979.

[3] C. M. Ronckers, C. E. Land, J. S. Miller, M. Stovall, J. E. Lonstein, and M.M. Doody, "Cancer mortality among women frequently exposed to radiographic examinations for spinal disorders," *Radiation Research*, vol. 174, no. 1, pp. 83–90, 2010.

[4] N. J. Oxborrow, "Assessing the child with scoliosis: the role of surface topography," *Archives of Disease in Childhood*, vol. 83, pp. 453–455, 2000.

[5] P. Knott, S. Mardjetko, M. Rollet, S. Baute, M. Riemenschneider, and L. Muncie, "Evaluation of the reproducibility of the formetric 4D measurements for scoliosis," *Scoliosis*, vol. 5, article O10, 2010.

[6] J. D. Pearson, P. H. Dangerfield, J. T. Atkinson et al., "Measurement of body surface topography using an automated imaging system," *Acta Orthopaedica Belgica*, vol. 58, supplement 1, pp. 73–79, 1992.

[7] M. Batouche, R. Benlamri, and M. K. Kholladi, "A computer vision system for diagnosing scoliosis using moiré images," *Computers in Biology and Medicine*, vol. 26, no. 4, pp. 33–53, 1996.

[8] A. M. Macdonald, C. J. Griffiths, F. J. MacArdle, and M. J. Gibson, "The effect of posture on Quantec measurements," *Studies in Health Technology and Informatics*, vol. 91, pp. 190–193, 2002.

[9] D. L. Hill, D. C. Berg, V. J. Raso et al., "Evaluation of a laser scanner for surface topography," *Studies in Health Technology and Informatics*, vol. 88, pp. 90–94, 2002.

[10] S. Treuillet, Y. Lucas, G. Crepin, B. Peuchot, and J. C. Pichaud, "SYDESCO: a laser-video scanner for 3D scoliosis evaluations," *Studies in Health Technology and Informatics*, vol. 88, pp. 70–73, 2002.

[11] X. C. Liu, J. G. Thometz, R. M. Lyon, and L. McGrady, "Effects of trunk position on back surface-contour measured by raster stereophotography," *The American Journal of Orthopedics*, vol. 31, no. 7, pp. 402–406, 2002.

[12] V. Pazos, F. Cheriet, L. Song, H. Labelle, and J. Dansereau, "Accuracy assessment of human trunk surface 3D reconstructions from an optical digitizing system," *Medical & Biological Engineering & Computing*, vol. 43, no. 1, pp. 11–15, 2005.

[13] P. Knott, S. Mardjetko, D. Nance, and M. Dunn, "Electromagnetic topographical technique of curve evaluation for adolescent idiopathic scoliosis," *Spine*, vol. 31, no. 24, pp. E911–E916, 2006.

[14] C. J. Goldberg, D. Grove, D. P. Moore, E. E. Fogarty, and F. E. Dowling, "Surface Topography and vectors: a new measure for the three dimensional quantification of scoliotic deformity," *Studies in Health Technology and Informatics*, vol. 123, pp. 449–455, 2006.

[15] H. Mitchell, S. Pritchard, and D. Hill, "Surface alignment to unmask scoliotic deformity in surface topography," *Studies in Health Technology and Informatics*, vol. 123, pp. 109–116, 2006.

[16] A. Zubovic, N. Davies, F. Berryman et al., "New method of scoliosis deformity assessment: ISIS2 system," *Studies in Health Technology and Informatics*, vol. 140, pp. 157–160, 2008.

[17] T. M. Shannon, "Development of an apparatus to evaluate Adolescent Idiopathic Scoliosis by dynamic surface topography," *Studies in Health Technology and Informatics*, vol. 140, pp. 121–127, 2008.

[18] F. Berryman, P. Pynsent, and J. Fairbank, "Measuring the rib hump in scoliosis with ISIS2," *Studies in Health Technology and Informatics*, vol. 140, pp. 65–67, 2008.

[19] C. Fortin, D. E. Feldman, F. Cherlet, and H. Labelle, "Validity of a quantitative clinical measurement tool of trunk posture in idiopathic scoliosis," *Spine*, vol. 35, no. 19, pp. E988–E994, 2010.

[20] E. C. Parent, S. Damaraju, D. L. Hill, E. Lou, and D. Smetaniuk, "Identifying the best surface topography parameters for detecting idiopathic scoliosis curve progression," *Studies in Health Technology and Informatics*, vol. 158, pp. 78–82, 2010.

[21] J. M. Frerich, K. Hertzler, P. Knott, and S. Mardjetko, "Comparison of radiographic and surface topography measurements in

adolescents with scoliosis," *The Open Orthopaedic Journal*, vol. 6, pp. 261–265, 2012.

[22] C. Goodvin, E. J. Park, K. Huang, and K. Sakaki, "Development of a real-time three-dimensional spinal motion measurement system for clinical practice," *Medical Biological Engineering & Computing*, vol. 44, pp. 1061–1075, 2006.

[23] J. L. McGinley, R. Baker, R. Wolfe, and M. Morris, "The reliability of three-dimensional kinematic gait measurements: a systematic review," *Gait & Posture*, vol. 29, no. 3, pp. 360–369, 2009.

[24] P. Knott, S. Mardjetko, and S. Thompson, "A comparison of automatic vs. manual detection of anatomical landmarks during surface topography evaluation using the formetric 4D system," *Scoliosis*, vol. 7, supplement 1, article O19, 2012.

[25] P. Knott, S. Mardjetko, D. Tager, R. Hund, and S. Thompson, "The influence of body mass index (BMI) on the reproducibility of surface topography measurements," *Scoliosis*, vol. 7, supplement 1, p. O18, 2012.

[26] H. R. Weiss and S. Seibel, "Can surface topography replace radiography in the management of patients with scoliosis?" *Hard Tissue*, vol. 2, no. 2, article 19, 2013.

9

Evaluation of HLA-G 14 bp Ins/Del and +3142G>C Polymorphism with Susceptibility and Early Disease Activity in Rheumatoid Arthritis

Mohammad Hashemi,[1,2] **Mahnaz Sandoughi,**[3] **Seyed Amirhossein Fazeli,**[3]
Gholamreza Bahari,[2] **Maryam Rezaei,**[2] **and Zahra Zakeri**[4]

[1]*Cellular and Molecular Research Center, Zahedan University of Medical Sciences, Zahedan 98167-43181, Iran*
[2]*Department of Clinical Biochemistry, School of Medicine, Zahedan University of Medical Sciences, Zahedan 98167-43181, Iran*
[3]*Department of Internal Medicine, School of Medicine, Zahedan University of Medical Sciences, Zahedan 98167-43181, Iran*
[4]*Department of Internal Medicine, School of Medicine, Shahid Beheshti University of Medical Sciences, Tehran 19857-17443, Iran*

Correspondence should be addressed to Zahra Zakeri; zah_zakeri@yahoo.com

Academic Editor: Maja Krajinovic

Purpose/Background. Mounting evidence designates that HLA-G plays a role in the regulation of inflammatory processes and autoimmune diseases. There are controversial reports concerning the impact of *HLA-G* gene polymorphism on rheumatoid arthritis (RA). This study was aimed at examining the impact of 14 bp ins/del and +3142G>C polymorphism with susceptibility and early disease activity in RA patients in a sample of the Iranian population. *Methods.* This case-control study was done on 194 patients with RA and 158 healthy subjects. The *HLA-G* rs1063320 (+3142G>C) and rs66554220 (14 bp ins/del) variants were genotype by polymerase chain reaction-restriction fragment length polymorphism (PCR-RFP) and PCR method, respectively. *Results.* The *HLA-G* +3142G>C polymorphism significantly decreased the risk of RA in codominant (OR = 0.61, 95% CI = 0.38–0.97, $p = 0.038$, GC versus GG; OR = 0.36, 95% CI = 0.14–0.92, $p = 0.034$, CC versus GG), dominant (OR = 0.56, 95% CI = 0.36–0.87, $p = 0.011$, GC + CC versus GG), and allele (OR = 0.58, 95% CI = 0.41–0.84, $p = 0.004$, C versus G) inheritance models tested. Our finding did not support an association between *HLA-G* 14 bp ins/del variant and risk/protection of RA. In addition, no significant association was found between the polymorphism and early disease activity. *Conclusion.* In summary, our results showed that *HLA-G* +3142G>C gene polymorphism significantly decreased the risk of RA in a sample of the Iranian population.

1. Introduction

Rheumatoid arthritis (RA) is the most common autoimmune disease of unknown etiology affecting approximately 0.5–1% of the human population worldwide [1, 2]. The disease is 2-3 times more common in females than in males. It has been proposed that both genetic and environmental factors are involved in the expression and complications of the disease [3–8]. Genetic factors are assumed to contribute to up to 60% of the risk of developing RA [2].

Human leucocyte antigen-G (HLA-G), a nonclassical major HLA class Ib molecule, may suppress functions of natural killer (NK) cells, CD4+, CD8+ lymphocytes, and dendritic cell [9–11]. HLA-G protein potentially exists as seven isoforms including four membrane-bound (HLA-G1, -G2, -G3, and -G4) as well as three secreted soluble (HLA-G5, -G6, and -G7) proteins [12].

HLA-G gene, which is located on chromosome 6 (6p21.31), contains a 14 bp insertion (ins)/deletion (del) and a +3142G>C (rs1063320) polymorphism in 3′-untranslated region (3′UTR) of HLA-G. HLA-G expression rate and plasma level are influenced by polymorphism in the promoter region as well as 3′-untranslated region (UTR) variants [13–15].

A 14 bp ins/del polymorphism in exon 8 in the 3′UTR of *HLA-G* was found to be associated with the stability and splicing patterns of *HLA-G* mRNA isoforms. The homozygous deletion of 14 bp confers a more stable mRNA as compared to the homozygous insertion genotype [13, 14, 16]. Low levels of membrane bound and sHLA-G levels are associated with the ins allele [13].

+3142G>C polymorphism influences the affinity of HLA-G mRNA targeted by different microRNAs as demonstrated by an in silico study [17]. +3142G allele has a binding site with higher affinity for miR-148a, miR-148b, and miR-152 downregulating the expression of HLA-G [15, 18].

The common polymorphism of the *HLA-G* seems to affect its level of expression and may have an impact on disease susceptibility in autoimmune disorders. It has been reported that plasma soluble HLA-G (sHLA-G) levels were lower in RA patients than in controls [19].

Several studies investigated the impact of common polymorphism of HLA-G (+3142G>C and 14 bp ins/del) on RA risk in various population, but the findings have been controversial [20–24]. Therefore, the present study was aimed at examining whether rs1063320 (+3142G>C) and rs66554220 (14 bp ins/del) polymorphism in the *HLA-G* gene were associated with susceptibility to RA in a sample of Iranian population.

2. Material and Methods

2.1. Patients. A total of 352 subjects including 194 patients with RA fulfilling the 2010 American College of Rheumatology/European League Against Rheumatism for RA [25] and 158 unrelated healthy subjects were enrolled in the study. The cases were selected from RA patients admitted to the Rheumatology Clinic of university-affiliated hospital (Ali-Ebne-Abitaleb Hospital, Zahedan, Iran). The control group consisted of 158 whose age and sex matched healthy individuals with no clinical symptoms or family histories of RA, and they were unrelated to RA patients, had no known autoimmune diseases, and were from the same geographical origin as the patients with RA (Zahedan, Iran). The project was approved by local ethics committee of Zahedan University of Medical Sciences and informed consent was obtained from all participants. Genomic DNA was extracted from peripheral blood samples using salting out method as described previously [26].

Among all the participant patients, 30 early RA subjects who were symptomatic for ≤1 year enrolled for subsequent follow-up study. All the patients were on standard therapeutic regimen. The disease activity was determined by disease activity score 28 (DAS-28) at the beginning and the end of the follow-up study (at least 18 months) by the same specialist rheumatologist. At the end of the study, the patients were stratified into remitting (DAS-28 < 2.6) and nonremitting (DAS-28 ≥ 2.6) patients.

Genotyping of HLA-G rs1063320 (+3142G>C) variant was performed by PCR-RFLP methods. The set of forward and reverse primers were 5′-CATGCTGAACTGCATTCC-TTCC-3′ and 5′-CTGGTGGGACAAGGTTCTACTG-3′ [27]. Amplification was done with an initial denaturation step at 95°C for 5 min, followed by 30 cycles of 30 s at 95°C, 30 s at 65°C, and 30 s at 72°C with a final step at 72°C for 10 min. 10 μL of PCR products was digested with BaeGI restriction enzyme (Fermentas). G allele digested and produced 316 bp

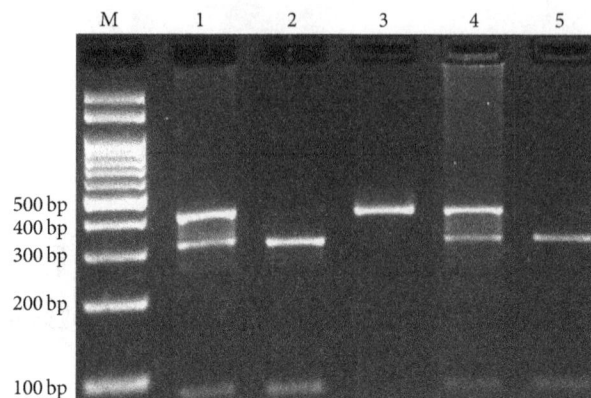

FIGURE 1: Photograph of the PCR products of HLA-G +3142G>C polymorphism by polymerase chain reaction-restriction fragment length polymorphism method (PCR-RFLP). G allele digested by BaeGI restriction enzyme and produced 316 bp and 90 bp while C allele undigested 406 bp. M: DNA Marker; Lanes 1 and 4: GC; Lanes 2 and 5: GG; Lane 3: CC.

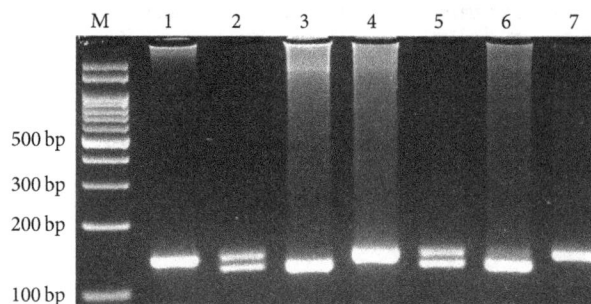

FIGURE 2: Photograph of the PCR products of *HLA-G* 14 bp ins/del polymorphism by polymerase chain reaction (PCR). Product sizes were 127 bp for del and 141 bp for ins allele. M: DNA Marker; Lanes 1, 4, and 7: ins/ins; Lanes 2 and 5: ins/del; Lanes 3 and 6: del/del.

and 90 bp (digested), while C allele undigested and produced 406 bp (Figure 1).

Genotyping of HLA-G rs66554220 (14 bp ins/del) variant was done by polymerase chain reaction [28]. The forward and reverse primers were 5′-TCACCCCTCACTGTGACTGATA-3′ and 5′-GCACAAAGAGGAGTCAGGGTT-3′, respectively. In each 0.20 mL PCR reaction tube, 1 μL of genomic DNA (~100 ng/mL), 1 μL of each primer (10 μM), 10 μL of 2x Prime Taq Premix (Genet Bio, Korea), and 5 μL ddH$_2$O were added. The PCR cycling conditions were as follows: an initial denaturation step of 5 min at 95°C followed by 30 cycles of 30 s at 95°C, annealing at 56°C for 30 s, and extension at 72°C for 30 s, with final extension at 72°C for 5 min. The PCR products were separated by electrophoresis in 2% agarose gels and observed under ultraviolet light. Product sizes were 127 bp for del and 141 bp for ins allele (Figure 2).

2.2. Statistical Analysis. Statistical analysis of the data was done using statistical software package SPSS 20 software. Independent sample *t*-test for continuous data and χ^2 test for categorical data were used. The associations between

TABLE 1: Association of HLA-G polymorphisms and the risk of RA.

HLA-G polymorphisms	Case n (%)	Control n (%)	OR (95% CI)	p	p^c
14-bp ins/del (rs66554220)					
Codominant					
Ins/ins	36 (18.6)	34 (21.5)	1.00	—	
Ins/del	123 (63.4)	97 (61.4)	1.20 (0.70–2.05)	0.582	1.00
Del/del	35 (18.0)	27 (17.1)	1.22 (0.62–2.43)	0.603	1.00
Dominant					
Ins/ins	36 (18.6)	34 (21.5)	1.00		
Ins/del + del/del	158 (81.4)	124 (78.5)	1.20 (0.71–2.03)	0.505	1.00
Recessive					
Ins/ins + ins/del	159 (82.0)	131 (82.9)	1.00		
Del/del	35 (18.0)	27 (17.1)	1.07 (0.61–1.86)	0.888	1.00
Allele					
Ins	195 (50.3)	165 (52.2)	1.00	—	
Del	193 (49.7)	151 (47.8)	1.08 (0.80–1.46)	0.649	1.00
+3142G>C (rs1063320)					
Codominant					
GG	135 (69.6)	89 (56.3)	1.00	—	
GC	52 (26.8)	56 (35.4)	0.61 (0.38–0.97)	0.038	0.076
CC	7 (3.6)	13 (8.2)	0.36 (0.14–0.92)	0.034	0.068
Dominant					
GG	135 (69.6)	89 (56.3)	1.00		
GC + CC	59 (30.4)	69 (43.7)	0.56 (0.36–0.87)	0.011	0.022
Recessive					
GG + GC	187 (96.4)	145 (91.8)	1.00		
CC	7 (3.6)	13 (8.2)	0.42 (0.16–1.07)	0.068	1.00
Allele					
G	322 (83.0)	234 (74.0)	1.00	—	
C	66 (17.0)	82 (26.0)	0.58 (0.41–0.84)	0.004	0.005

p^c: Bonferroni-corrected p.

genotypes of *HLA-G* gene and RA were assessed by computing the odds ratio (OR) and 95% confidence intervals (95% CI) from logistic regression analyses. Haplotype analysis was performed using SNPStats software (a web tool for the analysis of association studies). p value less than 0.05 was considered statistically significant. The Bonferroni correction was applied by multiplying p values by the number of SNPs analyzed.

3. Results

In this study, we recruited 194 RA patients (180 female and 14 male; mean age 45.3 ± 14.1 years) and 158 unrelated healthy subjects (140 female and 18 male; mean age: 46.1 ± 12.3 years). There was no significant difference between the groups concerning sex and age ($p = 0.815$ and $p = 0.465$, resp.).

The genotype and allele frequencies of *HLA-G* polymorphism in RA patients and in controls are shown in Table 1. *HLA-G* rs1063320 (+3142G>C) variant decreased the risk of

RA in codominant (OR = 0.61, 95% CI = 0.38–0.97, $p = 0.038$, GC versus GG; OR = 0.36, 95% CI = 0.14–0.92, $p = 0.034$, CC versus GG) and dominant (OR = 0.56, 95% CI = 0.36–0.87, $p = 0.011$, GC + CC versus GG) tested inheritance models. *HLA-G* rs1063320 C allele significantly decreased the risk of RA (OR = 0.58, 95% CI = 0.41–0.84, $p = 0.004$) compared to G allele.

Overall, both chi-square comparison and logistic regression analysis (which was calculated in each model of inheritance) did not reveal an association between *HLA-G* rs66554220 polymorphism and RA risk (Table 1).

In the combined analysis of two *HLA-G* variants, subjects carrying deldel/GG genotypes had significantly higher risk of RA than 14 bp deldel/+3142GG (Table 2).

Haplotype analysis is shown in Table 3. Haplotype +3142G/14 bp del significantly increased the risk of RA (OR = 1.77, 95% CI = 1.14–2.75, $p = 0.012$), while +3142C/14 bp del decreased the risk of RA (OR = 0.52, 95% CI = 0.30–0.90, $p = 0.019$) compared to +3142G/14 bp ins.

TABLE 2: Interaction of 14 bp ins/del and +3142G>C polymorphism of *HLA-G* gene on rheumatoid arthritis (RA) risk.

14 bp ins/del	+3142G>C	RA cases n (%)	Controls n (%)	OR (95% CI)	p	p^c
Ins/ins	GG	27 (13.9)	27 (17.1)	1.00	—	—
Ins/del	GG	84 (43.3)	56 (35.4)	1.50 (0.79–2.82)	0.257	1.000
Del/del	GG	24 (12.4)	6 (3.8)	4.00 (1.41–11.34)	0.010	0.039
Ins/del	GC	34 (17.5)	35 (22.2)	0.97 (0.48–1.98)	0.890	1.000
Del/del	GC	10 (5.2)	14 (8.9)	0.71 (0.27–1.89)	0.624	0.992
Ins/ins	GC	8 (4.1)	7 (4.4)	1.14 (0.36–3.60)	0.922	1.000
Del/del	CC	1 (0.5)	7 (4.4)	0.14 (0.02–1.24)	0.063	0.240
Ins/del	CC	5 (2.6)	6 (3.8)	0.83 (0.23–3.06)	0.927	1.000
Ins/ins	CC	1 (0.5)	0 (0.0)	—	—	—

p^c: Bonferroni-corrected p.

TABLE 3: Haplotype association of *HLA-G* +3142G>C and 14 bp ins/del variants with rheumatoid arthritis (RA) risk.

+3142G>C	14 bp ins/del	RA cases (frequency)	Controls (frequency)	OR (95% CI)	p
G	Ins	0.4250	0.4652	1.00	—
G	Del	0.4049	0.2753	1.77 (1.14–2.75)	0.012
C	Del	0.0925	0.2026	0.52 (0.30–0.90)	0.019
C	Ins	0.0776	0.0569	1.74 (0.75–4.05)	0.200

Baseline demographic and clinical characteristics of total follow-up cohort and the remitting and nonremitting subgroups are shown in Table 4. We determined the association of HLA-G polymorphism with early disease activity. Our results revealed no significant association between *HLA-G* +3142G>C and HLA-G 14 bp ins/del variant and early disease activity (Table 5).

The genotype frequency of the HLA-G polymorphism was examined for Hardy-Weinberg equilibrium (HWE). +3142G>C polymorphism in cases and controls was in HWE ($\chi^2 = 0.50$, $p = 0.480$ and $\chi^2 = 0.96$, $p = 0.328$, resp.), while the 14 bp I/D variant in cases and controls was not in HWE ($\chi^2 = 13.94$, $p = 0.0002$ and $\chi^2 = 8.38$, $p = 0.004$, resp.).

4. Discussion

HLA-G is a nonclassical HLA class I molecule that can bind to immune cells and inhibit their function [29, 30]. It is involved in several immunoregulatory processes and may potentially be involved in the pathogenesis of RA. Genetic variants in coding and noncoding regions of the *HLA-G* may affect biological features of the molecule. Expression rate of *HLA-G* gene and plasma level are affected by variants in the promoter region as well as 3'UTR [12].

In the present study, we investigated the impact of *HLA-G* 14 bp ins/del and +3142G>C polymorphism on risk of RA in a sample of Iranian population. The findings of our study showed an association between *HLA-G* +3142G>C polymorphism and RA in our population. The GC as well as C allele decreased the risk of RA in our population. Regarding *HLA-G* 14 bp ins/del variant, we did not find any statistically significant difference in either genotype or allele distribution between patients and controls. The deldel/GG genotypes significantly increased the risk of RA compared to insins/GG. In addition, we did not find an association between *HLA-G* variants and disease activity. In contrast to our findings, Rizzo et al. [31] investigated 23 early rheumatoid arthritis (ERA) patients during a 12-month follow-up disease treatment period. They found that the frequency of 14 bp del allele was associated with disease remission. They concluded that HLA-G may be a candidate biomarker to evaluate early prognosis and disease activity in ERA patients.

A meta-analysis performed by Lee et al. [32] revealed no significant association between *HLA-G* 14 bp I/D and +3142G/C polymorphism and RA risk. Similar negative findings have been reported in Brazilian [24] and Indian population [22]. Although Veit et al. [23] have observed no differences in allelic and genotypic frequencies of the *HLA-G* 14 bp ins/del polymorphism between RA patients and controls, the 14 bp ins/del polymorphism was associated with juvenile idiopathic arthritis in Brazilian population. In another study, Veit et al. [33] reported that +3142GG genotype significantly increased the risk of RA (odds ratio (OR) = 1.45, 95% confidence interval (CI) = 1.075–1.95, $p = 0.030$). Kim et al. [20] investigated the impact of rs1736936 (-1202T/C) and rs2735022 (-586C/T) promoter polymorphism of *HLA-G* gene on RA in Korean population. They found no significant differences in distributions of genotypes and haplotypes between RA patients and control subjects.

Verbruggen et al. [19] found that the levels of sHLA-G in patients with RA were significantly lower than healthy controls. They suggested that patients with low sHLA-G levels were unable to suppress self-reactive cells leading to development of autoimmunity. The 3'-untranslated region (UTR) has a major role in HLA-G regulation [17, 34]. It has been proposed that polymorphism exerts a significant effect in the

TABLE 4: Baseline demographic and clinical characteristics of total follow-up cohort and the remitting and nonremitting subgroups.

Parameters	Total patients ($n = 30$)	Remitting patients ($n = 15$)	Nonremitting patients ($n = 15$)	p
Age (mean ± SD)	45.56 ± 16.99	46.26 ± 17.22	44.86 ± 17.34	NS[*]
Gender (%)				
Male	2 (6.7)	2 (13.3)	0 (0.0)	NS
Female	28 (93.3)	13 (86.6)	15 (100.0)	
BMI (Kg/m^2) (mean ± SD)	25.18 ± 5.24	24.87 ± 3.34	25.52 ± 6.84	NS
Cigarette (pack/years; mean ± SD)	0.33 ± 1.82	0.00 ± 0.00	0.66 ± 2.58	
Hookah (%)	4 (13.3)	1 (6.6)	3 (20)	NS
Education				NS
Illiterate (%)	12 (40.0)	6 (40.0)	6 (40.0)	
Less than diploma (%)	5 (16.7)	1 (6.6)	4 (26.7)	
Diploma (%)	8 (26.6)	4 (26.7)	4 (26.7)	
Higher education (%)	5 (16.7)	4 (26.7)	1 (6.6)	
Length of symptom prior to study (months; mean ± SD)	8.20 ± 4.22	8.20 ± 4.63	8.20 ± 3.94	NS
Positive rheumatoid factor (%)	26 (86.7)	12 (80)	14 (93.3)	NS
Comorbidity				NS
No comorbidity (%)	17 (56.6)	7 (80.0)	10 (66.6)	
Type 2 diabetes mellitus (%)	3 (10.0)	1 (6.6)	2 (13.3)	
Hypertension (%)	6 (20.0)	5 (33.3)	1 (6.6)	
Dyslipidemia (%)	6 (20)	2 (13.3)	4 (26.6)	
Other factors (%)	5 (16.6)	4 (26.6)	1 (6.6)	

[*]Nonsignificant.

TABLE 5: Association of *HLA-G* polymorphism in remitting and nonremitting RA patients.

Genotypes	Remitting patients n (%)	Nonremitting patients n (%)	OR (95% CI)	p
14-bp ins/del				
Genotype				
Ins/ins	1 (50.0)	1 (50.0)	1.00	—
Ins/del	10 (43.5)	13 (56.5)	0.76 (0.04–13.88)	0.897
Del/del	4 (80.0)	1 (20.0)	4.00 (0.12–137.10)	0.912
Allele				
Ins	12 (40.0)	15 (50.0)	1.00	—
Del	18 (60.0)	15 (50.0)	1.50 (0.54–4.17)	0.602
+3142G>C				
Genotype				
GG	11 (45.8)	13 (54.2)	1.00	—
CG	4 (66.7)	2 (33.3)	2.36 (0.36–15.46)	0.651
CC	0 (0.0)	0 (0.0)	—	—
Allele				
G	26 (63.4)	28 (65.1)	1.00	—
C	15 (36.6)	15 (34.9)	0.90 (0.38–2.14)	0.826

HLA-G function and may have an impact on the expression of sHLA-G [35–37]. The HLA-G expression is influenced by 14 bp ins/del as well as +3142G/C polymorphism in the 3′-untranslated region (3′UTR) of HLA-G gene and may have possible implications of clinical significance [37].

The discrepancy in findings among studies may be due to genetic and environmental differences between the different populations being investigated.

The limitation of our study is that we have no data regarding anti-CCP antibodies, RF antibody, HLA-DRB1 shared epitope, and smoking history. Consequently, we could not evaluate the association between *HLA-G* variants and these factors. However, we believe that our findings provide an important input into the debate concerning the clinical relevance of studied variants. There is no clear explanation for deviation from HWE in our population. The possible reason is that the HLA-G gene is under balancing selection [34].

In summary, we found a significant association between *HLA-G* +3142G>C variant and susceptibility to RA in a sample of Iranian population. Further association studies with large sample size and different ethnicities are required to verify our findings.

Competing Interests

No competing financial interests exist.

Acknowledgments

This work was supported by a dissertation grant (MD thesis of SAF no. 6840) from Zahedan University of Medical Sciences.

References

[1] M. C. Hochberg and T. D. Spector, "Epidemiology of rheumatoid arthritis: update," *Epidemiologic Reviews*, vol. 12, no. 1, pp. 247–252, 1990.

[2] C. Turesson and E. L. Matteson, "Genetics of rheumatoid arthritis," *Mayo Clinic Proceedings*, vol. 81, no. 1, pp. 94–101, 2006.

[3] A. M. Ghelani, A. Samanta, A. C. Jones, and S. S. Mastana, "Association analysis of TNFR2, VDR, A2M, GSTT1, GSTM1, and ACE genes with rheumatoid arthritis in South Asians and Caucasians of East Midlands in the United Kingdom," *Rheumatology International*, vol. 31, no. 10, pp. 1355–1361, 2011.

[4] M. Hashemi, A. K. Moazeni-Roodi, A. Fazaeli et al., "The L55M polymorphism of paraoxonase-1 is a risk factor for rheumatoid arthritis," *Genetics and Molecular Research*, vol. 9, no. 3, pp. 1735–1741, 2010.

[5] M. F. Seldin, C. I. Amos, R. Ward, and P. K. Gregersen, "The genetics revolution and the assault on rheumatoid arthritis," *Arthritis and Rheumatism*, vol. 42, no. 6, pp. 1071–1079, 1999.

[6] M. Hashemi, Z. Zakeri, H. Taheri, G. Bahari, and M. Taheri, "Association between peptidylarginine deiminase type 4 rs1748033 polymorphism and susceptibility to rheumatoid arthritis in Zahedan, Southeast Iran," *Iranian Journal of Allergy, Asthma and Immunology*, vol. 14, no. 3, pp. 255–260, 2015.

[7] M. Hashemi, Z. Zakeri, E. Eskandari-Nasab et al., "CD226 rs763361 (Gly307ser) polymorphism is associated with susceptibility to rheumatoid arthritis in Zahedan, southeast Iran," *Iranian Biomedical Journal*, vol. 17, no. 4, pp. 194–199, 2013.

[8] M. Hashemi, E. Eskandari-Nasab, Z. Zakeri et al., "Association of pre-miRNA-146a rs2910164 and pre miRNA-499 rs3746444 polymorphisms and susceptibility to rheumatoid arthritis," *Molecular Medicine Reports*, vol. 7, no. 1, pp. 287–291, 2013.

[9] D. R. J. Bainbridge, S. A. Ellis, and I. L. Sargent, "HLA-G suppresses proliferation of CD^{4+} T-lymphocytes," *Journal of Reproductive Immunology*, vol. 48, no. 1, pp. 17–26, 2000.

[10] A. Dorling, N. Monk, and R. Lechler, "HLA-G inhibits the transendothelial cell migration of human NK cells: a strategy

[11] A. Dorling, N. J. Monk, and R. I. Lechler, "HLA-G inhibits the transendothelial migration of human NK cells," *European Journal of Immunology*, vol. 30, no. 2, pp. 586–593, 2000.

[12] E. A. Donadi, E. C. Castelli, A. Arnaiz-Villena, M. Roger, D. Rey, and P. Moreau, "Implications of the polymorphism of HLA-G on its function, regulation, evolution and disease association," *Cellular and Molecular Life Sciences*, vol. 68, no. 3, pp. 369–395, 2011.

[13] P. Rousseau, M. Le Discorde, G. Mouillot, C. Marcou, E. D. Carosella, and P. Moreau, "The 14 bp deletion-insertion polymorphism in the 3′ UT region of the HLA-G gene influences HLA-G mRNA stability," *Human Immunology*, vol. 64, no. 11, pp. 1005–1010, 2003.

[14] T. V. F. Hviid, S. Hylenius, C. Rørbye, and L. G. Nielsen, "HLA-G allelic variants are associated with differences in the HLA-G mRNA isoform profile and HLA-G mRNA levels," *Immunogenetics*, vol. 55, no. 2, pp. 63–79, 2003.

[15] T. D. Veit and J. A. B. Chies, "Tolerance versus immune response—microRNAs as important elements in the regulation of the HLA-G gene expression," *Transplant Immunology*, vol. 20, no. 4, pp. 229–231, 2009.

[16] X.-Y. Chen, W.-H. Yan, A. Lin, H.-H. Xu, J.-G. Zhang, and X.-X. Wang, "The 14 bp deletion polymorphisms in HLA-G gene play an important role in the expression of soluble HLA-G in plasma," *Tissue Antigens*, vol. 72, no. 4, pp. 335–341, 2008.

[17] E. C. Castelli, P. Moreau, A. O. E. Chiromatzo et al., "In silico analysis of microRNAS targeting the *HLA-G* 3′ untranslated region alleles and haplotypes," *Human Immunology*, vol. 70, no. 12, pp. 1020–1025, 2009.

[18] Z. Tan, G. Randall, J. Fan et al., "Allele-specific targeting of microRNAs to HLA-G and risk of asthma," *American Journal of Human Genetics*, vol. 81, no. 4, pp. 829–834, 2007.

[19] L. A. Verbruggen, V. Rebmann, C. Demanet, S. De Cock, and H. Grosse-Wilde, "Soluble HLA-G in rheumatoid arthritis," *Human Immunology*, vol. 67, no. 8, pp. 561–567, 2006.

[20] S. K. Kim, J. H. Chung, D. H. Kim, D. H. Yun, S. J. Hong, and K. H. Lee, "Lack of association between promoter polymorphisms of *HLA-G* gene and rheumatoid arthritis in Korean population," *Rheumatology International*, vol. 32, no. 2, pp. 509–512, 2012.

[21] Y. H. Lee and S. C. Bae, "Association between a functional HLA-G 14-bp insertion/deletion polymorphism and susceptibility to autoimmune diseases: a meta-analysis," *Cellular and Molecular Biology*, vol. 61, no. 8, pp. 24–30, 2015.

[22] C. M. Mariaselvam, A. B. Chaaben, S. Salah et al., "Human leukocyte antigen-G polymorphism influences the age of onset and autoantibody status in rheumatoid arthritis," *Tissue Antigens*, vol. 85, no. 3, pp. 182–189, 2015.

[23] T. D. Veit, P. Vianna, I. Scheibel et al., "Association of the HLA-G 14-bp insertion/deletion polymorphism with juvenile idiopathic arthritis and rheumatoid arthritis," *Tissue Antigens*, vol. 71, no. 5, pp. 440–446, 2008.

[24] E. Catamo, C. Addobbati, L. Segat et al., "HLA-G gene polymorphisms associated with susceptibility to rheumatoid arthritis disease and its severity in Brazilian patients," *Tissue Antigens*, vol. 84, no. 3, pp. 308–315, 2014.

[25] J. Funovits, D. Aletaha, V. Bykerk et al., "The 2010 American College of Rheumatology/European league against rheumatism classification criteria for rheumatoid arthritis: methodological report phase I," *Annals of the Rheumatic Diseases*, vol. 69, no. 9, pp. 1589–1595, 2010.

[26] M. Hashemi, H. Hanafi Bojd, E. Eskandari Nasab et al., "Association of adiponectin rs1501299 and rs266729 gene polymorphisms with nonalcoholic fatty liver disease," *Hepatitis Monthly*, vol. 13, no. 5, Article ID e9527, 2013.

[27] E. A. Cordero, T. D. Veit, M. A. da Silva, S. M. Jacques, L. M. Silla, and J. A. Chies, "HLA-G polymorphism influences the susceptibility to HCV infection in sickle cell disease patients," *Tissue Antigens*, vol. 74, no. 4, pp. 308–313, 2009.

[28] E. Eskandari-Nasab, M. Hashemi, S.-S. Hasani, M. Omrani, M. Taheri, and M.-A. Mashhadi, "Association between HLA-G 3′UTR 14-bp ins/del polymorphism and susceptibility to breast cancer," *Cancer Biomarkers*, vol. 13, no. 4, pp. 253–259, 2013.

[29] E. Alegre, R. Rizzo, D. Bortolotti, S. Fernandez-Landázuri, E. Fainardi, and A. González, "Some basic aspects of HLA-G biology," *Journal of Immunology Research*, vol. 2014, Article ID 657625, 10 pages, 2014.

[30] N. Rouas-Freiss, P. Moreau, J. Lemaoult, and E. D. Carosella, "The dual role of HLA-G in cancer," *Journal of Immunology Research*, vol. 2014, Article ID 359748, 10 pages, 2014.

[31] R. Rizzo, I. Farina, D. Bortolotti et al., "HLA-G may predict the disease course in patients with early rheumatoid arthritis," *Human Immunology*, vol. 74, no. 4, pp. 425–432, 2013.

[32] Y. H. Lee, S.-C. Bae, and G. G. Song, "Meta-analysis of associations between functional HLA-G polymorphisms and susceptibility to systemic lupus erythematosus and rheumatoid arthritis," *Rheumatology International*, vol. 35, no. 6, pp. 953–961, 2014.

[33] T. D. Veit, C. P. S. de Lima, L. C. Cavalheiro et al., "HLA-G +3142 polymorphism as a susceptibility marker in two rheumatoid arthritis populations in Brazil," *Tissue Antigens*, vol. 83, no. 4, pp. 260–266, 2014.

[34] Z. Tan, A. M. Shon, and C. Ober, "Evidence of balancing selection at the HLA-G promoter region," *Human Molecular Genetics*, vol. 14, no. 23, pp. 3619–3628, 2005.

[35] C. Ober, C. L. Aldrich, I. Chervoneva et al., "Variation in the HLA-G promoter region influences miscarriage rates," *American Journal of Human Genetics*, vol. 72, no. 6, pp. 1425–1435, 2003.

[36] E. C. Castelli, C. T. Mendes-Junior, N. H. S. Deghaide et al., "The genetic structure of 3′untranslated region of the *HLA-G* gene: polymorphisms and haplotypes," *Genes & Immunity*, vol. 11, no. 2, pp. 134–141, 2010.

[37] T. V. F. Hviid, R. Rizzo, O. B. Christiansen, L. Melchiorri, A. Lindhard, and O. R. Baricordi, "HLA-G and IL-10 in serum in relation to HLA-G genotype and polymorphisms," *Immunogenetics*, vol. 56, no. 3, pp. 135–141, 2004.

10

Use of Virtual Reality Tools for Vestibular Disorders Rehabilitation

Mathieu Bergeron,[1] Catherine L. Lortie,[1,2] and Matthieu J. Guitton[1,2]

[1]Department of Oto-Rhino-Laryngology and Ophthalmology, Faculty of Medicine, Laval University, Quebec City, QC, Canada G1V 0A6
[2]Institut Universitaire en Santé Mentale de Québec, Quebec City, QC, Canada G1J 2G3

Correspondence should be addressed to Matthieu J. Guitton; matthieu.guitton@fmed.ulaval.ca

Academic Editor: Ingo Todt

Classical peripheral vestibular disorders rehabilitation is a long and costly process. While virtual reality settings have been repeatedly suggested to represent possible tools to help the rehabilitation process, no systematic study had been conducted so far. We systematically reviewed the current literature to analyze the published protocols documenting the use of virtual reality settings for peripheral vestibular disorders rehabilitation. There is an important diversity of settings and protocols involving virtual reality settings for the treatment of this pathology. Evaluation of the symptoms is often not standardized. However, our results unveil a clear effect of virtual reality settings-based rehabilitation of the patients' symptoms, assessed by objectives tools such as the DHI (mean decrease of 27 points), changing symptoms handicap perception from moderate to mild impact on life. Furthermore, we detected a relationship between the duration of the exposure to virtual reality environments and the magnitude of the therapeutic effects, suggesting that virtual reality treatments should last at least 150 minutes of cumulated exposure to ensure positive outcomes. Virtual reality offers a pleasant and safe environment for the patient. Future studies should standardize evaluation tools, document putative side effects further, compare virtual reality to conventional physical therapy, and evaluate economical costs/benefits of such strategies.

1. Introduction

"Vertigo," symptoms of body balance disorders of vestibular origins, such as benign paroxysmal positional vertigo (BPPV) or Ménière's disease associated vertigo, has a lifetime prevalence of 7.4% [1, 2]. As 80% of sufferers consult for their vertigo, often resulting in work interruptions, peripheral vestibular disorders represent an important cost for society [1, 3]. Most of vertigo-related expenses are due to unnecessary diagnostic measures and ineffective treatments, for example, in the case of BPPV [3].

The classical therapeutic approach for vestibular disorders relies on vestibular rehabilitation and symptomatic medication [4, 5]. Vestibular rehabilitation uses central mechanisms of neuroplasticity (adaptation, habituation, and substitution) to increase static and dynamic postural stability and to improve visuovestibular interactions in situations that generate conflicting sensory information [2, 4, 6]. Vestibular rehabilitation can improve static and dynamic balance and gait, reduce symptoms of dizziness of comorbid depression and of anxiety, and ultimately result in an increase of self-confidence and quality of life of sufferers [7].

However, many factors may negatively affect the outcome of vestibular rehabilitation, including incorrect performance of exercises and the necessity of active efforts and interest from the patient [4, 8]. Due to the variability of patients' response to therapy, there is only moderate evidence to support that vestibular rehabilitation enables symptoms recovery and improves functioning in the medium term for unilateral peripheral vestibular dysfunction [9]. Thus, more efficient and cost-effective therapeutic tools are yet to come for vestibular rehabilitation. In this context, virtual reality-based treatment could represent an interesting potential candidate.

Virtual environments are interactive simulations of real world generated by computers and presented to users through media of varying degrees of complexity (e.g., computer screen, 360° circular screen, head-mounted display, etc.). Hardware devices can be added to the equipment in order to monitor movement kinematics or provide simulations of force and haptic feedback to participants [10–13]. Given that motor skills can be learned in a virtual environment and later on applied into the real world and that virtual settings can provide controlled and/or augmented feedback on motor performance, it is not surprising that medical rehabilitation began to use heavily such settings as therapeutic tools [10]. For instance, virtual settings have been used for rehabilitation of upper extremities motor control [14–17], gaits and lower extremities control [18, 19], spatial and perceptual motor training [20–22], or balance training [23].

Although the suitability of virtual reality in balance training of participant with vestibular disorders has already been demonstrated [24], neither homogeneous data on the optimal conditions to perform virtual reality-based vestibular rehabilitation therapy nor general recommendations are currently available. Therefore, we reviewed the existing literature on virtual reality and vestibular rehabilitation to fill this gap, document this particular form of technology-enhanced medical practice, and propose recommendations for future studies and clinical applications of virtual reality tools for vestibular disorders.

2. Materials and Methods

A comprehensive analysis was conducted to compare the efficiency of virtual reality-based rehabilitation on peripheral vestibular disorders. Following a PICOS standardized format, this study investigates patient > 18 years with old peripheral vestibular disorders (population) in the context of virtual reality rehabilitation (intervention). We compared the impact of peripheral vestibular symptoms using validated vestibular disorder questionnaires. This was performed for different virtual reality designs and protocols (comparison), quantifying the clinical improvement of dizziness (outcome). Results of individual studies were combined under the form of a meta-analysis to quantify the improvement of vestibular disorder with virtual reality (study design).

2.1. Selection of Relevant Primary Studies. Studies—papers published in peer-reviewed journals excluding conference abstracts—using virtual reality-based settings for vestibular disorders rehabilitation were gathered according to the following strategy. A comprehensive search was conducted in MedLine with the following keywords: "vestibular system," "vestibular dysfunction," "vertigo," "equilibrium," "balance," "virtual reality," "virtual treatment," and "virtual rehabilitation." Keywords "treatment" or "rehabilitation" were parts of all keyword strategy to optimize the search. Articles in English, French, Spanish, and Portuguese published from 1946 to August 2013 were included in the search. The search was independently performed twice, and references were cross-checked. In addition, references from all identified studies were systematically looked for to find any supplementary sources and ensure that all relevant studies were selected. Titles and abstracts of the 489 articles identified by the search were assessed for pertinence. Of the 489 articles found on MedLine, 316 articles were duplicates and 143 articles were ignored, mainly because they did not assess our primary subject (no rehabilitation and/or no virtual therapy and/or no vestibular disorder). Studies dealing with rehabilitation on geriatric population only were also excluded, since many confounding factors may be involved in balance disorders in this particular population. Articles about a one-time diagnostic test using virtual reality without a rehabilitation or treatment process were also excluded (12 articles). Finally, we also excluded studies on vertigo of central, neurological, and/or psychiatric origin (13 articles). Three more articles were excluded for not presenting their results or having incomplete results. An initial sample of 5 articles was thus selected for further analyses from the MedLine database. The exact same procedures using an identical selection strategy were used on Google Scholar and on the Cochrane Central Register of Controlled Trials databases. These subsequent searches provided 2 supplementary articles. Therefore, the final sample was composed of 7 studies.

2.2. Data Extraction. Data from studies meeting inclusion criteria were extracted into a standardized database and cross-checked for accuracy. Information regarding the type of balance disorder and age of the patient was extracted from the text and the tables or obtained from the figures.

When possible, three measures of efficiency were extracted from the studies. First, the percentage of improvement on the DHI (score after rehabilitation, baseline) after the rehabilitation compared to the baseline on the Dizziness Handicap Index (DHI). Second, the percentage of improvement on another scale used by the authors (e.g., Tinetti questionnaire, Vertigo Analytic Scale; score after rehabilitation, baseline). In case of multiple scales other than the DHI, the most standardized one was favored. Third and last, the average efficiency (mean improvement of the DHI and the other scale used) was computed in order to provide a more global evaluation of the improvements and to attenuate the potential differences between the assessment tools used across the different studies.

The nature of the device used to deliver the virtual reality exposure to patients was recorded (screen in front/around the patient, goggles, head-mounted display, . . .) together with the potential addition of a force platform or a treadmill. Studies were further divided into either "passive" or "active" in terms of virtual reality-based rehabilitation. Passive rehabilitation required only eyes or head movements or staying immobile during the treatment. In contrast, active rehabilitation requested complete motions of the body or muscle groups in order to perform demanding movements (walking on a treadmill, doing steps, or yoga).

When available, tolerability of the rehabilitation and side effects were noted. Finally, the level of validity of each study was assessed with the Oxford grading scale [25]. The Oxford grading scale rating could range from a score of 0 (bad) to a score of 5 (good). Randomization gives a maximum of 2 points: 1 if randomization is mentioned and an additional point if the method of randomization is appropriate (1 point is deduced if inappropriate). A maximum of 2 points is given for blinding: 1 if blinding is mentioned and one additional point if the method is appropriate (1 point is deduced if inappropriate). Finally, 1 point is given if withdrawal and drop-out are described for all patients.

2.3. Statistical Analysis. Spearman rank tests were performed to observe whether total exposure time to virtual therapy and the number of treatment sessions were associated with the efficiency of the rehabilitation process, as measured by the DHI, other scales, and the average efficiency. Studies were also subdivided into either "low efficiency" (<20% of improvement on average efficiency) or "high efficiency" (>20% of improvement). This threshold of 20% represents in most dizziness assessment tools an improvement equivalent to a change of handicap category (no handicap/mild handicap/moderate handicap/severe handicap). Nonparametric Mann-Whitney U tests were then used to compare the average efficiency, total exposure time, and the number of sessions between "low efficiency" and "high efficiency" studies as well as between studies using "active" versus "passive" virtual reality settings. When normality test successfully passed, Student's t-tests were used. The average efficiency was analyzed as a function of total exposure time and the number of sessions using simple linear regressions.

3. Results

3.1. Characteristics of the Selected Studies. Seven studies fulfilled our criteria (Table 1), for a total of 176 subjects (including 115 patients) who underwent a protocol of virtual reality-based vestibular rehabilitation. The studies included 8 to 71 subjects with patient groups formed by 8 to 37 individuals (see the paragraph "Reliability of the Studies" for the ratio of studies having a control group). Age of the subjects ranged from 18 to 84 years. Other demographic data were impossible to extract from the studies analyzed due to a lack of information in the texts. All the following data presented here rely only on patients suffering from vestibular disorders who underwent virtual reality rehabilitation. Subjects were exposed to 6 to 12 sessions of virtual reality rehabilitation, spread over 1 to 8 weeks. Each session lasted 24 to 45 minutes, for a total of 144 to 540 minutes spent in virtual reality-based rehabilitation. Two main categories of devices were used to expose subjects to virtual reality: either screen/projection or headset/goggles. Out of the 7 studies, 5 used goggles or a head-mounted device (71%), while the other 2 used screens in front of or around the subject (28%). In addition, in the vast majority of studies (5 out of 7, 71%), a treadmill or a force platform was added to enhance the rehabilitation process.

3.2. Impact of Interactive Involvement. Efficacy of the virtual rehabilitation was compared regarding the type of device used. Average efficiency varied from 4.65% to 43.5% for goggles/headset and from 4.4% to 42.61% for screen/projection.

The type of device used did not have an effect on efficiency (U tests, P = 0.86 for average efficiency, P = 0.53 for DHI evaluations and P = 0.86 for other scales). Efficacy of the virtual rehabilitation was also compared regarding active versus passive settings. Four studies (57%) used a passive approach, while 3 studies (43%) used a more active setting. However, no difference was observed between passive and active settings on average efficiency (U test, P = 0.63), DHI scores (U test, P = 0.53) and other scales scores (U test, P = 0.23).

3.3. Efficiency and Impact of Treatment Duration. A clear improvement following virtual reality-based therapy was observed in all studies whatever the assessment tool used. After completing all sessions, the average efficiency across studies varied between 4.4 to 43.5% (DHI score (4–63%) and other scales (4.4–51%)). In studies using the DHI, the mean decrease was 26 points over 100 on the scale, allowing patients to lessen their handicap either from severe to moderate or from moderate to mild.

Despite statistical trends, efficiency was not directly associated neither with total exposure time in virtual reality-based rehabilitation (Spearman rank tests, P = 0.24 for DHI evaluation, P = 0.09 for other scales and for average efficiency) nor with the number of sessions (Spearman rank tests, P = 0.36 for DHI evaluation, P = 0.09 for other scales and for average efficiency). Time per session was not related to efficiency either (Spearman rank tests, P = 0.17 for DHI evaluation, P = 0.78 for other scales and P = 0.60 for average efficiency). However, simple linear regressions revealed that the average efficiency was significantly explained by total exposure time (r^2 = 0.5975, P < 0.05, Figure 1(a)) and in a lesser extent by the number of sessions (r^2 = 0.5164, P = 0.07, Figure 1(b)).

As stated earlier, studies were divided into either "low efficiency" (<20% of improvement on average efficiency) or "high efficiency" (>20% of improvement, t-test, P < 0.001), (Table 2). Studies with lower efficiency had shorter total time spent in rehabilitation (t-test, P < 0.05, Figure 2(a)) and fewer sessions than more efficient studies (t-test, P < 0.05, Figure 2(b)).

3.4. Occurrence of Side Effects. Surprisingly, although a majority of studies mentioned that the rehabilitation was well tolerated, the side effects were almost never documented. Particularly, none of the studies evaluated motion sickness and/or cybersickness with a validated questionnaire. When mentioned, side effects and tolerability were only briefly described (5 of the 7 studies). In terms of tolerability, no study reported major issues following the use of virtual reality and no significant incident or fall was reported.

3.5. Reliability of the Studies. Only 4 out of the 7 studies had a control group, with only one study randomized (Table 3). Ratings using the Oxford grading scale [25] to evaluate the methodological quality of clinical trials revealed significant weaknesses. The studies ranged from 1 (3 studies out of 7; 43%) to 2 (3 studies out of 7; 43%), with only one study

TABLE 1: Main characteristics of the studies.

Study	Patients/ages	Vestibular problem	Type of virtual reality device	Measurements of efficacy
dos Santos et al. (2009) ACTA ORL [31]	n = 8 (18–60 years, mean 41 years)	Chronic vestibular dysfunction	Balance Rehabilitation Unit (BRU) with virtual reality glasses projecting visual stimuli	(i) Dizziness Handicap Index (DHI) (ii) Vertigo analogic Scale (VAS) (iii) Stabilisation limits (LOS) (iv) Audiometer (tonal, vocal) (v) Impedance (vi) Vectonystagmography (vii) Posturography
Rodrigues et al. (2009) Rev Equilibro Corporal e Saude [32]	n = 10 (24–76 years, mean 51 years)	Chronic vestibular disorder secondary to Ménière's disease	Balance Rehabilitation Unit (BRU) with visual stimuli (glasses)	(i) DHI (ii) VAS (iii) LOS (iv) Computerized Posturography
Viirre and Sitarz (2002) Laryngoscope [33]	n = 15 (age n/a) (i) n = 9 patients (ii) n = 6 controls	Vertigo symptoms for more than 6 months (with no improvement for at least 6 months)	Head-mounted Display (HMD) much like a visor with mounted video screens	(i) DHI (ii) Vestibuloocular reflex (VOR)
Pavlou et al. (2012) J Vestib Res [34]	n = 16 (18–75 years, mean 40 years) (i) n = 11 (Group S = static virtual reality) (ii) n = 5 (Group D = dynamic virtual reality) (iii) n = 5 Group D1 (5 patients from Group S who had also dynamic treatment)	Confirmed peripheral vestibular deficit (caloric test and/or rotational test on ENG)	ReaCtoR in the Department of Computer Science: immersive projection theatre (IPT). 3 rear-projected vertical screens (3 m × 2.2 m)	(i) Situational Vertigo Questionnaire (ii) Beck Depression Inventory (iii) Beck Anxiety Inventory (iv) Fear Questionnaire (v) Dynamic Gait Index (DGI) (vi) Virtual reality exercise symptom scores (VRCESS)
Sparrer et al. (2013) Acta Otolaryngol [35]	n = 71 (28–84 years, mean 43 years) (i) n = 37 patients (ii) n = 34 controls	Acute vestibular neuritis (sudden, spontaneous, and unilateral loss of peripheral vestibular function within 48 h of the onset of vertigo)	Wii Fit balance board with image on screen	(i) DHI (ii) Wii Fit age (iii) Sensory Organization Test (SOT) (iv) Vertigo Symptom Scale (VSS) (v) Tinetti questionnaire
Whitney et al. (2009) Physical Therapy Reviews [36]	n = 12 (18–80 years, mean 52 years)	Vestibular disorders with dizziness and loss of balance	Treadmill in a virtual grocery store on a screen	(i) DHI (ii) Activities-specific Balance Confidence Scale (ABC) (iii) Dynamic Gait Index (DGI) (iv) Timed Up and Go (TUG) (v) Sensory Organization Test (SOT)
Garcia et al. (2013) Braz J Otorhinolaryngol [37]	n = 44 (18–60 years, mean 48 years) (i) n = 23 cases (ii) n = 21 controls	Unilateral or Bilateral Ménière's disease	Balance Rehabilitation Unit (BRU) with virtual reality glasses projecting visual stimuli	(i) DHI (ii) Analog dizziness scale (iii) ENT examination (iv) PTA audiometry; impedance (v) Functional vestibular examination (vi) Speech intelligibility testing (vii) Posturography

(a)

(b)

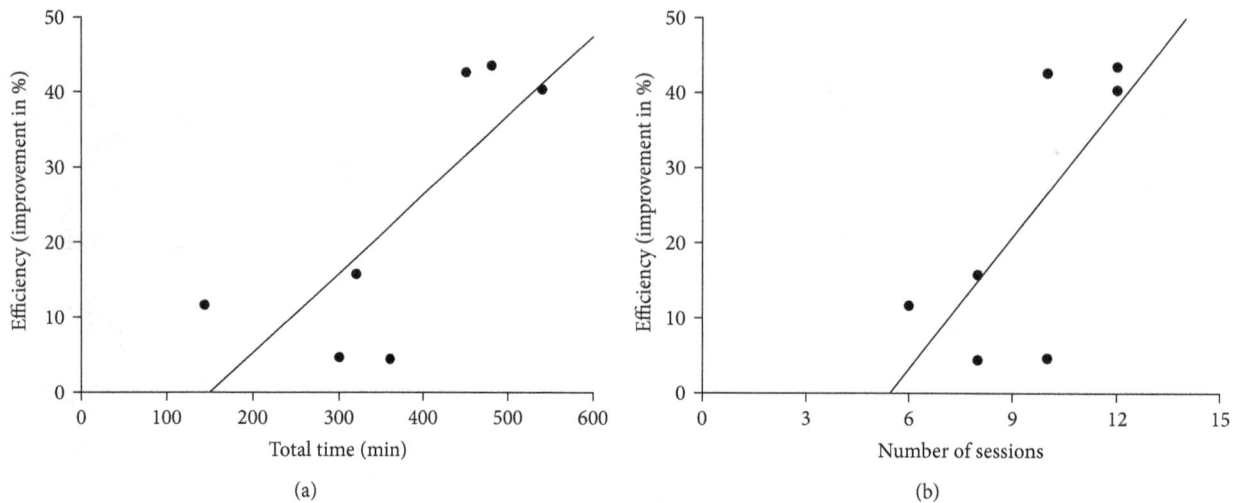

FIGURE 1: Impact of the duration of virtual reality exposure on treatment efficiency. (a) Average efficiency in terms of symptoms' improvement as a function of the total time spent in virtual reality-based therapy (linear regression, $r^2 = 0.5975$, $P < 0.05$). (b) Average efficiency in terms of symptoms' improvement as a function of the total number of sessions of virtual reality-based treatment ($r^2 = 0.5164$, $P = 0.07$).

TABLE 2: Efficiency of rehabilitation regarding the type of device.

Study	Efficiency	Active versus passive	Average efficiency
dos Santos et al. (2009) [31] ACTA ORL	Low	Passive	15.75%
Rodrigues et al. (2009) [32] Equilíbrio Corporal e Saúde	High	Passive	43.50%
Viirre and Sitarz (2002) [33] Laryngoscope	Low	Passive	4.65%
Pavlou et al. (2012) [34] J Vestib Res	Low	Active	4.40%
Sparrer et al. (2013) [35] Acta Otolaryngol	High	Active	42.61%
Whitney et al. (2009) [36] Physical Therapy Reviews	Low	Active	11.67%
Garcia et al. (2013) [37] Braz J Otorhinolaryngol	High	Passive	40.35%

reaching a score of 3 out of a maximum score of 5 (14%)—the minimum score for a study to be considered as acceptable.

4. Discussion

This comprehensive analysis confirmed that the utilization of virtual reality in the context of vestibular disorders could be a very valuable approach. Indeed, an improvement of the patients' symptoms has been documented in all the studies examined. With an average evaluation of the vertigo-related handicap going from moderate to mild at the end of the virtual reality-based rehabilitation, these emerging tools should not be neglected among the therapeutic arsenal when dealing with patients suffering from vestibular disorders. However, despite these promising results, further research is needed to document the exact parameters of an optimal protocol and to define the most cost-effective strategies.

4.1. Protocol Design and Assessment. In the context of defining an evidence-based strategy of virtual reality-based therapies for vestibular disorders, the relative methodological weakness of the studies examined was a major issue. Indeed, none of the selected studies ranked more than 3 on the Oxford grading scale. More worrying, the majority of studies ranked 1 or 2 (i.e., low methodological quality). These low ratings were mostly due to the absence of control groups, randomized conditions, and blind experiments. However, it should be noted here that, due to the nature of the diseases and of the rehabilitation interventions, blinding of the protocols is almost impossible to reach, partly explaining the relatively low score observed. Unfortunately, the small size of most of the cohorts combined with nonsystematic evaluations made it also difficult to reach absolute conclusions.

While increasing the group sizes or multiplying control groups could be difficult to do in the context of costly

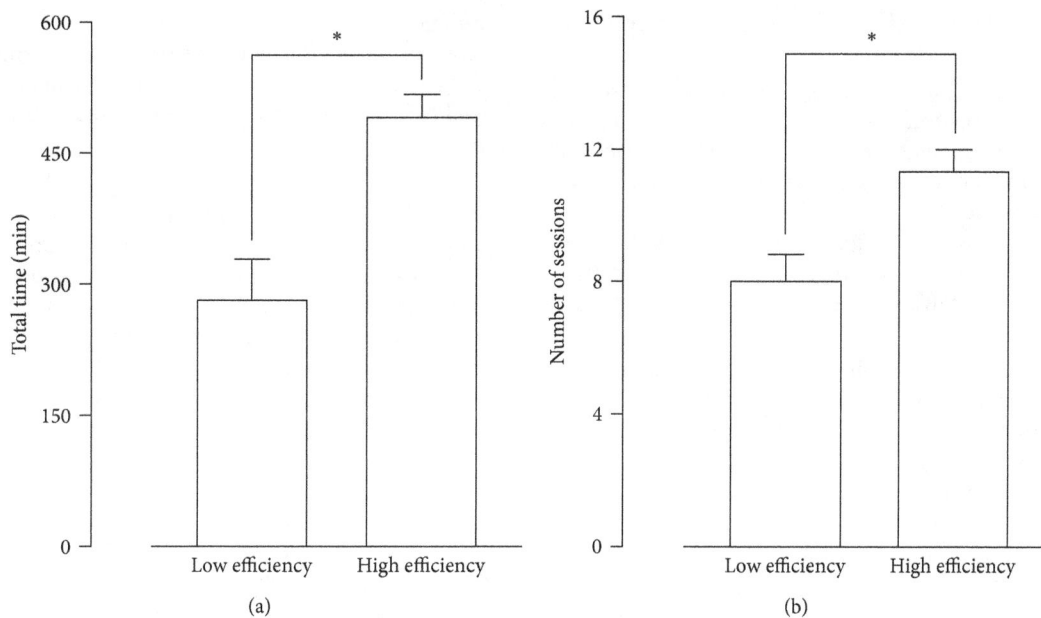

FIGURE 2: Differential characteristics of virtual reality protocols according to average efficiency. (a) Time spent in virtual reality-based treatment. (b) Number of sessions depending on the clinical impact of the treatment ("low efficiency" defining studies with less than 20% of improvement on average efficiency and "high efficiency" studies with more than 20% of improvement). $^{*}P < 0.05$.

TABLE 3: Studies reliability assessed according to the Oxford grading scale.

Study	Oxford scale	Control group	Limitations
dos Santos et al. (2009) [31] ACTA ORL	1	N	Limited number of patients
Rodrigues et al. (2009) [32] Equilíbrio Corporal e Saúde	1	N	Limited number of patients No control
Viirre and Sitarz (2002) [33] Laryngoscope	2	Y	Limited number of patients Limited demographic data
Pavlou et al. (2012) [34] J Vestib Res	2	Y	Unique and specific virtual reality device
Sparrer et al. (2013) [35] Acta Otolaryngol	2	Y	Limited number of patients
Whitney et al. (2009) [36] Physical Therapy Reviews	1	N	Limited number of patients No control
Garcia et al. (2013) [37] Braz J Otorhinolaryngol	3	Y	Patients also on medication (betahistine)

experiments involving patients and important resources, efforts should be done regarding the rigorousness and standardization of evaluation. For instance, the DHI was not systematically used. While many scales or questionnaires could be used to document vestibular disorder-related handicaps, the DHI still remains one of the most standard and easy to administer assessment tools [26]. A few studies preferred using nonvalidated "homemade" questionnaires. These questionnaires do not allow a direct and standardized comparison with the literature. Thus, they should be avoided or used only in conjunction with validated tools such as the DHI.

4.2. Practical Optimization. In a practical point of view, a very important issue is which of time spent in virtual reality-based training and the number of session is the key factor to increase the therapeutic effect. Interestingly, the present meta-analysis seemed to suggest that time spent in virtual reality-based therapy contributed more to the average efficiency than the number of sessions. Results unveil that a minimum exposure time of 120–150 minutes is required to detect a quantifiable benefit for the patient. However, the time spent and the number of sessions are intimately related. Furthermore, the effect of intertrial time (time between two consecutive sessions) has been so far overlooked. This parameter should be documented in future studies.

Given that time spent in virtual therapy is clearly of importance, longer sessions in a short period of time could be effective and convenient. However, the total duration of a session is strongly depending on the physical state of the patient. Of note, some of the results of this study might appear contradictory. However, that might be explained by the very size of our sample (only 7 studies met our criterions), limiting the overall power of a few analyses.

4.3. Clinical Applicability. Peripheral vestibular disorders can be heterogeneous in terms of etiology [27]. One of the strengths of this meta-analysis is that the studies examined gathered diverse populations of patients presenting various peripheral vestibular disorders similar to ones found in clinical settings.

Virtual reality settings are extremely useful for various pathologies [14]. However, one of the main limitations of using such protocols as clinical tools is the related cost. In the context of important attempts in cost reductions in health care systems, this issue could be a major argument against the implementation of virtual reality settings in clinical facilities. Although more studies have to be dedicated to answer the question on cost/efficiency of virtual reality in clinical situations, the case of vestibular rehabilitation seems encouraging. Indeed, our evidence-based data suggest that there is no need for the most expensive devices to obtain significant improvement in patients. Instead, very positive outcomes can be evidenced with affordable devices such as a Nintendo Wii. Furthermore, even if we did not observe a difference in efficiency between active and passive protocols, technological devices allowing active mobilization of muscular groups can be acquired with limited cost. Self-utilization of virtual reality devices by patients could in fact reduce the rehabilitation costs.

This leads us to a second limitation. None of the studies analyzed answered the question of whether virtual reality-based vestibular rehabilitation should be done alone or in combination with conventional vestibular rehabilitation. Intuitively, one could expect that the combination of various therapeutic protocols would have optimal results. However, this has to be demonstrated.

Another consideration limiting the use of virtual reality-based settings in rehabilitation medicine is cybersickness. Indeed, due to unnatural and sometimes conflicting multisensory stimuli, exposure to interactive virtual environments can cause discomfort during or after the session, which is referred to as cybersickness [28–30]. Symptoms reported are motion sickness-like, including nausea, vomiting, headache, somnolence, loss of balance, and altered eye-hand coordination [29]. These undesirable events, which can be distinguished from classical motion sickness caused by vestibular stimulation alone, are particularly worrying in participants with impaired vestibular function. While, to date, most studies have underlooked this issue, the occurrence of cybersickness should be systematically documented before virtual rehabilitation could be used on larger scales for these populations of patients. However, despite these limits, the absence of reported side effects or adverse events (e.g., falls) so far tends to support the notion that virtual rehabilitation is well tolerated and could be safely used in a rehabilitation setting.

4.4. Conclusions and Recommendations. The present meta-analysis demonstrates the promising potential of virtual reality-based treatment for peripheral vestibular disorders. Despite significant differences in terms of protocol used and outcomes evaluation, all studies demonstrated that virtual reality-based rehabilitation strategies had a positive effect and were seemingly well tolerated. The main criterion predicting treatment success and magnitude of symptoms improvement is the total time spent in virtual reality training. The complexity of the setting used does not seem to have a direct impact on efficiency, as important results are possible with inexpensive settings. Thus, virtual reality-based rehabilitation represents a potentially promising new avenue to reduce the costs of peripheral vestibular disorders rehabilitation.

In conclusion, some recommendations are proposed for future studies to standardize intervention protocols and evaluation tools, document side effects, determine if virtual reality-based rehabilitation should be combined with classical rehabilitation, and define profiles of patients susceptible to benefit from a virtual reality-based rehabilitation as follows.

Recommendations for Virtual Reality-Based Treatment Applied to Peripheral Vestibular Disorders

   (i) Use only validated assessment tool, including the DHI as primary assessing tool.

   (ii) Document clearly the time and number of sessions spent in rehabilitation and time between sessions.

   (iii) Document virtual reality-related side effects (cybersickness) with validated questionnaire, such as Simulator Sickness Questionnaire (SSQ).

   (iv) Document complications of virtual reality rehabilitation such as falls and fractures.

   (v) Document symptomatic medication taken by the patient.

   (vi) If possible, document the cost of the device and each session.

Conflict of Interests

The authors declare that there is no conflict of interests regarding the publication of this paper.

Acknowledgments

Matthieu J. Guitton holds a Career Grant from the "Fonds de Recherche du Québec-Santé" (FRQS). This work was supported by the Oto-Rhino-Laryngology-Head and Neck Surgery Research fund of the "Fondation de l'Université Laval".

References

[1] H. K. Neuhauser, M. Von Brevern, A. Radtke et al., "Epidemiology of vestibular vertigo: a neurotologic survey of the general population," *Neurology*, vol. 65, no. 6, pp. 898–904, 2005.

[2] B. T. Crane, D. A. Schessel, J. Nedzelski, and L. B. Minor, "Peripheral vestibular disorders," in *Cummings Otolaryngology: Head and Neck Surgery*, P. W. Flint, B. H. Haughey, V. J. Lund et al., Eds., pp. 2328–2345, Mosby Elsevier, Philadelphia, Pa, USA, 5th edition, 2010.

[3] J. C. Li, C. J. Li, J. Epley, and L. Weinberg, "Cost-effective management of benign positional vertigo using canalith repositioning," *Otolaryngology: Head and Neck Surgery*, vol. 122, no. 3, pp. 334–339, 2000.

[4] D. E. Bamiou and L. M. Luxon, "Vertigo: clinical management and rehabilitation," in *Scott-Brown's Otorhinolaryngology, Head and Neck Surgery*, M. Gleeson and L. M. Luxon, Eds., pp. 3791–3817, CRC Press, New York, NY, USA, 7th edition, 2008.

[5] I. S. Curthoys and G. M. Halmagyi, "Vestibular compensation," in *Vestibular Dysfunction and Its Therapy. Advances in Otorhinolaryngology*, U. Buttner, Ed., pp. 195–227, Karger, Basel, Switzerland, 1999.

[6] R. E. Gans, "Vestibular rehabilitation: critical decision analysis," *Seminars in Hearing*, vol. 23, no. 2, pp. 149–159, 2002.

[7] N. A. Ricci, M. C. Aratani, F. Doná, C. Macedo, H. H. Caovilla, and F. F. Ganança, "A systematic review about the effects of the vestibular rehabilitation in middle-age and older adults," *Revista Brasileira de Fisioterapia*, vol. 14, no. 5, pp. 361–371, 2010.

[8] M. E. Norré and W. De Weerft, "Treatment of vertigo based on habituation. II. 2. Technique and results of habituation training," *Journal of Laryngology and Otology*, vol. 94, no. 9, pp. 971–977, 1980.

[9] S. L. Hillier and M. McDonnell, "Vestibular rehabilitation for unilateral peripheral vestibular dysfunction," *Cochrane Database of Systematic Reviews*, vol. 2, Article ID CD005397, 2011.

[10] F. D. Rose, E. A. Attree, B. M. Brooks, D. M. Parslow, P. R. Penn, and N. Ambihaipahan, "Training in virtual environments: transfer to real world tasks and equivalence to real task training," *Ergonomics*, vol. 43, no. 4, pp. 494–511, 2000.

[11] M. K. Holden, "Virtual environments for motor rehabilitation: review," *Cyberpsychology and Behavior*, vol. 8, no. 3, pp. 187–211, 2005.

[12] R. P. Hawkins, J.-Y. Han, S. Pingree, B. R. Shaw, T. B. Baker, and L. J. Roberts, "Interactivity and presence of three eHealth interventions," *Computers in Human Behavior*, vol. 26, no. 5, pp. 1081–1088, 2010.

[13] M. P. Fried, J. I. Uribe, and B. Sadoughi, "The role of virtual reality in surgical training in otorhinolaryngology," *Current Opinion in Otolaryngology and Head and Neck Surgery*, vol. 15, no. 3, pp. 163–169, 2007.

[14] S. Hesse, H. Schmidt, C. Werner, and A. Bardeleben, "Upper and lower extremity robotic devices for rehabilitation and for studying motor control," *Current Opinion in Neurology*, vol. 16, no. 6, pp. 705–710, 2003.

[15] M. S. Cameirão, S. B. I. Badia, E. Duarte, A. Frisoli, and P. F. M. J. Verschure, "The combined impact of virtual reality neurorehabilitation and its interfaces on upper extremity functional recovery in patients with chronic stroke," *Stroke*, vol. 43, no. 10, pp. 2720–2728, 2012.

[16] Y. J. Kang, H. K. Park, H. J. Kim et al., "Upper extremity rehabilitation of stroke: facilitation of corticospinal excitability using virtual mirror paradigm," *Journal of NeuroEngineering and Rehabilitation*, vol. 9, no. 1, article 71, 2012.

[17] S. K. Subramanian, C. B. Lourenço, G. Chilingaryan, H. Sveistrup, and M. F. Levin, "Arm motor recovery using a virtual reality intervention in chronic stroke: randomized control trial," *Neurorehabilitation and Neural Repair*, vol. 27, no. 1, pp. 13–23, 2013.

[18] D. L. Jaffe, D. A. Brown, C. D. Pierson-Carey, E. L. Buckley, and H. L. Lew, "Stepping over obstacles to improve walking in individuals with poststroke hemiplegia," *Journal of Rehabilitation Research & Development*, vol. 41, no. 3, pp. 283–292, 2004.

[19] J. E. Deutsch, J. Latonio, G. C. Burdea, and R. Boian, "Poststroke rehabilitation with the Rutgers Ankle system: a case study," *Presence*, vol. 10, no. 4, pp. 416–430, 2001.

[20] J. S. Webster, P. T. McFarland, L. J. Rapport, B. Morrill, L. A. Roades, and P. S. Abadee, "Computer-assisted training for improving wheelchair mobility in unilateral neglect patients," *Archives of Physical Medicine and Rehabilitation*, vol. 82, no. 6, pp. 769–775, 2001.

[21] L. J. Buxbaum, M. A. Palermo, D. Mastrogiovanni et al., "Assessment of spatial attention and neglect with a virtual wheelchair navigation task," *Journal of Clinical and Experimental Neuropsychology*, vol. 30, no. 6, pp. 650–660, 2008.

[22] Y. M. Kim, M. H. Chun, G. J. Yun, Y. J. Song, and H. E. Young, "The effect of virtual reality training on unilateral spatial neglect in stroke patients," *Annals of Rehabilitation Medicine*, vol. 35, no. 3, pp. 309–315, 2011.

[23] K. H. Cho, K. J. Lee, and C. H. Song, "Virtual-reality balance training with a video-game system improves dynamic balance in chronic stroke patients," *Tohoku Journal of Experimental Medicine*, vol. 228, no. 1, pp. 69–74, 2012.

[24] H. S. Cohen, "Disability and rehabilitation in the dizzy patient," *Current Opinion in Neurology*, vol. 19, no. 1, pp. 49–54, 2006.

[25] A. R. Jadad, R. A. Moore, D. Carroll et al., "Assessing the quality of reports of randomized clinical trials: is blinding necessary?" *Controlled Clinical Trials*, vol. 17, no. 1, pp. 1–12, 1996.

[26] G. P. Jacobson and C. W. Newman, "The development of the Dizziness Handicap Inventory," *Archives of Otolaryngology—Head and Neck Surgery*, vol. 116, no. 4, pp. 424–427, 1990.

[27] K. Kroenke, R. M. Hoffman, and D. Einstadter, "How common are various causes of dizziness? A critical review," *Southern Medical Journal*, vol. 93, no. 2, pp. 160–167, 2000.

[28] F. Bonato, A. Bubka, and S. Palmisano, "Combined pitch and roll and cybersickness in a virtual environment," *Aviation, Space, and Environmental Medicine*, vol. 80, no. 11, pp. 941–945, 2009.

[29] P. A. Nolin, A. Stipanicic, M. Henry, C. C. Joyal, and P. Allain, "Virtual reality as a screening tool for sports concussion in adolescents," *Brain Injury*, vol. 26, no. 13-14, pp. 1564–1573, 2012.

[30] T. Kiryu and R. H. Y. So, "Sensation of presence and cybersickness in applications of virtual reality for advanced rehabilitation," *Journal of NeuroEngineering and Rehabilitation*, vol. 4, article 34, 2007.

[31] P. R. dos Santos, A. Manso, C. F. Ganança, A. P. B. de Avila Pires, N. W. Okai, and T. S. Pichelli, "Reabilitação vestibular com realidade virtual em pacientes com disfunção vestibular," *Acta Otorhinolaryngologica Italica*, vol. 27, no. 4, pp. 148–152, 2009.

[32] T. P. Rodrigues, C. F. Ganança, A. P. Garcia, H. H. Caovilla, M. M. Ganança, and F. F. Ganança, "Reabilitação vestibular com realidade virtual em pacientes com Doença de Ménière," *Revista Equilíbrio Corporal e Saúde*, vol. 1, no. 1, pp. 9–20, 2009.

[33] E. Viirre and R. Sitarz, "Vestibular rehabilitation using visual displays: preliminary study," *Laryngoscope*, vol. 112, no. 3, pp. 500–503, 2002.

[34] M. Pavlou, R. G. Kanegaonkar, D. Swapp, D. E. Bamiou, M. Slater, and L. M. Luxon, "The effect of virtual reality on visual vertigo symptoms in patients with peripheral vestibular dysfunction: a pilot study," *Journal of Vestibular Research: Equilibrium and Orientation*, vol. 22, no. 5-6, pp. 273–281, 2012.

[35] I. Sparrer, T. A. Duong Dinh, J. Ilgner, and M. Westhofen, "Vestibular rehabilitation using the Nintendo Wii Balance Board—a user-friendly alternative for central nervous compensation," *Acta Oto-Laryngologica*, vol. 133, no. 3, pp. 239–245, 2013.

[36] S. L. Whitney, P. J. Sparto, K. Alahmari, M. S. Redfern, and J. M. Furman, "The use of virtual reality for people with balance and vestibular disorders: the Pittsburgh experience," *Physical Therapy Reviews*, vol. 14, no. 5, pp. 299–306, 2009.

[37] A. P. Garcia, M. M. Ganança, F. S. Cusin, A. Tomaz, F. F. Ganança, and H. H. Caovilla, "Vestibular rehabilitation with virtual reality in Ménière's disease," *Brazilian Journal of Otorhinolaryngology*, vol. 79, no. 3, pp. 366–374, 2013.

11

Stroke Recovery: Surprising Influences and Residual Consequences

Argye E. Hillis[1,2,3] **and Donna C. Tippett**[1,2,4]

[1] *Department of Neurology, Johns Hopkins University School of Medicine, Baltimore, MD 21287, USA*
[2] *Department of Physical Medicine and Rehabilitation, Johns Hopkins University School of Medicine, Baltimore, MD 21287, USA*
[3] *Department of Cognitive Science, Krieger School of Arts and Sciences, Johns Hopkins University, Baltimore, MD 21218, USA*
[4] *Department of Otolaryngology-Head and Neck Surgery, Johns Hopkins University School of Medicine, Baltimore, MD 21287, USA*

Correspondence should be addressed to Argye E. Hillis; argye@jhmi.edu

Academic Editor: Matteo Paci

There is startling individual variability in the degree to which people recover from stroke and the duration of time over which recovery of some symptoms occurs. There are a variety of mechanisms of recovery from stroke which take place at distinct time points after stroke and are influenced by different variables. We review recent studies from our laboratory that unveil some surprising findings, such as the role of education in chronic recovery. We also report data showing that the consequences that most plague survivors of stroke and their caregivers are loss of high level cortical functions, such as empathy or written language. These results have implications for rehabilitation and management of stroke.

1. Introduction

Stroke is among the leading causes of serious, long-term disability worldwide; 15 million people suffer a stroke each year. Almost six million people die of stroke annually, and another five million people have permanent disability due to stroke (http://www.world-heart-federation.org/cardiovascular-health/stroke). Yet, physicians are notoriously weak in predicting who will recover from stroke, how much they will recover, and when they will recover. It is widely recognized that there is a great deal of individual variability in stroke recovery. Even two individuals with very similar appearing ischemic strokes may show very different outcomes one year later. In this paper, we review recent studies from our research group, the Stroke Cognitive Outcomes and Recovery (SCORE) Lab, revealing new insights into sequelae of stroke that are most important to survivors and caregivers and the variables that influence cognitive recovery after stroke. These data have implications for both acute management of stroke and the need to explore new avenues of rehabilitation.

1.1. Why Focus on Cognitive Recovery? The human brain is responsible for all of the functions that define who we are

and how we relate to one another—our talents, our intellect, our creativity, our ability to participate in sports, our ability to communicate, and our ability to understand and share in the emotions of others. Stroke can interfere with any or all of these functions. Most of the brain, in fact, supports cognitive and integrative processes underlying complex systems, such as attention, working memory, cognitive control, and language that are critical for these activities. Yet, stroke outcomes research traditionally has focused on recovery of very basic activities of daily living, such as feeding oneself and walking. Consider the most commonly used outcome measures for stroke intervention trials, the Modified Rankin Scale (MRS) [1], the Barthel Index (BI) [2], and the National Institutes of Health Stroke Scale (NIHSS; http://www.ninds.nih .gov/doctors/nih_stroke_scale.pdf). An MRS score of 3 corresponds to moderate disability, defined as "requires some help, but able to walk without assistance." An MRS score of 2, slight disability, is defined as "unable to carry out all previous activities, but able look after own affairs without assistance." A score of 2 encompasses the status of all of those individuals who are unable to go back to their previous work because of mild or moderate language or cognitive deficits (e.g., affecting spelling, grammar, and executive function), loss of creativity, impaired emotional regulation, or loss of empathy that interferes with interpersonal relationships, as long as these deficits are not severe enough to interfere with looking after one's own affairs. Artists, executives, physicians, lawyers, and so on might be disabled from returning to previous vocations by deficits that would not interfere with some other vocations. Thus, a given higher level cortical deficit might yield an MRS score of 2 in one person and a score of 1 (no significant disability despite symptoms) in another. Furthermore, an individual might show substantial, meaningful recovery in higher cortical function over time without showing any change in the MRS scale. Likewise, the BI captures only the status of feeding, bathing, grooming, dressing, bowel function, bladder function, toilet use, transfers, mobility on level surfaces, and mobility on stairs. While this scale may measure how easy or difficult it is to care for someone after a large stroke, many people recover completely in all of these functions but remain unable to return to work or previous social roles because of residual deficits in higher cortical functions. Moreover, recovery of these basic functions is not what makes stroke survivors or their caregivers happy. A recent longitudinal study of 399 stroke survivors and their caregivers found that caregivers reported greater sense of well-being when the stroke survivor had more severe stroke, but fewer symptoms of depression and better cognitive function [3]. Individuals with cognitive impairment after stroke have poorer functional recovery, higher rates of depression, and even higher mortality after stroke [4, 5].

The NIHSS also has only a few items that evaluate cognitive function (particularly right hemisphere cognitive functions), but many more points that evaluate motor function (e.g., 8 points for holding up the arm and the leg on one side). This limitation has important consequences for evaluating both candidates for treatment and outcomes of treatment. For example, several studies have shown that the NIHSS score underestimates the volume of ischemia in patients with right hemisphere stroke relative to left hemisphere stroke [6–8]. Because of this limitation, the NIHSS may underestimate response to reperfusion of the cortex, particularly after right hemisphere stroke, as illustrated in Section 2.1.1 [9]. To address this limitation, Gottesman and colleagues [10] evaluated whether adding greater weight to right hemisphere cortical dysfunction (hemispatial neglect and extinction) would improve its correlation with volume of infarct. In a study of 200 individuals with acute stroke with concurrent NIHSS, cognitive testing, and MRI, they showed that adding a few simple quantitative tests of neglect and extinction to the NIHSS improved its detection of right and left hemisphere ischemia and its correlation with volume of infarct.

Thus, it is possible that some of the treatments that have failed to show benefit in acute stroke trials have "failed" simply because they have not measured changes in cognitive function. Often, in large vessel stroke, there is early infarct in the deep subcortical areas (e.g., lenticulostriate territory) with surrounding hypoperfused cortex that may be salvageable. The motor deficits due to deep infarct may not recover. But if there is reperfusion of the cortex, cognitive function may

be restored (as discussed later in Section 2.1.2). Therefore, it is crucial to include adequate evaluation of cortical function to measure the effects of acute intervention. Recent clinical trials in stroke are just beginning to include cognitive endpoints (e.g., [11]), but trials aiming at reperfusion typically have not included such endpoints.

1.2. Surprising Sequelae of That Stymie Stroke Survivors. Previous studies that have investigated quality of life (QOL) or health related quality of life QOL (HRQOL) after stroke have focused on motor function, communication, and activities of daily living, using instruments that survey participants about stroke sequelae which typically are evaluated by medical personnel [12, 13]. Studies have found that age, nonwhite race, impaired upper-extremity function, and greater number of comorbidities are all associated with reduced HRQOL within the physical domain. A larger number of comorbidities are also associated with poorer HRQOL in the domain of memory and thinking, and stroke survivors whose hemiparesis affected the dominant side or had ischemic (rather than hemorrhagic) stroke reported poorer HRQOL in the domain of communication (QOL) [12]. Several studies have shown that depression is strongly correlated with QOL measured with traditional HRQOL instruments for stroke [14, 15].

We carried out a pilot study to identify the sequelae that were most important to stroke survivors and caregivers. This study was motivated by the observation that individuals who were recovering from stroke sometimes assigned surprisingly different values to various consequences of stroke, compared to values assigned by their family members or professionals. An additional motivation was the observation that stroke survivors or their caregivers frequently reported problems that are not typically measured by stroke scales—difficulty in sleep or sex, overwhelming fatigue, change in personality, and so on. As it is critical to understand what sequelae have the greatest impact on QOL of survivors and their caregivers to focus poststroke interventions, we created new questionnaires, including questions about all the sequelae noted above, as a preliminary investigation of the impact of various consequences of stroke. The appendix includes a list of these items.

We surveyed 33 stroke patients and 28 caregivers of the same stroke patients in our Stroke Prevention and Recovery Center (SPARC) using questionnaires about possible stroke sequelae [16]. They were asked to rate residual problems in two ways: (1) from most to least important in terms of the impact on QOL and (2) as severe, moderate, mild, or not a problem. Symptoms included change in personality or behavior, motor function (weakness, clumsiness, etc.), motor speech, word retrieval, reading, writing, memory, attention, spatial perception (neglect of one side), other cognitive problems, sensation (vision, numbness/tingling, pain, etc.), mood, walking, swallowing, sleep, empathy (understanding emotions of others and expressing emotion through tone of voice and facial expression), pain, fatigue, and sexual function (see the appendix).

Stroke survivors were on average 66 (31–83) years old and were surveyed at an average of 22.2 months after stroke;

TABLE 1: Sequelae reported by stroke survivors and their caregivers (in percent) who reported impairment as one of the "top 5" most important problems or moderate/important problems (n = 14 each group)*.

Domain**	Left hemisphere stroke survivor	Right hemisphere stroke survivor	Caregiver of left stroke survivor	Caregiver of right stroke survivor
Word retrieval	43	0	57	0
Reading	50	21	50	36
Writing/spelling	71	0	71	43
Memory	21	0	50	43
Energy (fatigue)	43	21	50	43
Mood	29	21	57	43
Walking	50	14	36	29
Right motor function	57	0	7	0
Left motor function	0	21	0	29
Prosody	0	0	0	29
Empathy	0	14	0	50
Spatial attention	0	0	0	29
Other cognitive	0	7	0	43
Personality/behavior	0	0	0	43
Sexual function	36	21	0	0

*Results from bilateral and brainstem stroke patients and their caregivers are not included as there were only 2 or 3 participants in each group.
**Other domains were not rated as moderate/important or in "top 5" most important problems by any participant (see the appendix for complete list of domains/symptoms).

42% were women. Diagnoses included 14 left hemisphere, 14 right hemisphere, 3 bilateral, and 2 brainstem strokes. We identified symptoms that were rated as the top 5 most important residual problems and/or at least "moderate" problems. The single most frequently reported important/moderate consequence by both survivors of left hemisphere stroke and their caregivers was difficulty in spelling and/or writing (identified by 71% of each) (see Table 1). Word-retrieval and mood problems were also frequently reported (by 57% of caregivers), as was right-sided weakness (by 57% of survivors). Right hemisphere stroke survivors themselves reported few residual deficits, but equally common were: fatigue, left-sided weakness, problems with mood, reading, writing, memory, and sexual function (with symptoms in each of these domains rated as important/moderate problem by 21% of right hemisphere stroke survivors). The most frequently reported important/moderate consequence by caregivers of right hemisphere stroke survivors was impaired recognition of the emotions of others (loss of emotional empathy), identified by 50% of caregivers, followed by "other cognitive problems," "change in personality and behavior," and "walking" (Table 1).

These results reveal that deficits in spelling/writing after left hemisphere stroke and loss of empathy after right hemisphere stroke are probably underestimated as residual consequences of stroke. Spelling has taken on new importance in a community that relies on email, texting, and online shopping and banking. The importance of empathy in communication and social relationship has been understood by social scientists for decades, but little attention has been given to impairments of empathy after stroke [17]. Efforts to understand the variables that mediate these deficits and

interventions to alleviate these problems are essential to improve QOL after stroke.

2. Mechanisms of Stroke Recovery

In general, the deficits caused by stroke are the most severe at onset and gradually improve over time although the most rapid recovery (especially in motor function) often occurs in the first three months [18]. In a large study of chronic aphasia recovery described below, Hope and colleagues [19] found that the single most important determinant of recovery of speech production was time since onset of stroke, indicating that improvement continues over time, even in the chronic stage. The brain recovers from a focal lesion like stroke through a variety of mechanisms that take place at different times after onset [20, 21]. Here we briefly review some of these mechanisms, focusing on restoring blood flow to critical brain regions and reorganization of structure-function relationships.

2.1. Early Cognitive Recovery Depends on Degree and Location of Reperfusion

2.1.1. Restoring Blood Flow Improves Cognitive Function, Even When There Is No Change in NIHSS. The focus of acute stroke interventions, such as thrombolysis, embolectomy, stenting, and transcranial Doppler ultrasound-augmented clot disruption, is to restore blood flow to ischemic tissue that is receiving enough blood to survive, but not enough to function (the so-called "ischemic penumbra"). In most cases, the ischemic tissue that is salvageable is largely limited to the cortex. Yet, most acute stroke trials have measured response to treatment using scales that are insensitive to change in cortical function, such as the MRS and BI, or are heavily weighted toward assessment of motor function, such as the NIHSS as described earlier.

In an initial investigation, we studied 10 patients with acute, nondominant hemisphere stroke who were candidates for intervention to restore perfusion, based on having a small acute stroke (measured on diffusion-weighted imaging or DWI), but a larger area of hypoperfusion (measured on perfusion-weighted imaging or PWI), and a visualized clot or area of stenosis in cerebral vessel. They underwent DWI, PWI, NIHSS, and a simple line cancellation test (a test of hemispatial neglect) on Days 1 and 3. We calculated correlations between change in volume of stroke, change in perfusion abnormality (defined as time to peak delay of contrast in a region of interest relative to the homologous region of interest in the opposite hemisphere), and change in functional tests. Initial NIHSS score ranged from 1 to 16 (mean = 9). Initial score on the line cancellation test was ranged from 12% to 93% (mean = 55.5%) errors. Volume of infarct on DWI ranged from 3 to 31 cm^3 (mean = 8.9 cm^3). Volume of PWI abnormality ranged from 55 to 284 cm^3 (mean = 156 cm^3). Notably, all of these patients had large areas of hypoperfusion beyond the infarct and were considered candidates for intervention to restore blood flow. Intervention included endovascular treatment, urgent endarterectomy, and temporarily induced blood pressure elevation [22]. With intervention, change in NIHSS score ranged from −5 to 0 (mean = −1.7). Change in line cancellation ranged from −39.6 to +14.6 (mean = −14.3 cm^3). Change in infarct volume ranged from −4 to 32 cm^3 (mean = 4.3 cm^3). Change in PWI abnormality ranged from −209 to 0 cm^3 (mean = −70.2 cm^3). Change in volume of hypoperfused tissue on PWI correlated with change in line cancellation performance ($r = 0.83$; $P = 0.003$) but did not correlate with change in NIHSS score ($r = 0.26$; $P = NS$). This study provided evidence that improvement in perfusion was associated with improvement in a simple measure of cognitive function, even when it was not associated with improvement in the NIHSS score [9].

2.1.2. Restoring Blood Flow to Specific Areas Results in Early Recovery of Specific Cognitive Function. In a series of studies, we tested the hypothesis that improvement in cortical function depends not only on how much tissue is reperfused but also on the location of the cortex that is reperfused.

In one recent study, we evaluated the hypothesis that restoring blood flow to specific cortical regions in the right hemisphere after acute stroke results in improvement in distinct variants of hemispatial neglect (viewer-centered neglect versus stimulus-centered neglect) [23]. These two forms of neglect are shown in Figure 1. Previous studies have shown that these two forms of neglect result from different locations of stroke [24–26]. Twenty-five patients with acute right stroke were evaluated at Day 1 and Days 3–5 with a battery of neglect tests and diffusion- and perfusion-weighted MR Imaging.

We used multivariate linear regression analysis to identify areas where reperfusion predicted degree of improvement in scores on each type of neglect, independently of reperfusion of other areas, total change in the volume of infarct or hypoperfusion (defined as >4 second delay in time to peak arrival of contrast, relative to homologous voxels on the left), and age. The stroke patients were on average 65.5 (± SD 16.1) years old. At onset, 8 (30%) had viewer-centered neglect; 6 (22%) had stimulus-centered neglect plus viewer-centered neglect. Mean infarct DWI at onset was 23.1 (±27.2) cc. The mean volume of hypoperfusion on PWI was 94.6 (±85.5) cc. They received a variety of interventions to restore blood flow, including carotid stenting, urgent endarterectomy, endovascular therapy, thrombolysis, and temporarily induced blood pressure elevation. The mean change in volume of ischemia on DWI was 3.2 (±18.5) cc increase (growth in infarct); the mean change in volume of hypoperfusion on PWI was −35.1 (±55.0) cc or improvement in perfusion. Multivariate linear regression analysis revealed specific Brodmann areas (BA) where reperfusion was associated with improvement in viewer- or stimulus-centered neglect, independently of reperfusion of other regions and independently of age and change in volume of infarct and hypoperfusion. Analyses revealed that reperfusion of dorsal frontoparietal cortex (right BA 46, 4, 40) independently predicted improvement in viewer-centered neglect, such as detecting stimuli on the left side of the page and copying left stimuli in the scene ($r = 0.951$; $P < 0.0001$), as illustrated in Figure 2. Reperfusion of right temporooccipital cortex (right BA 37, 18, 38) independently contributed to improvement in stimulus-centered neglect, measured by detecting left gaps in circles on both sides of the page ($r = 0.926$; $P < 0.0001$), as illustrated in Figure 3. These results confirmed that restoring blood flow to specific cortical regions yields improvement in different types of neglect [23].

Likewise, in several additional studies, we tested the hypothesis that reperfusion of the distinct cortical regions of the left hemisphere, in the absence of infarct in that region, would restore the associated language function [27]. In one study, we investigated five patients with impaired word meaning associated with poor perfusion, but not infarction, in superior temporal cortex, and one patient with a superimposed deficit in word retrieval, associated with poor perfusion of left inferior temporal cortex. Each patient was treated to increase perfusion of the ischemic and dysfunctional tissue. Daily testing of naming and comprehension, with stimuli matched for difficulty, showed improvement in word meaning in the patients who showed reperfusion of left superior temporal cortex and showed improvement in oral naming (but not word meaning) in the patient who showed reperfusion of left inferior temporal cortex [27]. In another study, reperfusion of inferior temporal cortex (within BA 37) was the area most strongly associated with improvement in naming in patients with acute left hemisphere stroke [28]. Yet another study showed that reperfusion of left inferior frontal cortex was associated with improvement specific to writing verbs [29]. These results illustrate that reperfusion of specific brain regions results in recovery of distinct language functions.

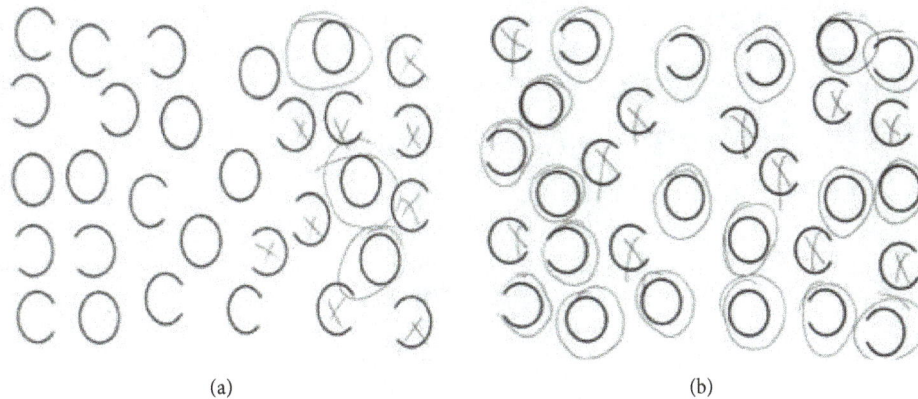

(a)   (b)

FIGURE 1: Contrasting performance of patients with viewer-centered and stimulus-centered neglect on the gap-detection test [24] (in this task the patient is asked to circle all the complete circles and put an X over circles that have a gap on the left or right side). (a) Performance by a patient with a right frontoparietal stroke and viewer-centered neglect on the gap-detection test. Note that he misses all of the stimuli on the left side of the view but detects left gaps in circles on the right view. (b) Performance by a patient with a right temporal stroke and stimulus-centered neglect on the gap-detection test. Note that he fails to detect the left gaps in circles on the right and left sides of the view.

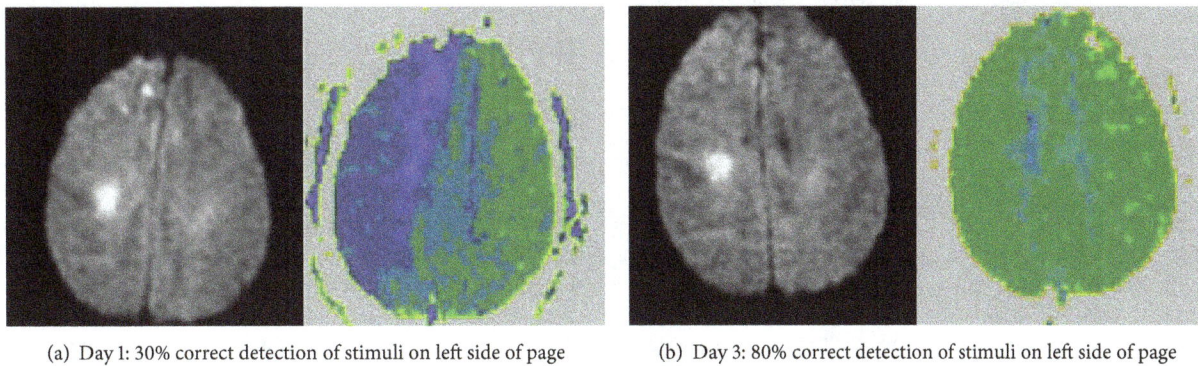

(a) Day 1: 30% correct detection of stimuli on left side of page   (b) Day 3: 80% correct detection of stimuli on left side of page

FIGURE 2: (a) Diffusion-weighted image (DWI; left), showing small subcortical infarct and perfusion-weighted image (PWI; right) of a patient with severe viewer-centered neglect at Day 1. (b) DWI and PWI of the same patient at Day 3, after viewer-centered neglect recovered, as indicated by recovery of detecting stimuli on the left and copying stimuli on the left of a scene. PWI shows that reperfusion of the right frontoparietal cortex was associated with recovery of viewer-centered neglect. In this case, reperfusion was brought about with induced blood pressure elevation.

3. Surprising Patient Variables That Influence Cognitive Recovery

Several studies have demonstrated that motor or language recovery is significantly associated with volume of infarct, although the association is relatively weak [30]. A great deal of variance in recovery of cognitive functions remains unexplained, even after accounting for lesion volume. For example, in a study of 270 (mostly left hemisphere) stroke patients, recovery of speech production (a composite score) correlated with volume of infarct ($r^2 = 0.35$, $F = 144.73$, $P < 0.001$) [19]. In that study, the correlation improved when information about site of lesion was added. Recovery of speech production was best predicted by subset of 37 variables ($r^2 = 0.59$, $F = 38.38$, $P < 0.001$), including time after stroke (which was the most significant, single predictor), volume of stroke, and involvement of 35 different brain regions. Recovery of speech production was not predicted by

a combination of time since stroke, age at stroke, premorbid handedness, and gender. The role of education was not evaluated in that study. We hypothesized that education might have a role in recovery from cognitive sequelae of stroke, based on previous studies indicating that education may promote neuroplasticity or may have a neuroprotective effect against cognitive decline [31]. The proposal that education provides "cognitive reserve" that reduces the risk of dementia has received support from a variety of sources [32–35]. That is, higher education may provide more general cognitive resources on which to rely and thus delay the onset of dementia. However, the role of education in recovery from stroke has been less well studied. One study did find that the highest educational levels were associated with lower rates of poststroke cognitive deficits and dementia and higher rates of long-term survival, independently of stroke severity, age, sex, marital status, and white matter lesions in individuals with mild/moderate ischemic stroke [36]. Results were interpreted

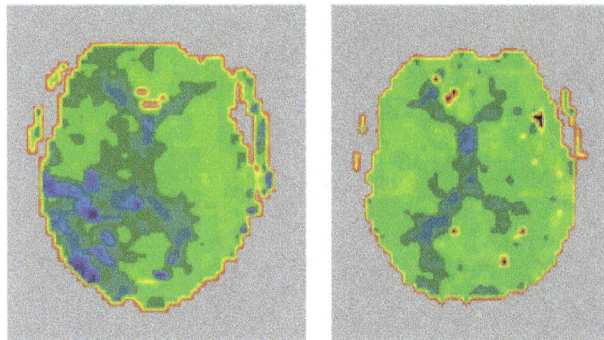

(a) Day 1: 86% correct detection of gaps on left side of stimuli

(b) Day 3: 99% correct detection of gaps on left side of stimuli

FIGURE 3: (a) PWI of a patient with severe stimulus-centered neglect at Day 1. (b) PWI of the same patient at Day 6, after stimulus-centered neglect recovered, as indicated by recovery of detecting gaps on the left sides of circles (irrespective of their location w.r.t. the viewer) and copying the left halves of stimuli on both sides of a scene. PWI shows that reperfusion of the right temporal cortex was associated with recovery of stimulus-centered neglect. In this case, reperfusion was brought about by urgent carotid endarterectomy.

as support for the hypothesis that high education, a proxy for cognitive reserve, protects against poststroke cognitive impairment.

3.1. The Effects of Education and Antidepressant Use on Language Recovery.
We tested the hypothesis that degree of recovery beyond 3 months is influenced not only by lesion volume but also independently by education. We tested 45 acute left hemisphere ischemic stroke patients. Their mean age was 54.9 years; range was 18 to 90 years; mean education was 14.7 years; range was 6 to 20 years. They were studied on average for 35.4 months after onset of stroke on the Western Aphasia Battery (WAB). The primary outcome variable was a summary score of comprehension, repetition, and naming summary scores from the WAB. "Spontaneous speech" fluency and content scores were omitted, because these scores are subjective rating scores and have a lower interrater reliability in scoring than the objective scores on the other subtests. Infarct volume was measured on follow-up MRI obtained at the time of testing. We determined variables associated with WAB Quartile (because scores were not normally distributed) using multivariable logistic regression, with antidepressant use (from onset of stroke through recovery) as cofactor, and age, education, infarct volume, and time postonset (TPO) as covariates. Individuals who were prescribed antidepressants at onset consistently stayed on the medication, although doses were adjusted. Nearly all antidepressants were selective serotonin reuptake inhibitors (SSRIs); a small percentage consisted of venlafaxine (which has SSRI and tricyclic properties) or tricyclic antidepressants.

We found that final WAB Quartile was significantly predicted by a model that included education, age, volume of infarct, and antidepressant use but did not include time since onset (chi-square for goodness of fit = 207; $P < 0.0001$;

Cox and Snell $r^2 = 0.47$). Education had the highest Wald statistic of 17.3 ($P < 0.0001$) [df = 1], followed by volume of infarct (Wald = 7.0; $P = 0.008$), antidepressant use (Wald = 5.2; $P = 0.022$), and age (Wald = 5.0; $P = 0.023$). Compared to individuals who had never taken antidepressants, those taking antidepressants had higher repetition scores (mean 9.4 versus 7.6; $P = 0.039$), even though they had larger infarct (mean 225 versus 82 cc; $P = 0.008$); they were no differences in age, education, TPO, or total WAB (mean 28.4 versus 22.9). These results show that better chronic aphasia recovery is associated with higher education and current antidepressant use, as well as smaller lesion size and younger age (independently of one another). Although our study was smaller than the study by Hope and colleagues [19], the effects of education and antidepressant use were so powerful, that, even with lower power, they had a highly significant effect independently of lesion size [37]. The positive effect of antidepressant use (mostly SSRIs) is consistent with a recent clinical trial showing positive effects of fluoxetine on motor recovery after acute stroke, independently of the effects on depression [38], as well as a recent study of the effects of SSRIs on dependence, overall neurological impairment, depression, and anxiety after stroke [39].

The effect of education on very simple language tests is somewhat surprising. The WAB tests can be performed easily by healthy individuals with a grade school education; they include tasks of naming familiar objects, following simple commands (e.g., pointing to body parts). But education may be a marker for something else that allows good recovery, such as discipline or determination (that led to a high education and may lead to greater participation in rehabilitation) or cognitive reserve. Alternatively, education may be a marker of economic resources (e.g., access to more rehabilitation) or may be correlated with healthy life style (lower rates of smoking, more exercise, and greater compliance with medications).

One previous study narrowed down the potential accounts of the effects of education. Education not only is associated with better recovery from aphasia but (to a lesser degree) is also associated with incidence and severity of impairment at onset in language tasks, even with 5th grade level of difficulty [40]. We studied 173 stroke patients within 24 hours of symptom development and hospitalized controls matched for age, education, and socioeconomic status (SES) with MRI and nine language tasks (auditory and written comprehension, naming (oral, written, and tactile), oral reading, oral spelling, written spelling, and repetition). Education was recorded in years, and SES was obtained from census tract data and assessed by mean neighborhood household income and family income. We found that the error rate for patients with 12th grade education or higher was significantly lower for auditory and written comprehension, written naming, oral reading, and spelling of fifth grade vocabulary words, even after adjusting for age, sex, stroke volume, and SES. These results indicate that even once learned, language performance may become less vulnerable to disruption by stroke with increasing years of education; and the effects of education cannot be explained by SES (a rough estimate of economic resources).

3.2. The Effects of Education on Recovery of Simple Attention to Space. In light of observed effect of education on language performance, we hypothesized that higher education might also be associated with better recovery of other focal cognitive functions. We evaluated the effect of education on hemispatial neglect, because it is a common but devastating impairment in spatial attention after right hemisphere stroke. We used a test that (1) can be performed easily by healthy children in first grade and (2) distinguishes between two forms of left hemispatial neglect failure to attend to the left side of the view (viewer-centered neglect) and failure to attend to the left side of individual objects on both sides of the view (stimulus-centered neglect), as shown in Figure 1.

To identify predictors of recovery of viewer-centered and stimulus-centered hemispatial neglect after acute right hemisphere stroke, we tested 35 patients with acute right hemisphere ischemic stroke at Day 1 and mean 32 weeks after stroke on the test shown in Figure 1, which distinguishes between viewer- and stimulus-centered neglect. They completed this task of detecting gaps in left or right sides of circles scattered across a page and MRI with PWI at Day 1 and then completed the same task at follow-up. Initial volumes of infarct and hypoperfusion were measured by a technician, who was masked to neglect scores. We identified variables associated with recovery of viewer-centered neglect (error rate in marking stimuli on left side of view) and stimulus-centered neglect (error rate in detecting left gaps in circles, irrespective of side of viewer) using multivariable regression. Age, education, volume of infarct, volume of hypoperfusion, initial error rate in marking stimuli on the left, initial error rate in detecting left-sided gaps in circles, and interval between onset and follow-up were entered as independent variables.

For the entire group of 35 patients, the average age was 58.4 years; and average education was 12.6 years. A total of 14 patients had viewer-centered neglect; 12 had stimulus-centered neglect; and 9 had both at onset. The degree of recovery in stimulus-centered neglect was associated with education and initial severity of stimulus-centered neglect (error rate in detecting left gaps at onset; $r^2 = 0.59$; $P = 0.045$). The degree of recovery in viewer-centered neglect was associated with education and initial severity of egocentric neglect; $r^2 = 0.66$; $P < 0.0001$, independently of other factors. Furthermore, the univariate (Pearson) correlation between education in years and accuracy in stimulus detection (egocentric neglect) was significant at follow-up ($r = 0.57$; $P = 0.0003$), but not at onset ($r = 0.32$; NS). These data show that the degree of recovery of both variants of neglect was positively correlated with higher education and lower initial severity of the specific type of neglect, independently of volume of infarct, volume of hypoperfusion, age, and time after onset of stroke [41].

Once again the effect of education on recovery may be somewhat surprising, particularly in this case, as the outcome we measured at follow-up does not require any formal education. Furthermore, better performance on the task at onset was not associated with higher education, while better *recovery* of performance was associated with higher education. These results indicate that people with

higher education tend to show greater cognitive recovery after stroke. It will be important to identify the factors that mediate this association.

4. Conclusions

In this paper, we review a series of studies evaluating the consequences of stroke that have the greatest impact on quality of life and important variables that influence the degree of cognitive recovery after stroke. We unveil some surprising findings. First, while stroke treatment and outcome research to date has largely focused on recovery of very basic activities of daily living and motor function, survivors and their caregivers are more concerned with recovery of higher level cognitive functions, such as the ability to use written language and to empathize with others. Secondly, the degree to which an individual recovers even simple cognitive functions (which do not normally require formal education) is influenced by changes in blood flow in the early period and by their education level, as well as the size of their stroke or initial severity. That is, people with higher education make better recovery, although it is not yet clear whether this is a direct effect of education or whether a higher education is a marker for "cognitive reserve," healthier lifestyle, or something else that might positively influence recovery. Independently of the positive effects of education, antidepressant use, particularly SSRIs, may also have positive effects on stroke recovery. Many of the studies reviewed here are relatively small, and so the findings need to be confirmed in large prospective studies and clinical trials, some of which are currently underway.

Appendix

Items Included in the Questionnaire for Stroke Survivors and Caregivers

Domain: Symptom(s) Rated by Survivor and Caregiver

Right motor function:

weakness in right arm;
weakness in right leg;
clumsiness/difficulty in using right hand;
clumsiness/difficulty in using right leg.

Left motor function:

weakness in left arm;
weakness in left leg;
clumsiness/difficulty in using left hand;
clumsiness/difficulty in using left leg.

Walking/gait:

difficulty in walking.

Swallowing:

difficulty in swallowing.

Motor speech:

difficulty in speaking.

Word retrieval:

difficulty in word retrieval.

Auditory comprehension:

difficulty in comprehending what other people say.

Spelling/writing:

difficulty in spelling;
difficulty in writing.

Reading:

difficulty in reading.

Calculation:

difficulty in calculating.

Music:

difficulty in singing or in other aspects of music.

Empathy:

difficulty in understanding the feelings of other people (loss of emotional empathy);
difficulty in understanding the thoughts of other people (loss of cognitive empathy).

Prosody:

difficulty in recognizing tone of voice and facial expressions in others;
impaired use of tone of voice and facial expression to show emotion.

Spatial attention:

difficulty in perceiving things on one side of space ("neglect").

Attention:

inattention.

Memory:

impaired memory.

Other cognitive functions:

other cognitive problems.

Other cognitive functions:

other motor problems.

Vision:

visual problems.

Extraocular movements:

eye movement problems.

Mood:

mood problems (circle one: depressed bipolar irritable manic other:_____).

Energy/fatigue:

fatigue.

Sexual function:

sexual dysfunction.

Personality/behavior:

change in personality or behavior.

Sleep:

impaired sleep.

Pain:

pain (specify where:_____).

Sensation:

sensory problems (specify where:_____ _____).

Conflict of Interests

The authors declare that there is no conflict of interests regarding to the publication of this paper.

Acknowledgment

The research reported in this paper was supported by NIH, through Grants R01 DC05375, R01 NS47691, and R01 DC03681.

References

[1] B. Farrell, J. Godwin, S. Richards, and C. Warlow, "The United Kingdom transient ischaemic attack (UK-TIA) aspirin trial: final results," *Journal of Neurology Neurosurgery and Psychiatry*, vol. 54, no. 12, pp. 1044–1054, 1991.

[2] D. Wade and C. Collin, "The Barthel ADL index: a standard measure of physical disability?" *Disability & Rehabilitation*, vol. 10, no. 2, pp. 64–67, 1988.

[3] J. I. Cameron, D. E. Stewart, D. L. Streiner, P. C. Coyte, and A. M. Cheung, "What makes family caregivers happy during the first 2 years post stroke?" *Stroke*, vol. 45, no. 4, pp. 1084–1089, 2014.

[4] M. Acler, E. Robol, A. Fiaschi, and P. Manganotti, "A double blind placebo RCT to investigate the effects of serotonergic modulation on brain excitability and motor recovery in stroke patients," *Journal of Neurology*, vol. 256, no. 7, pp. 1152–1158, 2009.

[5] G. Nys, M. Van Zandvoort, P. De Kort et al., "Domain-specific cognitive recovery after first-ever stroke: A follow-up study of 111 cases," *Journal of the International Neuropsychological Society*, vol. 11, no. 7, pp. 795–806, 2005.

[6] D. Woo, J. P. Broderick, R. U. Kothari et al., "Does the National Institutes of Health Stroke Scale favor left hemisphere strokes?" *Stroke*, vol. 30, no. 11, pp. 2355–2359, 1999.

[7] P. Lyden, L. Claesson, S. Havstad, T. Ashwood, and M. Lu, "Factor analysis of the National Institutes of Health Stroke Scale in patients with large strokes," *Archives of Neurology*, vol. 61, no. 11, pp. 1677–1680, 2004.

[8] M. M. Glymour, L. F. Berkman, K. A. Ertel, M. E. Fay, T. A. Glass, and K. L. Furie, "Lesion characteristics, NIH stroke scale, and functional recovery after stroke," *The American Journal of Physical Medicine and Rehabilitation*, vol. 86, no. 9, pp. 725–733, 2007.

[9] A. E. Hillis, R. J. Wityk, P. B. Barker, J. A. Ulatowski, and M. A. Jacobs, "Change in perfusion in acute nondominant hemisphere stroke may be better estimated by tests of hemispatial neglect than by the national institutes of health stroke scale," *Stroke*, vol. 34, no. 10, pp. 2392–2396, 2003.

[10] R. F. Gottesman, J. T. Kleinman, C. Davis, J. Heidler-Gary, M. Newhart, and A. E. Hillis, "The NIHSS-plus: improving cognitive assessment with the NIHSS," *Behavioural Neurology*, vol. 22, no. 1-2, pp. 11–15, 2010.

[11] L. A. Pearce, L. A. McClure, D. C. Anderson, C. Jacova, M. Sharma, and O. R. Benavente, "Effects of long-term blood pressure lowering and dual antiplatelet therapy on cognition in patients with recent lacunar stroke: secondary prevention of small subcortical strokes (SPS3) trial," *Lancet Neurology*. In press.

[12] K. Hilari, J. J. Needle, and K. L. Harrison, "What are the important factors in health-related quality of life for people with aphasia? A systematic review," *Archives of Physical Medicine and Rehabilitation*, vol. 93, no. 1, pp. S86–S95, 2012.

[13] D. S. Nichols-Larsen, P. C. Clark, A. Zeringue, A. Greenspan, and S. Blanton, "Factors influencing stroke survivors' quality of life during subacute recovery," *Stroke*, vol. 36, no. 7, pp. 1480–1484, 2005.

[14] M.-L. Niemi, R. Laaksonen, M. Kotila, and O. Waltimo, "Quality of life 4 years after stroke," *Stroke*, vol. 19, no. 9, pp. 1101–1107, 1988.

[15] J. Carod-Artal, J. A. Egido, J. L. González, and E. V. Seijas, "Quality of life among stroke survivors evaluated 1 year after stroke: experience of a stroke unit," *Stroke*, vol. 31, no. 12, pp. 2995–3000, 2000.

[16] V. Urrutia, B. Johnson, and A. Hillis, "Relative importance of stroke sequelae according to patients and caregivers," in *Abstract Presented at the Annual Meeting of the American Academy of Neurology*, Philadelphia, Pa, USA, April 2014.

[17] P. J. Eslinger, K. Parkinson, and S. G. Shamay, "Empathy and social-emotional factors in recovery from stroke," *Current Opinion in Neurology*, vol. 15, no. 1, pp. 91–97, 2002.

[18] E. Zarahn, L. Alon, S. L. Ryan et al., "Prediction of motor recovery using initial impairment and fMRI 48 h poststroke," *Cerebral Cortex*, vol. 21, no. 12, pp. 2712–2721, 2011.

[19] T. M. H. Hope, M. L. Seghier, A. P. Leff, and C. J. Price, "Predicting outcome and recovery after stroke with lesions extracted from MRI images," *NeuroImage: Clinical*, vol. 2, no. 1, pp. 424–433, 2013.

[20] S. Jarso, M. Li, A. Faria et al., "Distinct mechanisms and timing of language recovery after stroke," *Cognitive Neuropsychology*, vol. 30, no. 7-8, pp. 454–475, 2013.

[21] S. R. Zeiler and J. W. Krakauer, "The interaction between training and plasticity in the poststroke brain," *Current Opinion in Neurology*, vol. 26, no. 6, pp. 609–616, 2013.

[22] A. E. Hillis, J. A. Ulatowski, P. B. Barker et al., "A pilot randomized trial of induced blood pressure elevation: effects on function and focal perfusion in acute and subacute stroke," *Cerebrovascular Diseases*, vol. 16, no. 3, pp. 236–246, 2003.

[23] S. Khurshid, L. A. Trupe, M. Newhart et al., "Reperfusion of specific cortical areas is associated with improvement in distinct forms of hemispatial neglect," *Cortex*, vol. 48, no. 5, pp. 530–539, 2012.

[24] H. Ota, T. Fujii, K. Suzuki, R. Fukatsu, and A. Yamadori, "Dissociation of body-centered and stimulus-centered representations in unilateral neglect," *Neurology*, vol. 57, no. 11, pp. 2064–2069, 2001.

[25] A. E. Hillis, M. Newhart, J. Heidler, P. B. Barker, E. H. Herskovits, and M. Degaonkar, "Anatomy of spatial attention: insights from perfusion imaging and hemispatial neglect in acute stroke," *The Journal of Neuroscience*, vol. 25, no. 12, pp. 3161–3167, 2005.

[26] J. Medina, V. Kannan, M. A. Pawlak et al., "Neural substrates of visuospatial processing in distinct reference frames: evidence from unilateral spatial neglect," *Journal of Cognitive Neuroscience*, vol. 21, no. 11, pp. 2073–2084, 2009.

[27] A. E. Hillis, A. Kane, E. Tuffiash et al., "Reperfusion of specific brain regions by raising blood pressure restores selective language functions in subacute stroke," *Brain and Language*, vol. 79, no. 3, pp. 495–510, 2001.

[28] A. E. Hillis, J. T. Kleinman, M. Newhart et al., "Restoring cerebral blood flow reveals neural regions critical for naming," *Journal of Neuroscience*, vol. 26, no. 31, pp. 8069–8073, 2006.

[29] A. E. Hillis, R. J. Wityk, P. B. Barker, and A. Caramazza, "Neural regions essential for writing verbs," *Nature Neuroscience*, vol. 6, no. 1, pp. 19–20, 2003.

[30] E. Plowman, B. Hentz, and C. Ellis, "Post-stroke aphasia prognosis: a review of patient-related and stroke-related factors," *Journal of Evaluation in Clinical Practice*, vol. 18, no. 3, pp. 689–694, 2012.

[31] EClipSE Collaborative Members, C. Brayne, P. G. Ince et al., "Education, the brain and dementia: neuroprotection or compensation?" *Brain*, vol. 133, part 8, pp. 2210–2216, 2010.

[32] C. M. Roe, C. Xiong, J. P. Miller, and J. C. Morris, "Education and Alzheimer disease without dementia: support for the cognitive reserve hypothesis," *Neurology*, vol. 68, no. 3, pp. 223–228, 2007.

[33] Y. Stern, S. Albert, M.-X. Tang, and W.-Y. Tsai, "Rate of memory decline in AD is related to education and occupation: cognitive reserve?" *Neurology*, vol. 53, no. 9, pp. 1942–1947, 1999.

[34] Y. Stern, "Cognitive reserve and Alzheimer disease," *Alzheimer Disease & Associated Disorders*, vol. 20, no. 2, pp. 112–117, 2006.

[35] G. E. Alexander, M. L. Furey, C. L. Grady et al., "Association of premorbid intellectual function with cerebral metabolism in Alzheimer's disease: implications for the cognitive reserve hypothesis," *The American Journal of Psychiatry*, vol. 154, no. 2, pp. 165–172, 1997.

[36] J. Ojala-Oksala, H. Jokinen, V. Kopsi et al., "Educational history is an independent predictor of cognitive deficits and long-term survival in postacute patients with mild to moderate ischemic stroke," *Stroke*, vol. 43, no. 11, pp. 2931–2935, 2012.

[37] A. M. Suneja, M. Gonzalez-Fernandez, and A. E. Hillis, "Predictors of recovery of chronic aphasia," in *Proceedings of the Annual Meeting of the American Academy of Neurology*, Philadelphia, Pa, USA, April 2014.

[38] F. Chollet, J. Tardy, J.-F. Albucher et al., "Fluoxetine for motor recovery after acute ischaemic stroke (FLAME): a randomised placebo-controlled trial," *The Lancet Neurology*, vol. 10, no. 2, pp. 123–130, 2011.

[39] G. E. Mead, C.-F. Hsieh, and M. Hackett, "Selective serotonin reuptake inhibitors for stroke recovery," *JAMA—Journal of the American Medical Association*, vol. 310, no. 10, pp. 1066–1067, 2013.

[40] M. González-Fernández, C. Davis, J. J. Molitoris, M. Newhart, R. Leigh, and A. E. Hillis, "Formal education, socioeconomic status, and the severity of aphasia after stroke," *Archives of Physical Medicine and Rehabilitation*, vol. 92, no. 11, pp. 1809–1813, 2011.

[41] J. Posner, L. A. Trupe, C. L. Davis, Y. Gomez, D. Tippett, and A. E. Hillis, "Predictors of recovery of allocentric and egocentric neglect: the role of education," in *Proceedings of the Annual Meeting of the American Academy of Neurology*, Philadelphia, Pa, USA, April 2014.

12

Topical Colchicine Gel versus Diclofenac Sodium Gel for the Treatment of Actinic Keratoses: A Randomized, Double-Blind Study

Gita Faghihi,[1] **Azam Elahipoor,**[2] **Fariba Iraji,**[1] **Shadi Behfar,**[3] **and Bahareh Abtahi-Naeini**[4]

[1]*Skin Diseases and Leishmaniasis Research Center, Isfahan University of Medical Sciences, Isfahan, Iran*
[2]*Department of Dermatology, Qom University of Medical Sciences, Qom, Iran*
[3]*Department of Dermatology, School of Medicine, Rafsanjan University of Medical Sciences, Rafsanjan, Iran*
[4]*Cancer Research Center, Semnan University of Medical Sciences, Semnan, Iran*

Correspondence should be addressed to Azam Elahipoor; azaam.elahipoor@gmail.com

Academic Editor: Jacek Cezary Szepietowski

Introduction. Actinic keratoses (AKs), a premalignant skin lesion, are a common lesion in fair skin. Although destructive treatment remains the gold standard for AKs, medical therapies may be preferable due to the comfort and reliability .This study aims to compare the effects of topical 1% colchicine gel and 3% diclofenac sodium gel in AKs. *Materials and Methods.* In this randomized double-blind study, 70 lesions were selected. Patients were randomized before receiving either 1% colchicine gel or 3% diclofenac sodium cream twice a day for 6 weeks. Patients were evaluated in terms of their lesion size, treatment complications, and recurrence at 7, 30, 60, and 120 days after treatment. *Results.* The mean of changes in the size was significant in both groups both before and after treatment (<0.001). The mean lesion size before treatment and at 30, 60, and 120 days was not different between the two groups ($p > 0.05$). No case of erythema was seen in the colchicine group, while erythema was seen in 22.9% (eight cases) of patients in the diclofenac sodium group ($p = 0.005$). *Conclusions.* 1% colchicine gel was a safe and effective medication with fewer side effects and lack of recurrence of the lesion.

1. Introduction

Actinic keratoses (AKs), also known as premalignant lesions, are a common skin lesion in most communities and are observed in the form of erythematous, scaly lesions in the exposed areas of the skin. It seems that AKs occur where they can develop toward squamous cell carcinoma (SCC), particularly on the head, face, ears, lips, arms, and hands; they are a precancerous lesion [1, 2]. The common symptoms of AKs include painless brown or red scaly macule on sun-exposed areas [1]. Prolonged exposure to sun rays, resulting from outdoor working environments (such as those working in the agricultural sector or engaged in regular outdoor sporting activities), in particular those who have fair skin and are subjected to sun exposure, and compromised immune system by disease or drug have been identified as risk factors affecting the disease, while, so far, the actual etiology of the

disease is unknown [3]. AKs will disappear by treatment but new lesions may appear again (particularly at the edges of the treated area) [3]. The possible complication of this disease is the possibility of SCC formation [4].

Surgical or invasive procedures represent the main approach for the treatment of AKs, but noninvasive, tissue-sparing, and topical self-administered treatments may be a highly desirable alternative in both aged and unhealthy patients (who may be poor surgical candidates) as well as for lesions located on cosmetically sensitive areas [5, 6]. While destructive methods of treatment of actinic keratosis remain the gold standard for the eradication of visible and palpable AKs, medical therapies may be able to accomplish this goal with more comfort and reliability for the patient [7].

In the management of multiple AKs, topical therapies include 5% fluorouracil (5-FU), 5% imiquimod (IQ), and 3%

diclofenac sodium (DS) gels, which should be preferred over more destructive treatments including surgery, cryotherapy, and curettage surgery and/or invasive treatments [8, 9]. Topical therapy allows the treatment of both visible and subclinical lesions [8]. These treatments showed similar efficacies with different adverse events and cosmetic outcomes. Consequently, it can be seen that guidelines are difficult to construct [8].

Newer topical medications, such as colchicine, ingenol mebutate, and retinoids, are used, but no comparative study has yet been conducted on these drugs with more popular drugs such as DS [10, 11]. Therefore, this study aims to compare the efficacy and safety of topical 1% colchicine gel versus 3% DS gel in the treatment when treating AKs.

2. Materials and Methods

2.1. Participants. This randomized double-blind study was conducted in Al-Zahra and Noor University Hospitals, Isfahan University of Medical Sciences, Isfahan, Iran, from 2013 to 2014. The protocol of study was approved by the Institutional Review Board of Isfahan University of Medical Sciences and carried out in agreement with the Declaration of Helsinki and its subsequent revisions. After complete explanation of the study details, written informed consent was obtained from eligible patients. This trial was registered at the Iranian Registry of Clinical Trials (IRCT registration number: IRCT2015040721645N1, http://www.irct.ir/searchresult.php?keyword=&id=21645&number=1&prt=8369&total=10&m=1.

The diagnosis of AK was confirmed by two blinded dermatologists before participants were entered into the study. All AKs were located on the face and/or back of the hands and/or scalp in the subjects who were over 18 years of age. The study excluded pregnant or lactating women, patients taking investigational medication, and patients who had received treatment for their lesions within the 8 weeks preceding the study. In addition, patients who had other skin diseases in the area that was to be treated and known sensitivity to any component of the medications under investigation and patients who failed to follow up for various reasons were excluded.

2.2. Study Design. Patients underwent a standard clinical assessment and necessary laboratory evaluation 1 week after the onset of the treatment (so that all possible drug complications could be monitored). Overall, 70 patients were selected. Patients were randomized to receive 1% colchicine gel or 3% diclofenac sodium cream in a 1 : 1 ratio using a computer-generated code. Patients underwent a 6-week treatment with one of the two medications. Dermatologist and patients were not informed on the type of treatment and subjects received either treatment A or treatment B by chance. The randomization and allocation process was undertaken by a pharmacist at Al-Zahra Hospital. All patients were instructed to avoid direct sunlight exposure and to use sunscreen. The duration of treatment was twice daily for 6 weeks for both groups.

2.2.1. Medication Preparation. To prepare 1% colchicine gel, the pure colchicine powder (Modava Pharmaceutical Company, Iran) was readied and after being dissolved in water reached the desired volume and percentage on the base of hydroxypropyl methyl cellulose [12].

To prepare the 3% diclofenac cream, the pure powder (Modava Pharmaceutical Company, Iran) was dissolved in water and hydroxypropyl methyl cellulose and 2.5% hyaluronic acid was added to the gel to increase the drug's influence [13].

2.2.2. Outcome Assessment. Two dermatologists conducted a blind evaluation of patients 1 week and 30 and 60 days after the end of treatment and recorded new photographic images (under the same conditions of light and distance in which the first ones were taken).

These dermatologists also conducted a blind evaluation of before and after photographs at the beginning and the end of the treatment. The rate of recovery was considered as complete recovery (complete disappearance of erythema and desquamation) and partial recovery (reduction of erythema, desquamation, and lesion diameter by the scale ruler for dermatology).

Side effects of treatment were systematically recorded throughout the study and were assessed with the use of a checklist, which included pruritus, burning, erythema, and gastrointestinal complication on days 7, 30, 60, and 120.

2.3. Statistical Analysis. Statistical analysis was performed using SPSS version 22.0 for Windows; results were presented as mean ± SD. To compare the demographic data and frequency of side effects between the protocols, t-test, Fisher's exact test, and chi-square test were performed. Differences were considered significant if $p \leq 0.05$.

3. Results

No significant difference was found between those patients that had been randomly assigned to each group with regard to the basic demographic data including age, gender, and location of lesions. The distributions of age and sex and lesion site are given in Table 1. Also CONSORT flow diagram of the study is given in Figure 1.

The mean of the changes in the size of lesion was significant in both groups both before and after treatment (<0.001).

The mean (±SD) of size of lesions was shown at the start of the treatment and one and two months after the treatment (Table 2).

According to t-test, mean (±SD) of surface of lesions had no significant difference between the two groups before treatment ($p = 0.84$) (Table 2).

One month after the treatment, the size of surface of lesions in both groups was reduced to $0.45 \pm 0.39 \, \text{cm}^2$ in the group treated by colchicine and $0.39 \pm 0.21 \, \text{cm}^2$ in the group treated by diclofenac. According to t-test, no significant difference was observed between two groups ($p = 0.42$) (Table 2).

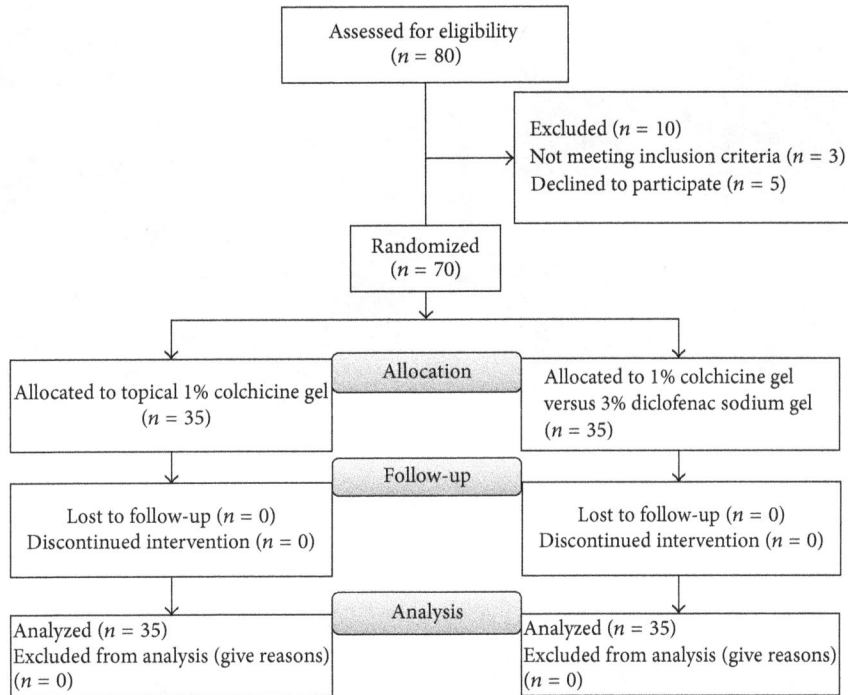

FIGURE 1: CONSORT flow diagram: topical 1% colchicine gel versus 3% diclofenac sodium gel for the treatment of actinic keratosis.

TABLE 1: Distribution of age and sex and location of the lesion in two groups separately.

| Variables | | Groups | | |
		Colchicine gel	Diclofenac gel	p value
Mean (±SD) of age		63.7 ± 9.2	62.3 ± 8.4	0.48
Sex N (%)	Male	26 (74.3)	30 (85.7)	0.23
	Female	9 (25.7)	5 (14.3)	
Location N (%)	Face	27 (77.1)	29 (82.9)	0.55
	Scalp	8 (22.9)	6 (17.1)	

TABLE 2: Mean (±SD) of surface of lesion: before and after the treatment.

| Time | Groups | | |
	Colchicine gel	Diclofenac gel	p value
Before treatment	0.65 ± 0.37	0.65 ± 0.21	0.84
30 days later	0.39 ± 0.21	0.45 ± 0.39	0.42
60 days later	0.21 ± 0.11	0.23 ± 0.11	0.62
p value	<0.001	<0.001	—

Two months after treatment, the size of surface of lesions in both groups was reduced to 0.23 ± 0.11 cm^2 in the group treated by colchicine and 0.21 ± 0.11 cm^2 in the group treated by diclofenac. According to the previously mentioned test, there was no difference between the two groups ($p = 0.42$) (Table 2).

The clinical efficacy of topical colchicine gel in a representative patient at baseline and at the end of follow-up can be seen in Figure 2.

Although the surface of the lesions was reduced in both groups at 30 and 60 days after treatment, there was no significant difference between the two groups at 30 and 60 days following treatment (Figure 3).

The two groups had no significant difference in terms of distribution of age, sex, and site of lesion (>0.05) (Figure 4).

Table 3 shows the percentage of frequency of drug complications as shown in both groups. Overall, 15 cases in colchicine group and 16 cases of the diclofenac sodium group suffered complications as a result of their treatment (42.9% versus 45.7%). According to Fisher's exact test, the complications were the same for both groups ($p = 0.99$).

No case of erythema was seen in colchicine group, while erythema was seen in 22.9% ($n = 8$) of patients in the diclofenac sodium group. This difference was significant ($p = 0.005$). No patient in either group chose to stop their treatment as a result of side effects.

Four months following the end of treatment, the lesions recurred in 2 (5.7%) lesions of the group treated with diclofenac, while no case of recurrence was seen in the group treated by colchicine. According to Fisher's exact test, there was no significant difference in the incidence of recurrence between two groups ($p = 0.49$).

4. Discussion

In our studies, colchicine gel was shown to be effective in treating AKs with a 1% concentration gel being applied twice daily for 8 weeks to the face, scalp, trunk, or extremities. Treatment with colchicine and diclofenac led to a significant improvement in the lesions; although a considerable percentage of patients suffered from the complications of

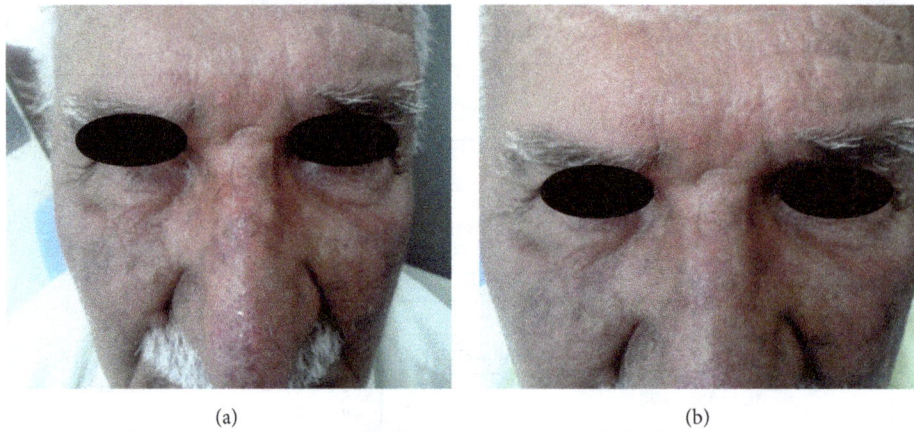

FIGURE 2: Large AKs on the nose of a participant in the colchicine group (a) at baseline and (b) at the end of the study (8 weeks of treatment).

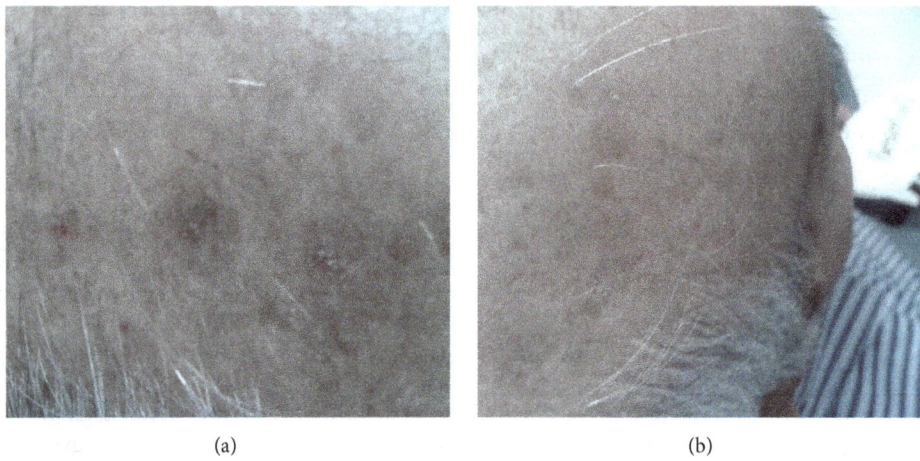

FIGURE 3: AKs on the scalp of a participant in the diclofenac group (a) at baseline and (b) at the end of the study (8 weeks of treatment).

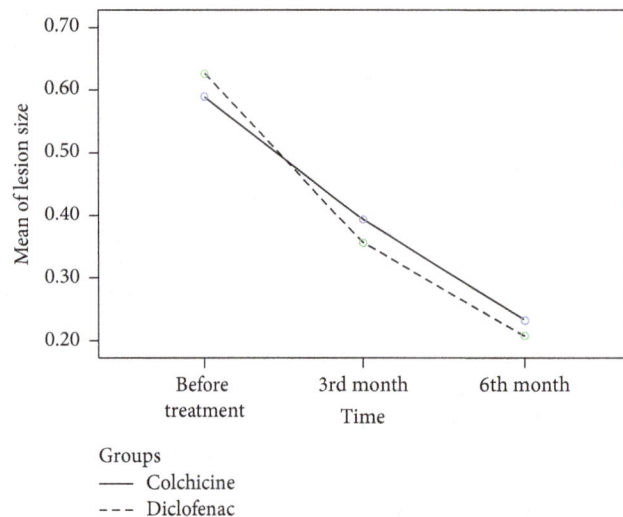

FIGURE 4: Mean of size of lesions: before and after the treatment. Covariates appearing in the model are evaluated at the following values: sex = 1.2128, age = 63.9362, and place = 1.1702.

TABLE 3: Frequency of the incidence of complications during treatment in both groups.

Side effects (n)		Colchicine (n/%)	Diclofenac (n/%)	p value
Pruritus	Yes (15)	7 (20)	8 (22.9)	0.99
	No (55)	28 (80)	27 (77.1)	
Burning	Yes (17)	10 (28.5)	7 (20)	0.57
	No (53)	25 (71.5)	28 (80)	
Erythema	Yes (8)	0 (0)	8 (22.9)	0.005
	No (62)	35 (100)	27 (77.1)	
Infection	Yes (0)	0 (0)	0 (0)	
	No (70)	35 (100)	35 (100)	
Gastrointestinal complication	Yes (31)	15 (42.9)	16 (45.7)	0.99
	No (39)	20 (57.1)	19 (54.3)	

treatment, the complications were both mild and tolerable. Colchicine had the capacity to interrupt mitosis and linkage to dimers of tubulin [14]. Such microtubular toxicity results in the cessation of mitosis in metaphase and interference in cellular mobility [15]. This mechanism can explain the clinical effect of colchicine on the treatment of AKs.

In the study by Grimaître et al., the application of a 1% colchicine gel for AKs in double-blind placebo-controlled trials was evaluated. The result of their study showed no recurrence after two months of follow-up. Burning and itching only occurred in patients in the colchicine group two or three days after application, with an inflammatory reaction being seen on those areas where the gel had been applied [12].

Within this study that used colchicine gel, no irritation or erythema was seen in the study participants, and there was no recurrence of lesion up to four months after treatment.

Akar et al. (2001) evaluated the efficacy of different concentrations of topical colchicine applied to AKs. Eight cases were treated with 1% topical colchicine and eight cases with 0.5% topical colchicine. Akar et al.'s (2001) results showed that topical colchicine is an effective and safe alternative agent for the treatment of AKs. Cream containing 0.5% colchicine is equally effective as 1% colchicine cream when treating AKs [16].

A meta-analysis of three studies for treatment of AKs with diclofenac 3% gel in 2.5% hyaluronic acid with a total of 364 patients revealed complete remission in 39.1% of patients [17].

Systemic toxicity with colchicine is a concern, and it is known that colchicine and its analogs interfere with microtubule growth within nerve cells, ciliated cells, leukocytes, and sperm [18].

Colchicine forms high-affinity complexes with tubulin and inhibits this protein's polymerization. Microtubule assembly and elongation are, therefore, disrupted, limiting the chemotactic and phagocytic activity of polymorphonuclear lymphocytes [19, 20].

Although the patients in this study only received topical colchicine, they were monitored closely for clinical signs of systemic toxicity such as hematologic side effects, including pancytopenia.

None of our patients demonstrated any systemic adverse events.

Our experiences with colchicine suggest that this effective treatment modality is a useful option for patients with AKs. There appears to be a low risk of systemic or local toxicity with this regimen. The data suggest that a more randomized, blinded, and controlled clinical trial using a larger sample size was needed in order to establish the true efficacy of colchicine.

Our study had some limitations, including small sample size and short duration of follow-up. Consequently, further comparative studies for clinical evaluation are recommended.

5. Conclusion

The results of the study show the use of topical 1% colchicine gel and 3% diclofenac sodium gel for the treatment of AKs to be both safe and effective treatment for AKs. The lack of long-term erythema and recurrence of the lesion is encouraging for use of topical colchicine gel.

Disclosure

The authors alone are responsible for the content and writing of the manuscript.

Competing Interests

The authors declare that there are no competing interests.

Acknowledgments

The authors thank all the subjects who contributed in clinical data gathering but not complete authorship criteria in this study.

References

[1] D. L. Stulberg, N. Clark, and D. Tovey, "Common hyperpigmentation disorders in adults: part II. Melanoma, seborrheic keratoses, acanthosis nigricans, melasma, diabetic dermopathy, tinea versicolor, and postinflammatory hyperpigmentation," *American Family Physician*, vol. 68, no. 10, pp. 1963–1968, 2003.

[2] D. L. Stulberg, N. Clark, and D. Tovey, "Common hyperpigmentation disorders in adults: part i. diagnostic approach, café au lait macules, diffuse hyperpigmentation, sun exposure, and phototoxic reactions," *American Family Physician*, vol. 68, no. 10, pp. 1955–1960, 2003.

[3] W. J. McIntyre, M. R. Downs, and S. A. Bedwell, "Treatment options for actinic keratoses," *American Family Physician*, vol. 76, no. 5, pp. 667–671, 2007.

[4] R. S. Stern, "Treatment of Photoaging," *The New England Journal of Medicine*, vol. 350, no. 15, pp. 1526–1534, 2004.

[5] J. F. McGuire, N. N. Ge, and S. Dyson, "Nonmelanoma skin cancer of the head and neck I: histopathology and clinical behavior," *American Journal of Otolaryngology—Head and Neck Medicine and Surgery*, vol. 30, no. 2, pp. 121–133, 2009.

[6] R. Werner and A. Nast, "Treating actinic keratosis," *British Journal of Dermatology*, vol. 174, no. 2, pp. 260–261, 2016.

[7] S. Silapunt, L. H. Goldberg, and M. Alam, "Topical and light-based treatments for actinic keratoses," *Seminars in Cutaneous Medicine and Surgery*, vol. 22, no. 3, pp. 162–170, 2003.

[8] G. Micali, F. Lacarrubba, M. R. Nasca, S. Ferraro, and R. A. Schwartz, "Topical pharmacotherapy for skin cancer: part II. Clinical applications," *Journal of the American Academy of Dermatology*, vol. 70, no. 6, pp. 979.e1–979.e12, 2014.

[9] I. Fariba, A. Ali, S. A. Hossein, S. Atefeh, and A. Z. B. S. Afshin, "Efficacy of 3% diclofenac gel for the treatment of actinic keratoses: a randomized, double-blind, placebo controlled study," *Indian Journal of Dermatology, Venereology and Leprology*, vol. 72, no. 5, pp. 346–349, 2006.

[10] W. D. Tutrone, R. Saini, S. Caglar, J. M. Weinberg, and J. Crespo, "Topical therapy for actinic keratoses, II: diclofenac, colchicine, and retinoids," *Cutis*, vol. 71, no. 5, pp. 373–379, 2003.

[11] M. Lebwohl, N. Swanson, L. L. Anderson, A. Melgaard, Z. Xu, and B. Berman, "Ingenol mebutate gel for actinic keratosis," *The New England Journal of Medicine*, vol. 366, no. 11, pp. 1010–1019, 2012.

[12] M. Grimaître, A. Etienne, M. Fathi, P.-A. Piletta, and J.-H. Saurat, "Topical colchicine therapy for actinic keratoses," *Dermatology*, vol. 200, no. 4, pp. 346–348, 2000.

[13] J. E. Wolf Jr., J. R. Taylor, E. Tschen, and S. Kang, "Topical 3.0% diclofenac in 2.5% hyaluronan gel in the treatment of actinic keratoses," *International Journal of Dermatology*, vol. 40, no. 11, pp. 709–713, 2001.

[14] M. Levy, M. Spino, and S. E. Read, "Colchicine: a state-of-the-art review," *Pharmacotherapy*, vol. 11, no. 3, pp. 196–211, 1991.

[15] C. Konda and A. G. Rao, "Colchicine in dermatology," *Indian Journal of Dermatology, Venereology and Leprology*, vol. 76, no. 2, pp. 201–205, 2010.

[16] A. Akar, H. B. Taştan, H. Erbil, E. Arca, Z. Kurumlu, and A. R. Gür, "Efficacy and safety assessment of 0.5% and 1% colchicine cream in the treatment of actinic keratoses," *Journal of Dermatological Treatment*, vol. 12, no. 4, pp. 199–203, 2001.

[17] D. Pirard, P. Vereecken, C. Mélot, and M. Heenen, "Three percent diclofenac in 2.5% hyaluronan gel in the treatment of actinic keratoses: a meta-analysis of the recent studies," *Archives of Dermatological Research*, vol. 297, no. 5, pp. 185–189, 2005.

[18] L. Margulis, "Colchicine-sensitive microtubules," *International Review of Cytology*, vol. 34, pp. 333–361, 1973.

[19] E. Dallaverde, P. T. Fan, and Y. H. Chang, "Mechanism of action of colchicine. V. Neutrophil adherence and phagocytosis in patients with acute gout treated with colchicine," *Journal of Pharmacology and Experimental Therapeutics*, vol. 223, no. 1, pp. 197–202, 1982.

[20] M. Ehrenfeld, M. Levy, M. Bar Eli, R. Gallily, and M. Eliakim, "Effect of colchicine on polymorphonuclear leucocyte chemotaxis in human volunteers," *British Journal of Clinical Pharmacology*, vol. 10, no. 3, pp. 297–300, 1980.

13

Dietary Energy Density, Renal Function, and Progression of Chronic Kidney Disease

Mohammad Hossein Rouhani,[1] **Mojgan Mortazavi Najafabadi,**[2]
Ahmad Esmaillzadeh,[1,3] **Awat Feizi,**[4] **and Leila Azadbakht**[1,3,5]

[1]*Food Security Research Center and Department of Community Nutrition, School of Nutrition and Food Science,*
Isfahan University of Medical Sciences, Isfahan, Iran

[2]*Department of Nephrology, Isfahan Kidney Diseases Research Center, Isfahan, Iran*

[3]*Department of Community Nutrition, School of Nutritional Sciences and Dietetics, Tehran University of Medical Sciences,*
Tehran, Iran

[4]*Faculty of Epidemiology and Biostatistics, Isfahan University of Medical Sciences, Isfahan, Iran*

[5]*Diabetes Research Center, Endocrinology and Metabolism Clinical Sciences Institute, Tehran University of Medical Sciences,*
Tehran, Iran

Correspondence should be addressed to Leila Azadbakht; azadbakht@hlth.mui.ac.ir

Academic Editor: Denis A. Cozzi

Background. There is evidence of the association between dietary energy density and chronic diseases. However, no report exists regarding the relation between DED and chronic kidney disease (CKD). *Objective.* To examine the association between dietary energy density (DED), renal function, and progression of chronic kidney disease (CKD). *Design.* Cross-sectional. *Setting.* Three nephrology clinics. *Subjects.* Two hundred twenty-one subjects with diagnosed CKD. *Main Outcome Measure.* Dietary intake of patients was assessed by a validated food frequency questionnaire. DED (in kcal/g) was calculated with the use of energy content and weight of solid foods and energy yielding beverages. Renal function was measured by blood urea nitrogen (BUN), serum creatinine (Cr), and estimated glomerular filtration rate (eGFR). *Results.* Patients in the first tertile of DED consumed more amounts of carbohydrate, dietary fiber, potassium, phosphorus, zinc, magnesium, calcium, folate, vitamin C, and vitamin B2. After adjusting for confounders, we could not find any significant trend for BUN and Cr across tertiles of DED. In multivariate model, an increased risk of being in the higher stage of CKD was found among those in the last tertile of DED (OR: 3.15; 95% CI: 1.30, 7.63; $P = 0.01$). *Conclusion.* We observed that lower DED was associated with better nutrient intake and lower risk of CKD progression.

1. Introduction

Chronic kidney disease (CKD) refers to a group of disorders in kidney structure and function [1]. Although CKD had been 27th cause of global total mortality in 1990, it moved up to 18th cause in 2010 [2]. Estimated global prevalence of CKD was 8–16% in 2013 [2]. Reports from a cross-sectional study published in 2009 showed that 18.9% of Iranian adults were diagnosed with CKD [3]. Dietary intake has an important role in prevention and treatment of CKD [4]. Although nutritional recommendations for patients with CKD have focused on limiting protein, sodium, potassium, and phosphorous

intake [5], the importance of other aspects of diet (e.g., diet quality indices) should not be neglected. The association between diet quality indices and CKD was partially assessed previously. Findings of a research showed that nutritional quality of individuals with CKD was not adequate [6]. A recent study reported that there was a favorable association between a modified Alternative Healthy Eating Index score and progression of CKD [7]. Also, unhealthy dietary patterns were positively related to progression of CKD [8].

Dietary energy density, one of the most used diet quality indices, shows energy content of a given weight of diet [9]. There is a large body of evidence showing that DED is positively related to the risk of chronic diseases such as obesity [10], metabolic syndrome [11], and diabetes [12]. Also, DED was directly associated with chronic inflammation [13]. Moreover, previous study reported an increased oxidative stress among subjects who consumed high energy-dense meals [14]. A higher grade of inflammation and oxidative stress was observed among patients with CKD [15]. It was suggested that inflammation was directly related to CKD progression [16]. Therefore, we hypothesized that there was a relation between DED and biomarkers of renal function and CKD progression. As this association was not assessed previously, the aim of current study was to assess the relation between DED and markers of kidney function and progression of CKD.

2. Methods

2.1. Subjects. Two hundred twenty-one patients with diagnosed CKD were recruited for this study. Estimated glomerular filtration rate (eGFR) lower than $60 \, \text{mL/min/1.73} \, \text{m}^2$ was determined as diagnostic criteria of CKD [17]. eGFR was calculated by Modification of Diet in Renal Disease (MDRD) method [18]. CKD was classified as stage 3 ($30 \leq \text{eGFR} \leq 59 \, \text{mL/min/1.73} \, \text{m}^2$), stage 4 ($15 \leq \text{eGFR} \leq 29 \, \text{mL/min/1.73} \, \text{m}^2$), and stage 5 ($\text{eGFR} < 15 \, \text{mL/min/1.73} \, \text{m}^2$) [17]. Other diseases (e.g., diabetes and nephrolithiasis) had been controlled by related specialist. Patients who signed written consent were recruited for this cross-sectional study. Therefore, we included patients with diagnosed CKD (eGFR $< 60 \, \text{mL/min/1.73} \, \text{m}^2$) who signed written consent form. Subjects who needed dialysis treatment were excluded.

2.2. Dietary Assessment and DED. An interviewer-administered food frequency questionnaire (FFQ) was used to assess dietary intake of patients during the previous year. The frequency of consumption of 168 food items was measured by foresaid FFQ. The validity and reliability of this semiquantitative FFQ were reported elsewhere [19]. Energy and nutrient content of consumed foods were analyzed by Nutritionist IV software (N-Squared Computing, Salem, OR). Daily energy intake <800 or >4200 kcal/d was considered as under- and overreporting, respectively. Under- and overreported data were excluded.

DED (in kcal/g) was calculated with the use of energy content and weight of solid foods and energy yielding beverages.

2.3. Biochemical Measures. After 12-hour overnight fasting, a blood sample was collected and then centrifuged at 3000 ×g for 10 min. Blood urea nitrogen (BUN) was measured by incubation of the blood sample with urease (intra-assay coefficient was 3.75 and interassay coefficient was 2.74). Serum creatinine (Cr) was determined by colorimetric reflectance spectrophotometry (intra-assay coefficient was 3.22 and interassay coefficient was 1.78). All kits were produced by Pars Azmoon Inc.

2.4. Other Variables. Demographic characteristics were assessed by oral questions. Subjects were asked regarding income, occupation, education, and region of residence to assess socioeconomic status. Weight was measured by digital scale to the nearest 0.1 kg. Height was assessed by self-reported measures. Participants were asked to report their sedentary time and activities to measure physical activity [20]. A trained assistance measured systolic and diastolic blood pressure by a standard mercury sphygmomanometer.

2.5. Statistical Analysis. Normality of the variables was tested using Kolmogorov-Smirnov test and histogram curve. We reported CKD stage, physical activity level (low, moderate, and high), marital status, sex ratio, and socioeconomic status (low, moderate, and high) as percentage frequency. Chi-square test was performed to detect difference in these variables. Continues variables (age, body mass index, biomarkers, and dietary intakes of nutrients) were presented as mean ± standard deviation. We used analysis of variance (ANOVA) to compared biochemical variables across the tertiles of DED. Analysis of covariance (ANCOVA) was performed to report energy-adjusted nutrient intakes across the tertiles of DED. Odds ratio and 95% confidence interval of the being in the higher stages of CKD were obtained using logistic regression. The risk was reported in crude and 2 adjusted models. The firs model was adjusted for age, physical activity, socioeconomic status, height, weight, and systolic and diastolic blood pressure. Further adjustment was performed for dietary intake of sodium, potassium, phosphorus, and animal protein per body weight in model 2. We considered $P < 0.05$ as significance level. Also, we used SPSS version 20 (IBM) to analyze this data.

3. Results

Demographic characteristics of patients with CKD across tertiles of DED are presented in Table 1. We did not observe any significant difference in demographic characteristics across tertiles of DED. The mean age of the patients in all three tertiles was more than 50 years. Most percentage of the subjects had middle socioeconomic status and low physical activity level. Also, most patients fell within stage 3 of CKD.

Nutrient intake of patients with CKD across tertiles of DED is reported in Table 2. The findings showed that patients in the first tertile of DED consumed more amounts of carbohydrate ($P < 0.01$), dietary fiber ($P < 0.01$), potassium ($P < 0.01$), phosphorus ($P = 0.02$), zinc ($P = 0.02$), magnesium ($P < 0.01$), calcium ($P = 0.04$), folate ($P < 0.01$), vitamin C ($P < 0.01$), and vitamin B2 ($P < 0.01$). In contrast, the intake of vitamin B3 in top tertile was significantly more than lower tertiles ($P = 0.01$).

Mean of renal function variables reported by tertiles of DED is presented in Table 3. We could not find any significant trend for BUN and Cr across tertiles of DED in crude and 3 adjusted models.

Odds ratios for being in the higher stage of CKD according to tertiles of DED are shown in Table 4. We did not observe a significant trend for risk of higher stage of CKD in crude model (P for trend = 0.18) and in model 1 (P for trend = 0.13). After adjusting for dietary confounders, an increased

TABLE 1: Demographic characteristics of patients with chronic kidney disease across tertiles of dietary energy density.

Variables	Tertiles of dietary energy density			P^2
	T1 (≤0.7 kcal/g) (n = 74)	T2 (0.8–0.9 kcal/g) (n = 73)	T3 >0.9 kcal/g (n = 74)	
Age (year)	56.53 ± 14.70[1]	58.04 ± 13.82	55.16 ± 17.02	0.52
Male (%)	64.9	67.1	75.7	0.32
Height (cm)	168.26 ± 8.81	167.16 ± 7.70	169.35 ± 9.76	0.32
BMI (kg/m^2)	25.49 ± 3.66	25.96 ± 4.21	26.08 ± 5.10	0.68
Physical activity (%)				
Low	60.8	63.0	62.2	
Moderate	36.5	34.2	33.8	
High	2.7	2.7	4.1	0.98
Socioeconomic status (%)				
Low	9.5	20.5	24.3	
Middle	74.3	63.0	59.5	
High	16.2	16.4	16.2	0.18
CKD stage (%)				
Stage 3	67.6	74.0	59.5	
Stage 4	29.7	24.7	40.5	
Stage 5	2.7	1.4	0.0	0.18

BMI: body mass index; CKD: chronic kidney disease.
[1]Mean ± SD.
[2]Calculated by Chi-square and analysis of variance for qualitative and quantitative variables, respectively.

TABLE 2: Nutrient intake of patients with chronic kidney disease across tertiles of dietary energy density.

Variables	Tertiles of dietary energy density			P^2
	T1 (≤0.7 kcal/g) (n = 74)	T2 (0.8–0.9 kcal/g) (n = 73)	T3 >0.9 kcal/g (n = 74)	
Carbohydrate (g)	198.31 ± 61.68[1]	171.26 ± 67.22	133.14 ± 80.15	<0.01
Protein (g)	30.05 ± 11.34	29.36 ± 8.61	30.58 ± 13.85	0.81
Fat (g)	24.41 ± 7.99	24.01 ± 8.61	25.58 ± 13.85	0.27
Saturated fatty acid (g)	7.75 ± 7.99	7.40 ± 3.82	8.84 ± 4.79	0.10
Cholesterol (g)	147.56 ± 45.71	149.02 ± 42.89	153.40 ± 52.46	0.74
Dietary fiber (g)	15.07 ± 4.86	14.62 ± 6.92	13.68 ± 3.21	<0.01
Sodium (mg)	2425.38 ± 340.38	2334.14 ± 253.63	2439.59 ± 505.21	0.19
Potassium (mg)	1909.82 ± 853.64	1488.08 ± 444.86	1101.94 ± 531.74	<0.01
Phosphorus (mg)	770.78 ± 287.62	676.95 ± 196.15	651.99 ± 317.48	0.02
Zinc (mg)	6.42 ± 1.68	5.91 ± 1.35	5.67 ± 1.74	0.02
Magnesium (mg)	214.48 ± 55.43	185.00 ± 33.29	158.51 ± 42.65	<0.01
Calcium (mg)	910.35 ± 358.81	818.68 ± 214.23	790.68 ± 295.39	0.04
Folate (μg)	264.92 ± 110.96	210.29 ± 46.64	184.66 ± 97.15	<0.01
Vitamin E (mg)	13.39 ± 6.67	12.78 ± 6.37	12.84 ± 5.79	0.81
Vitamin C (mg)	110.42 ± 103.95	88.78 ± 44.65	70.79 ± 39.80	<0.01
Vitamin B1 (mg)	1.49 ± 0.17	1.49 ± 16	1.51 ± 0.34	0.80
Vitamin B2 (mg)	1.46 ± 0.46	1.25 ± 0.28	1.19 ± 0.40	<0.01
Vitamin B3 (mg)	15.12 ± 2.27	16.07 ± 3.11	16.80 ± 4.67	0.01

[1]All values are mean ± SD and adjusted for total energy intake.
[2]Calculated by multivariate analysis of variance.

TABLE 3: Mean of renal function variables reported by tertiles of dietary energy density among patients with chronic kidney disease.

| Variables | Tertiles of dietary energy density | | | P^2 |
	T1 ($\leq$0.7 kcal/g) ($n = 74$)	T2 (0.8–0.9 kcal/g) ($n = 73$)	T3 (>0.9 kcal/g) ($n = 74$)	
BUN (mg/dL)				
Crude	26.72 ± 12.90^1	28.15 ± 13.50	29.12 ± 12.90	0.45
Model 1	28.97 ± 13.33	30.98 ± 13.32	31.77 ± 13.33	0.42
Model 2	28.89 ± 13.07	30.75 ± 13.06	32.06 ± 13.16	0.42
Model 3	28.95 ± 13.50	30.72 ± 12.98	32.04 ± 13.93	0.42
Creatinine (mg/dL)				
Crude	1.85 ± 1.40	1.87 ± 1.36	2.02 ± 1.37	0.20
Model 1[3]	1.97 ± 0.69	1.98 ± 0.68	2.12 ± 0.69	0.38
Model 2[4]	1.97 ± 0.67	1.97 ± 0.72	2.12 ± 0.67	0.38
Model 3[5]	1.97 ± 0.76	1.98 ± 0.72	2.13 ± 0.78	0.40

BUN: blood urea nitrogen.
[1] Mean ± SD.
[2] Calculated by multivariate analysis of variance (in crude model) and multivariate analysis of covariance (in adjusted model).
[3] Model 1: adjusted for age, sex, physical activity, and socioeconomic status.
[4] Model 2: model 1 + systolic and diastolic blood pressure.
[5] Model 3: model 2 + weight, height, sodium, potassium, phosphorus, and animal protein intake per body weight.

TABLE 4: Odds ratios and 95% confidence intervals for being in the higher stage of chronic kidney disease according to tertiles of dietary energy density among patients with chronic kidney disease.

| Models | Tertiles of dietary energy density | | | P for trend[1] |
	T1 ($\leq$0.7 kcal/g) ($n = 74$)	T2 (0.8–0.9 kcal/g) ($n = 73$)	T3 >0.9 kcal/g ($n = 74$)	
Crude	1	0.73 (0.36, 1.50)	1.42 (0.72, 2.48)	0.18
Model 1[2]	1	0.71 (0.34, 1.51)	1.52 (0.74, 3.12)	0.13
Model 2[3]	1	3.48 (1.55, 7.79)	3.15 (1.30, 7.63)	0.01

[1] P value was calculated by logistic regression.
[2] Model 1: adjusted for age, physical activity, socioeconomic status, height, weight, and systolic and diastolic blood pressure.
[3] Model 2: model 1 + sodium, potassium, phosphorus, and animal protein intake per body weight.

risk of being in the higher stage of CKD was found among those in the higher tertiles of DED (P for trend = 0.01).

4. Discussion

The results of the current study suggest that patients in the higher tertiles of DED had increased risk of being in the higher stage of CKD. To the best of our knowledge, this is the first study regarding the association between DED and risk of being in the higher stage of CKD. Furthermore, those in the lowest tertile of DED consumed higher amounts of different nutrients.

The results of the present study showed that patients in the first tertile of DED consumed more amounts of carbohydrate. We used energy-adjusted nutrient intake in the current study. Similar finding was observed in a large population-based study in which energy-adjusted nutrient intake was reported [21]. Also, results of an Iranian study conducted in young females supported our findings regarding carbohydrate [22]. Moreover, previous study reported that subjects who had

low energy-dense diet consumed higher amounts of zinc, calcium, vitamin C, and vitamin B2 [23]. As patients in the first tertile of DED consumed more amounts of dietary fiber, it was suggested that large amounts of consumed carbohydrate were from fruits, vegetables, and whole grains. This hypothesis justifies our findings regarding higher intake of nutrients found in these foods (i.e., potassium, phosphorus, magnesium, folate, vitamin C, and vitamin B2).

Previous studies reported that high energy-dense diets may be associated with lower nutrient intake [22–24]. A large cross-sectional study reported that dietary fiber was related to reduction of inflammation and mortality among patients with CKD [25]. Therefore, beneficial effects of a low energy-dense diet on renal function may be mediated by dietary fiber and its effect on inflammation. Higher intake of dietary fiber may inhibit rapid digestion of carbohydrates which results in lower production of inflammatory mediators [26]. Recent evidence focused on higher consumption of dietary fiber in patients with CKD [27]. Intake of dietary fiber has been restricted in these patients because phosphorus content of foods rich in dietary fiber is high [5]. It should be noted that phosphorus is in phytate form in whole grains and legumes and its bioavailability is low [28]. Therefore, patients with CKD have been suggested to consume high amounts of dietary fiber found in whole grains and legumes.

An increased risk of being in a higher stage of CKD was observed among those in higher tertiles of DED in multivariable-adjusted model. Previous observational study reported that risk of incidence of CKD was higher among those who consumed more amounts of energy-dense, nutrient-poor sources of carbohydrate [29].

Our finding was adjusted for general (age, physical activity, socioeconomic status, height, weight, and blood pressure) and dietary (sodium, potassium, phosphorus, and animal protein intake) confounders. These confounders were selected according to the existing evidence. There was a significant association between age and outcomes of CKD [30]. Also, Cr might be affected by high physical activity level [31]. Socioeconomic status [32], anthropometric measurements [33], and blood pressure [34] were related to renal function and CKD. Moreover, kidney function may be affected by sodium intake [35] and animal protein [36, 37]. An elevated serum Cr was observed after meat consumption in a feeding study [38]. Moreover, a positive relation between meat intake and urea nitrogen was reported in clinical trials [39]. Also, nutritional recommendations for patients with CKD have focused on limiting potassium and phosphorous intake [5]. Therefore, we included all these confounder variables in our analysis.

Added sugars and fat are two means to achieve a high energy-dense diet [29]. Evidence showed that high sugar intake resulted in increased serum uric acid [40]. There is a positive association between elevated serum uric acid and hypertension which may lead to higher risk of renal damage [41]. On the other hand, observational studies reported a direct relation between high dietary fat intake and proteinuria [42]. It was suggested that the association between renal damage and dietary fat was mediated by inflammatory markers [42]. A positive relation between inflammatory marker (e.g., high sensitivity C-reactive protein) and saturated fatty acid was reported by an observational study [43]. Also, there is a significant positive association between high sensitivity C-reactive protein and proteinuria [44]. Therefore, inflammation can mediate the association between dietary fat (especially saturated fatty acid) and renal damage.

We should acknowledge a number of limitations. First, this was a cross-sectional study, and therefore we could not find a casual relationship. It is strongly recommended that future prospective cohort studies assess the association between DED and renal dysfunction. Second, we evaluate renal dysfunction by measuring BUN and creatinine. Future studies should measure other renal biochemical variables such as proteinuria. Third, we did not focus on a specific group of patients with CKD (e.g., diabetic nephropathy).

The strengths of present study are that we reported a new finding regarding the association between DED and chronic diseases. As mentioned, most previous studies focused on the relation between DED and cardiovascular diseases, diabetes and obesity. Therefore, this is the first study regarding the association between DED and kidney disease.

In conclusion, we observed that lower DED was associated with better nutrient intake and lower risk of CKD progression.

Abbreviations

ANOVA: Analysis of variance
BUN: Blood urea nitrogen
CKD: Chronic kidney disease
Cr: Creatinine
DED: Dietary energy density
eGFR: Estimated glomerular filtration rate
FFQ: Food frequency questionnaire.

Additional Points

Practical Application. Dietitians should recommend a low energy-dense diet to patients with CKD to delay progression of CKD.

Competing Interests

The authors declare that there are no competing interests.

Authors' Contributions

Leila Azadbakht, Ahmad Esmaillzadeh, Awat Feizi, and Mojgan Mortazavi Najafabadi designed the study. Mohammad Hossein Rouhani and Mojgan Mortazavi Najafabadi collected data. Mohammad Hossein Rouhani, Leila Azadbakht, and Awat Feizi performed statistical analysis. Mohammad Hossein Rouhani and Leila Azadbakht wrote manuscript.

Acknowledgments

The authors appreciate the financial support provided by the Research Council of the Food Security Research Center, Isfahan University of Medical Sciences, Isfahan, Iran.

References

[1] A. S. Levey and J. Coresh, "Chronic kidney disease," *The Lancet*, vol. 379, no. 9811, pp. 165–180, 2012.

[2] V. Jha, G. Garcia-Garcia, K. Iseki et al., "Chronic kidney disease: global dimension and perspectives," *The Lancet*, vol. 382, no. 9888, pp. 260–272, 2013.

[3] F. Hosseinpanah, F. Kasraei, A. A. Nassiri, and F. Azizi, "High prevalence of chronic kidney disease in Iran: a large population-based study," *BMC Public Health*, vol. 9, article 44, 2009.

[4] J. M. Turner, C. Bauer, M. K. Abramowitz, M. L. Melamed, and T. H. Hostetter, "Treatment of chronic kidney disease," *Kidney International*, vol. 81, no. 4, pp. 351–362, 2012.

[5] US National library of Medicine, "Diet—chronic kidney disease," February 2015, https://medlineplus.gov/ency/article/002442.htm.

[6] H. Kim, H. Lim, and R. Choue, "Compromised diet quality is associated with decreased renal function in children with

chronic kidney disease," *Clinical Nutrition Research*, vol. 3, no. 2, pp. 142–149, 2014.

[7] D. Dunkler, M. Kohl, K. K. Teo et al., "Dietary risk factors for incidence or progression of chronic kidney disease in individuals with type 2 diabetes in the European Union," *Nephrology Dialysis Transplantation*, vol. 30, supplement 4, pp. iv76–iv85, 2015.

[8] O. M. Gutiérrez, P. Muntner, D. V. Rizk et al., "Dietary patterns and risk of death and progression to ESRD in individuals with CKD: a cohort study," *American Journal of Kidney Diseases*, vol. 64, no. 2, pp. 204–213, 2014.

[9] J. H. Ledikwe, H. M. Blanck, L. K. Khan et al., "Dietary energy density is associated with energy intake and weight status in US adults," *The American Journal of Clinical Nutrition*, vol. 83, no. 6, pp. 1362–1368, 2006.

[10] R. Pérez-Escamilla, J. E. Obbagy, J. M. Altman et al., "Dietary energy density and body weight in adults and children: a systematic review," *Journal of the Academy of Nutrition and Dietetics*, vol. 112, no. 5, pp. 671–684, 2012.

[11] A. Esmaillzadeh and L. Azadbakht, "Dietary energy density and the metabolic syndrome among Iranian women," *European Journal of Clinical Nutrition*, vol. 65, no. 5, pp. 598–605, 2011.

[12] J. Lindström, M. Peltonen, J. G. Eriksson et al., "High-fibre, low-fat diet predicts long-term weight loss and decreased type 2 diabetes risk: the Finnish Diabetes Prevention Study," *Diabetologia*, vol. 49, no. 5, pp. 912–920, 2006.

[13] M. B. Schulze, K. Hoffmann, J. E. Manson et al., "Dietary pattern, inflammation, and incidence of type 2 diabetes in women," *The American Journal of Clinical Nutrition*, vol. 82, no. 3, pp. 675–684, 2005.

[14] S. Devaraj, J. Wang-Polagruto, J. Polagruto, C. L. Keen, and I. Jialal, "High-fat, energy-dense, fast-food-style breakfast results in an increase in oxidative stress in metabolic syndrome," *Metabolism: Clinical and Experimental*, vol. 57, no. 6, pp. 867–870, 2008.

[15] S. H. Rangwala, R. F. Finn, C. E. Smith et al., "High-level production of active HIV-1 protease in *Escherichia coli*," *Gene*, vol. 122, no. 2, pp. 263–269, 1992.

[16] D. M. Silverstein, "Inflammation in chronic kidney disease: role in the progression of renal and cardiovascular disease," *Pediatric Nephrology*, vol. 24, no. 8, pp. 1445–1452, 2009.

[17] National Kidney Foundation, "K/DOQI clinical practice guidelines for chronic kidney disease: evaluation, classification, and stratification," *American Journal of Kidney Diseases*, vol. 39, no. 2, supplement 1, pp. S1–S266, 2002.

[18] A. S. Levey, J. P. Bosch, J. B. Lewis, T. Greene, N. Rogers, and D. Roth, "A more accurate method to estimate glomerular filtration rate from serum creatinine: a new prediction equation. Modification of Diet in Renal Disease Study Group," *Annals of Internal Medicine*, vol. 130, no. 6, pp. 461–470, 1999.

[19] L. Azadbakht and A. Esmaillzadeh, "Red meat intake is associated with metabolic syndrome and the plasma c-reactive protein concentration in women," *Journal of Nutrition*, vol. 139, no. 2, pp. 335–339, 2009.

[20] A. J. Atkin, T. Gorely, S. A. Clemes et al., "Methods of measurement in epidemiology: sedentary behaviour," *International Journal of Epidemiology*, vol. 41, no. 5, pp. 1460–1471, 2012.

[21] A. K. Kant and B. I. Graubard, "Energy density of diets reported by American adults: association with food group intake, nutrient intake, and body weight," *International Journal of Obesity*, vol. 29, no. 8, pp. 950–956, 2005.

[22] L. Azadbakht and A. Esmaillzadeh, "Dietary energy density is favorably associated with dietary diversity score among female university students in Isfahan," *Nutrition*, vol. 28, no. 10, pp. 991–995, 2012.

[23] L. Azadbakht, F. Haghighatdoost, and A. Esmaillzadeh, "Dietary energy density is inversely associated with the diet quality indices among Iranian young adults," *Journal of Nutritional Science and Vitaminology*, vol. 58, no. 1, pp. 29–35, 2012.

[24] M. H. Rouhani, M. Mirseifinezhad, N. Omrani, A. Esmaillzadeh, and L. Azadbakht, "Fast food consumption, quality of diet, and obesity among Isfahanian adolescent girls," *Journal of Obesity*, vol. 2012, Article ID 597924, 8 pages, 2012.

[25] V. M. R. Krishnamurthy, G. Wei, B. C. Baird et al., "High dietary fiber intake is associated with decreased inflammation and all-cause mortality in patients with chronic kidney disease," *Kidney International*, vol. 81, no. 3, pp. 300–306, 2012.

[26] L. Qi, R. M. van Dam, S. Liu, M. Franz, C. Mantzoros, and F. B. Hu, "Whole-grain, bran, and cereal fiber intakes and markers of systemic inflammation in diabetic women," *Diabetes Care*, vol. 29, no. 2, pp. 207–211, 2006.

[27] C. Williams, C. Ronco, and P. Kotanko, "Whole grains in the renal diet—is it time to reevaluate their role?" *Blood Purification*, vol. 36, no. 3-4, pp. 210–214, 2013.

[28] C. Sullivan, S. S. Sayre, J. B. Leon et al., "Effect of food additives on hyperphosphatemia among patients with end-stage renal disease: a randomized controlled trial," *JAMA-Journal of the American Medical Association*, vol. 301, no. 6, pp. 629–635, 2009.

[29] B. Gopinath, D. C. Harris, V. M. Flood, G. Burlutsky, J. Brand-Miller, and P. Mitchell, "Carbohydrate nutrition is associated with the 5-year incidence of chronic kidney disease," *The Journal of Nutrition*, vol. 141, no. 3, pp. 433–439, 2011.

[30] A. M. O'Hare, A. I. Choi, D. Bertenthal et al., "Age affects outcomes in chronic kidney disease," *Journal of the American Society of Nephrology*, vol. 18, no. 10, pp. 2758–2765, 2007.

[31] M. Samra and A. C. Abcar, "False estimates of elevated creatinine," *The Permanente journal*, vol. 16, no. 2, pp. 51–52, 2012.

[32] S. D. S. Fraser, P. J. Roderick, G. Aitken et al., "Chronic kidney disease, albuminuria and socioeconomic status in the Health Surveys for England 2009 and 2010," *Journal of Public Health*, vol. 36, no. 4, pp. 577–586, 2014.

[33] B. Afsar, R. Elsurer, E. Güner, and A. Kirkpantur, "Which anthropometric parameter is best related with urinary albumin excretion and creatinine clearance in type 2 diabetes: body mass index, waist circumference, waist-to-hip ratio, or conicity index?" *Journal of Renal Nutrition*, vol. 21, no. 6, pp. 472–478, 2011.

[34] M. Ravera, M. Re, L. Deferrari, S. Vettoretti, and G. Deferrari, "Importance of blood pressure control in chronic kidney disease," *Journal of the American Society of Nephrology*, vol. 17, no. 4, supplement 2, pp. S98–S103, 2006.

[35] H. J. Lambers Heerspink, G. Navis, and E. Ritz, "Salt intake in kidney disease-a missed therapeutic opportunity?" *Nephrology Dialysis Transplantation*, vol. 27, no. 9, pp. 3435–3442, 2012.

[36] B. A. Ince, E. J. Anderson, and R. M. Neer, "Lowering dietary protein to U.S. Recommended dietary allowance levels reduces urinary calcium excretion and bone resorption in young women," *The Journal of Clinical Endocrinology & Metabolism*, vol. 89, no. 8, pp. 3801–3807, 2004.

[37] W. F. Martin, L. H. Cerundolo, M. A. Pikosky et al., "Effects of dietary protein intake on indexes of hydration," *Journal of the American Dietetic Association*, vol. 106, no. 4, pp. 587–589, 2006.

[38] S. Nair, S. V. O'Brien, K. Hayden et al., "Effect of a cooked meat meal on serum creatinine and estimated glomerular filtration rate in diabetes-related kidney disease," *Diabetes Care*, vol. 37, no. 2, pp. 483–487, 2014.

[39] L. O. Dragsted, "Biomarkers of meat intake and the application of nutrigenomics," *Meat Science*, vol. 84, no. 2, pp. 301–307, 2010.

[40] R. J. Johnson, M. S. Segal, Y. Sautin et al., "Potential role of sugar (fructose) in the epidemic of hypertension, obesity and the metabolic syndrome, diabetes, kidney disease, and cardiovascular disease1–3," *American Journal of Clinical Nutrition*, vol. 86, no. 4, pp. 899–906, 2007.

[41] S. Watanabe, D.-H. Kang, L. Feng et al., "Uric acid, hominoid evolution, and the pathogenesis of salt-sensitivity," *Hypertension*, vol. 40, no. 3, pp. 355–360, 2002.

[42] J. Lin, S. Judd, A. Le et al., "Associations of dietary fat with albuminuria and kidney dysfunction," *The American Journal of Clinical Nutrition*, vol. 92, no. 4, pp. 897–904, 2010.

[43] J. A. Nettleton, L. M. Steffen, E. J. Mayer-Davis et al., "Dietary patterns are associated with biochemical markers of inflammation and endothelial activation in the Multi-Ethnic Study of Atherosclerosis (MESA)," *The American Journal of Clinical Nutrition*, vol. 83, no. 6, pp. 1369–1379, 2006.

[44] J. Lin, F. B. Hu, C. Mantzoros, and G. C. Curhan, "Lipid and inflammatory biomarkers and kidney function decline in type 2 diabetes," *Diabetologia*, vol. 53, no. 2, pp. 263–267, 2010.

14

Treatment Alternatives to Negotiate Peri-Implantitis

Eli E. Machtei

Department of Periodontology, School of Graduate Dentistry, Rambam Health Care Campus and Faculty of Medicine, Technion (Israel Institute of Technology), Rambam HCC, 8 Ha'alia Hashnia Street, 31096 Haifa, Israel

Correspondence should be addressed to Eli E. Machtei; machtei@rambam.health.gov.il

Academic Editor: Silvana Barros

Peri-implant diseases are becoming a major health issue in dentistry. Despite the magnitude of this problem and the potential grave consequences, commonly acceptable treatment protocols are missing. Hence, the present paper reviews the literature treatment of peri-implantitis in order to explore their benefits and limitations. Treatment of peri-implantitis may include surgical and nonsurgical approaches, either individually or combined. Nonsurgical therapy is aimed at removing local irritants from the implants' surface with or without surface decontamination and possibly some additional adjunctive therapies agents or devices. Systemic antibiotics may also be incorporated. Surgical therapy is aimed at removing any residual subgingival deposits and additionally reducing the peri-implant pockets depth. This can be done alone or in conjunction with either osseous respective approach or regenerative approach. Finally, if all fails, explantation might be the best alternative in order to arrest the destruction of the osseous structure around the implant, thus preserving whatever is left in this site for future reconstruction. The available literature is still lacking with large heterogeneity in the clinical response thus suggesting possible underlying predisposing conditions that are not all clear to us. Therefore, at present time treatment of peri-implantitis should be considered possible but not necessarily predictable.

1. Introduction

Peri-implantitis is becoming an ever growing oral health concern that is frequently encountered in the dental office. The number of dental implants that are currently placed annually is somewhat elusive; however, the best estimate available puts this figure at around fifteen million new implants (worldwide) every year [1]. Of these, how many will eventually develop peri-implant diseases is also debatable. Zitzmann and Berglundh on behalf of the VI workshop of the European Federation of Periodontology have suggested that 80 percent of the patients and 50 percent of the implants will develop peri-implant mucositis during the years. These corresponding figures for peri-implantitis are 28–56 percent of the patients and 12–43 percent of the implants [2]. To the contrary, Mombelli et al., on behalf of the 3rd European academy of osteointegration workshop in 2012, have suggested somewhat lower numbers for peri-implantitis: 20 percent of the subjects and 10% of the implants [3]. More recently, Atieh and coworkers [4] in a meta-analysis of 504 studies which included 1497 patients with 6293 implants

reported the prevalence of peri-implant mucositis to be 63.4 percent (of the patients) and 30.7 percent (of the implants). A higher frequency of occurrence of peri-implant diseases was recorded for smokers with a summary estimate of 36.3 percent.

The reason for this large variation in the reported literature might be associated with patients variables such as smoking [5, 6], preexisting periodontal disease [7, 8], oral hygiene [9, 10], quality of prosthetic reconstruction [11, 12], and some systemic conditions and medications [13, 14]. Koldsland and coworkers [15] have suggested a different approach to explain this variability. Using different threshold levels to define peri-implantitis (i.e., bone loss of >2 mm or >3 mm and implants probing depth of >4 mm and >6 mm), the prevalence of peri-implantitis varied significantly from 11.3 to 47.1 percent. Thus, with the current lack of universally accepted criteria for the definition of peri-implantitis, the use of different thresholds is likely to produce different prevalence rates. However, even with the more conservative estimates, the number of new implants that are likely to be affected by peri-implant diseases every year is the high million range, of

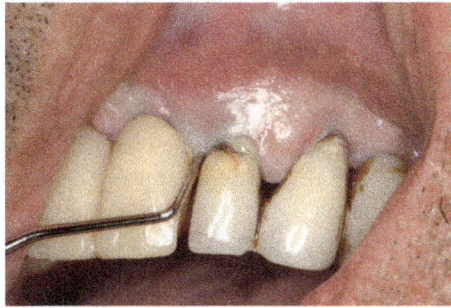

FIGURE 1: Peri-implantitis with suppuration.

which 7-8 million are likely to develop peri-implant mucositis while about 3-4 million will develop peri-implantitis.

Nevertheless, despite the magnitude of this problem and the potential grave consequences that may result from a non-responsive peri-implantitis condition, a commonly accept-able treatment protocols are yet to be agreed upon. Hence, the purpose of this paper is to review the available literature pertaining to both surgical and nonsurgical therapies of peri-implantitis in order to explore their benefits and limitations (Figure 1).

2. Body

The treatment of peri-implantitis may include each of the following modalities, either individually or combined: non-surgical therapy is aimed at removing local irritants from the implants' surface with or without surface decontamination and possibly some additional adjunctive therapies. Surgi-cal therapy is aimed at removing any residual subgingival deposits and additionally reducing the peri-implant pockets depth. This can be done alone or in conjunction with either osseous respective therapy or the contrary regenerative approach. Finally, if all fails, explantation of the affected nonresponsive implant might be the best alternative in order to arrest the destruction of the osseous structure around the implant, thus preserving whatever is left in this site for future reconstruction.

2.1. Nonsurgical Treatment of Peri-Implantitis

2.1.1. Implant's Debridement. The microbial origin of peri-implantitis has been previously established [16]. Shibli et al. [17] in an experimental peri-implantitis study in the canine model have found *Prevotella intermedia/nigrescens* in 13.89% of implants at baseline and 100% of implants at other periods. *Porphyromonas gingivalis* was not detected at base-line, but after 20 and 40 days it was detected in 33.34% of implants and at 60 days it was detected in 29.03% of dental implants. *Fusobacterium* spp. were detected in all time points. Streptococci were detected in 16.67% of implants at baseline and in 83.34%, 72.22%, and 77.42% of implants at 20, 40, and 60 days, respectively. *Campylobacter* spp. and *Candida* spp. were detected in low proportions. Total viable count analysis showed significant difference after ligature

placement ($P < 0.0014$). However, there was no significant qualitative difference, in spite of the difference among the periods. The same authors (2008) have compared the micro-bial biofilm of healthy and peri-implantitis implants; they found significantly higher mean counts of *Porphyromonas gingivalis*, *Treponema denticola*, and *Tannerella forsythia* in the peri-implantitis sites, both supra- and subgingivally. Also, the proportions of the pathogens from the red complex were elevated, while host-compatible beneficial microbial complexes were reduced in diseased compared with healthy implants. The microbiological profiles of supra- and subgin-gival environments did not differ substantially within each group [18]. Thus, the need for implant debridement in order to eliminate bacterial flora that is likely associated with the peri-implant disease is obvious.

However, the clinical efficacy of this treatment modality has been shown to be relatively limited. Persson et al. [19] in a single-blinded randomized longitudinal clinical study of mechanical nonsurgical treatment of peri-implantitis reported that the most prevalent bacteria were *Fusobac-terium nucleatum* sp., *Staphylococcus* sp., *Aggregatibacter actinomycetemcomitans*, *Helicobacter pylori*, and *Tannerella forsythia*. 30 min after treatment (with curettes only), *Aggre-gatibacter actinomycetemcomitans* (serotype a), *Lactobacillus acidophilus*, *Streptococcus anginosus*, and *Veillonella parvula* were found at lower counts ($P < 0.001$). However, at 6 months, microbiological differences between baseline and 6-month samples were not significant for any species or between treatment methods in these peri-implantitis sites. Renvert et al. in a corresponding clinical report of this study [20] have shown minimal pocket reduction between baseline (5.1 mm) and 6-month (4.9 mm) measurements; $P = 0.30$. These minimal changes were attained in both groups (ultrasonic instruments and the hand held curettes). Plaque scores at treated implants decreased from 73% to 53% ($P < 0.01$). Bleeding scores also decreased ($P < 0.01$), again with no group differences.

2.1.2. Surface Decontamination. To try improving the out-come of nonsurgical therapy of peri-implantitis site, the use of surface decontamination has been studied extensively. This is usually being performed mechanically via the use of air abrasive devices or chemical agents.

In vitro studies have confirmed the potency of this device to remove plaque and biofilm. Tastepe et al. [21] have studied the cleaning and modification of intraorally contaminated medium roughness titanium discs using calcium phosphate powder abrasive treatment. They have concluded that air powder abrasive methods using various agents were all efficient in removing the biofilm from contaminated titanium discs. Nonetheless, clinical studies of the efficacy of this treatment approach had produced mixed results. In a recent prospective, randomized, controlled clinical study, Sahm and coworkers [22] compared the efficacy of nonsurgical treatment of peri-implantitis using an air abrasive device versus mechanical debridement and local application of chlorhexidine solution. After six months, the air abrasive group revealed significantly higher changes in mean BOP scores when compared with mechanically treated sites (43.5 ± 27.7% versus 11.0 ± 15.7%). However, pocket reduction was minimal (0.6 mm) in both treatment groups. Likewise, clinical attachment level gains were minimal and very similar in both groups (0.4 ± 0.7 mm and 0.5 ± 0.8 mm, resp.). Likewise, Renvert et al. [23] in a nonsurgical treatment study of peri-implantitis patients have reported a mean pocket reduction after 6 months to be 0.9 mm following this intervention. While this seems to be slightly greater than that reported for debridement only, still the magnitude of these changes is not sufficient. Thus, none surprisingly, Tastepe et al. [24] in a recent review of the literature have concluded that the *in vivo* data on air powder abrasive treatment as an implant surface cleaning method is not sufficient to draw definitive conclusions.

2.1.3. The Use of Lasers.

The efficacy of different laser wavelength to eliminate bacteria from implants' surface had been demonstrated *in vitro*. Deppe and coworkers [25] used a XeCl 308 nm excimer laser irradiation with a constant energy of 0.8 J/cm and a constant frequency of 20 Hz on peri-implantitis-associated bacteria *in vitro*. They have been able to show that 200 pulses were sufficient to reduce the replication of these anaerobic microorganisms for more than 99.9%. Likewise, Kreisler and coworkers [26], using an Er:YAG laser on different implant surfaces contaminated with *Streptococcus sanguinis*, were able to report that, compared to nonirradiated specimens, mean bacterial reductions ranged from 99.51% to 99.6% at a pulse energy of 60 mJ and from 99.92% to 99.94% (TPS) at 120 mJ. The adjunctive effect of photodynamic therapy in conjunction with soft laser therapy was also studied *in vitro* by Haas et al. [27]. After contaminating these rough surface implants with *Actinobacillus actinomycetemcomitans* or *Porphyromonas gingivalis* or *Prevotella intermedia*, these surfaces were then treated with a toluidine blue solution and irradiated with a diode soft laser with a wave length of 905 nm for 1 min. None of the smears obtained from the thus treated surfaces showed any bacterial growth, whereas the smears obtained from the controls showed unchanged growth of every target organism tested. Likewise, Salmeron et al. [28] in a preclinical rat model have studied laser therapy alone or with photodynamic therapy and compared them to both negative and positive controls for implant surface decontamination. The results of this histomorphometric study were then followed longitudinally: while photodynamic therapy showed some improved early (7 days) results; over longer time periods (>14 days), all methods produced similar results.

Here again, clinical studies have failed to support the *in vitro* microbiological results. Renvert [23] in his clinical study which explored different treatment modalities for peri-implantitis reported minimal (0.8 mm) pocket reduction around implants treated with Er:YAG laser. Likewise, Schwarz et al. [29] in a clinical and histological study using Er:YAG laser in peri-implantitis patients reported that while patients exhibited some improvements in the clinical parameter this amounted to approximately 0.5 mm for all time intervals (up to 24 months); furthermore, histopathological

examination of tissue biopsies revealed a mixed chronic inflammatory cell infiltrate (macrophages, lymphocytes, and plasma cells) which seemed to be encapsulated by deposition of irregular bundles of fibrous connective tissue showing increased proliferation of vascular structures. Thus, they have concluded that a single course of nonsurgical treatment of peri-implantitis using ERL may not be sufficient for the maintenance of failing implants. These authors in yet another study [30] reported that mean value of BOP decreased in the Er:YAG treated group from 83% at baseline to 31% after 6 months while in the C group from 80% at baseline to 58% after 6 months. The sites treated with Er:YAG demonstrated a mean CAL change from 5.8 ± 1 mm at baseline to 5.1 ± 1.1 mm after 6 months; similarly, the C sites demonstrated a mean CAL gain from 6.2 ± 1.5 mm at baseline to 5.6 ± 1.6 mm at 6 months (the difference between the two groups being statistically insignificant). Most recently, Esposito and coworkers [31] in a one-year multicenter pragmatic randomized controlled clinical trial of the adjunctive use of light-activated disinfection (LAD) in the treatment of peri-implantitis have concluded that LAD therapy (FotoSan) with mechanical cleaning of implants affected by peri-implantitis did not improve any clinical outcomes when compared to mechanical cleaning alone up to 1 year after treatment.

2.1.4. The Adjunctive Effect of Local Delivery of Antibacterial Agents.

To further improve the response to nonsurgical treatment of peri-implantitis, the use of local delivery of antibacterial agents has been advocated. As early as 2001, Mombelli and coworkers [32] explored the adjunctive effect of tetracycline fibers in the nonsurgical treatment of peri-implantitis. After twelve months, a significant decrease in frequency of detection was noted for *Prevotella intermedia/nigrescens*, *Fusobacterium* sp., *Bacteroides forsythus*, and *Campylobacter rectus*. Clinically, mean pocket reduction was 1.2–1.9 mm which was maintained up to 12 months postop. However, three subjects have shown continuous deterioration in the clinical parameters and were thus removed from the study and are not included in the results.

Renvert and coworkers [33] in a 12-month clinical study of 32 patients with peri-implantitis were treated with minocycline microspheres or chlorhexidine gel as adjunct to mechanical debridement: At one year, pocket reduction amounted to only 0.6 mm with no difference between the two treatment groups. Salvi and coworkers [34] in a similar study reported some greater pocket reduction (1.6 mm) in implants treated with minocycline microspheres. However, 6 implants in six subjects (of the original 31 implants) required rescue treatment or were exited from the study all together, due to continuing attachment level loss despite this treatment. More recently, Schär et al. [35] reported that, 3 months following treatment with either minocycline microspheres of photodynamic therapy, implants of both groups yielded a statistically significant reduction in the number of BOP-positive sites compared with baseline. Changes in implants probing depth, while statistically significantly different from baseline, amounted to only 0.4 mm. One should keep in mind that the initial pocket depth in these sites was moderate. Likewise, CAL gain was approximately 0.25 mm.

The use of chlorhexidine irrigation was studied in a preclinical canine study by Porras et al. [36]. Subjects received dental prophylaxis and were randomly assigned to the control group (mechanical debridement and oral hygiene instructions) or to the test group (antiseptic therapy which included mechanical cleansing and oral hygiene instructions supplemented by local irrigation with chlorhexidine 0.12%, using a plastic syringe, and topical application of a 0.12% chlorhexidine gel). Both treatment modalities were effective in reducing peri-implant infection and implants probing depths and in improving attachment levels with no inter-group differences. Similarly, Sahm and coworkers [22] in a clinical trial of nonsurgical treatment of peri-implantitis sites reported that implants' mean pocket reduction was 0.8 mm and attachment level gain was also 0.8 mm when using mechanical debridement and adjunctive subgingival irrigation with CHX solution and gel application into the pockets. Likewise, Renvert et al. [37] have used chlorhexidine gel in conjunction with mechanical debridement for the treatment of moderate pocket sites around dental implants. Only moderate pocket reduction (0.43 mm) could be attained; however, bleeding on probing was significantly reduced from 86% of the sites at screening to 30% at the end of the study, one year later.

Büchter and coworkers [38] in a randomized clinical trial were using doxycycline gel in the peri-implant pockets as an adjunct implants mechanical therapy. Pocket reduction (1.15 mm) and CAL gain (1.17 mm) were significantly greater than those of the mechanical treatment only (0.56 mm for both outcomes).

More recently, our group has reported in a randomized double blind placebo controlled multicenter clinical trial on the use of chlorhexidine containing chips (Periochip) in the treatment of peri-implantitis [39]. In this study of moderate to severe peri-implantitis sites, chlorhexidine containing chips were repeatedly inserted into the peri-implant pockets every other week (unless pockets were already reduced to 5 mm or less) for a period of up to 3 months. This novel approach of repeated placement of chlorhexidine chips has resulted in a significant improvement of the peri-implant soft tissue parameters six months postop: pocket reduction (mean 2.29 mm) and attachment level gain (2.21 mm) were significantly better than those previously reported for non-surgical treatment of peri-implantitis. Furthermore, 73% of these sites had had pocket reduction of 2 mm or greater, while 40 percent had pocket reduction of at least 3 mm.

Conversely, Renvert et al. [40] in a similar nonsurgical treatment study of moderate peri-implantitis sites used repeated subgingival application of minocycline microspheres (Arestin) once a month for up to three months. Mean pocket reduction in the deepest sites amounted to 0.9 mm in the experimental group.

2.1.5. Systemic Antibiotics.
The use of systemic antibiotics as an adjunctive tool in nonsurgical periodontal therapy had been shown to have small but statistically significant added benefit over scaling and root planning alone [41]. Thus, the use of such protocols in the nonsurgical treatment of peri-implantitis would seem like a logical course to take. Hallström et al. [42] have compared, in a randomized clinical trial design, nonsurgical treatment of peri-implant mucositis with or without systemic antibiotics. Forty-eight subjects received nonsurgical debridement with or without systemic Azithromycin for four days and were followed during 6 months. Pocket reduction was 0.9 mm in the antibiotics group (1.4 mm in the deepest sites) and 0.5 mm in the debridement only group (0.8 mm in its deepest sites). However, these differences between the antibiotics and control group were not statistically significant.

Lindhe and Meyle [43] on behalf of the VI European workshop in periodontology have concluded that there was limited evidence that nonsurgical treatment of peri-implantitis with the adjunctive use of systemic antibiotics could resolve a number of peri-implantitis lesions. Most recently, Javed et al. [44] in a systematic review of the use of antibiotics in the treatment protocol of peri-implantitis concluded that the significance of adjunctive antibiotic therapy in the treatment of peri-implantitis remains controversial. A potential explanation for this minimal adjunctive effect for these systemic antibiotics comes from a recent study by Rams and coworkers [45]. In this study, a hundred and six peri-implantitis sites in 120 patients were sampled microbiologically and tested for potential antibiotic resistance. They found that one or more cultivable submucosal bacterial pathogens (most often *Prevotella intermedia/nigrescens* or *Streptococcus constellatus*) were resistant *in vitro* to clindamycin, amoxicillin, doxycycline, or metronidazole in 46.7%, 39.2%, 25%, and 21.7% of the peri-implantitis subjects, respectively. Overall, 71.7% of the 120 peri-implantitis subjects exhibited submucosal bacterial pathogens resistant *in vitro* to one or more of the tested antibiotics.

Another important issue that needs to be discussed *vis-a-vis* the use of systemic antibiotics for the treatment of peri-implantitis is the risk for antibiotic resistance as a worldwide health hazard. The wide spread use of antibiotics in medicine at large in the past fifty years is now back firing at our profession with the ever increasing prevalence of resistant bacterial strains [46, 47]. This phenomenon is causing a medical crisis that might have severe and far reaching repercussions on the population. Thus, the use of antibiotics should be restricted to patients and conditions where it has been clearly shown to have significant benefits which outweigh the risks that are involved [48, 49]. Thus, current research has not yet substantiated such benefits and consequently systemic antibiotics should be limited to acute phase of peri-implant infection rather than to be the treatment of choice for peri-implantitis [50].

2.2. Surgical Treatment of Peri-Implantitis

2.2.1. Open Flap Debridement.
The clinical scenario in humans differs significantly from that in animals. The greatest difference is the inability, in most cases, to remove the prosthetic super structure in order to allow for a submerged

healing of the regenerated sites. Thus, the results of many of the human clinical trials are less favorable and more diverse than these reported in animals models. Still, open flap debridement is the treatment of choice by many clinicians. Lagervall and Jansson [51] in a retrospective study of treatment outcome in patients with peri-implantitis performed in a private practice based clinical setting have reported that open flap debridement was selected for 47 percent of the sites affected by peri-implantitis. Albouy et al. [52] in a preclinical experimental peri-implantitis study in canines have compared responses to open flap debridement surgery (as a stand-alone procedure) in four different implants design and surface topographies. Two of the four TiUnite implants were lost after surgical therapy. Radiographic bone gain occurred at implants with turned, TiOblast, and SLA surfaces, while at TiUnite implants additional bone loss was found after treatment. Resolution of peri-implantitis was achieved in tissues surrounding implants with turned and TiOblast surfaces. Thus, they concluded that resolution of peri-implantitis following treatment without systemic or local antimicrobial therapy is possible, but the outcome of treatment is influenced by implant surface characteristics. Similarly, Persson et al. [53] have studied the effect of implants surface topography on reosseointegration in an experimental peri-implantitis model in the canines. Implants with turned surface were compared with SLA implants when treated with systemic antibiotics followed by open flap debridement. Treatment resulted in a 72% bone fill of the bone defects at turned sites and 76% at SLA sites. The amount of reosseointegration was 22% at turned sites and 84% at SLA sites. Nonetheless, while these variations do exist, open flap debridement offers a useful tool to negotiate peri-implant disease. Máximo et al. [54] in a short term clinical study were able to show that three months following access flap surgery all clinical parameters have improved. For the peri-implantitis groups, mean reduction in CAL was 2.3 ± 1.6 mm and mean implants pocket reduction was 3.1 ± 1.7 mm. Levels of *Treponema denticola*, *Tannerella forsythia*, and *Parvimonas micra* and of *Fusobacterium nucleatum* were significantly reduced after peri-implantitis therapy. In addition, counts of *Porphyromonas gingivalis* and *Treponema socranskii* and the proportions of red complex were also reduced. These same authors in a subsequent report have shown that TNF-alpha levels, initially much greater than healthy controls, were significantly reduced achieving the same level as the healthy group at 3 months after therapy [55]. Mechanical therapies alone were effective in treating mucositis and peri-implantitis over a period of 3 months. The open debridement procedure showed clinical and microbiological benefits on the treatment of peri-implantitis and could be safely used as a standard control group for future studies.

2.2.2. The Supplementary Use of Osseous Resection.
The use of osteoplasty and/or ostectomy to allow for better adaptation of the surgical flap and thus further improve the surgical outcome has been studied extensively. de Waal and coworkers [56] reported on thirty patients (79 implants) with peri-implantitis that were treated with apically repositioned flap, bone recontouring, and surface debridement and decontamination with 0.12% chlorhexidine gluconate + 0.05% cetylpyridinium chloride or placebo. Nine implants in two patients in the placebo-group were lost due to severe persisting peri-implantitis. The test group showed a significantly greater reduction in bacterial load, but clinical improvement (i.e., bleeding, suppuration, implants pocket depth, and radiographic bone loss) was sizeable however similar in both groups.

Serino and Turri [57] reported on their two-year prospective clinical trial of thirty-one subjects (86 implants) treated for peri-implantitis using a surgical procedure based on pocket elimination and bone recontouring. Two years following treatment, 15 (48%) subjects had no signs of recurrent peri-implant disease; 24 patients (77%) had no implants with a probing pocket depth of 0.6 mm associated with bleeding and/or suppuration following probing. Nevertheless, 36 implants (42%) out of the original 86 had had persistent peri-implant disease despite this treatment. The proportion of implants that remained healthy following treatment was higher for those with minor initial bone loss (2–4 mm bone loss as assessed during surgery) compared with the implants with an initial bone loss of 0.5 mm (74% versus 40%). Among the eighteen implants with bone loss of 0.7 mm at baseline, seven were explanted.

2.2.3. The Complementary Use of Regenerative Techniques (Figure 2).
As early as 1993, Grunder et al. [58], in ligature-induced peri-implantitis study in canines using guided tissue regeneration with a nonresorbable ePTFE membrane and comparing it to flap surgery alone, reported that there were no differences between any of the clinical parameters in both the control and experimental sites from the submerged and non-submerged groups. Histologic and histomorphometric analyses also revealed no significant differences between groups with regard to new bone formation. Likewise, Nociti et al. [59] in a similar animal model compared different membranes, with and without additional bone graft, to flap surgery only for the treatment of peri-implantitis. Their results showed that debridement alone as well as grafting alone had the same effect as did either membrane. To the contrary, Hurzeler and coworkers [60] reported in a similar canine study that guided bone regeneration procedures resulted in the greatest amount of new bone formation, followed by bone grafts alone, and flap debridement. In humans, Roos-Jansåker et al. [61] were able to show similar response to therapy (implants pocket reduction of 2.9–3.4 mm and new bone fill of 1.4-1.5 mm) for peri-implantitis sites treated with either bone grafts alone or bone grafts in conjunction with resorbable collagen membrane. This same group [62], in a subsequent 3-year follow-up report, has found that this improvement was maintained almost unchanged three years later. Aghazadeh et al. have attempted to compare autogenous bone to bovine derived xenograft for the treatment of peri-implantitis [63]. At 12 months, bovine derived xenograft provided more radiographic bone fill than autogenous bone; however, the success for both surgical regenerative procedures was limited.

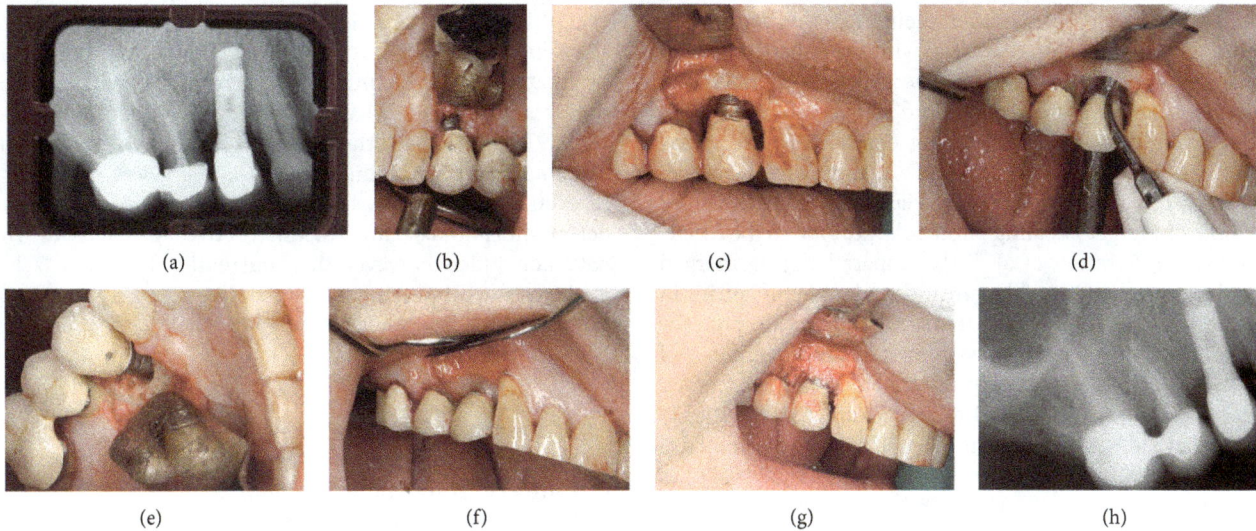

FIGURE 2: Treatment of peri-implantitis using a regenerative approach. (a) Preop, note the severe bone loss on implant at position #14. (b) Upon reflection of the flaps, note the granulation tissue but also excess cementum on the crown's margin. (c) Following degranulation, demonstrating the extent of bone loss. (d) Excess cement was removed and the implant surface was debrided using hand instruments and ultrasonic scaler. (e) Decortication was performed using diamond burs. (f) Surface decontamination was supplemented with the application of 24% EDTA for 3 minutes. (g) The defect was grafted with bovine derived Xenograft (BioOss). (h) 3 years later, complete resolution of the radiographic defect is evident.

More recently, Wiltfang et al. [64] have reported significant bone fill in a twelve-month clinical trial in which peri-implantitis sites were treated with surface decontamination and regenerative flap surgery that included a 1:1 ratio of autogenous and xenogeneic bone graft. Mean radiographic bone fill amounted to 3.5 mm. Schwarz et al. [65] presented a case series where twenty-two patients with moderate peri-implantitis were randomly treated with access flap surgery and the application of nanocrystalline hydroxyapatite (NHA) or a natural bone mineral in combination with a collagen membrane (NBM + CM). Clinical parameters were recorded at baseline and after 12, 18, and 24 months of nonsubmerged healing. After two years, both groups revealed clinically important probing depth reductions (NHA: 1.5 ± 0.6 mm; NBM + CM: 2.4 ± 0.8 mm) and clinical attachment level gains (NHA: 1.0 ± 0.4 mm; NBM + CM: 2.0 ± 0.8 mm). However, these clinical improvements seemed to be better in the NBM + CM.

Sahrmann et al. [66] in a recent systematic review have concluded that complete fill of the bony defect using GBR seems not to be a predictable outcome. The mucosal health status is left unconsidered in most studies. Well-controlled trials are needed to determine predictable treatment protocols for the successful regenerative treatment of peri-implantitis using GBR technique.

A possible explanation to this diversity in clinical response to regenerative surgical treatment around dental implants was suggested by Schwarz et al. [67]. In this study, three types of osseous defects around dental implants with peri-implantitis were treated with bone graft and resorbable collagen membranes. The circumferential defects sites yielded significantly better response than these sites with dehiscence type defect. Thus, defects' anatomy might affect

the outcome of these regenerative techniques. Nonetheless, regenerative approach to peri-implantitis may at time produce significant improvement in these sites. Froum et al. [68] reported on long-term follow-up of 51 consecutively treated peri-implantitis sites (using combination of platelet-derived growth factor with an organic bovine bone or mineralized freeze-dried bone coverage with a collagen membrane or a subepithelial connective tissue graft). Probing depth reductions at 3 to 7.5 years of follow-up were 5.1–5.4 mm. Concomitant bone level gain was from 3.0 to 3.75 mm. None of these implants lost bone throughout the duration of the study. Another source for this diversity in implants response to regenerative treatment could be associated with implants surface topography. Roccuzzo and coworkers [69] reported on twenty-six patients with one crater-like defect, around either TPS or SLA dental implants, with a probing depth (PD) of 0.6. Following flap approach, the implant surface was mechanically debrided and treated using a 24% EDTA gel and a 1% chlorhexidine gel and the osseous defect filled with a bovine-derived xenograft (BDX); all sites were left to heal in a nonsubmerged environment. At one-year follow-up mean implants pocket depth reduction was 2.1 ± 1.2 mm in the TPS implants compared to 3.4 ± 1.7 mm in the SLA group (these differences being statistically significant). Complete defect fill was never found around TPS group, while it occurred in three out of 12 SLA implants. Finally, submergence of the dental implants during the healing of the regenerative procedure might have a beneficial effect on the outcome. Roos-Jansåker and coworkers [70] reported on a one-year case series of twelve patients with a progressive loss of > or = 3 threads (1.8 mm) following the first year of healing. Following flap reflection, implants were decontaminated with 3% hydrogen peroxide and a bone substitute (Algipore) was grafted with a resorbable collagen membrane that was placed over the grafted defect and secured with the cover screw and covered by flaps for 6-month submerged healing; after that time, the abutment was reconnected to the suprastructure. At twelve months, implant probing depth was reduced by 4.2 mm and a mean defect fill of 2.3 mm was achieved. However, comparisons of human trials between submerged and nonsubmerged healing protocols are yet to be done. Nevertheless, Schwarz et al. [71] compared nonsubmerged and submerged healing of ligature induced peri-implantitis in 5 beagle dogs (30 implants). In this study, both treatment procedures resulted in statistically significant improvements of all clinical parameters at both nonsubmerged and submerged implants. However, radiological improvements were only observed at submerged implant sites. Histomorphometrical analysis revealed that all nonsubmerged implants exhibited low amounts of new BIC (1.0–1.2%), while mean BIC was statistically significantly higher in the respective submerged implant groups (8.7%–44.8%).

The best grafting material to be used in the surgical management of peri-implantitis is yet to be determined. Different studies have employed different materials; however, the diversity in clinical design, defect morphology, outcome variables, and follow-up period makes their comparison nearly impossible [66, 72–76]. One of the most likely regenerative materials that was least tested is autogenous bone graft. Romanos and Nentwig [77] reported on a comparative study of peri-implantitis sites treated with autogenous bone or a xenogeneic bone grafting material (BioOss) both covered with a collagen membrane. In this study, radiological resolution of the lesions was observed for most sites with no intergroup differences. Schou and coworkers used different decontamination agents and different regenerative materials for the treatment of experimental peri-implantitis in monkeys [78–80]. Autogenous bone alone was compared to autogenous bone plus membrane, membrane alone, or a conventional flap procedure alone as a negative control. The animals were sacrificed 6 months after treatment. Healthy peri-implant tissue was established irrespective of the applied surgical procedure. A mean bone gain of 4.7 mm was identified around implants treated with autogenous bone plus membrane, while 4.0 mm, 3.0 mm, and 1.9 mm of bone gain were recorded for the bone only, membrane only, and conventional flap only groups, respectively. Quantitative digital subtraction radiography confirmed considerable bone gain within defects treated with autogenous bone with or without membrane coverage. The bone gain, especially for defects treated with combined bone-membrane approach, seemed to be almost at the level before development of peri-implantitis. By contrast, 38 and 25% of the defect were on average characterized by bone gain when treated with membrane only or flaps only, respectively. Thus, the present studies demonstrate considerable bone regeneration after treatment of experimental peri-implantitis with autogenous bone graft particles in this monkey model.

Despite this ample piece of evidence showing good regenerative response with the use of regenerative materials, the superiority of this approach over a conventional open flap debridement is yet to be established. Khoshkam et al. [81] in a systematic review and meta-analysis aimed at evaluating the effectiveness of reconstructive procedures for treating peri-implantitis revealed that the weighted mean radiographic defect fill was 2.17 mm, probing depth reduction was 2.97 mm, clinical attachment level gain was 1.65 mm, and bleeding on probing reduction was 45.8%. Great variability in reparative outcomes was found attributed to patient factors, defect morphology, and reconstructive agents used. They have concluded however that, currently, there is a lack of evidence for supporting additional benefit of reconstructive procedures to the other treatment modalities for managing peri-implantitis.

2.2.4. Systemic Antibiotics to Supplement Surgical Flap Approach. Systemic antibiotics as adjunct to peri-implant flap surgery treatment are commonly used. Heitz-Mayfield and coworkers [82] have recently reported on a prospective clinical trial of thirty-six implants in 24 partially dentate patients with moderate to advanced peri-implantitis that were treated using an anti-infective surgical protocol incorporating open flap debridement and implant surface decontamination, with adjunctive systemic amoxicillin and metronidazole. At twelve months, mean pocket reduction was 2.6 mm with all treated implants having a mean PD < 5 mm. 47% of the implants had complete resolution of inflammation with no bleeding on probing. 92% of implants had stable crestal bone levels or bone gain. There were no significant effects of smoking on any of the treatment outcomes. Leonhardt et al. [83] reported on a five-year clinical, microbiological, and radiological study into the treatment of peri-implantitis. Surgical exposure of the lesions and cleaning of the implants were performed using hydrogen peroxide. The patients were than given systemic antibiotics according to a susceptibility test of target bacteria that were previously cultured. The treatment was evaluated clinically, microbiologically, and radiographically at 6 months, 1 year, and 5 years. Seven out of 26 implants with peri-implantitis at baseline were lost during the 5-year follow-up period despite a significant reduction in the presence of plaque and gingival bleeding. Four implants continued to lose bone, 9 had an unchanged bone level, and 6 gained bone. Five of the patients were treated with antibiotics directed against putative periodontopathogens, that is, *A. actinomycetemcomitans, P. intermedia,* or *P. gingivalis*; three patients were treated for presence of enterics (*E. coli* and *E. cloacae*); and, in one patient, treatment was directed against *S. aureus.*

2.3. Explantation (Figure 3). The management of peri-implantitis may at time be unpredictable especially for the more advanced lesion associated with severe bone loss [84, 85]. This may in turn lead to further bone loss, increase in pocket depth and suppuration, and consequently severe damage to the alveolar bone. Thus, explantation as a treatment option that will help arrest the progression of the destructive process is sometime advocated [86]. Moreover, severely compromised dental implants might be at greater risk for mechanical fracture [87] which may lead to further peri-implant bone loss. However, explantation of

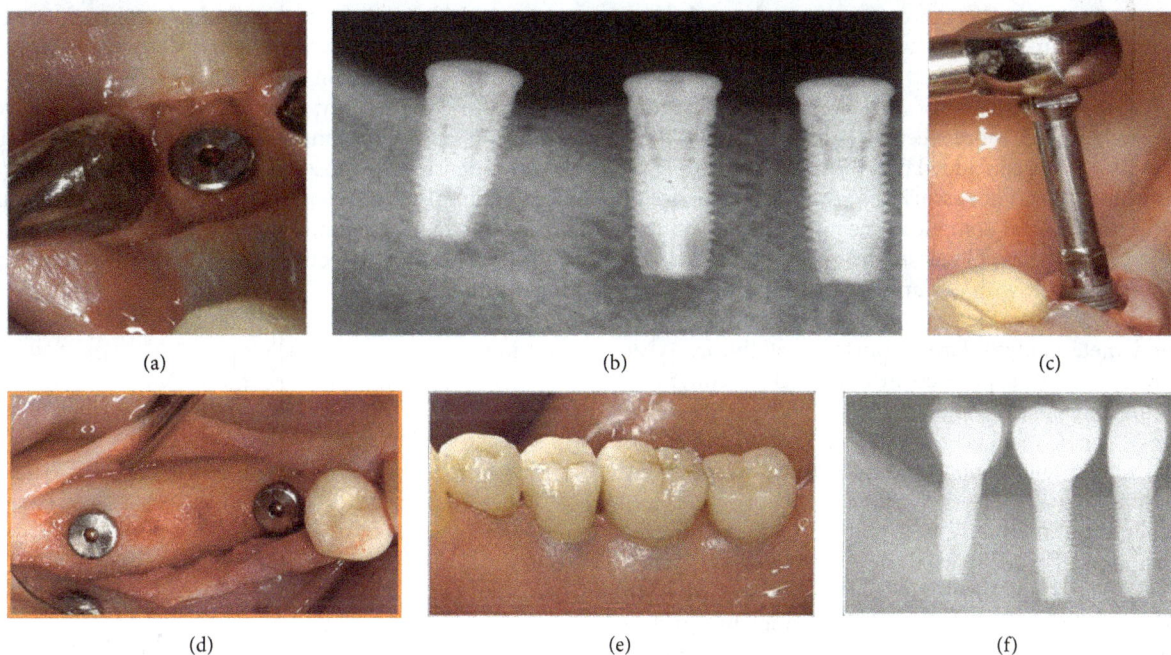

(a)   (b)   (c)

(d)   (e)   (f)

FIGURE 3: Explantation of dental implant.

such compromised implant will require additional treatment to replace the now missing implants. Reimplantation of a new implant in the sites of the previously diseased implant is the most logical treatment option [88]; however, this treatment approach is not without limitation: bone loss that has occurred around the diseased implant might not allow for straightforward reimplantation. Instead, sometimes an elaborate augmentation procedure will be required before this site is ready for a redo implant placement [89]. Mardinger et al. [90] in a retrospective analysis of the factors affecting the decision to replace failed implants after they have been removed reported that the chances of a patient with minor bone loss undergoing reimplantation were 20 times greater (odds ratio, 20.4) than those of a patient with severe bone loss. The main patient-related reasons for avoiding reimplantation were the additional costs (27%), fear of additional pain (17.7%), and fear of a second failure (16.2%).

The survival and success rates of dental implants in previously failed implant sites were first reported by Alsaadi and coworkers [91]. A total of 41 patients (58 implants) experienced the nonintegration. Of those, seven implants (in seven subjects) have failed again (which represents a survival rate of 87.9%). Similarly, Grossmann and Levin (2007) reported on the success and survival of single dental implants placed in sites of previously failed implants [92]. Seventy five patients (with a total of 96 implants) experienced failure of one or more implants. Of those, 31 implants in 28 patients were replaced with a similar implant placed in the same location. Nine of the replacement implants failed, resulting in an overall survival rate of 71%. Follow-up ranged from 6 to 46 months. Replacement of maxillary and mandibular failed implants was similar. All failures

occurred during the first year after implant replacement. In a similar retrospective study, we have shown that of fifty-six patients with a total of 79 redo implants that were followed for three years, thirteen implants failed and that resulted in an overall survival rate of 83.5%. Successful implants had greater diameter (4.05 ± 0.52 mm) than failed implants (3.72 ± 0.56 mm) did; however, these differences were only marginal ($P = 0.06$). Conversely, smoking habits, implants length and location, mode of placement, and spontaneous exposure did not have a significant effect on the outcome of this procedure [93]. Kim and coworkers [94] were able to report somewhat better results for redo of dental implants into previously contaminated sites where an implant was removed. The survival rate of the second implant after removal of failed implant was 88.3%. The marginal bone loss at the final (two years) follow-up was minimal (0.33 ± 0.49 mm). No significant difference in the failure rate of the second implant was observed between the immediate and delayed replacement groups ($P > 0.05$). This slightly greater survival rate the second time around (compare to other studies) might be attributed to the use of smoking (a strong confounding condition) as an exclusion criterion. Even slightly higher figure (92.3% CSR) was reported by Mardinger and coworkers [95] in a private practice based clinical study.

Alternatively, sites where previous implants were retrieved might be rehabilitated using fixed partial denture anchored to proximal implants, natural teeth, or combination of the above. The dogma of one implant per one missing tooth can no longer be supported automatically. Eliasson et al. [96] in an eighteen-year retrospective study of 123 implant patients have shown that survival rates for dental prostheses supported by 2 and 3 implants were 96.8% and

97.6%, respectively. Furthermore, the mean bone loss at 5 years was 0.3 mm for the two groups. No significant differences in bone loss ($P > 0.05$), implant failure rate ($P > 0.05$), or incidence of mechanical complications ($P > 0.05$) were found. More recently, Salvi and Brägger [97] in a systematic review concluded that the number of implants supporting an FDP was not associated with the prevalence of mechanical or technical complications nor with the implant survival or success rates. Likewise, the option of replacing a lost/removed implant with a 3-unit tooth-supported FPD is also a solid alternative. Pjetursson et al. [98] in a literature review and meta-analysis have reported that the five-year survival rate of tooth-supported FPD was 93.8% compared to 95.2% for an implant-supported FPD (with no statistical differences). The 10-year survival rates were 89.2% and 86.7% for teeth- and implant-supported prostheses, respectively ($P > 0.05$).

Another valid alternative will be to do a hybrid tooth-implant-supported fixed partial denture. In a systematic review, Weber and Sukotjo [99] have shown that, after an observation period of at least six years, implant survival and prosthetic success were similar for implant supported and tooth to implant supported prostheses. Likewise, Lang et al. [100] in their systematic review on the survival and complications of combined tooth-implant-supported FPD reported 90.1% implants' survival after 5 years and 82.1% after 10 years. The corresponding figures for the FPD survival were 94.1% and 77.8% after five and ten years, respectively. These results are very similar (both for survival and success) to what was reported for teeth-born and implants-born fixed prosthesis. Thus, such rehabilitation may be considered in cases where a potential abutment tooth is present across an edentulous site where one of the implants has failed.

Contrary to common beliefs, the use of nonrigid connection in such hybrid prostheses is not recommended. Nickening et al. [101] in a five-year follow-up of eighty-four hybrid fixtures have shown low rate of complications in these prostheses with rigid connection (5.3%) while these restorations with nonrigid connection exhibited significantly greater rate of complications (28.5%). Another risk associated with nonrigid connection increases the risk for intrusion of the abutment teeth [102].

3. Conclusions

In the present review, we went through the literature pertaining to treatment alternatives to peri-implant diseases and the great diversity that is being reflected from this data. Both nonsurgical and surgical treatment strategies have shown to yield some beneficial effect on the peri-implant disease. However, while some implants/patients seemed to have benefited greatly from these treatment regiments, others have responded less favorably.

The most frustrating piece of information is the heterogeneity in the clinical response of peri-implantitis sites that were treated similarly as it was reported in the different studies.

Good independent randomized control trials are scarce, and the need for such well-designed studies was highlighted by Tonetti et al. [103] on behalf of the VIII European workshop in periodontology. Likewise, Esposito and coworkers [104] in a recent systematic review and meta-analysis that tried to identify the most effective interventions for treating peri-implantitis around osseointegrated dental implants have concluded that there is no reliable evidence suggesting which could be the most effective interventions for treating peri-implantitis.

We are still in the dark when it comes to the following questions.

(i) Which is the best decontaminating agent (or do we really need it all together)?

(ii) Can nonsurgical therapies solve the mild to moderate peri-implantitis condition without a need to resort to access flaps?

(iii) Are regenerative procedures superior to access flap only approach?

(iv) Which of the regenerative techniques is most suitable in cases with peri-implantitis?

With the ever growing prevalence of peri-implant diseases, the need to address these questions is both real and urgent. Until that time when these data are available, treatment of peri-implantitis should be considered as possible but not necessarily predictable.

Conflict of Interests

The author declares the following potential conflict of interests: research grants and lecturing fees from Dexcel Pharma (manufacturer of PerioChip), free material samples from HA Systems (distributor of Arestin), research grant from GABA International (manufacturer of a variety of anti-infective medications), and research grant from Silonit, manufacturer of high-pressure implant irrigating device.

References

[1] http://www.idataresearch.com/research-categories/dental/dental-implants-market-research-reports/.

[2] N. U. Zitzmann and T. Berglundh, "Definition and prevalence of peri-implant diseases," *Journal of Clinical Periodontology*, vol. 35, no. 8, supplement, pp. 286–291, 2008.

[3] A. Mombelli, N. Müller, and N. Cionca, "The epidemiology of peri-implantitis," *Clinical Oral Implants Research*, vol. 23, supplement 6, pp. 67–76, 2012.

[4] M. A. Atieh, N. H. Alsabeeha, C. M. Faggion Jr., and W. J. Duncan, "The frequency of peri-implant diseases: a systematic review and meta-analysis," *Journal of Periodontology*, vol. 84, no. 11, pp. 1586–1598, 2013.

[5] S. Rinke, S. Ohl, D. Ziebolz, K. Lange, and P. Eickholz, "Prevalence of periimplant disease in partially edentulous patients: a practice-based cross-sectional study," *Clinical Oral Implants Research*, vol. 22, no. 8, pp. 826–833, 2011.

[6] O. F. Rodriguez-Argueta, R. Figueiredo, E. Valmaseda-Castellon, and C. Gay-Escoda, "Postoperative complications in

smoking patients treated with implants: a retrospective study," *Journal of Oral and Maxillofacial Surgery*, vol. 69, no. 8, pp. 2152–2157, 2011.

[7] J. Cho-Yan Lee, N. Mattheos, K. C. Nixon, and S. Ivanovski, "Residual periodontal pockets are a risk indicator for peri-implantitis in patients treated for periodontitis," *Clinical Oral Implants Research*, vol. 23, no. 3, pp. 325–333, 2012.

[8] M. Roccuzzo, F. Bonino, M. Aglietta, and P. Dalmasso, "Ten-year results of a three arms prospective cohort study on implants in periodontally compromised patients—part 2: clinical results," *Clinical Oral Implants Research*, vol. 23, no. 4, pp. 389–395, 2012.

[9] O. Carcuac and L. Jansson, "Peri-implantitis in a specialist clinic of periodontology. Clinical features and risk indicators," *Swedish Dental Journal*, vol. 34, no. 2, pp. 53–61, 2010.

[10] G. Serino and C. Ström, "Peri-implantitis in partially edentulous patients: association with inadequate plaque control," *Clinical Oral Implants Research*, vol. 20, no. 2, pp. 169–174, 2009.

[11] C. Wadhwani, D. Rapoport, S. la Rosa, T. Hess, and S. Kretschmar, "Radiographic detection and characteristic patterns of residual excess cement associated with cement-retained implant restorations: a clinical report," *Journal of Prosthetic Dentistry*, vol. 107, no. 3, pp. 151–157, 2012.

[12] B. Balevi, "Implant-supported cantilevered fixed partial dentures," *Evidence-Based Dentistry*, vol. 11, no. 2, pp. 48–49, 2010.

[13] S. Renvert, A. Aghazadeh, H. Hallström, and G. R. Persson, "Factors related to peri-implantitis—a retrospective study," *Clinical Oral Implants Research*, vol. 25, no. 4, pp. 522–529, 2014.

[14] J. Lindhe and J. Meyle, "Peri-implant diseases: consensus Report of the Sixth European Workshop on Periodontology," *Journal of Clinical Periodontology*, vol. 35, no. 8, supplement, pp. 282–285, 2008.

[15] O. C. Koldsland, A. A. Scheie, and A. M. Aass, "Prevalence of peri-implantitis related to severity of the disease with different degrees of bone loss," *Journal of Periodontology*, vol. 81, no. 2, pp. 231–238, 2010.

[16] Å. Leonhardt, S. Renvert, and G. Dahlén, "Microbial findings at failing implants," *Clinical Oral Implants Research*, vol. 10, no. 5, pp. 339–345, 1999.

[17] J. A. Shibli, M. C. Martins, R. F. M. Lotufo, and E. Marcantonio Jr., "Microbiologic and radiographic analysis of ligature-induced peri-implantitis with different dental implant surfaces," *The International Journal of Oral & Maxillofacial Implants*, vol. 18, no. 3, pp. 383–390, 2003.

[18] J. A. Shibli, L. Melo, D. S. Ferrari, L. C. Figueiredo, M. Faveri, and M. Feres, "Composition of supra- and subgingival biofilm of subjects with healthy and diseased implants," *Clinical Oral Implants Research*, vol. 19, no. 10, pp. 975–982, 2008.

[19] G. R. Persson, E. Samuelsson, C. Lindahl, and S. Renvert, "Mechanical non-surgical treatment of peri-implantitis: a single-blinded randomized longitudinal clinical study. II. Microbiological results," *Journal of Clinical Periodontology*, vol. 37, no. 6, pp. 563–573, 2010.

[20] S. Renvert, E. Samuelsson, C. Lindahl, and G. R. Persson, "Mechanical non-surgical treatment of peri-implantitis: a double-blind randomized longitudinal clinical study. I: clinical results," *Journal of Clinical Periodontology*, vol. 36, no. 7, pp. 604–609, 2009.

[21] C. S. Tastepe, Y. Liu, C. M. Visscher, and D. Wismeijer, "Cleaning and modification of intraorally contaminated titanium discs with calcium phosphate powder abrasive treatment," *Clinical Oral Implants Research*, 2012.

[22] N. Sahm, J. Becker, T. Santel, and F. Schwarz, "Non-surgical treatment of peri-implantitis using an air-abrasive device or mechanical debridement and local application of chlorhexidine: a prospective, randomized, controlled clinical study," *Journal of Clinical Periodontology*, vol. 38, no. 9, pp. 872–878, 2011.

[23] S. Renvert, C. Lindahl, A.-M. R. Jansåker, and R. G. Persson, "Treatment of peri-implantitis using an Er:YAG laser or an air-abrasive device: a randomized clinical trial," *Journal of Clinical Periodontology*, vol. 38, no. 1, pp. 65–73, 2011.

[24] C. S. Tastepe, R. van Waas, Y. Liu, and D. Wismeijer, "Air powder abrasive treatment as an implant surface cleaning method: a literature review," *The International Journal of Oral & Maxillofacial Implants*, vol. 27, no. 6, pp. 1461–1473, 2012.

[25] H. Deppe, H.-H. Horch, V. Schrödl, C. Haczek, and T. Miethke, "Effect of 308-nm excimer laser light on peri-implantitis-associated bacteria—an in vitro investigation," *Lasers in Medical Science*, vol. 22, no. 4, pp. 223–227, 2007.

[26] M. Kreisler, W. Kohnen, C. Marinello et al., "Bactericidal effect of the Er:YAG laser on dental implant surfaces: an in vitro study," *Journal of Periodontology*, vol. 73, no. 11, pp. 1292–1298, 2002.

[27] R. Haas, O. Dörtbudak, N. Mensdorff-Pouilly, and G. Mailath, "Elimination of bacteria on different implant surfaces through photosensitization and soft laser: an in vitro study," *Clinical Oral Implants Research*, vol. 8, no. 4, pp. 249–254, 1997.

[28] S. Salmeron, M. L. R. Rezende, A. Consolaro et al., "Laser therapy as an effective method for implant surface decontamination: a histomorphometric study in rats," *Journal of Periodontology*, vol. 84, no. 5, pp. 641–649, 2013.

[29] F. Schwarz, K. Bieling, E. Nuesry, A. Sculean, and J. Becker, "Clinical and histological healing pattern of peri-implantitis lesions following non-surgical treatment with an Er:YAG laser," *Lasers in Surgery and Medicine*, vol. 38, no. 7, pp. 663–671, 2006.

[30] F. Schwarz, A. Sculean, D. Rothamel, K. Schwenzer, T. Georg, and J. Becker, "Clinical evaluation of an Er:YAG laser for nonsurgical treatment of periimplantitis: a pilot study," *Clinical Oral Implants Research*, vol. 16, no. 1, pp. 44–52, 2005.

[31] M. Esposito, M. G. Grusovin, N. de Angelis, A. Camurati, M. Campailla, and P. Felice, "The adjunctive use of light-activated disinfection (LAD) with FotoSan is ineffective in the treatment of peri-implantitis: 1-year results from a multicentre pragmatic randomised controlled trial," *European Journal of Oral Implantology*, vol. 6, no. 2, pp. 109–119, 2013.

[32] A. Mombelli, A. Feloutzis, U. Brägger, and N. P. Lang, "Treatment of peri-implantitis by local delivery of tetracycline: clinical, microbiological and radiological results," *Clinical Oral Implants Research*, vol. 12, no. 4, pp. 287–294, 2001.

[33] S. Renvert, J. Lessem, G. Dahlén, C. Lindahl, and M. Svensson, "Topical minocycline microspheres versus topical chlorhexidine gel as an adjunct to mechanical debridement of incipient peri-implant infections: a randomized clinical trial," *Journal of Clinical Periodontology*, vol. 33, no. 5, pp. 362–369, 2006.

[34] G. E. Salvi, G. R. Persson, L. J. A. Heitz-Mayfield, M. Frei, and N. P. Lang, "Adjunctive local antibiotic therapy in the treatment of peri-implantitis II: clinical and radiographic outcomes," *Clinical Oral Implants Research*, vol. 18, no. 3, pp. 281–285, 2007.

[35] D. Schär, C. A. Ramseier, S. Eick, N. B. Arweiler, A. Sculean, and G. E. Salvi, "Anti-infective therapy of peri-implantitis with adjunctive local drug delivery or photodynamic therapy: six-month outcomes of a prospective randomized clinical trial," *Clinical Oral Implants Research*, vol. 24, no. 1, pp. 104–110, 2013.

[36] R. Porras, G. B. Anderson, R. Caffesse, S. Narendran, and P. M. Trejo, "Clinical response to 2 different therapeutic regimens to treat peri-implant mucositis," *Journal of Periodontology*, vol. 73, no. 10, pp. 1118–1125, 2002.

[37] S. Renvert, J. Lessem, G. Dahlén, H. Renvert, and C. Lindahl, "Mechanical and repeated antimicrobial therapy using a local drug delivery system in the treatment of peri-implantitis: a randomized clinical trial," *Journal of Periodontology*, vol. 79, no. 5, pp. 836–844, 2008.

[38] A. Büchter, U. Meyer, B. Kruse-Lösler, U. Joos, and J. Kleinheinz, "Sustained release of doxycycline for the treatment of peri-implantitis: randomised controlled trial," *British Journal of Oral and Maxillofacial Surgery*, vol. 42, no. 5, pp. 439–444, 2004.

[39] E. E. Machtei, S. Frankenthal, G. Levi et al., "Treatment of peri-implantitis using multiple applications of chlorhexidine chips: a double-blind, randomized multi-centre clinical trial," *Journal of Clinical Periodontology*, vol. 39, no. 12, pp. 1198–1205, 2012.

[40] S. Renvert, J. Lessem, C. Lindahl, and M. Svensson, "Treatment of incipient peri-implant infections using topical minocycline microspheres versus topical chlorhexidine gel as an adjunct to mechanical debridement," *Journal of the International Academy of Periodontology*, vol. 6, no. 4, supplement, pp. 154–159, 2004.

[41] F. Sgolastra, R. Gatto, A. Petrucci, and A. Monaco, "Effectiveness of systemic amoxicillin/metronidazole as adjunctive therapy to scaling and root planing in the treatment of chronic periodontitis: a systematic review and meta-analysis," *Journal of Periodontology*, vol. 83, no. 10, pp. 1257–1269, 2012.

[42] H. Hallström, G. R. Persson, S. Lindgren, M. Olofsson, and S. Renvert, "Systemic antibiotics and debridement of peri-implant mucositis. A randomized clinical trial," *Journal of Clinical Periodontology*, vol. 39, no. 6, pp. 574–581, 2012.

[43] J. Lindhe and J. Meyle, "Peri-implant diseases: consensus Report of the Sixth European Workshop on Periodontology," *Journal of Clinical Periodontology*, vol. 35, no. 8, supplement, pp. 282–285, 2008.

[44] F. Javed, A. S. T. Alghamdi, A. Ahmed, T. Mikami, H. B. Ahmed, and H. C. Tenenbaum, "Clinical efficacy of antibiotics in the treatment of peri-implantitis," *International Dental Journal*, vol. 63, no. 4, pp. 169–176, 2013.

[45] T. E. Rams, J. E. Degener, and A. J. van Winkelhoff, "Antibiotic resistance in human peri-implantitis microbiota," *Clinical Oral Implants Research*, vol. 25, no. 1, pp. 82–90, 2014.

[46] A. J. van Winkelhoff, D. Herrera Gonzales, E. G. Winkel, N. Dellemijn-Kippuw, C. M. J. E. Vandenbroucke-Grauls, and M. Sanz, "Antimicrobial resistance in the subgingival microflora in patients with adult periodontitis: a comparison between the Netherlands and Spain," *Journal of Clinical Periodontology*, vol. 27, no. 2, pp. 79–86, 2000.

[47] G. L. French, "The continuing crisis in antibiotic resistance," *International Journal of Antimicrobial Agents*, vol. 36, supplement 3, pp. S3–S7, 2010.

[48] D. B. Havard and J. M. Ray, "How can we as dentists minimize our contribution to the problem of antibiotic resistance?" *Oral and Maxillofacial Surgery Clinics of North America*, vol. 23, no. 4, pp. 551–555, 2011.

[49] M. Esposito, M. G. Grusovin, V. Loli, P. Coulthard, and H. V. Worthington, "Does antibiotic prophylaxis at implant placement decrease early implant failures? A Cochrane systematic review," *European Journal of Oral Implantology*, vol. 3, no. 2, pp. 101–110, 2010.

[50] A. J. van Winkelhoff, "Antibiotics in the treatment of peri-implantitis," *European Journal of Oral Implantology*, vol. 5, supplement, pp. S43–S50, 2012.

[51] M. Lagervall and L. E. Jansson, "Treatment outcome in patients with peri-implantitis in a periodontal clinic: a retrospective study," *Journal of Periodontology*, vol. 84, no. 10, pp. 1365–1373, 2013.

[52] J.-P. Albouy, I. Abrahamsson, L. G. Persson, and T. Berglundh, "Implant surface characteristics influence the outcome of treatment of peri-implantitis: an experimental study in dogs," *Journal of Clinical Periodontology*, vol. 38, no. 1, pp. 58–64, 2011.

[53] L. G. Persson, T. Berglundh, L. Sennerby, and J. Lindhe, "Re-osseointegration after treatment of peri-implantitis at different implant surfaces—an experimental study in the dog," *Clinical Oral Implants Research*, vol. 12, no. 6, pp. 595–603, 2001.

[54] M. B. Máximo, A. C. de Mendonça, V. Renata Santos, L. C. Figueiredo, M. Feres, and P. M. Duarte, "Short-term clinical and microbiological evaluations of peri-implant diseases before and after mechanical anti-infective therapies," *Clinical Oral Implants Research*, vol. 20, no. 1, pp. 99–108, 2009.

[55] P. M. Duarte, A. C. de Mendonça, M. B. B. Máximo, V. R. Santos, M. F. Bastos, and F. H. Nociti Jr., "Effect of anti-infective mechanical therapy on clinical parameters and cytokine levels in human peri-implant diseases," *Journal of Periodontology*, vol. 80, no. 2, pp. 234–243, 2009.

[56] Y. C. M. de Waal, G. M. Raghoebar, J. J. R. Huddleston Slater, H. J. A. Meijer, E. G. Winkel, and A. J. van Winkelhoff, "Implant decontamination during surgical peri-implantitis treatment: a randomized, double-blind, placebo-controlled trial," *Journal of Clinical Periodontology*, vol. 40, no. 2, pp. 186–195, 2013.

[57] G. Serino and A. Turri, "Outcome of surgical treatment of peri-implantitis: results from a 2-year prospective clinical study in humans," *Clinical Oral Implants Research*, vol. 22, no. 11, pp. 1214–1220, 2011.

[58] U. Grunder, M. B. Hürzeler, P. Schüpbach, and J. R. Strub, "Treatment of ligature-induced peri-implantitis using guided tissue regeneration: a clinical and histologic study in the beagle dog," *The International Journal of Oral & Maxillofacial Implants*, vol. 8, no. 3, pp. 282–293, 1993.

[59] F. H. Nociti Jr., M. Â. N. Machado, C. M. Stefani, and E. A. Sallum, "Absorbable versus nonabsorbable membranes and bone grafts in the treatment of ligature-induced peri-implantitis defects in dogs: a histometric investigation," *The International Journal of Oral & Maxillofacial Implants*, vol. 16, no. 5, pp. 646–652, 2001.

[60] M. B. Hürzeler, C. R. Quiñoncs, P. Schüpback, E. C. Morrison, and R. G. Caffesse, "Treatment of peri-implantitis using guided bone regeneration and bone grafts, alone or in combination, in beagle dogs—part 2: histologic findings," *The International Journal of Oral & Maxillofacial Implants*, vol. 12, no. 2, pp. 168–175, 1997.

[61] A.-M. Roos-Jansåker, H. Renvert, C. Lindahl, and S. Renvert, "Surgical treatment of peri-implantitis using a bone substitute with or without a resorbable membrane: a prospective cohort study," *Journal of Clinical Periodontology*, vol. 34, no. 7, pp. 625–632, 2007.

[62] A.-M. Roos-Jansåker, C. Lindahl, G. R. Persson, and S. Renvert, "Long-term stability of surgical bone regenerative procedures of peri-implantitis lesions in a prospective case-control study over 3 years," *Journal of Clinical Periodontology*, vol. 38, no. 6, pp. 590–597, 2011.

[63] A. Aghazadeh, G. Rutger Persson, and S. Renvert, "A single-centre randomized controlled clinical trial on the adjunct treatment of intra-bony defects with autogenous bone or a xenograft: results after 12 months," *Journal of Clinical Periodontology*, vol. 39, no. 7, pp. 666–673, 2012.

[64] J. Wiltfang, O. Zernial, E. Behrens, A. Schlegel, P. H. Warnke, and S. T. Becker, "Regenerative treatment of peri-implantitis bone defects with a combination of autologous bone and a demineralized xenogenic bone graft: a series of 36 defects," *Clinical Implant Dentistry and Related Research*, vol. 14, no. 3, pp. 421–427, 2012.

[65] F. Schwarz, A. Sculean, K. Bieling, D. Ferrari, D. Rothamel, and J. Becker, "Two-year clinical results following treatment of peri-implantitis lesions using a nanocrystalline hydroxyapatite or a natural bone mineral in combination with a collagen membrane," *Journal of Clinical Periodontology*, vol. 35, no. 1, pp. 80–87, 2008.

[66] P. Sahrmann, T. Attin, and P. R. Schmidlin, "Regenerative treatment of peri-implantitis using bone substitutes and membrane: a systematic review," *Clinical Implant Dentistry and Related Research*, vol. 13, no. 1, pp. 46–57, 2011.

[67] F. Schwarz, N. Sahm, K. Schwarz, and J. Becker, "Impact of defect configuration on the clinical outcome following surgical regenerative therapy of peri-implantitis," *Journal of Clinical Periodontology*, vol. 37, no. 5, pp. 449–455, 2010.

[68] S. J. Froum, S. H. Froum, and P. S. Rosen, "Successful management of peri-implantitis with a regenerative approach: a consecutive series of 51 treated implants with 3- to 7.5-year follow-up," *The International Journal of Periodontics & Restorative Dentistry*, vol. 32, no. 1, pp. 11–20, 2012.

[69] M. Roccuzzo, F. Bonino, L. Bonino, and P. Dalmasso, "Surgical therapy of peri-implantitis lesions by means of a bovine-derived xenograft: comparative results of a prospective study on two different implant surfaces," *Journal of Clinical Periodontology*, vol. 38, no. 8, pp. 738–745, 2011.

[70] A.-M. Roos-Jansåker, H. Renvert, C. Lindahl, and S. Renvert, "Submerged healing following surgical treatment of peri-implantitis: a case series," *Journal of Clinical Periodontology*, vol. 34, no. 8, pp. 723–727, 2007.

[71] F. Schwarz, S. Jepsen, M. Herten, M. Sager, D. Rothamel, and J. Becker, "Influence of different treatment approaches on non-submerged and submerged healing of ligature induced peri-implantitis lesions: an experimental study in dogs," *Journal of Clinical Periodontology*, vol. 33, no. 8, pp. 584–595, 2006.

[72] J. C. Wohlfahrt, S. P. Lyngstadaas, H. J. Rønold et al., "Porous titanium granules in the surgical treatment of peri-implant osseous defects: a randomized clinical trial," *The International Journal of Oral & Maxillofacial Implants*, vol. 27, no. 2, pp. 401–410, 2012.

[73] A. Y. Gamal, K. A. Abdel-Ghaffar, and V. J. Iacono, "A novel approach for enhanced nanoparticle-sized bone substitute adhesion to chemically treated peri-implantitis-affected implant surfaces: an in vitro proof-of-principle study," *Journal of Periodontology*, vol. 84, no. 2, pp. 239–247, 2013.

[74] F. Schwarz, K. Bieling, T. Latz, E. Nuesry, and J. Becker, "Healing of intrabony peri-implantitis defects following application of a nanocrystalline hydroxyapatite (Ostim) or a bovine-derived xenograft (Bio-Oss) in combination with a collagen membrane (Bio-Gide). A case series," *Journal of Clinical Periodontology*, vol. 33, no. 7, pp. 491–499, 2006.

[75] M. Baron, R. Haas, O. Dörtbudak, and G. Watzek, "Experimentally induced peri-implantitis: a review of different treatment methods described in the literature," *The International Journal of Oral & Maxillofacial Implants*, vol. 15, no. 4, pp. 533–544, 2000.

[76] A.-M. Roos-Jansåker, "Long time follow up of implant therapy and treatment of peri-implantitis," *Swedish Dental Journal. Supplement*, no. 188, pp. 7–66, 2007.

[77] G. E. Romanos and G. H. Nentwig, "Regenerative therapy of deep peri-implant lnfrabony defects after CO_2 laser implant surface decontamination," *International Journal of Periodontics and Restorative Dentistry*, vol. 28, no. 3, pp. 245–255, 2008.

[78] S. Schou, P. Holmstrup, T. Jørgensen et al., "Anorganic porous bovine-derived bone mineral (Bio-Oss) and ePTFE membrane in the treatment of peri-implantitis in cynomolgus monkeys," *Clinical Oral Implants Research*, vol. 14, no. 5, pp. 535–547, 2003.

[79] S. Schou, P. Holmstrup, L. T. Skovgaard, K. Stoltze, E. Hjørting-Hansen, and H. J. G. Gundersen, "Autogenous bone graft and ePTFE membrane in the treatment of peri-implantitis. II. Stereologic and histologic observations in cynomolgus monkeys," *Clinical Oral Implants Research*, vol. 14, no. 4, pp. 404–411, 2003.

[80] S. Schou, P. Holmstrup, T. Jørgensen et al., "Implant surface preparation in the surgical treatment of experimental peri-implantitis with autogenous bone graft and ePTFE membrane in cynomolgus monkeys," *Clinical Oral Implants Research*, vol. 14, no. 4, pp. 412–422, 2003.

[81] V. Khoshkam, H. Chan, G. Lin et al., "Reconstructive procedures for treating peri-implantitis: a systematic review," *Journal of Dental Research*, vol. 92, no. 12, supplement, pp. 131S–138S, 2013.

[82] L. J. A. Heitz-Mayfield, G. E. Salvi, A. Mombelli, M. Faddy, and N. P. Lang, "Anti-infective surgical therapy of peri-implantitis. A 12-month prospective clinical study," *Clinical Oral Implants Research*, vol. 23, no. 2, pp. 205–210, 2012.

[83] Å. Leonhardt, G. Dahlén, and S. Renvert, "Five-year clinical, microbiological, and radiological outcome following treatment of peri-implantitis in man," *Journal of Periodontology*, vol. 74, no. 10, pp. 1415–1422, 2003.

[84] G. Charalampakis, P. Rabe, Å. Leonhardt, and G. Dahlén, "A follow-up study of peri-implantitis cases after treatment," *Journal of Clinical Periodontology*, vol. 38, no. 9, pp. 864–871, 2011.

[85] S. D. Horvath and R. J. Kohal, "Rehabilitation of an extensive anterior explantation defect—a case report," *Quintessence International*, vol. 42, no. 7, pp. 539–545, 2011.

[86] E. E. Machtei, "What do we do after an implant fails? A review of treatment alternatives for failed implants," *The International Journal of Periodontics & Restorative Dentistry*, vol. 33, no. 4, pp. e111–e119, 2013.

[87] B. Manzoor, M. Suleiman, and R. M. Palmer, "The effects of simulated bone loss on the implant-abutment assembly and likelihood of fracture: an in vitro study," *The International Journal of Oral & Maxillofacial Implants*, vol. 28, no. 3, pp. 729–738, 2013.

[88] S. G. Kolonidis, S. Renvert, C. H. F. Hämmerle, N. P. Lang, D. Harris, and N. Claffey, "Osseointegration on implant surfaces previously contaminated with plaque: an experimental study in the dog," *Clinical Oral Implants Research*, vol. 14, no. 4, pp. 373–380, 2003.

[89] S. D. Horvath and R. J. Kohal, "Rehabilitation of an extensive anterior explantation defect—a case report," *Quintessence International*, vol. 42, no. 7, pp. 539–545, 2011.

[90] O. Mardinger, O. Oubaid, Y. Manor, J. Nissan, and G. Chaushu, "Factors affecting the decision to replace failed implants: a

retrospective study," *Journal of Periodontology*, vol. 79, no. 12, pp. 2262–2266, 2008.

[91] G. Alsaadi, M. Quirynen, and D. van Steenberghe, "The importance of implant surface characteristics in the replacement of failed implants," *The International Journal of Oral & Maxillofacial Implants*, vol. 21, no. 2, pp. 270–274, 2006.

[92] Y. Grossmann and L. Levin, "Success and survival of single dental implants placed in sites of previously failed implants," *Journal of Periodontology*, vol. 78, no. 9, pp. 1670–1674, 2007.

[93] E. E. Machtei, D. Mahler, O. Oettinger-Barak, O. Zuabi, and J. Horwitz, "Dental implants placed in previously failed sites: survival rate and factors affecting the outcome," *Clinical Oral Implants Research*, vol. 19, no. 3, pp. 259–264, 2008.

[94] Y.-K. Kim, J.-Y. Park, S.-G. Kim, and H.-J. Lee, "Prognosis of the implants replaced after removal of failed dental implants," *Oral Surgery, Oral Medicine, Oral Pathology, Oral Radiology and Endodontology*, vol. 110, no. 3, pp. 281–286, 2010.

[95] O. Mardinger, Y. Ben Zvi, G. Chaushu, J. Nissan, and Y. Manor, "A retrospective analysis of replacing dental implants in previously failed sites," *Oral Surgery, Oral Medicine, Oral Pathology and Oral Radiology*, vol. 114, no. 3, pp. 290–293, 2012.

[96] A. Eliasson, T. Eriksson, A. Johansson, and A. Wennerberg, "Fixed partial prostheses supported by 2 or 3 implants: a retrospective study up to 18 years," *The International Journal of Oral & Maxillofacial Implants*, vol. 21, no. 4, pp. 567–574, 2006.

[97] G. E. Salvi and U. Brägger, "Mechanical and technical risks in implant therapy," *The International Journal of Oral & Maxillofacial Implants*, vol. 24, supplement, pp. 69–85, 2009.

[98] B. E. Pjetursson, U. Brägger, N. P. Lang, and M. Zwahlen, "Comparison of survival and complication rates of tooth-supported fixed dental prostheses (FDPs) and implant-supported FDPs and single crowns (SCs)," *Clinical Oral Implants Research*, vol. 18, supplement 3, pp. 97–113, 2007.

[99] H.-P. Weber and C. Sukotjo, "Does the type of implant prosthesis affect outcomes in the partially edentulous patient?" *The International Journal of Oral & Maxillofacial Implants*, vol. 22, supplement, pp. 140–172, 2007.

[100] N. P. Lang, B. E. Pjetursson, K. Tan, U. Brägger, M. Egger, and M. Zwahlen, "A systematic review of the survival and complication rates of fixed partial dentures (FPDs) after an observation period of at least 5 years: II. Combined tooth-implant-supported FPDs," *Clinical Oral Implants Research*, vol. 15, no. 6, pp. 643–653, 2004.

[101] H.-J. Nickenig, C. Schäfer, and H. Spiekermann, "Survival and complication rates of combined tooth-implant-supported fixed partial dentures," *Clinical Oral Implants Research*, vol. 17, no. 5, pp. 506–511, 2006.

[102] C. Hita-Carrillo, M. Hernández-Aliaga, and J.-L. Calvo-Guirado, "Tooth-implant connection: a bibliographic review," *Medicina Oral, Patologia Oral y Cirugia Bucal*, vol. 15, no. 2, pp. e387–e394, 2010.

[103] M. Tonetti and R. Palmer, "Clinical research in implant dentistry: study design, reporting and outcome measurements: consensus report of Working Group 2 of the VIII European Workshop on Periodontology," *Journal of Clinical Periodontology*, vol. 39, no. 12, pp. 73–80, 2012.

[104] M. Esposito, M. G. Grusovin, and H. V. Worthington, "Treatment of peri-implantitis: what interventions are effective? A Cochrane systematic review," *European Journal of Oral Implantology*, vol. 5, supplement, pp. S21–S41, 2012.

15

Intestinal Parasite Profile in the Stool of HIV Positive Patients in relation to Immune Status and Comparison of Various Diagnostic Techniques with Special Reference to *Cryptosporidium* at a Tertiary Care Hospital in South India

Vishnu Kaniyarakkal,[1] **Nizamuddin Mundangalam,**[1]
Anitha Puduvail Moorkoth,[1] **and Sheela Mathew**[2]

[1]*Department of Microbiology, Government Medical College Kozhikode, Kozhikode 673016, India*
[2]*Department of Infectious Diseases, Government Medical College Kozhikode, Kozhikode 673016, India*

Correspondence should be addressed to Vishnu Kaniyarakkal; drkvishnu@gmail.com

Academic Editor: Lucia Lopalco

Acquired immunodeficiency syndrome and related opportunistic infections are a significant cause of morbidity and mortality in susceptible population. This study aims to negate the paucity of data regarding the relation between CD4 levels, prevalence of enteric parasites, and the outcome of treatment with HAART (highly active antiretroviral therapy) and Cotrimoxazole in Kerala, India. Multiple stool samples from 200 patients in a cross-sectional study were subjected to microscopy and *Cryptosporidium* stool antigen ELISA. Parasites were identified in 18 samples (9%). *Cystoisospora* and *Cryptosporidium* spp. were seen in 9 cases (4.5%) and 5 cases (2.5%), respectively. *Microsporidium* spores and *Chilomastix mesnili* cysts were identified in 1 case each (0.5% each). Seven cases of *Cystoisospora* diarrhoea recovered after treatment with Cotrimoxazole. Diarrhoea due to *Cryptosporidium* spp. in all 5 cases subsided after immune reconstitution with HAART. This study concludes that a positive association was seen between low CD4 count (<200 cells/μL) and overall parasite positivity (P value < 0.01). ELISA is a more sensitive modality for the diagnosis of *Cryptosporidium* diarrhoea. *Chilomastix mesnili*, generally considered a nonpathogen, may be a cause of diarrhoeal disease in AIDS. Immune reconstitution and Cotrimoxazole prophylaxis remain to be the best therapeutic approach in AIDS-related diarrhoea.

1. Introduction

Infection with human immunodeficiency virus (HIV) and its end stage, acquired immunodeficiency syndrome (AIDS), is a major public health challenge of modern times. Diarrhoea caused by parasites is one of the major opportunistic illnesses in HIV/AIDS resulting in significant morbidity. It diminishes patients' quality of life and if persistent causes dehydration, poor nutrition, and weight loss. Diarrhoea has been associated with 50% of HIV/AIDS patients in the developed world and in up to 100% of patients residing in developing countries [1]. The etiological enteric parasitic agents vary from patient to patient and from country to country depending on the geographical distribution, endemicity, seasonal variation of pathogens, and also the immune status of the patient [1].

HIV and parasitic infections may interact and mutually affect one another and parasitoses may facilitate the progression from asymptomatic HIV infection to AIDS. The common immunopathogenetic basis for the deleterious effects that parasitic diseases may have on the natural history of HIV infection involves a preferential activation of the T helper (Th2) type process. Thus the control of parasitic diseases is also necessary to aid in combating the HIV pandemic [2].

Since the start of the HIV epidemic, around 78 million people have become infected and 39 million have died of

TABLE 1: Results.

Patient characteristics	All patients (n = 200)	Patients with intestinal parasites (n = 18)	Patients without intestinal parasites (n = 182)	P value
Gender male, n (%)	136 (68%)	17 (94.4%)	119 (65.4%)	0.012
WHO staging of HIV, n (%)				0.076
Stage 1	11 (5.5%)	0 (0%)	11 (6%)	
Stage 2	34 (17%)	2 (11%)	32 (17.6%)	
Stage 3	145 (72.5%)	13 (72.2%)	132 (72.5%)	
Stage 4	10 (5%)	3 (16.7%)	7 (3%)	
Diarrhoea, n (%)	91 (45.5%)	15 (83.3%)	76 (41.8%)	0.001
Immune status, n (%)				0.000
No immunosuppression (CD4 > 500 cells/μL)	76 (38%)	1 (5.6%)	75 (41.2%)	
Mild immunosuppression (CD4 350–499 cells/μL)	40 (20%)	3 (16.7%)	37 (20.3%)	
Advanced immunosuppression (CD4 200–349 cells/μL)	34 (17%)	2 (11.1%)	32 (17.6%)	
Severe immunosuppression (CD4 < 200 cells/μL)	50 (25%)	12 (66.7%)	38 (20.9%)	
HAART, n (%)	147 (73.5%)	13 (72.2%)	134 (73.6%)	0.898
Cotrimoxazole prophylaxis, n (%)	57 (28.5%)	5 (27.8%)	52 (28.6%)	0.943
Drinking water, n (%)				0.004
Boiled water	87 (43.5%)	2 (11.1%)	85 (46.7%)	
Tap water	113 (56.5%)	16 (88.9%)	97 (53.3%)	

WHO, World Health Organisation; HAART, highly active antiretroviral therapy.

AIDS-related illnesses [3]. In 2013, of the 4.8 million people living with HIV in Asia and the Pacific, 250 000 died of AIDS-related causes [3]. India accounts for 51% of all AIDS-related deaths in the region [3].

There is paucity of data on relationship of CD4 levels and HIV/AIDS status with prevalence of enteric parasites among the HIV patients from Kerala, India. The present study therefore aims to determine the profile of enteric parasites and to study their association with immune status in HIV patients registered at the antiretroviral treatment centre of a tertiary care hospital in Kerala. Emphasis is also given on the comparison between various diagnostic techniques.

2. Materials and Methods

The study was conducted among 200 HIV seropositive patients registered at the antiretroviral treatment centre of Government Medical College Kozhikode, over a period of one year from January 2013 to December 2013. A clinical workup comprising history, WHO staging of the disease, antiretroviral treatment status, presence or absence of diarrhoea, Cotrimoxazole prophylaxis, and source of drinking water was constructed using a structured questionnaire. Flow cytometry (CyFlow Counter, Partec) was used to assess the CD4 T cell count and expressed as cells per cubic millimetre of blood (cells/μL).

A minimum of three feces samples were obtained from each patient on separate days. Concentration was done by formol ether sedimentation technique. Microscopy of wet mount and smear preparation was carried out before and after concentration. Smears were stained by Kinyoun's acid-fast method, rapid field stain, and modified trichrome stain (Ryan Blue method) for detection of trophozoites and cyst forms of parasites including the spores of Microsporidia. Cryptosporidium antigen stool ELISA (DRG Instruments GmbH, Frauenbergstr. 18, 35039 Marburg) was performed on samples with CD4 T cell count <200. Bacterial and fungal culture was done on all samples to rule out nonparasitic infectious causes of diarrhoea.

3. Results

Of the 200 HIV positive stool samples studied, 136 (68%) were of males and 64 (32%) were of females. 91 patients (45.5%) had acute or chronic diarrhoea and 109 (54.5%) patients did not have diarrhoea. 147 patients (73.5%) included in the study were on ART and 53 patients (26.5%) were ART naive. 58 (29%) were on Cotrimoxazole prophylaxis and the rest of the subjects were not on Cotrimoxazole prophylaxis. 37 subjects (74%) with severe immunosuppression (CD4 count <200) presented with diarrhoea and 26 subjects (34.2%) with no immunosuppression (CD4 count >500) presented with diarrhoea (Table 1).

Parasites were identified in 18 samples (9%). Cystoisospora oocysts (Figures 1–3) were identified in 9 cases (4.5%) and Cryptosporidium oocysts (Figures 4 and 5) in 5 cases (2.5%). Enterobius vermicularis worm (Figures 6 and 7) and ova (Figure 8) were identified in 2 cases (1%) and hookworm ova (Figure 9), Microsporidium spores (Figures 10 and 11), and Chilomastix mesnili cysts (Figure 12) in 1 case each

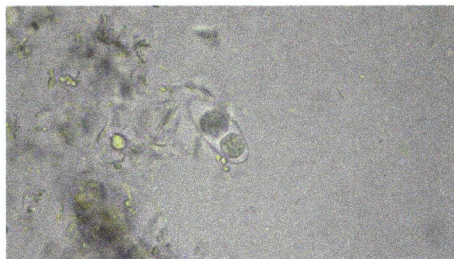

FIGURE 1: Mature *Cystoisospora* oocyst on normal saline wet mount, under high power.

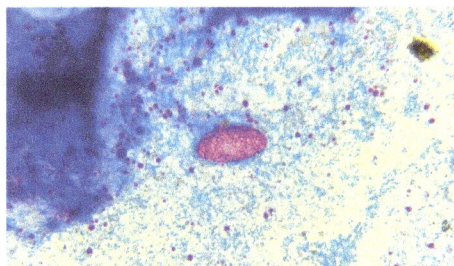

FIGURE 2: Immature *Cystoisospora* oocyst on modified acid-fast stain, under oil immersion.

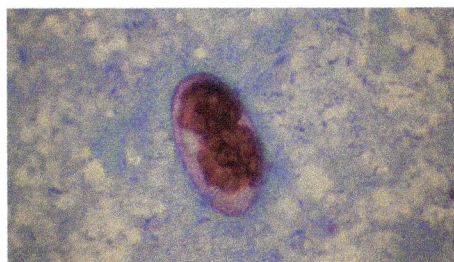

FIGURE 3: Mature *Cystoisospora* oocyst with two sporoblasts on modified acid-fast stain, under oil immersion.

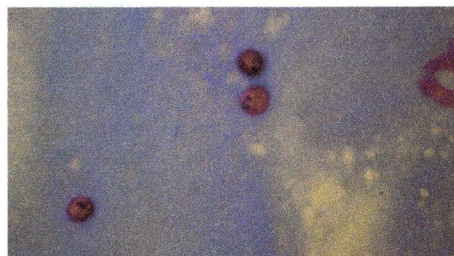

FIGURE 4: *Cryptosporidium* oocysts on modified acid-fast stain, under oil immersion.

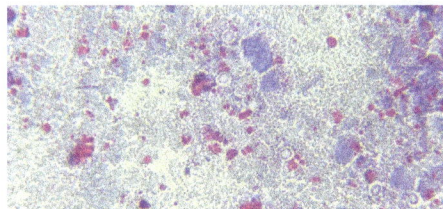

FIGURE 5: *Cryptosporidium* oocysts appearing as unstained structures on modified trichrome stain, under oil immersion.

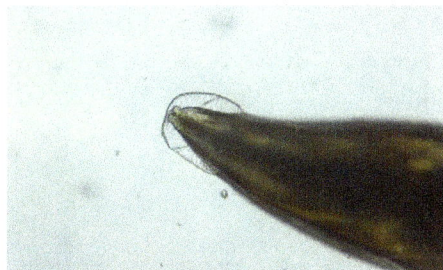

FIGURE 6: Cervical alae of *Enterobius vermicularis*, under low power.

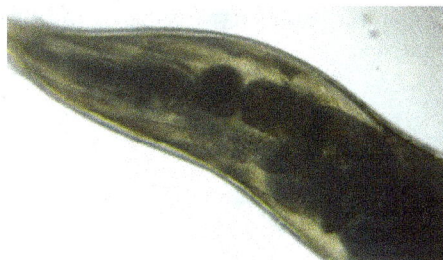

FIGURE 7: Double bulb oesophagus of *Enterobius vermicularis*, under low power.

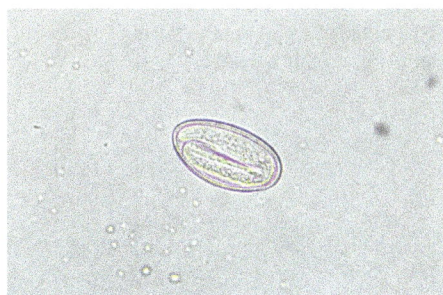

FIGURE 8: Non-bile-stained ovum of *Enterobius vermicularis* with larva inside on normal saline wet mount, under high power.

(0.5% each). One subject had mixed infection with both *Cryptosporidium* spp. and *Microsporidium* spp. (Figure 13). This study shows a positive association of low CD4 count with diarrhoea and parasite positivity (both with *P* value < 0.01). Also majority of the parasite positive cases (83.3%) presented with diarrhoea (*P* value = 0.001).

All *Cryptosporidium* oocyst positive cases in this study were seen in subjects with a CD4 cell count <200 (severe immunosuppression). Thus there is a positive association between *Cryptosporidium* positivity in stool and a CD4 cell count of <200 (*P* value = 0.002). On the other hand, there is no significant association between CD4 cell count <200 (severe immunosuppression) and *Cystoisospora* positivity in this study (*P* value of 0.06).

Only 2 cases of *Cryptosporidium* diarrhoea were diagnosed by modified acid-fast staining of stool samples, whereas 5 cases were diagnosed to have *Cryptosporidium*

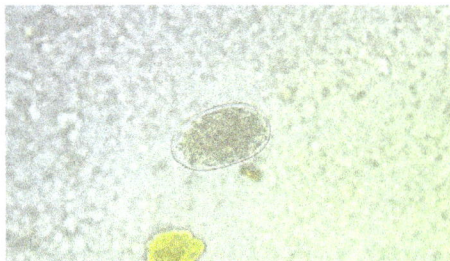

FIGURE 9: Non-bile-stained ovum of hookworm with segmented embryo inside on normal saline wet mount, under high power.

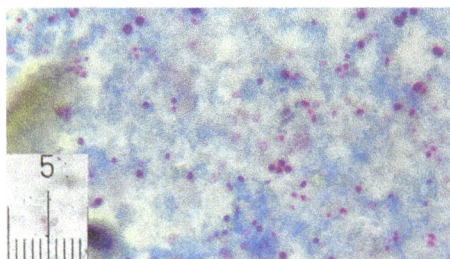

FIGURE 13: Variably acid-fast *Cryptosporidium* oocysts and microsporidial spores on modified acid-fast stain, under oil immersion.

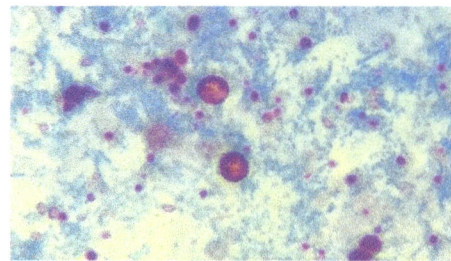

FIGURE 10: Microsporidial spores stained reddish pink with horizontal stripe measuring 1.9 μm (inset) on modified acid-fast stain, under oil immersion.

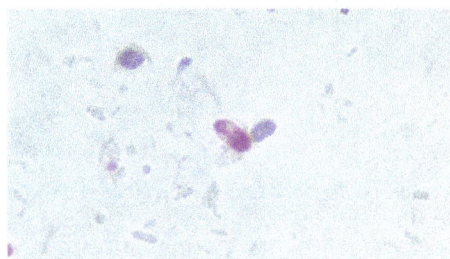

FIGURE 11: Magnified view of microsporidial spore on modified trichrome stain, under oil immersion.

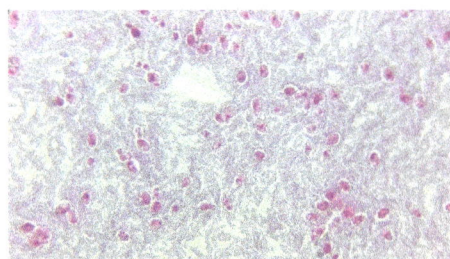

FIGURE 12: Cysts of *Chilomastix mesnili* on modified trichrome stain, under oil immersion.

diarrhoea by stool antigen ELISA (Table 2). The study shows that stool ELISA is a better diagnostic modality than stool modified acid-fast stain for the diagnosis of *Cryptosporidium* (P value < 0.01). The 9 cases of *Cystoisospora* infection in this study were demonstrated by both wet mount and modified acid-fast stain. In all the 9 cases, *Cystoisospora*

oocysts were demonstrated in modified acid-fast stain on primary examination itself. But in only 5 cases, oocysts were demonstrated at preliminary examination by wet mount, the other 4 being demonstrated in wet mount on retrospective examination. The *Cystoisospora* oocysts in these 5 cases, 2 cases of *Enterobius vermicularis,* and 1 case of hook worm were the only parasites demonstrated on wet mount before concentration. In all the other cases, parasites were demonstrated either on wet mount or by staining of concentrated samples only.

One of the *Cryptosporidium* positive cases and 6 of the *Cystoisospora* positive cases (38.9%) were identified on repeated stool sample examination only. One case positive for *Cystoisospora* was identified on examination of the sixth stool sample.

Of the five patients diagnosed to have *Cryptosporidium* infection, diarrhoea subsided in four, after a change of ART regimen from ZLN (Zidovudine, Lamivudine, and Nevirapine) to TLE (Tenofovir, Lamivudine, and Efavirenz). Fifth patient had complete remission of symptoms after he was started on first-line ART. No other treatment specific for *Cryptosporidium* was instituted in these patients.

Two patients out of nine who were diagnosed with *Cystoisospora* infection succumbed to the disease and expired. Out of these two patients, Cotrimoxazole could not be given to one because of hypersensitivity reactions and the other continued to have diarrhoea despite therapy with Cotrimoxazole. The rest of the seven patients became symptom-free after they were started on Cotrimoxazole prophylaxis as per National AIDS Control Organisation guidelines.

In this study bacterial culture for *Salmonella*, *Shigella*, and *Vibrio cholerae* yielded no pathogen. Fungal culture was also negative for opportunistic fungi causing diarrhoea.

4. Discussion

In Asia, the highest numbers of HIV-infected individuals belong to India and China [4]. The most common parasites causing diarrhoea in HIV-infected individuals include *Cryptosporidium parvum*, *Isospora belli*, *Microsporidium* spp., *Giardia intestinalis*, *Entamoeba histolytica,* and *Strongyloides stercoralis* [4]. This study determined the profile of intestinal parasites among HIV positive individuals and attempted to

TABLE 2: *Cryptosporidium* positive cases.

Age & sex	*Cryptosporidium* stool antigen ELISA positivity	Modified acid-fast positivity	CD4 count (cells/μL)
35/male	Yes	No	40
54/male	Yes	Yes	17
38/male	Yes	No	132
38/male	Yes	No	32
69/male[*]	Yes	Yes	54

[*]This case presented as mixed infection along with *Microsporidium* spp.

investigate whether the distribution of parasites was affected by immune status. Also, different diagnostic techniques were compared to determine the more effective and practical one to be used in resource poor settings.

Majority of the subjects in the study were males (68%). Studies from other parts of India also show a higher proportion of males among HIV-infected population (61%–64%) [5, 6]. This male preponderance should be because of the propensity of males to travel outside hometown for work and greater exposure to promiscuous and unprotected sex. Diarrhoea was seen in 45.5% of the subjects which is consistent with the data available from developing countries [7–9]. Overall parasite positivity in the study was 9%. The prevalence of intestinal parasitic infections in HIV-infected patients from developing countries ranges from 12% to 38% [9–12]. The lower prevalence of parasites reported in this study could be due to the fact that stool examinations were performed whether or not the patients had diarrhoea. In this study, among patients with diarrhoea, the parasite positivity was 16%.

Cystoisospora was identified in maximum number of cases followed by *Cryptosporidium* in this study. In various studies conducted in north India and other countries, the most common parasite was *Cryptosporidium* [13, 14]. But studies from south India had findings similar to the one in this study [15, 16]. This difference may be attributed to the variation in geographical habitat of parasites and climate. Mixed infection with *Cryptosporidium* and *Microsporidium* was seen in one patient identified by both modified acid-fast staining and modified trichrome staining. Studies substantiate the fact that mixed infection with *Cryptosporidium* spp. and *Microsporidium* spp. is indeed common among HIV positive population [17–19]. Positive association between a CD4 count of <200 (severe immunosuppression) and parasite positivity in general was seen in this study (P value < 0.01). This association was not seen in case of *Cystoisospora* positive cases. These findings are corroborated in studies conducted worldwide [9, 14, 20, 21]. *Chilomastix mesnili* cysts were identified in one patient with CD4 count <200 cells/μL, showing the pathogenic nature of this otherwise nonpathogenic parasite in HIV patients [22]. The nature of periodic shedding of parasites necessitates multiple stool sample examinations for accurate diagnosis [23].

Immune reconstitution with HAART is the best therapeutic approach in diarrhoea due to *Cryptosporidium*. Even though treatment with Cotrimoxazole is effective for diarrhoea caused by *Cystoisospora*, a possibility of Cotrimoxazole resistant cystoisosporiasis should be borne in mind [24, 25].

This study shows a positive association between consumption of tap water and parasite positivity (P value = 0.004). Two subjects consuming boiled water at home also were diagnosed with parasitosis. This can be attributed to the unreliability of quality of water and food that one is exposed to, while travelling in a developing country like India. In a study conducted in Nepal, although a statistically significant association between the source of drinking water and parasite positivity was not seen, 20% of those taking direct tap water for drinking purposes and 12.5% of those using bore well water had intestinal parasitosis [10].

5. Conclusions

This study underscores the importance of routine screening for intestinal parasites in the stool of HIV patients with severe immunosuppression and diarrhoeal symptoms. Diarrhoea due to *Cystoisospora* is more common in south Indian settings. Mixed infections with *Cryptosporidium* and *Microsporidium* are not uncommon, necessitating a high index of suspicion and the use of different staining methods. While there was a positive association between severe immunosuppression and *Cryptosporidium* positivity, no such association was seen in case of cystoisosporiasis. ELISA is a better modality for the diagnosis of Cryptosporidial diarrhoea and should be included in the diagnostic depository where possible. *Chilomastix mesnili*, generally considered a nonpathogen, may be a cause of diarrhoeal disease in HIV positive population. The association of *Cystoisospora* infection with mortality necessitates the prompt institution of Cotrimoxazole prophylaxis and effective supportive therapy. In diarrhoea due to *Cryptosporidium*, treatment should always be aimed at immune reconstitution.

Competing Interests

The authors declare that there is no conflict of interests regarding the publication of this paper.

References

[1] A. K. Jha, B. Uppal, S. Chadha et al., "Clinical and microbiological profile of HIV/AIDS cases with diarrhea in North India," *Journal of Pathogens*, vol. 2012, Article ID 971958, 7 pages, 2012.

[2] W. Winn Jr., S. Allen, W. Janda et al., *Koneman's Color Atlas and Textbook of Diagnostic Microbiology*, chapter 22, Lippincott Williams & Wilkins, 6th edition, 2006.

[3] UN AIDS Fact Sheet 2014.

[4] N. S. Chavan and S. N. Chavan, "Intestinal parasitic infections in HIV infected patients," *International Journal of Current Microbiology and Applied Sciences*, vol. 3, no. 2, pp. 265–270, 2014.

[5] A. Pandey, D. Sahu, T. Bakkali et al., "Estimate of HIV prevalence and number of people living with HIV in India 2008-2009," *BMJ Open*, vol. 2, no. 5, Article ID e000926, 2012.

[6] S. Bishnu, D. Bandyopadhyay, S. Samui et al., "Assessment of clinico-immunological profile of newly diagnosed HIV patients presenting to a teaching hospital of eastern India," *Indian Journal of Medical Research*, vol. 139, no. 6, pp. 903–912, 2014.

[7] S. Gupta, S. Narang, V. Nunavath, and S. Singh, "Chronic diarrhoea in HIV patients: prevalence of coccidian parasites," *Indian Journal of Medical Microbiology*, vol. 26, no. 2, pp. 172–175, 2008.

[8] S. R. Framm and R. Soave, "Agents of diarrhea," *Medical Clinics of North America*, vol. 81, no. 2, pp. 427–447, 1997.

[9] B. R. Tiwari, P. Ghimire, S. Malla, B. Sharma, and S. Karki, "Intestinal parasitic infection among the HIV-infected patients in Nepal," *Journal of Infection in Developing Countries*, vol. 7, no. 7, pp. 550–555, 2013.

[10] R. Amatya, R. Shrestha, N. Poudyal, and S. Bhandari, "Opportunistic intestinal parasites and CD4 count in HIV infected people," *Journal of Pathology of Nepal*, vol. 1, pp. 118–121, 2011.

[11] J. Pavie, J. Menotti, R. Porcher et al., "Prevalence of opportunistic intestinal parasitic infections among HIV-infected patients with low CD4 cells counts in France in the combination antiretroviral therapy era," *International Journal of Infectious Diseases*, vol. 16, no. 9, pp. e677–e679, 2012.

[12] I. Asma, S. Johari, L. H. S. Benedict, and A. L. L. Yvonne, "How common is intestinal parasitism in HIV-infected patients in Malaysia?" *Tropical Biomedicine*, vol. 28, no. 2, pp. 400–410, 2011.

[13] O. O. Oguntibeju, "Prevalence of intestinal parasites in HIV-positive/AIDS patients," *Malaysian Journal of Medical Sciences*, vol. 13, no. 1, pp. 68–73, 2006.

[14] A. Missaye, M. Dagnew, A. Alemu, and A. Alemu, "Prevalence of intestinal parasites and associated risk factors among HIV/AIDS patients with pre-ART and on-ART attending dessie hospital ART clinic, Northeast Ethiopia," *AIDS Research and Therapy*, vol. 10, no. 1, article 7, 2013.

[15] A. Mukhopadhya, B. S. Ramakrishnan, G. Kang et al., "Enteric pathogens in southern Indian HIV-infected patients with and without diarrhoea," *Indian Journal of Medical Research*, vol. 109, pp. 85–89, 1999.

[16] S. S. Kumar, S. Ananthan, and P. Saravanan, "Role of coccidian parasites in causation of diarrhoea in HIV infected patients in Chennai," *Indian Journal of Medical Research*, vol. 116, pp. 85–89, 2002.

[17] L. S. Garcia, R. Y. Shimizu, and D. A. Bruckner, "Detection of microsporidial spores in fecal specimens from patients diagnosed with cryptosporidiosis," *Journal of Clinical Microbiology*, vol. 32, no. 7, pp. 1739–1741, 1994.

[18] A. De, K. Patil, and M. Mathur, "Detection of enteric parasites in HIV positive patients with diarrhea," *Indian Journal of Sexually Transmitted Diseases*, vol. 30, no. 1, pp. 55–56, 2009.

[19] R. Weber, B. Sauer, R. Lüthy, and D. Nadal, "Intestinal coinfection with *Enterocytozoon bieneusi* and *Cryptosporidium* in a human immunodeficiency virus-infected child with chronic diarrhea," *Clinical Infectious Diseases*, vol. 17, no. 3, pp. 480–483, 1993.

[20] L. Tuli, A. K. Gulati, S. Sundar, and T. M. Mohapatra, "Correlation between CD4 counts of HIV patients and enteric protozoan in different seasons—an experience of a tertiary care hospital in Varanasi (India)," *BMC Gastroenterology*, vol. 8, article 36, 2008.

[21] A. B. Janagond, G. Sasikala, D. Agatha, T. Ravinder, and P. R. Thenmozhivalli, "Enteric parasitic infections in relation to diarrhoea in HIV infected individuals with CD4 T cell counts <1000 cells/μl in Chennai, India," *Journal of Clinical and Diagnostic Research*, vol. 7, no. 10, pp. 2160–2162, 2013.

[22] N. Morimoto, M. Korenaga, and C. Komatsu, "A case report of an overseas-traveller's diarrhoea probably caused by *Chilomastix mesnili* infection," *Japanese Journal of Tropical Medicine and Hygiene*, vol. 24, no. 3, pp. 177–180, 1996.

[23] C. P. Cartwright, "Utility of multiple-stool-specimen ova and parasite examinations in a high-prevalence setting," *Journal of Clinical Microbiology*, vol. 37, no. 8, pp. 2408–2411, 1999.

[24] Y. M. Miao and B. G. Gazzard, "Management of protozoal diarrhoea in HIV disease," *HIV Medicine*, vol. 1, no. 4, pp. 194–199, 2000.

[25] V. G. Mudholkar and R. D. Namey, "Heavy infestation of Isospora belli causing severe watery diarrhea," *Indian Journal of Pathology and Microbiology*, vol. 53, no. 4, pp. 824–825, 2010.

16

Knowledge and Attitude of Obstetric Care Providers on Partograph and Its Associated Factors in East Gojjam Zone, Northwest Ethiopia

Desalegne Amare Zelellw,[1] **Teketo Kassaw Tegegne,**[2] **and Girma Alem Getie**[3]

[1]*Department of Nursing, College of Medicine and Health Sciences, Bahir Dar University, P.O. Box 79, Bahir Dar, Ethiopia*
[2]*Department of Public Health, College of Medicine and Health Sciences, Debre Markos University, Debre Markos, Ethiopia*
[3]*Department of Nursing, College of Medicine and Health Sciences, Debre Markos University, Debre Markos, Ethiopia*

Correspondence should be addressed to Desalegne Amare Zelellw; desa2001@yahoo.com

Academic Editor: Françoise Vendittelli

Introduction. Universal use of partograph is recommended during labor, to improve maternal and fetal outcome. The aim was to assess knowledge and attitude of obstetric caregivers about partograph and associated factors. *Methods.* Facility based cross-sectional study was conducted on 273 study participants. Study facilities and study units were selected using simple random sampling technique. Midwives, Nurses, Public Health Officers, Medical Doctors, and masters in Emergency Surgery and Obstetric were included in the study. Epi-data and SPSS statistical software were used. *Results.* About 153 (56.04%) and 150 (54.95%) of the obstetric caregivers had good knowledge and favorable attitude about partograph, respectively. Knowledge of partograph was significantly higher among obstetric caregivers that learnt about partograph during their College and who had received partograph on job training (AOR: 2.14, 95% C.I (1.17–3.93)) and (AOR: 2.25, 95% C.I (1.21–4.19)), respectively. Favorable attitude towards partograph was significantly higher among obstetrical caregivers who had training and learnt about partograph during their college (AOR: 3.37, 95% C.I (1.49–5.65)) and (AOR: 2.134, 95% C.I (1.175–3.877)), correspondingly. *Conclusion.* Above half of obstetric caregivers had good knowledge and a favorable attitude on partograph. The provision of on preservice and job training is necessary to improve caregivers' knowledge and attitude.

1. Background

The 2013-world health organization (WHO) report showed that over 289,000 mothers died globally, of which developing countries accounted for 99% and sub-Saharan Africa region alone accounted for about 62% [1]. The majority, 70% of death cases, occurred due to obstructed labor and ruptured uterus [2]. The 2011 Ethiopian demographic and health survey (EDHS) indicated that maternal mortality ratio was at 676 maternal deaths per 100,000 live births [3]. In addition, the 2013 WHO report also showed that maternal mortality in Ethiopia was 420 per 100,000 [1].

Prolonged and obstructed labor is one of the five major causes of maternal death which was responsible for 8% of all maternal deaths. An estimated 6.5 million women in the world have obstructed labor each year (2–15 cases/1000 births). It is the most common cause of complications like death and fistula. Approximately, 2–5% of women who experience a prolonged or obstructed labor can develop fistula [3].

WHO report showed that the global maternal deaths resulted from complications of pregnancy and childbirth, especially, in developing countries [4, 5]. From survive childbirth, at least 8 million develop serious morbidities and a further 50 million suffer minor complications [5]. Out of the causes of deaths and complications, obstetric hemorrhage and obstructed labor are common causes and easily preventable by using partograph [6]. Senegal and Mali indicate that the most common reported causes of maternal death were postpartum hemorrhage. Furthermore, obstructed labor was the cause for maternal death [7].

The World Health Organization recommends the universal use of the partograph during labor [8]. It is a cost-effective and affordable tool used to improve monitoring of the progress of labor and maternal and fetal well-being, which later on is used to reduce maternal deaths and complications due to obstructed and prolonged labor conditions [9, 10]. Physicians should set reasonable expectations for labor progress to avoid unnecessary interventions and anxiety [11]. Prolonged latent phase of labor is associated with a higher risk of postpartum hemorrhage, chorioamnionitis, neonatal admission to the intensive care unit, and long hospital stay [12]. Therefore, early detection of abnormal progress and prevention of prolonged labor can significantly reduce maternal mortality and morbidity [2].

Previously, partograph was introduced to illustrate cervical dilation graphically during labor [13] and later it incorporates the action and alert lines [14]. Currently, the Modified WHO Partograph comprises different variables; therefore, the current partograph was designed to monitor not only the progress of labor but also the condition of the mother and fetus during labor. It involves various parameters to assess progress of labor and maternal and fetal conditions during labor. The progress of labor is assessed through cervical dilatation and descent of the head and uterine contractions. On the other hand, fetal condition is monitored by fetal heart rate, color of liquor, and the moulding of the fetal skull. Furthermore, the maternal condition is also assessed through monitoring maternal pulse rate, blood pressure, temperature and urine for volume, protein, and ketone bodies and additional crucial factor in active management of labor is the timing of interventions as and when needed, such as amniotomy, augmentation with oxytocin, caesarean section, or transfer to a higher center [15].

A study done in Southwest Nigeria revealed that obstetric care providers from tertiary level of care were significantly more knowledgeable about the assessments that could be inferred from the partograph. In addition, most of them had received prior training about partograph In addition, most of them had received prior training about partograph and they knew at least one component of the partograph [16]. However, knowledge of the functions of alert line and action line was generally poor as only 16.6% and 24.3% of them had explained the function of alert line and action line, respectively. A higher proportion of study participants from tertiary level of care perceived that partograph utilization can reduce maternal/perinatal morbidity and mortality and it improves the quality of care [12].

There was a differing knowledge level between healthcare providers working in general hospitals and university teaching hospital, the first having a higher level of knowledge [16]. Previous training on partograph was independently associated with the knowledge of obstetrical care providers about the components of the partograph [17]. In North Shoa, Central Ethiopia obstetric caregivers had a good level of knowledge on the partograph and their level of knowledge was significantly associated with working in hospitals and having on-the-job training about partograph [18].

Knowledge of obstetric caregivers' about the partograph at public health facilities of Addis Ababa, Ethiopia, was fair; 96.6% of the study participants correctly mentioned at least one component of it. In this study, 53.3% and 82.6% of the caregivers properly explained the function of alert line and action line, respectively [19]. A study done in Nigeria indicated that at tertiary and general hospitals healthcare providers' knowledge and previous training on partograph were significantly associated with its utilization during labor. Furthermore, lack of detailed knowledge of it, nonavailability of the partograph, and shortage of staff were the militating factors against the use of partograph [16]. Therefore, this study was aimed to assess knowledge and attitude of partograph and its associated factors among obstetric care providers.

2. Methods and Materials

2.1. Study Setting. The study was conducted from March to July 2015 at Public Health Facilities (health centers and a hospital) in East Gojjam Zone, Amhara Regional State, and Northwest Ethiopia. Debre Markos is the capital of East Gojjam Zone, which is located at 299 Kilometer Northwest of Addis Ababa. In the zone, there are 19 districts/woreda, 101 health centers, and two hospitals.

Health center is a primary healthcare unit (PHCU) with each health center having five satellite health posts. Health centers comprise (1/15,000–25,000 population) and their satellite health posts (1/3,000–5,000 population) that are connected to each other by a referral system. Hospitals can be district/a primary hospital (with population coverage of 60,000–100,000 people), general hospital with population coverage of 1–1.5 million people, and thirdly a specialized hospital that covers population of 3.5–5 million [20].

2.2. Study Design. A health facility based cross-sectional study was conducted at public health facilities in East Gojjam Zone.

2.3. Study Population. In governmental health facilities of East Gojjam Zone, estimated 1417 health workers (Nurses, Midwives, Public Health Officers, Medical Doctors, and M.S. in Emergency Surgery and Obstetric) were found.

2.4. Sampling. The sample size was determined using a single population proportion, assuming a 95% confidence interval and with 5% margin of error and 26.6% of the proportion of proper knowledge on components of partograph taken from a study done in Amhara Region [21]. Based on this $n = z^2(p(1-p))/d^2$ formula: the sample size was obtained 300. Since the entire population was below 10,000 a reduction formula was used and the sample size was reduced to 248. The final sample size with a 10% nonresponse rate was obtained, 273.

2.5. Sampling Techniques. From the total 103 public health facilities in the zone, that is, 101 health centers and two hospitals, 29 health centers and one hospital were selected by simple random sampling technique. The 273 study participants in the sampled health facilities were selected using simple random sampling method with proportionate allocation to size after getting the list of health workers working in labor and delivery care on either a routine or duty program.

2.6. Inclusion and Exclusion Criteria. The survey was conducted among all healthcare professionals: that is, all Midwives, Nurses, Public Health Officers, Medical Doctors, and masters in Emergency Surgery and Obstetric who were working in labor and delivery on a regular and/or duty program were included in this study. However, health workers that had a workload during the visit were excluded from this study.

2.7. Variables. Sociodemographic characteristics (age, sex, religion, and marital status), working department, health professional qualification, health facility type, training partograph and obstetrics care, and experience are independent variables while knowledge and attitude of the participants on the partographs are the dependent variables.

2.8. Data Collection Process. Questionnaires were adapted and modified from related articles to collect data through self-administered questionnaire. The questionnaire mainly focused on sociodemographic characteristics, qualification, types of health facilities, current working department, knowledge and attitude about partograph, and previous obstetric care training. The study participants were instructed how to fill the questionnaire and the data collection took an average of 30–50 minutes. The data were collected by Nurses, Midwives, and Public Health Officer. A total of three Nurses, two midwifes, and one public health officers were involved in the data collection process.

2.9. Data Quality Assurance. The questionnaire was pretested on 5% of non-sampled hospitals and health centers. Based on the pretest findings modification was made. Data collectors and supervisors were trained for two days on data collection instruments and sample collection. All selected data collectors had Bachelor of Science degree in their perspective professions to enhance the quality of the data. The investigators and supervisors were made on site supervision during the whole period of data collection. Data were checked for completeness and consistency after each day of data collection by holding a meeting with the data collectors. Data double entry was made for all the questionnaires to enhance data quality.

2.10. Measurements. Knowledge of obstetric caregivers about the partograph was measured based on eight knowledge specific questions. Each correct response earned one point, whereas any wrong response attracted no mark and thus the sum score of knowledge was calculated (8 points). The mean score of partograph knowledge (4.44 ± 2.18) was used to decide cutoffs of the rank. Respondents who scored 0–4 points were adjudged as having poor knowledge, whereas those that scored 5–8 points were adjudged as having a good knowledge, respectively (Table 1).

On the other hand, the attitude towards partograph was assessed using attitude scoring method. The attitude score for each of the personnel was obtained by adding up the scores for correct answers given to the ten questions. Based on the

TABLE 1: Criteria for the partograph knowledge score.

Parameters	No	Yes
Correct definition of partograph	0	1
Mention at least one component of partograph	0	1
The use of partograph	0	1
Know functions of alert line	0	1
Know functions of action line	0	1
Know when to start plotting on partograph	0	1
Importance of partograph	0	1
Know satisfactory labor progress	0	1

TABLE 2: Criteria for the partograph attitude score.

Parameters	Disagree	Agree
Like to use partograph	0	1
Partograph is important to monitor labor	0	1
Partograph should be used in all labor	0	1
Partograph use reduces risks of maternal and/neonatal morbidity and mortality	0	1
Partograph helps for early detection for surgery or cesarean section	0	1
Wish to use partograph routinely	0	1
Not all normal labor needs partograph	1	0
Using partograph is the only responsibility of physicians	1	0
Partograph is not effective to monitor labor progress	1	0
Using partograph is time consuming	1	0

overall attitude scores, the respondents' level of attitude of the partograph was rated using a median score of 8.00 ± 3.49 as unfavorable (0–7) and favorable (8–10) (Table 2).

2.11. Data Analysis. Data were entered using Epi-data version 3.1, and analysis was performed using SPSS version 20.0 statistical software. Bivariate and multiple models were run to assess any relationship between each independent and the outcome variables. Crude and adjusted odd's ratios were used to identify any association between the dependent and independent variables. Pearson correlation coefficient was used to examine the effect of knowledge on the attitude of participants and vice versa. Level of significance was determined using 95% confidence intervals. Independent variables with p value less than or equal to 0.2 at the bivariate level were included in the multiple logistic regression models for the dependent variables to control potential confounding variables.

2.12. Ethical Consideration. Ethical approval and clearance were obtained from Debre Markos University, medicine and health science college Ethical Review Committee. A formal letter of permission and support was written to East Gojjam Zone Health Department. Also the zonal health department wrote a permission letter and support to the sampled health facilities. Then it was communicated at each level of the health facilities and each study participant. The purpose of the study was explained to participants, and written informed consent was obtained from each study subject. Confidentiality of information was maintained by omitting any personal identifier from the questionnaires.

3. Result

3.1. Characteristics of Obstetric Caregivers. In this study, 273 obstetric caregivers participated obtaining a response rate of 100%. More than half, 157 (57.5%), of them were males. The mean age of the study participants was 27.64 (±4.50) years and nearly half, 128 (46.9%), of them were within the age group of 25–29 years. About 198 (72.5%) of the healthcare providers had a diploma educational status.

The majority, 246 (90.1%) of obstetrics caregivers, were working in the health centers and more than one-fifth, 60 (22.0%), of them were Diploma Midwives. One hundred forty-one (51.6%) of the caregivers were working at delivery ward regularly while the rest were working during the night duty and/or on the weekend. Nearly half, 132 (48.4%) of obstetric caregivers, had a maximum of three years of clinical service and only 91 (33.3%) of them had training on obstetric care. However, only 78 (28.6%) of them received in-service or refresher training on partograph directly or indirectly (see Table 3).

3.2. Knowledge about Partograph. In this study, more than half, 153 (56.1%), of the obstetric caregivers had good knowledge about partograph. Even though nearly three-fourth, 200 (73.3%), of the obstetric caregivers knew the components of partograph, there was knowledge deficiency in some other aspects. Only the 57 (20.9%) obstetric caregivers exactly knew that plotting on the partograph is started when the cervical dilation is at four centimeters. Furthermore, 133 (48.7%) of them knew the correct function of the alert line on the partograph (see Table 4). To enhance their knowledge about partograph 161 (58.9%) of the care providers want to receive partograph training. About 53.8% of participants used the tool routinely.

With regard to obstetric caregivers' detail knowledge about the partograph components, 214 (78.4%) of them knew that fetal heart rate (FHR) is one of its components in monitoring the FHR condition. Furthermore, 195 (71.4%) and 186 (68.1%) knew that uterine contraction and urine volume, protein, and ketone bodies are its components in monitoring of the labor progress and maternal conditions, respectively (Figure 1).

3.3. Attitude of Obstetric Caregivers towards Partograph. Above half, 150 (55%), of the obstetric care providers in this study had a favorable attitude towards partograph. However, only 111 (40.7%) of the caregivers agreed to use partograph, but 171 (64.1%) of them had agreed that maternal and newborn morbidities and mortalities can be reduced by using partograph. Furthermore, 183 (67%) of the providers agreed that partograph is important, for early detection of labor abnormalities for surgery or caesarean section. A lower proportion, 83 (30.4%), of the caregivers believed that

TABLE 3: Characteristics of obstetric caregivers and public health institutions of East Gojjam Zone, Northwest Ethiopia, 2015 (*n* = 273).

Variables	Frequency	Percentage
Sex		
Male	157	57.5
Female	116	42.5
Age in years		
≤24	71	26
25–29	128	46.9
≥30	74	27.1
Health institution		
Health center	246	90.1
Hospital	27	9.9
Qualification level		
Diploma	198	72.5
Degree and above	75	27.5
Profession		
Nurse	155	56.8
Midwife	74	27.1
Public Health Officer	37	13.6
Others[†]	7	2.6
Regular working department		
Delivery ward	141	51.7
Antenatal care	47	17.2
Family planning	36	13.2
OPD (adult & or under-five)	49	17.9
Clinical service years		
≤3 years	132	48.4
4–6 years	87	31.9
≥7 years	54	19.8

[†]Others (medical doctors and M.S. in emergency surgery and obstetrics).

TABLE 4: Knowledge of obstetric caregivers on partograph and its use, East Gojjam Zone, Northwest Ethiopia, 2015 (*n* = 273).

Knowledge variables	Correct response (*n*)	Percentage
Definition of partograph	153	56
Components of partograph	200	73.3
The use of partograph	156	57.1
Functions of alert line	133	48.7
Functions of action line	197	72.2
When to start plotting on partograph	57	20.9
Importance of partograph	163	59.7
Satisfactory labor progress	152	55.7
Overall knowledge		
Good knowledge	153	56.1
Poor knowledge	120	43.9

partograph is used only for physicians (medical doctors). Similarly, 107 (39.2%) of them agreed that use of partograph

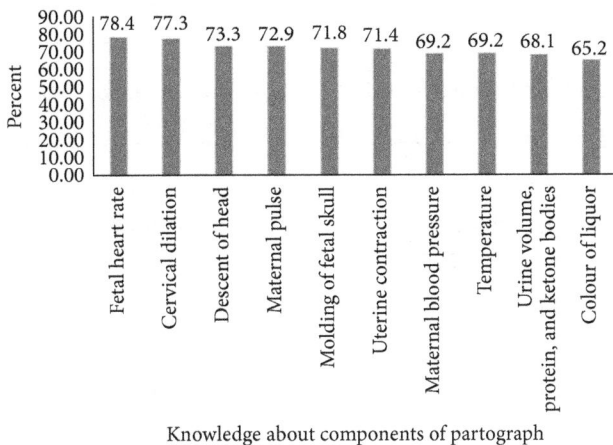

Figure 1: Obstetric caregivers knowledge about components of partograph, East Gojjam Zone, Northwest Ethiopia, 2015 ($n = 273$).

is time consuming and all normal labor does not need to use partograph, 89 (32.6%) (Table 5).

3.4. Factors Associated with Partograph Knowledge.

According to the multivariable analysis, obstetric care providers within the age of 25–29 years were 2.47 times more probable to have good knowledge about partograph than those below 25 years old (AOR (95% C.I): 2.47 (1.32–4.64)). Obstetric caregivers who were working at antenatal and family planning ward usually were 4.94 and 2.61 times more likely to have good partograph knowledge than those who were routinely working in outpatient department (AOR (95% C.I): 4.94 (1.97–12.40) and 2.61 (1.03–6.61)), respectively. Moreover, caregivers who had learnt about partograph during their college and/or university level of education were 2.14 times more likely to have good knowledge about partograph than their counterparts (AOR (95% C.I): 2.14 (1.17–3.93)). Similarly, obstetric caregivers who had received on-the-job training on partograph were also 2.25 times more likely to have good partograph knowledge than their counterparts (AOR (95% C.I): 2.25 (1.21–4.19)) (see Table 6). However, having obstetric training was a confounding factor on partograph knowledge.

3.5. Factors Associated with Attitude towards Partograph.

According to the multivariable analysis obstetric care providers, working in a hospital, were 5.04 times more likely to have a favorable attitude towards partograph than those working in health centers (AOR (95% C.I): 5.04 (1.60–15.80)). Similarly, obstetric caregivers who had received on-the-job training on partograph were also 3.37 times more likely to have a favorable attitude towards partograph than their counterparts (AOR (95% C.I): 3.37 (1.76–6.44)). Furthermore, care providers that learnt about partograph college and/or university were 2.13 times more likely to have a favorable attitude towards partograph (AOR (95% C.I): 2.13 (1.17–3.87)) (see Table 7).

Pearson correlation coefficient between knowledge and attitude was ($r = 0.370$). The degree of relationship between the two variables was moderate (see Table 8).

Table 5: Attitude of obstetric caregivers on partograph and its use, East Gojjam Zone, Northwest Ethiopia, 2015 ($n = 273$).

Attitude variables	Response (agreed) (n)	Percentage
Like to use partograph	111	40.7
Partograph is important to monitor labor	171	62.6
Partograph should be used in all labor	181	66.3
Partograph use reduces risks of maternal and/neonatal morbidity and mortality	175	64.1
Partograph helps early detection for surgery or CS	183	67.0
Wish to use partograph routinely	174	63.7
Not all normal labors need partograph	89	32.6
Using partograph is the only responsibility of physicians	83	30.4
Partograph is not effective to monitor labor	84	30.8
Using partograph is time consuming	107	39.2
Overall attitude		
Favorable attitude	150	55
Unfavorable attitude	123	45

4. Discussion

This study found that above half of the caregivers had good knowledge and favorable attitude about partograph and its use. Knowledge of partograph was higher among those within the age of 25–29 years old, regularly working in antenatal and family planning ward, who had partograph training and those who had learnt partograph at their college or university-level education. On the other hand, obstetric caregivers working in the hospital had good knowledge and training on partograph and had a favorable attitude towards partograph utilization. Overall utilization (53.8%) of the partograph was lower than the knowledge and attitude of the care providers.

In this study above half (56.1%) of the obstetric caregivers had good knowledge about partograph. But there is a knowledge gap in specific areas like when to start plotting on the partograph and the functions of the alert line on the partograph. The reported knowledge is closely related to a study done in Amhara Region, Ethiopia [21], but it was lower than another study done in North Shoa, Ethiopia [19]. This good knowledge score might be obtained due to training opportunities or supportive supervisions and the integration of partograph in routine intrapartum care. Moreover, it was true that on-the-job training on partograph had a positive influence on partograph knowledge [18].

In this study, 55% of the obstetric care providers had a favorable attitude towards partograph and its use. This finding was much lower than a study done in Port-Said and Ismailia Cities as more than 90% of the caregivers had positive attitude towards partograph [22]. A study done in Uganda found that the health workers perceived that use of partograph is useful in helping them to detect abnormal labor [23]. However, in Kenya obstetric caregivers had a negative

TABLE 6: Factors associated with knowledge of partograph, East Gojjam Zone, Northwest Ethiopia, 2015 ($n = 273$).

Variables	Partograph knowledge		Crude odds ratio (95% C.I)	Adjusted odds ratio (95% C.I)
	Poor	Good		
	n (%)	n (%)		
Age in years				
≤24	39 (54.93)	32 (45.07)	1.00	1.00
25–29	45 (35.16)	83 (64.84)	**2.25 (1.24–4.06)**[**]	**2.47 (1.32–4.64)**[**]
≥30	36 (48.65)	38 (51.35)	1.29 (0.67–2.47)	1.76 (0.86–3.59)
Regular working department				
Outpatient department	29 (59.18)	20 (40.82)	1.00	1.00
Delivery ward	63 (44.68)	78 (55.32)	1.80 (0.93–3.47)	1.74 (0.87–3.52)
Antenatal care	13 (27.66)	34 (72.34)	**3.79 (1.61–8.93)**[**]	**4.94 (1.97–12.40)**[**]
Family planning	15 (41.67)	21 (58.33)	2.03 (0.85–4.86)	**2.61 (1.03–6.61)**[*]
Obstetric training				
No	88 (48.35)	94 (51.65)	1.00	1.00
Yes	32 (35.16)	59 (64.84)	**1.73 (1.03–2.90)**[*]	0.98 (0.45–2.15)
Partograph training				
No	98 (50.26)	97 (49.74)	1.00	1.00
Yes	22 (28.21)	56 (71.79)	**2.57 (1.46–4.54)**[**]	**2.25 (1.21–4.19)**[*]
Learnt partograph				
No	48 (59.26)	33 (40.74)	1.00	1.00
Yes	72 (37.50)	120 (62.50)	**2.42 (1.43–4.12)**[**]	**2.14 (1.17–3.93)**[*]
Profession				
Nurse	70 (45.2)	85 (54.8)	1.00	
Midwifes	32 (43.2)	42 (56.8)	1.08 (0.61–1.88)	
Public Health Officer	15 (40.5)	22 (59.5)	1.20 (0.58–2.50)	
Others	3 (42.9)	4 (57.1)	1.09 (0.23–5.07)	
Clinical service years				
≤3 years	55 (41.7%)	77 (58.3%)	1	
4–6 years	35 (40.2%)	52 (59.8%)	1.06 (0.61–1.84)	
≥7 years	30 (55.6%)	24 (44.4%)	0.57 (0.30–1.08)	

Significant at [*] p value < 0.05 and [**] p value < 0.01. Others: medical doctor and masters of emergency and emergency obstetrics.

attitude towards using partograph [24]. These differences might be attributed to differences in study area, which might be explained by differing strategies and commitments in implementing the health policy at the various levels throughout the country and different levels of knowledge of the obstetric care providers towards partograph. In addition, the difference in study participants might have a difference in attitude towards partograph.

Knowledge about partograph was significantly higher among obstetric caregivers within the age group of 25–29 years old as compared to those below 25 years. It might be because as the age of individual increases, the probability of acquiring comprehensive knowledge of the partograph would also be increased. This could be related to experience or on-the-job training as refresher training on partograph or obstetric care had a positive relationship in the knowledge and use of the partograph [16]. Moreover, they might be the only one to be consulted by their junior obstetric caregivers and thus might update themselves.

Furthermore, knowledge about partograph was significantly higher among obstetric care providers who had ever received on-the-job training on partograph. In addition, those obstetrics care givers who have had favorable attitude likely to have better knowledge as compare to unfavorable knowledge. This finding was supported by another study done in Southwestern Nigeria, Addis Ababa and North Shoa, Ethiopia [17–19]. This might be due to the fact that obstetric care providers that received on-job training might enhance their better knowledge or understanding of the partograph than others that in turn improves their partograph utilization.

Knowledge of the partograph was significantly associated with participants that learnt partograph on their formal educational curriculum at university or college level, which was supported by a study done in Southwest Nigeria [12]. This University or college-level formal education on partograph might improve their knowledge and skills, later on improving utilization of partograph as supported by another study [16]. Therefore, this brings the need to introduce some form of obstetric/partograph training or continued professional development its value. Those participants who had been working at antenatal care and family planning department were independently associated with knowledge

TABLE 7: Factors associated with attitude towards partograph, East Gojjam Zone, Northwest Ethiopia, 2015 ($n = 273$).

Variables	Attitude towards partograph		Crude odds ratio (95% C.I)	Adjusted odds ratio (95% C.I)
	Unfavorable n (%)	Favorable n (%)		
Health facilities				
Health center	119 (48.37)	127 (51.63)	1.00	1.00
Hospital	4 (14.81)	23 (85.19)	**5.39 (1.81–16.04)****	**5.04 (1.60–15.80)****
Regular working department				
Outpatient department	31 (63.27)	18 (36.73)	1.00	1.00
Delivery ward	53 (37.59)	88 (62.41)	**2.86 (1.46–5.61)****	**2.26 (1.09–4.65)****
Antenatal care	23 (48.94)	24 (51.06)	1.80 (0.80–4.06)	1.97 (0.82–4.72)
Family planning	16 (44.44)	20 (55.56)	2.15 (0.90–5.18)	2.53 (0.99–6.43)
Obstetric training				
No	96 (52.75)	86 (47.25)	1.00	1.00
Yes	27 (29.67)	64 (70.33)	**2.65 (1.55–4.52)*****	1.32 (0.59–2.94)
Learnt partograph				
No	53 (65.43)	28 (34.57)	1.00	1.00
Yes	70 (35.46)	122 (63.54)	**3.30 (1.92–5.68)*****	**2.13 (1.17–3.87)****
Partograph training				
No	105 (53.85)	90 (46.15)	1.00	1.00
Yes	18 (23.08)	60 (76.92)	**3.89 (2.14–7.07)*****	**3.37 (1.76–6.44)*****
Profession				
Nurse	80 (51.6)	75 (48.4)	1.00	1.00
Midwifes	27 (36.5)	47 (63.5)	**1.85 (1.05, 3.27)***	0.58 (0.27–1.27)
Public health officer	15 (40.5)	22 (59.5)	1.56 (0.75–3.24)	1.62 (0.74–3.53)
Others	1 (14.3)	6 (85.7)	6.40 (0.75–54.41)	0.62 (0.04–8.11)
Clinical service years				
≤3 years	54 (40.9%)	78 (59.1%)	1	
4–6 years	44 (50.6%)	43 (49.4%)	0.68 (0.39–1.17)	
≥7 years	25 (46.3%)	29 (53.7%)	0.80 (0.42–1.52)	

Significant at *p value < 0.05, **p value < 0.01, and ***p value < 0.001.

TABLE 8: Degree of relationship between the knowledge and attitude of the obstetrics care providers.

	Pearson correlation		
	Knowledge	Attitude	p value
Knowledge	1	0.370**	0.000
Attitude	0.370**	1	0.000

**Correlation is significant at the 0.01 level (2-tailed).

of partograph, though the association was marginally significant in case of participants who worked at family planning department. This might be due to the fact that obstetric caregivers assigned in antenatal care and family planning departments could have a better chance of receiving training on partograph which might improve their knowledge about partograph than others.

Obstetric caregivers' attitude towards partograph was significantly higher among those who were working a hospital. The knowledge and attitude have positive correlation: that is, as the knowledge of the participants increased, the attitude also increased and vice versa. The likely explanation for this might be that obstetric caregivers working in the hospital might have good knowledge as it was corroborated by a study done in Addis Ababa [19]. Furthermore, as it is supported by this study's finding, they might have on-the-job training on partograph which builds a favorable attitude on partograph and the importance of its utilization.

5. Conclusion

More than half of the obstetric care providers had good knowledge and favorable attitude about partograph. Partograph knowledge was higher among obstetric caregivers within the age of 25–29 years old, had in-service partograph training, and those who had college and/or university-level education about partograph and who were regularly working at the antenatal care and family planning departments. Those who had on-the-job training on partograph and who had college and/or university-level education about partograph had significant association with favorable attitude. Knowledge had effects to have favorable attitude and vice versa. Therefore, a greater emphasis should be given for preservice and on-job training for obstetric caregivers to improve their knowledge and attitude about partograph.

Competing Interests

The authors declare that they have no competing interests.

Authors' Contributions

Desalegne Amare Zelellw and Teketo Kassaw Tegegne wrote the proposal, participated in data collection, analyzed the data, and wrote the paper. Girma Alem Getie was participated in data collection, data analysis, and paper writing. The authors revised drafts of the paper. All authors read and approved the final paper.

Acknowledgments

The authors would like to acknowledge and thank Debre Markos University for Financial and Technical Support. The authors would like to thank their data collectors and the supervisors for their invaluable effort; without them this study would not have come to be completed. The authors' deep gratitude also goes to their study participants who volunteered and took their time to give them all the relevant information for the study. Last but not least, the authors would like to thank all district health offices and health facilities for their cooperation and help during the data collection.

References

[1] WHO, UNICEF, UNFPA, and The World Bank and the United Nations Population Division, *Trends in Maternal Mortality: 1990 to 2013, "Estimates by WHO, UNICEF, UNFPA, The World Bank and the United Nations Population Division"*, World Health Organization, 2014.

[2] Maternal Mortality Rates, *A Tabulation of Available Information*, WHO document FHE/86-3, 2nd edition, 1996.

[3] USAID, Fistula Center, Engender Health for a Better Life, and Intra Health, *Prevention of Prolonged and Obstructed Labor*, 2004.

[4] World Health Organization, *Trends in Maternal Mortality: 1990-2008. Estimates Developed by WHO, UNICEF, UNFPA and The World Bank*, World Health Organization, Geneva, Switzerland, 2010.

[5] WHO/UNICEF/UNFPA, *Maternal Mortality in 2000: Estimates Developed by the WHO, UNICEF and UNFPA*, World Health Organization, Geneva, Switzerland, 2004.

[6] K. S. Khan, D. Wojdyla, L. Say, A. M. Gülmezoglu, and P. F. Van Look, "WHO analysis of causes of maternal death: a systematic review," *The Lancet*, vol. 367, no. 9516, pp. 1066–1074, 2006.

[7] V. Briand, A. Dumont, M. Abrahamowicz et al., "Maternal and perinatal outcomes by mode of delivery in senegal and mali: a cross-sectional epidemiological survey," *PLoS ONE*, vol. 7, no. 10, Article ID e47352, 2012.

[8] Central Statistical Agency and ORC Macro, *Ethiopia Demographic and Health Survey 2011*, Central Statistical Agency, Addis Ababa, Ethiopia; ORC Macro, Calverton, Md, USA, 2012.

[9] WHO, "World Health Organization partograph in management of labour," *The Lancet*, vol. 343, no. 8910, pp. 1399–1404, 1994.

[10] N. Magon, "Partograph revisited," *International Journal Clinical Cases Investigation*, vol. 3, no. 1, pp. 1–2, 2011.

[11] A. Ness, J. Goldberg, and V. Berghella, "Abnormalities of the first and second stages of labor," *Obstetrics and Gynecology Clinics of North America*, vol. 32, no. 2, pp. 201–220, 2005.

[12] A. O. Fawole, K. I. Hunyinbo, and D. A. Adekanle, "Knowledge and utilization of the partograph among obstetric care givers in south west Nigeria," *African Journal of Reproductive Health*, vol. 12, no. 1, pp. 22–29, 2008.

[13] E. Friedman, "The graphic analysis of labor," *American Journal of Obstetrics and Gynecology*, vol. 68, no. 6, pp. 1568–1575, 1954.

[14] R. H. Philpott and W. M. Castle, "Cervicographs in the management of labour in primigravidae. I. The alert line for detecting abnormal labour," *Journal of Obstetrics and Gynaecology of the British Commonwealth*, vol. 79, no. 7, pp. 592–598, 1972.

[15] WHO, *Preventing Prolonged Labor: A Pratcical Guide, "The Partograph Part I: Principles and Strategy. Maternal Health and Safemotherhood Programe Division of Family Health"*, World Health Ogranization, Geneva, Switzerland, 1994.

[16] B. O. Ita, E. A. Udeme, O. O. Afiong, J. E. Ekere, U. A. Thomas, and E. Monjok, "An evaluation of the knowledge and utilization of the partogragh in primary, secondary, and tertiary care settings in Calabar, South-South Nigeria," *International Journal of Family Medicine*, vol. 2014, Article ID 105853, 9 pages, 2014.

[17] A. O. Fawole, D. A. Adekanle, and K. I. Hunyinbo, "Utilization of the partograph in primary health care facilities in southwestern Nigeria," *Nigerian Journal of Clinical Practice*, vol. 13, no. 2, pp. 200–204, 2010.

[18] N. Wakgari, G. A. Tessema, and A. Amano, "Knowledge of partograph and its associated factors among obstetric care providers in North Shoa Zone, Central Ethiopia: a cross sectional study," *BMC Research Notes*, vol. 8, article 407, 2015.

[19] E. Yisma, B. Dessalegn, A. Astatkie, and N. Fesseha, "Knowledge and utilization of partograph among obstetric care givers in public health institutions of Addis Ababa, Ethiopia," *BMC Pregnancy and Childbirth*, vol. 13, article 17, 2013.

[20] Federal Democratic Republic of Ethiopia Ministry of Health, "Health Sector Development Program IV 2010/11–2014/15 Final Draft," 2010.

[21] F. Abebe, D. Birhanu, W. Awoke, and T. Ejigu, "Assessment of knowledge and utilization of the partograph among health professionals in Amhara region, Ethiopia," *Science Journal of Clinical Medicine*, vol. 2, no. 2, pp. 26–42, 2013.

[22] N. S. Salama, I. M. A. Allah, and M. F. Heeba, "The partograph: knowledge, attitude, and utilization by professional birth attendances in Port-Said and Ismailia cities," *Medical Journal of Cairo University*, vol. 78, no. 1, pp. 165–174, 2010.

[23] S. Gwang, Z. Karyabakabo, and E. Rutebemberwa, "Assessment of partogram use during labour in Rujumbura Health Sub District, Rukungiri District, Uganda," *African Health Sciences*, vol. 9, no. 1, 2009.

[24] Z. P. Qureshi, C. Sekadde-Kingondu, and S. M. Mutiso, "Rapid assessment of Partograph utilisation in selected maternity units in Kenya," *East African Medical Journal*, vol. 87, no. 6, pp. 235–241, 2010.

17

Prevalence of *Schistosoma mansoni* Infection in Four Health Areas of Kisantu Health Zone, Democratic Republic of the Congo

R. Khonde Kumbu,[1,2,3] **K. Mbanzulu Makola,**[4] **and Lu Bin**[1]

[1]*Key Laboratory of Environment and Health, Ministry of Education and Ministry of Environmental Protection and State Key Laboratory of Environmental Health (Incubating), School of Public Health, Tongji Medical College, Huazhong University of Science and Technology, Wuhan, Hubei 430030, China*

[2]*Department of Pediatrics, Faculty of Medicine, University of Kinshasa, P.O. Box 747, Kinshasa, Democratic Republic of the Congo*

[3]*Department of Pediatrics, Faculty of Medicine, Catholic University of Bukavu, P.O. Box 285, Bukavu, South Kivu, Democratic Republic of the Congo*

[4]*Department of Tropical Medicine, Infectious and Parasitic Diseases, Faculty of Medicine, University of Kinshasa, P.O. Box 747, Kinshasa, Democratic Republic of the Congo*

Correspondence should be addressed to Lu Bin; lubin@mails.tjmu.edu.cn

Academic Editor: Rashidul Haque

Background. Schistosomiasis is a public health problem in Democratic Republic of the Congo but estimates of its prevalence vary widely. The aim of this study was to determine prevalence of *Schistosoma mansoni* infection and associated risk factors among children in 4 health areas of Kisantu health zone. *Methods.* A cross-sectional study was carried out in 4 health areas of Kisantu health zone. 388 children randomly selected were screened for *S. mansoni* using Kato Katz technique and the sociodemographic data was collected. Data were entered and encoded using software EpiData version 3.1. Analysis was performed using SPSS version 21 software. *Results.* The prevalence of *S. mansoni* was 26.5% (103); almost two-thirds (63) (61.2%) had light infection intensity. A significant association was found between *S. mansoni* infection and age ($p = 0.005$), educational level ($p = 0.001$), and practices of swimming/bathing ($p < 0.001$) and using water from river/lake/stream for domestic use ($p < 0.001$). Kipasa health area had high prevalence of schistosomiasis (64.6%) (64/99; 95% CI 54.4–74.0) compared to other health areas. *Conclusion.* *Schistosoma mansoni* infection still remains a public health problem in these areas. There is a need to promote health education and promote behavioral changes in children towards schistosomiasis.

1. Introduction

Worldwide, schistosomiasis is still a global health problem in the 21st century. It continues to threaten millions of people, particularly in Sub-Saharan Africa [1, 2]. By its prevalence, schistosomiasis ranks 1st of diseases transmitted by water and has 2nd place for its public health importance in tropical and subtropical areas of the globe, behind malaria [3]. It is estimated that 600 million people are at risk of schistosomiasis. Among them 200 million people in 74 countries are infected, of whom 120 million are symptomatic and 20 million

people have severe disease; 85% live in Sub-Saharan Africa [4, 5].

School children constitute a high risk group and are the worst affected by schistosomiasis [6]. The standard curves of prevalence of age for *Schistosoma mansoni*, which are based on the excretion of eggs, show that the prevalence and intensity of infection peak are between 10 and 15 years, after which the prevalence decreases gradually over the years and intensity of infection declines more rapidly [7]. The age distribution of the prevalence and intensity of infection are usually attributed to the high levels of contact with contaminated water cercariae in school aged children and adolescents followed by less contact with water and the development of a protective acquired immunity against infection in older adolescents and in adulthood [8, 9].

Globally, in the African Region of WHO, 10 countries account for 67.4% of the total number of people that require preventive chemotherapy [10]. Democratic Republic of the Congo (DRC) is one of the endemic countries for schistosomiasis which WHO has ranked among countries where preventive chemotherapy is required [10]. Schistosomiasis has been found present in some provinces for over a century [11]. However, there is a particular lack of surveillance activity related to schistosomiasis in the DRC. Kongo Central (Bas-Congo) is one of the endemic provinces for schistosomiasis in the DRC as highlighted by Madinga et al. [12]. At present, there are only estimates of the disease burden of schistosomiasis which are inaccurate due to lack of studies and these authors emphasize that there is an urgent need to investigate the prevalence of neglected tropical diseases [13].

2. Materials and Methods

The pilot survey was carried out from January 2016 to February 2016 in Kisantu health zone (KHZ) situated in the province of Kongo Central in the western part of Democratic Republic of the Congo, with a rainy season from September 15 to May 15 and a dry season from May 15 to September 15 of each year. The population of KHZ is estimated at 183,749 inhabitants, whose principal activity is agriculture. The weakness of agriculture does not allow the population to cover the needs of 100% of the population of KHZ [14]. The major causes of morbidity remain the unhealthiness, promiscuity, lack of latrines, and social debridement with increasing of sexually transmitted infections [14]. KHZ is crossed by several rivers including the Inkisi River, Ngufu River, Lassa River, Wolokoso River, Luwuwa River, and Kiela River. These rivers contain snails, intermediate hosts of schistosomes. The most snail species found along these rivers are *Biomphalaria pfeifferi*; however *Bulinus forskalii* are also reported [14, 15]. The more prevalent water is free flowing, with a low flow rate, which promotes domestic use of this water. However, there is also stagnant water.

KHZ is composed of 15 health areas, rural, semirural, and urban. In total 4 health areas (HA) were selected based on the level of the degree of urbanization. These 4 HA were Kipasa rural HA crossed by rivers Kiela and Lassa, Nkandu semirural HA, Kitanu 1 urban HA, and Kitanu 2 semirural HA.

The study population was randomly selected within the community from these 4 health areas. A total of 388 children participated in the study by responding to a questionnaire and providing the required faeces samples.

The parasitological examination was performed by the method of Kato Katz [16] in the laboratory of Tropical Medicine/Faculty of Medicine of University of Kinshasa. It had a faeces sample obtained by means of a spatula. It was passed through a sieve to remove the coarse particles. 41.7 mg of these faeces was collected using a mold and placed on a slide glass and then covered with a piece of cellophane

that has kept for at least 24 hours in a glycerin solution with malachite green. The blade was turned so that the covered sample of cellophane is placed against a flat surface. It correctly makes straight smear; reading and counting were made at ×400 magnification of the optical microscope. The number of eggs found was multiplied by 24 in order to obtain the number of eggs per gram of feces (EPG). According to WHO guidelines, parasite egg counts were used to classify *Schistosoma mansoni* infection into light (1–99 EPG), moderate (100–399 EPG), or heavy infection intensity ($\geq$400 EPG) [6].

Data were entered and encoded using software Epidata version 3.1. Analysis was performed using SPSS version 21 software. Descriptive statistics were presented as mean ± standard deviation for the continuous data and percentages for categorical data. Pearson's chi-square was used to compare proportions. p values less than 0.05 were considered statistically significant.

2.1. Ethical Considerations. Ethical approval was provided by Ethics Committee of the School of Public Health of the Faculty of Medicine/University of Kinshasa (approbation number ESP/CE/077/15) in Democratic Republic of the Congo. Before inclusion, written informed consent was obtained from the parents or legal tutor. Each informed consent was signed. For those who did not know how to sign for any reason, we took a thumb print instead of the signature.

3. Results

In total, three hundred and eighty-eight (388) children from 10 to 18 years with a mean age of 12.7 ± 2.05 years were included in the study. Of the 388 children examined, 212 (54.8%) were males while 176 (45.2%) were females. From these 388 children examined, 103 (26.5%) were infected with *S. mansoni* and 54 (52.4%) children were males versus 49 (47.6%) females. Of 103 children infected by *S. mansoni*, almost two-thirds (66) (64%) were in the age group of 10–12 years, 31 (30%) were in the age group of 13–15 years, and 6 (6%) were in the age group of 16–18 years. Among these infected children, 63 (61.2%) were found with a light infection intensity while 25 (24.3%) had a moderate infection and only 15 (14.5%) children had a heavy infection intensity. Schistosomiasis was associated with age ($p = 0.005$) and educational level ($p = 0.001$). According to educational system of Democratic Republic of the Congo, primary school is from grade 1 to grade 6 and secondary school is from grade 7 to grade 12. The mean time taken by children from home to river/lake/stream was 16.68 minutes with minimum time of 1 minute and maximum of 120 minutes. Schistosomiasis was significantly associated ($p < 0.001$) with practices of swimming/bathing in open water ($p < 0.001$) and of using water from river/lake/stream for domestic use, but it was not associated with profession of father ($p = 0.09$) and mother ($p = 0.08$) who were largely farmers (Table 1). Children of Kipasa health area had high prevalence of schistosomiasis (64.6%) (64/99; 95% CI 54.4–74.0) compared to other health areas (Table 2).

TABLE 1: *Schistosoma mansoni* infection and associated factors in the four health areas of Kisantu health zone.

Variables	Schistosoma presence				Total number	Total percent	χ^2	p value
	Positive		Negative					
	Number	Percent	Number	Percent				
Gender								
Male	54	25.5	158	74.5	212	54.8	0.27	0.59
Female	49	27.8	127	72.2	176	45.2		
Age								
10–12	66	33.5	131	66.5	197	50.8		
13–15	31	20.8	118	79.2	149	38.4	10.64	0.005*
16–18	6	14.3	36	85.7	42	10.8		
Educational level								
Primary	90	31.7	194	68.3	284	73.2		
Secondary	12	12.2	86	87.8	98	25.3	14.43	0.001*
Not at school	1	16.7	5	83.3	6	1.5		
Swim/bath in open water								
Never	35	16.7	175	83.3	210	54.1		
Rarely	26	31.0	58	69.0	84	21.7	27.2	<0.001*
Always	42	44.7	52	55.3	94	24.2		
Using water from river/lake/stream for domestic use								
Never	26	24.3	81	75.7	107	27.6		
Rarely	30	18.0	137	82.0	167	43.0	19.18	<0.001*
Always	47	41.2	67	58.8	114	29.4		
Profession of father								
Farmer	73	29.70	173	70.30	246	63.40	2.95	0.09
Other	30	21.10	112	78.90	142	36.60		
Profession of mother								
Farmer	87	28.80	215	71.20	302	77.80	3.07	0.08
Other	16	18.60	70	81.40	86	22.20		
Total	103	26.5	285	73.5	388	100.0		

*Significant association $p < 0.05$.

TABLE 2: Prevalence of *Schistosoma mansoni* infection in the four health areas of Kisantu health zone.

Heath area	Number		Percent	95% CI
	Examined	Infected		
KIPASA	99	64	64.6	54.4–74.0
NKANDU	98	11	11.2	5.6–18.8
KITANU 1	95	21	22.1	14.2–31.9
KITANU 2	96	7	7.3	3.1–14.7
Total	388	103	26.5	22.3–31.3

4. Discussion

This descriptive study showed that schistosomiasis still remains a real public health problem in the four health areas. Schistosomiasis prevalence rate was 26.5% (103).

The findings are close to those reported in Songololo Territory, Democratic Republic of the Congo (31.2%) [17], and in Nigeria (32.2%) [18] while that is less than those found in several studies in Tanzania (64.3%) [19], (68%) in Mali [20], and (82.7%) in Kasansa health zone, Democratic Republic of the Congo [21]. However, that is higher than those found in other studies elsewhere, 6.4% in Mokali health area, Democratic Republic of the Congo [22], and 8.0% and 9.3% in Yemen [23, 24].

The prevalence was similar in both genders (25.5% for males and 27.8% for females) with $p = 0.59$. In DRC, especially in KHZ, males are more in contact with water due to their habits of swimming/bathing in this open water; however, females help their mother in household activities and usually go to water for domestic activities such as laundry and doing dishes. This could explain the fact that both male and female are equally infected. These findings are similar to those found by several authors, especially in Mali [20], in Kenya [25], in Ethiopia [26], and in Democratic Republic of the Congo [21]. However, the results differ from several studies where male predominance was reported in Yemen [24], in Ethiopia [27], and in Ghana [28].

The intensity infection showed that the largest number of infected children (61.2%) (63) had light intensity. The findings are similar to those reported in Ethiopia [27, 29], in Democratic Republic of the Congo [22], and in Yemen [23]. However, these results are opposite to those found in Nigeria [18] and in Ethiopia [26, 30].

The findings showed that schistosomiasis was associated with age and educational level. Montresor et al. emphasized that children are more vulnerable and susceptible to infection because of their poor hygiene and playing habits in the water [31]. Most infected children were in age group 10–12 years. Younger children are those who have most habits to play/swim/urinate/defecate into the water and being close to water river/lake/stream increases this risk of contracting schistosomiasis. These results are close to those in Nigeria [32], in Senegal [33], in Ethiopia [26], and in Tanzania [19]. However, other authors found different results in Ethiopia [34] and in Côte d'Ivoire [35]. Association between schistosomiasis and educational level was also reported in Ethiopia [29].

The mean time taken by children to reach river was 16.68 minutes; it means that they were close to the water and being close to water increases the risk of contracting schistosomiasis as that was reported in Zambia [36], in Côte d'Ivoire [37], and in Yemen [24].

The findings showed that schistosomiasis was significantly associated with practices of swimming/bathing in open water ($p < 0.001$); these results are similar to those found in Ghana [28], Nigeria [18], and Ethiopia [29].

The findings also showed that schistosomiasis was significantly associated with practices using water from river/lake/stream for domestic use ($p < 0.001$); just 27.6% never used this water at home. These results are similar to those found in Nigeria [18, 32], in Kenya [38], in Yemen [24], and in Ethiopia [27, 29, 30].

Although farming activities are often associated with schistosomiasis, the findings showed that the prevalence was not associated with farming activities of parents ($p = 0.09$ for father and $p = 0.08$ for mother); these results are similar to those found in Côte d'Ivoire [37] and in Yemen [24]. However, other studies found the opposite, as in Ethiopia [27, 34] and in Ghana [28].

Children of Kipasa health area had high prevalence of schistosomiasis (64.6%) (64/99; 95% CI 54.4–74.0) compared to other health areas. Unfortunately, this study did not assess the factors associated with infection that could explain this difference. However, this high rate could be explained by the fact that this health area is crossed by two rivers, the Lassa River and the Kiela River, which are incriminated as shelter for snails, intermediate hosts of *Schistosoma* [15], and children living there are more closely in contact with these rivers and therefore more at risk of being infected by schistosomiasis compared to children living in the other three health areas.

5. Conclusion

The study conducted among children in Kisantu health zone revealed that schistosomiasis remains a major public health problem. Schistosomiasis was associated with age, educational level, and the practices of swimming/bathing/using water from river for domestic use and Kipasa health area had a high prevalence.

Therefore, there is a need to promote health education of children and parents, to enhance communication for behavior change towards schistosomiasis and to promote the fight for the elimination of snails.

Competing Interests

The authors declare that there is no conflict of interests regarding the publication of this paper.

Acknowledgments

The authors' gratitude goes to the persons that permitted the realization of this project: David Lupande, Henrique Mathe, Maurice Khonde, Brigitte Muaka, Nissi Bafwa, and Ma Huiting.

References

[1] M. J. Van Der Werf, S. J. De Vlas, S. Brooker et al., "Quantification of clinical morbidity associated with schistosome infection in sub-Saharan Africa," *Acta Tropica*, vol. 86, no. 2-3, pp. 125–139, 2003.

[2] B. J. Vennervald and D. W. Dunne, "Morbidity in schistosomiasis: an update," *Current Opinion in Infectious Diseases*, vol. 17, no. 5, pp. 439–447, 2004.

[3] A. Rougemont and J. Brunet-Jailly, *Health Planning, Management, and Evaluation in Tropical Countries*, Doin Éditeurs, 1989.

[4] WHO, "Prevention and control of schistosomiasis and soil-transmitted helminthiasis," Technical Report Series 912, World Health Organization, Geneva, Switzerland, 2002.

[5] L. Chitsulo, D. Engels, A. Montresor, and L. Savioli, "The global status of schistosomiasis and its control," *Acta Tropica*, vol. 77, no. 1, pp. 41–51, 2000.

[6] A. Montresor, *Lutte Contre les Helminthiases Chez les Enfants D'âge Scolaire: Guide à L'intention des Responsables des Programmes de Lutte*, World Health Organization, Geneva, Switzerland, 2004.

[7] J. R. Verani, B. Abudho, S. P. Montgomery et al., "Schistosomiasis among young children in Usoma, Kenya," *The American Journal of Tropical Medicine and Hygiene*, vol. 84, no. 5, pp. 787–791, 2011.

[8] P. R. Dalton and D. Pole, "Water-contact patterns in relation to Schistosoma haematobium infection," *Bulletin of the World Health Organization*, vol. 56, no. 3, pp. 417–426, 1978.

[9] A. E. Butterworth, M. Capron, J. S. Cordingley et al., "Immunity after treatment of human schistosomiasis mansoni. II. Identification of resistant individuals, and analysis of their immune responses," *Transactions of the Royal Society of Tropical Medicine and Hygiene*, vol. 79, no. 3, pp. 393–408, 1985.

[10] WHO, *Schistosomiasis: Progress Report 2001–2011, Strategic Plan 2012–2020*, World Health Organization, Geneva, Switzerland, 2013.

[11] WHO, *Epidemiology and Control of Schistosomiasis: Report of a WHO Expert Committee*, World Health Organisation, Geneva, Switzerland, 1967.

[12] J. Madinga, S. Linsuke, L. Mpabanzi et al., "Schistosomiasis in the democratic Republic of Congo: a literature review," *Parasites & Vectors*, vol. 8, no. 1, article 601, pp. 1–10, 2015.

[13] A. W. Rimoin and P. J. Hotez, "NTDs in the heart of darkness: the Democratic Republic of Congo's unknown burden of neglected tropical diseases," *PLoS Neglected Tropical Diseases*, vol. 7, no. 7, Article ID e2118, 2013.

[14] Kisantu Health Zone, Central Office Archives, Kongo Central, Democratic Republic of Congo, 2015.

[15] J. Gillet and J. Wolfs, "Les bilharzioses humaines. au Congo Belge et au Ruanda-Urundi," *Bulletin of the World Health Organization*, vol. 10, no. 3, pp. 315–419, 1954.

[16] N. Katz, A. Chaves, and J. Pellegrino, "A simple device for quantitative stool thick-smear technique in *Schistosomiasis mansoni*," *Revista do Instituto de Medicina Tropical de São Paulo*, vol. 14, no. 6, pp. 397–400, 1972.

[17] C. Lengeler, J. Makwala, D. Ngimbi, and J. Utzinger, "Simple school questionnaires can map both *Schistosoma mansoni* and *Schistosoma haematobium* in the Democratic Republic of Congo," *Acta Tropica*, vol. 74, no. 1, pp. 77–87, 2000.

[18] O. A. Morenikeji and B. A. Idowu, "Studies on the prevalence of urinary schistosomiasis in Ogun State, South-Western Nigeria," *West African Journal of Medicine*, vol. 30, no. 1, pp. 62–65, 2011.

[19] H. D. Mazigo, R. Waihenya, G. Mkoji et al., "Intestinal schistosomiasis: prevalence, knowledge, attitude and practices among school children in an endemic area of north western Tanzania," *Journal of Rural and Tropical Public Health*, vol. 9, pp. 53–60, 2010.

[20] H. Sangho, A. Dabo, O. Sangho, A. Diawara, and O. Doumbo, "Prevalence and perception of schistosomiasis in irrigated rice field area in Mali," *Le Mali Medical*, vol. 20, no. 3, pp. 15–20, 2004.

[21] S. Linsuke, S. Nundu, S. Mupoyi et al., "High prevalence of *Schistosoma mansoni* in six health areas of—Kasansa health zone, Democratic Republic of the Congo: short report," *PLoS Neglected Tropical Diseases*, vol. 8, no. 12, Article ID e3387, 2014.

[22] J. R. Matangila, J. Y. Doua, S. Linsuke et al., "Malaria, schistosomiasis and soil transmitted helminth burden and their correlation with anemia in children attending primary schools in Kinshasa, Democratic Republic of Congo," *PLoS ONE*, vol. 9, no. 11, Article ID e110789, 2014.

[23] H. Sady, H. M. Al-Mekhlafi, W. M. Atroosh et al., "Knowledge, attitude, and practices towards schistosomiasis among rural population in Yemen," *Parasites & Vectors*, vol. 8, no. 1, pp. 1–13, 2015.

[24] H. Sady, H. M. Al-Mekhlafi, M. A. K. Mahdy, Y. A. L. Lim, R. Mahmud, and J. Surin, "Prevalence and associated factors of schistosomiasis among children in yemen: implications for an effective control programme," *PLoS Neglected Tropical Diseases*, vol. 7, no. 8, Article ID e2377, 2013.

[25] S. Nagi, E. A. Chadeka, T. Sunahara et al., "Risk factors and spatial distribution of schistosoma mansoni infection among primary school children in Mbita District, Western Kenya," *PLoS Neglected Tropical Diseases*, vol. 8, no. 7, article e2991, 2014.

[26] G. Alebie, B. Erko, M. Aemero, and B. Petros, "Epidemiological study on *Schistosoma mansoni* infection in Sanja area, Amhara region, Ethiopia," *Parasites and Vectors*, vol. 7, no. 1, article 15, 2014.

[27] A. Assefa, T. Dejenie, and Z. Tomass, "Infection prevalence of *Schistosoma mansoni* and associated risk factors among schoolchildren in suburbs of Mekelle city, Tigray, Northern Ethiopia," *Momona Ethiopian Journal of Science*, vol. 5, no. 1, pp. 174–188, 2013.

[28] F. Anto, V. Asoala, M. Adjuik et al., "Childhood activities and schistosomiasis infection in the Kassena-Nankana district of Northern Ghana," *Journal of Infectious Diseases and Therapy*, vol. 2, article 152, 2014.

[29] T. Essa, Y. Birhane, M. Endris, A. Moges, and F. Moges, "Current status of *Schistosoma mansoni* infections and associated risk factors among students in Gorgora town, Northwest Ethiopia," *ISRN Infectious Diseases*, vol. 2013, Article ID 636103, 7 pages, 2013.

[30] L. Worku, D. Damte, M. Endris, H. Tesfa, and M. Aemero, "Schistosoma mansoni infection and associated determinant factors among school children in Sanja Town, northwest Ethiopia," *Journal of Parasitology Research*, vol. 2014, Article ID 792536, 7 pages, 2014.

[31] A. Montresor, D. W. T. Crompton, A. Hall, D. A. P. Bundy, and L. Savioli, *Guidelines for the Evaluation of Soil-Transmitted Helminthiasis and Schistosomiasis at Community Level*, World Health Organization, Geneva, Switzerland, 1998.

[32] O. Adeyeba and S. Ojeaga, "Urinary schistosomiasis and concomitant urinary tract pathogens among school children in metropoitan Ibadan, Nigeria," *African Journal of Biomedical Research*, vol. 5, no. 3, 2010.

[33] B. Senghor, A. Diallo, S. N. Sylla et al., "Prevalence and intensity of urinary schistosomiasis among school children in the district of Niakhar, region of Fatick, Senegal," *Parasites and Vectors*, vol. 7, no. 1, article 5, 2014.

[34] S. Geleta, A. Alemu, S. Getie, Z. Mekonnen, and B. Erko, "Prevalence of urinary schistosomiasis and associated risk factors among Abobo Primary School children in Gambella Regional State, southwestern Ethiopia: a cross sectional study," *Parasites and Vectors*, vol. 8, no. 1, article 215, 2015.

[35] K. D. Adoubryn, J. Ouhon, C. G. Yapo, E. Y. Assoumou, K. M. L. Ago, and A. Assoumou, "Profil épidémiologique des schistosomoses chez les enfants d'âge scolaire dans la région de l'Agnéby (sud-est de la Côte-d'Ivoire)," *Bulletin de la Société de Pathologie Exotique*, vol. 99, no. 1, pp. 28–31, 2006.

[36] A. Lemma, "Background and historical review. Another development in schistosomiasis: the case of Endod for use as a molluscicide," in *Phytolacca Dodecandra (Endod): Final Report of the International Scientific Workshop, Lusaka, Zambia, March 1983/editors, Aklilu Lemma, Donald Heyneman, Sitali M. Silangwa*, Zambian Natl Council for Scientific Research by Tycooly Internatl Pub, Dublin, Republic of Ireland, 1984.

[37] B. Matthys, A. B. Tschannen, N. T. Tian-Bi et al., "Risk factors for *Schistosoma mansoni* and hookworm in urban farming communities in western Côte d'Ivoire," *Tropical Medicine & International Health*, vol. 12, no. 6, pp. 709–723, 2007.

[38] T. Handzel, D. M. S. Karanja, D. G. Addiss et al., "Geographic distribution of schistosomiasis and soil-transmitted helminths in Western Kenya: implications for anthelminthic mass treatment," *The American Journal of Tropical Medicine and Hygiene*, vol. 69, no. 3, pp. 318–323, 2003.

18

Antifungal Susceptibility Patterns of *Candida* Species Recovered from Endotracheal Tube in an Intensive Care Unit

Elham Baghdadi,[1] Sadegh Khodavaisy,[2,3] Sassan Rezaie,[3] Sara Abolghasem,[4] Neda Kiasat,[5] Zahra Salehi,[6] Somayeh Sharifynia,[7] and Farzad Aala[2]

[1]*Department of Microbiology, Faculty of Science, Islamic Azad University, Varamin-Pishva Branch, Tehran, Iran*

[2]*Department of Medical Parasitology and Mycology, Kurdistan University of Medical Sciences, P.O. Box 14155-6446, Sanandaj, Iran*

[3]*Division of Molecular Biology, Department of Medical Mycology and Parasitology, School of Public Health, Tehran University of Medical Sciences, Tehran, Iran*

[4]*Department of Microbiology, Faculty of Science, Islamic Azad University, North Tehran Branch, Tehran, Iran*

[5]*Department of Medical Mycology, Jondishapour University of Medical Sciences, Ahvaz, Iran*

[6]*Department of Medical Mycology, Tarbiat Modares University, Tehran, Iran*

[7]*Clinical Tuberculosis and Epidemiology Research Center, National Research Institute of Tuberculosis and Lung Diseases (NRITLD), Shahid Beheshti University of Medical Sciences, Tehran, Iran*

Correspondence should be addressed to Farzad Aala; farzadaala@yahoo.com

Academic Editor: Anastasia Kotanidou

Aims. Biofilms formed by *Candida* species which associated with drastically enhanced resistance against most antimicrobial agents. The aim of this study was to identify and determine the antifungal susceptibility pattern of *Candida* species isolated from endotracheal tubes from ICU patients. *Methods.* One hundred forty ICU patients with tracheal tubes who were intubated and mechanically ventilated were surveyed for endotracheal tube biofilms. Samples were processed for quantitative microbial culture. Yeast isolates were identified to the species level based on morphological characteristics and their identity was confirmed by PCR-RFLP. Antifungal susceptibility testing was determined according to CLSI document (M27-A3). *Results.* Ninety-five strains of *Candida* were obtained from endotracheal tubes of which *C. albicans* ($n = 34$; 35.7%) was the most frequently isolated species followed by other species which included *C. glabrata* ($n = 24$; 25.2%), *C. parapsilosis* ($n = 16$; 16.8%), *C. tropicalis* ($n = 12$; 12.6%), and *C. krusei* ($n = 9$; 9.4%). The resulting MIC_{90} for all *Candida* species were in increasing order as follows: caspofungin (0.5 μg/mL); amphotericin B (2 μg/mL); voriconazole (8.8 μg/mL); itraconazole (16 μg/mL); and fluconazole (64 μg/mL). *Conclusion.* *Candida* species recovered from endotracheal tube are the most susceptible to caspofungin.

1. Introduction

Nosocomial infections are an important cause of mortality and increasing hospital costs [1]. The infection is usually transmitted to susceptible patients through infected medical staff and equipment by pathogenic organisms [2]. Biofilms are microbial communities embedded in biopolymer matrix on living or nonliving substrates [3]. According to the National Institutes of Health America, approximately 80% of hospital infections are associated with microbial biofilms [4]. Important microorganisms involved in microbial biofilm formation predominantly consist of many species of both fungal and bacterial. Among pathogenic fungi, *Candida* species are the most common cause of superficial and systemic disease [5]. *Candida* species can aggregate on medical devices such as venous and urinary catheters, dentures, and ocular implants by biofilms [3, 6, 7]. *Candida* biofilms can identify in individuals with certain circumstances, such as immunocompromised patients, HIV infected, cancerous, and organ transplant recipients. Ventilator-associated pneumonia is the most frequent intensive care unit (ICU) acquired infection among patients ventilated through tracheostomy or endotracheal intubation [8]. This topic can provide the conditions such as prolonged hospitalization and use of a variety of devices for colonization and creating biofilms by *Candida* species. Biofilms formed by these fungal organisms are associated with drastically enhanced resistance against most antifungal therapy [8, 9]. Several studies show that antifungal agents, that is, amphotericin B, fluconazole, itraconazole, and ketoconazole, displayed less activity against *Candida albicans* biofilms formed on the PVC disk [10–12]. In addition, non-*C. albicans* have shown resistance to two new antifungal drugs (voriconazole and ravuconazole), but it seems that antibiofilm activity of amphotericin B lipid formulation and also echinocandins have existed [13]. Therefore the aim of the present study was to evaluate antifungal susceptibility testing of *Candida* spp. isolated from endotracheal tubes in ICU patients.

2. Materials and Methods

This study was carried out in the Intensive Care Unit of the Imam Khomeini and Golestan Hospitals, Ahvaz, during January–September 2015. One hundred forty ICU patients with tracheal tubes who were intubated and mechanically ventilated were surveyed for endotracheal tube biofilms. The length of hospitalization was at least two weeks prior to sampling. Collected endotracheal tubes of patients who had clinical manifestation of pneumonia including cough, purulent respiratory secretion, fever, and new or progressive infiltration of lung in CXR were placed in sealed sterile bottles and referred immediately to the laboratory for processing. From the central region of each endotracheal tube 1 cm section was cut and processed for quantitative microbial culture.

2.1. Morphological and Molecular Identification. The specimens were inoculated onto Sabouraud Dextrose Agar (SDA, Difco) supplemented with chloramphenicol and incubated at 37°C for two days. Primarily, yeast colonies were identified by conventional tools such as colony color on CHROMagar *Candida* medium (CHROMagar Company, Paris, France), germ tube tests in serum at 37°C for 2-3 h, and microscopic morphology on cornmeal agar (Difco Laboratories, Detroit, Mich., USA) with 1% Tween 80. Confirmation molecular approaches were adjusted. Genomic DNA was extracted, using the method of glass bead disruption, and the PCR-RFLP method was performed as described previously [14].

2.2. Antifungal Susceptibility Testing. MICs (minimum inhibitory concentrations) of identified *Candida* isolates were determined according to recommendations stated in the Clinical and Laboratory Standards Institute (CLSI) M27-A3 document [15]. Amphotericin B (Sigma, St. Louis, MO, USA), fluconazole (Pfizer, Groton, CT, USA), itraconazole (Janssen Research Foundation, Beerse, Belgium), voriconazole (Pfizer, Groton, CT, USA), and caspofungin (Merck, Whitehouse Station, NJ, USA) were obtained as reagent-grade powders from the respective manufacturers for preparation of the CLSI microdilution trays. Inoculum was prepared by gently scraping the surface of the fungal colonies with a sterile

cotton swab moistened with sterile physiological saline. Conidial suspensions were adjusted to transmission of 75% to 77% at 530 nm (approximate 1×10^6–5×10^6 CFU/mL). The inoculum suspensions, including mostly nongerminated conidia, were diluted 1 : 1000 in RPMI 1640 medium and the final inoculum in assay wells was between 0.5×10^3 and 5×10^3 CFU/mL. The microdilution trays were incubated at 35°C for 24–48 h. MICs were determined visually by comparison of the growth in the wells containing the drug with the drug-free control. *Candida parapsilosis* (ATCC 22019) and *Candida krusei* (ATCC 6258) reference strains were for quality control.

3. Results

Out of one hundred forty ICU patients hospitalized, ninety-five strains of *Candida* which were obtained from endotracheal tubes were studied. The positive specimens belonged to 67 male and 28 female hospitalized patients. The duration of being intubated had a median of 9 days and hospital stay duration average was 29 ± 3.6 days. The isolates were confirmed based on species level using PCR-RFLP of which *C. albicans* (n = 34; 35.7%) was the most frequently isolated species, followed by *C. glabrata* (n = 24; 25.2%), *C. parapsilosis* (n = 16; 16.8%), *C. tropicalis* (n = 12; 12.6%), and *C. krusei* (n = 9; 9.4%). Table 1 summarizes the results of *in vitro* antifungal susceptibility profiles (MIC range, geometric mean MIC, MIC_{50}, and MIC_{90}) of several antifungal drugs against all *Candida* species. The resulting MIC_{50} for all *Candida* species were in increasing order as follows: caspofungin (0.5 μg/mL); amphotericin B (1 μg/mL); voriconazole (0.25 μg/mL); itraconazole (0.75 μg/mL); and fluconazole (4 μg/mL). Results showed the widest range and the highest MICs for fluconazole (0.016–≥64 μg/mL), voriconazole (0.016–≥16 μg/mL), and itraconazole (0.016–≥16 μg/mL). Results revealed statistically significant differences when comparing the susceptibility of *C. albicans* and non-*albicans Candida* to fluconazole, voriconazole, and itraconazole ($P < 0.05$) with *C. albicans* being found to be the most susceptible to these antifungal agents. MIC results among all the isolates of *Candida* species showed that they were fully susceptible to caspofungin (Table 2).

4. Discussion

Candida is opportunistic pathogen which causes a life-threatening infection with high rates of mortality especially in immunocompromised individuals [16]. The pathogenicity of *Candida* species is attributed to certain virulence factors, mostly production of biofilm [17, 18]. *Candida* species are now recognized as major agents of hospital-acquired infection. Almost invariably, an implanted device such as an urinary catheter or endotracheal tube is associated with these infections [18]. *Candida* species can cause significant problems of medical settings as persistent and recurrent device related infections [19, 20]. This properties also differed among different species of *Candida* [17, 21]. In this study *C. albicans* (35.7%) was the most common species obtained from endotracheal tube, compatible with other studies that mentioned that *C. albicans* is considered as major etiologic

TABLE 1: *In vitro* susceptibilities of *Candida* spp. recovered from endotracheal tube to antifungal agents. MIC range, geometric mean, MIC_{50}, and MIC_{90} values are expressed in $\mu g/mL$.

Species (n)	Antifungal agents	Ranges	MIC_{50}	MIC_{90}	GM
Total *Candida* spp. (95)	Amphotericin B	0.062–4	1	2	0.420
	Itraconazole	0.016–≥16	0.75	4	0.847
	Voriconazole	0.016–≥16	0.25	4	0.381
	Fluconazole	0.016–≥64	4	64	2.881
	Caspofungin	0.008–2	0.5	0.5	0.294
C. albicans (34)	Amphotericin B	0.062–2	0.5	2	0.178
	Itraconazole	0.016–≥16	0.062	16	0.242
	Voriconazole	0.016–≥16	0.031	8	0.119
	Fluconazole	0.016–≥64	0.5	8	0.999
	Caspofungin	0.008–0.5	0.5	0.5	0.182
C. glabrata (24)	Amphotericin B	0.062–2	1	2	0.706
	Itraconazole	0.016–16	8	16	3.121
	Voriconazole	0.016–16	0.5	16	0.684
	Fluconazole	0.25–16	16	64	5.941
	Caspofungin	0.125–1	0.5	0.75	0.390
C. parapsilosis (16)	Amphotericin B	0.016–1	0.25	0.5	0.158
	Itraconazole	0.016–0.5	0.5	0.5	0.249
	Voriconazole	0.016–0.5	0.125	0.25	0.157
	Fluconazole	0.125–4	2	2	1
	Caspofungin	0.125–0.5	0.5	0.5	0.314
C. tropicalis (12)	Amphotericin B	1–4	2	4	2
	Itraconazole	1–≥64	16	16	7.245
	Voriconazole	0.125–4	2	2	1
	Fluconazole	4–≥64	16	—	19.02
	Caspofungin	0.008–2	0.5	0.5	0.458
C. krusei (9)	Amphotericin B	0.062–2	2	—	0.447
	Itraconazole	0.031–8	0.37	—	0.398
	Voriconazole	0.125–16	0.25	—	0.870
	Fluconazole	0.016–4	32	—	2.512
	Caspofungin	0.008–2	0.375	—	0.353

GM: geometric mean.

agent in candidiasis [16, 17, 20]. Other studies reported that the ability of biofilm production in *C. parapsilosis* and *C. glabrata* was significantly less than *C. albicans* [17, 21]. Biofilm phenotype in non-*C. albicans* species is the cause of the survival and well adapted to colonization of tissues and indwelling devices [20]. This difference in our results probably is due to variety of biofilms formation among *Candida* species from different sources. Mahmoudabadi et al. showed a higher percentage *C. albicans* (41.7%) which have recovered from blood samples in comparison with other sources [21]. In our investigation, other species of *Candida* included *C. glabrata* (25.2%), *C. parapsilosis* (16.8%), *C. tropicalis* (12.6%), and *C. krusei* (9.4%) obtained from endotracheal tubes. These data are in agreement with the findings of a previous study [22–25]. Also Shokohi et al., Richter et al., and Papon et al. mentioned *C. glabrata* as the most common non-*C. albicans* species in their investigation [24–27]. Deorukhkar et al.'s

study indicated *C. tropicalis* (29.4%) as the major non-*C. albicans* species isolate followed by *C. glabrata* (20.7%) that is incompatible with these studies [28, 29]. The obtained antifungal susceptibility patterns indicated that *C. albicans* isolates were highly susceptible to caspofungin (100%) (MIC $\leq 2\,\mu g/mL$). These findings are in agreements with other studies that reported [30, 31]. In this investigation 26.4% of *C. albicans* strains were resistant to fluconazole (MIC $\geq 64\,\mu g/mL$), whereas other studies reported the rates of this resistance as 45.83%, 11.9%, 74.2%, 2.7%, and 38.7%, respectively [27, 32–35]. Studies by Shokohi et al., Al-Mamari et al., Aher et al., Awari, and Roy et al. indicated the resistance of *C. albicans* to itraconazole as 5.4%, 10.3%, 36.9%, 35%, and 19.3%, respectively [26, 32, 36, 37]. However, in our finding 35.2% of *C. albicans* strains were shown to be resistant to itraconazole MIC $\geq 1\,\mu g/mL$. In our study 14.7% of *C. albicans* isolates were resistant to voriconazole (MIC

TABLE 2: MIC interpretation of five antifungal drugs against *Candida* spp. recovered from endotracheal tube.

Antifungal agents		C. albicans n = 34 (%)	C. glabrata n = 24 (%)	C. parapsilosis n = 16 (%)	C. tropicalis n = 12 (%)	C. krusei n = 9 (%)
Amphotericin B	S	28 (82.3)	20 (83.3)	16 (100)	10 (83.3)	7 (77.7)
	R	6 (17.6)	4 (16.6)	—	2 (16.7)	2 (22.2)
Itraconazole	S	20 (58.8)	12 (50)	6 (37.5)	4 (33.3)	3 (33.3)
	DD	2 (5.8)	6 (25)	10 (62.5)	—	5 (55.5)
	R	12 (35.2)	6 (25)	—	8 (66.6)	1 (11.1)
Voriconazole	S	27 (79.4)	11 (45.8)	12 (75)	4 (33.3)	6 (66.6)
	DD	2 (5.8)	5 (20.8)	4 (25)	3 (25)	2 (22.2)
	R	5 (14.7)	8 (33.3)	—	5 (41.6)	1 (11.1)
Fluconazole	S	22 (64.7)	3 (12.5)	14 (87.5)	3 (25)	5 (55.5)
	DD	3 (8.8)	2 (8.3)	2 (12.5)	4 (33.3)	2 (22.2)
	R	9 (26.4)	19 (79.1)	—	5 (41.6)	2 (22.2)
Caspofungin	S	34 (100)	24 (100)	16 (100)	12 (100)	9 (100)
	R	—	—	—	—	—

S: susceptible; R: resistance; DD: dose-dependent.

$\geq 1\,\mu g/mL$) that was different from results of Zang et al. and Badiee and Alborzi's studies [23, 38]. MIC range (0.016–$\geq 16\,\mu g/mL$) and MIC$_{90}$ ($8\,\mu g/mL$) for voriconazole in present study were different from results by Zhang et al. and Badiee and Alborzi which reported MIC range and MIC90 as 0.0313–$4\,\mu g/mL$ and $0.25\,\mu g/mL$ and 0.003–$16\,\mu g/mL$ and $4\,\mu g/mL$, respectively [23, 38]. In addition, 17.6% of *C. albicans* isolates in our study were indicated to be resistant to amphotericin B MIC $\geq 2\,\mu g/mL$. The result was to some extent similar to the result reported by of Aher et al. (13.8%) and differs from results by Njunda et al. (54.4%), Awari et al. (7.5%), and Zhang et al. (1.1%) [26, 33, 35, 37–39]. MIC range (0.062–$2\,\mu g/mL$) and MIC$_{90}$ ($2\,\mu g/mL$) for amphotericin B in present study differ from the data reported by Bosco-Borgeat et al. which reported MIC Range and MIC$_{90}$ as 0.13–$1\,\mu g/mL$ and $0.5\,\mu g/mL$, respectively [39]. Our data indicated that 79.1% of *C. glabrata* were resistance to itraconazole. These data are in disagreement with the rate of itraconazole resistance *C. glabrata* in studies by Shokohi et al. (12.5%), Haddadi et al. (21%), and Deorukhkar et al. (46.2%) [27, 29, 40]. Also Aher reported 46.4% and 40% resistance to fluconazole and itraconazole, respectively; these mentioned rates differ from the results of our investigation [26]. Our study has shown that fluconazole MIC$_{90}$ values (8, 64, and $2\,\mu g/mL$), itraconazole (16, 16, and $0.5\,\mu g/mL$), and voriconazole (8, 16, and 0.25) against *C. albicans*, *C. glabrata*, and *C. parapsilosis*, respectively, according to study by Badiee and Alborzi in regard to fluconazole rates are lower (16, 128, and 4) and itraconazole and voriconazole have higher amount (2, 16, and 0.25 and 4, 3, and 0.033), respectively [23]. In fact, MIC$_{90}$ in *C. glabrata* as the main non-*Candida albicans* to fluconazole, itraconazole, and voriconazole was higher than *C. albicans* and *C. parapsilosis*. MIC$_{90}$ fluconazole, itraconazole, and voriconazole for *C. glabrata* in our investigation were 64, 16, and 16. Long term fluconazole and itraconazole prophylaxis were accompanied with reduction in sensitivity to these

agents and recently *C. glabrata* known as naturally less susceptible to azoles compared to other *Candida* species [35, 41, 42]. Our study has shown that amphotericin B and caspofungin MIC$_{90}$ values were 2, 2, and $0.5\,\mu g/mL$ and 0.5, 0.75, and $0.5\,\mu g/mL$ against *C. albicans*, *C. glabrata*, and *C. parapsilosis*, respectively. However in other studies MIC$_{90}$ values of amphotericin B were lower (0.25, 0.5, and $0.25\,\mu g/mL$) [23]. In present study 87.5%, 37.5%, and 75% of *C. parapsilosis* strains were susceptible to fluconazole, itraconazole, and voriconazole, respectively. This result is similar to that by Shokohi et al. who found no resistance species among them. Badiee et al. obtained 6.9% and 3.5% resistance to fluconazole and itraconazole, respectively. In addition they find no voriconazole resistance *C. parapsilosis* among them. In addition Zhang et al.'s findings show 15.4% resistance to fluconazole; however there was no resistance to itraconazol and voriconazole [23, 27, 38]. In our study we find that 41.6%, 66.6%, and 41.6% of *C. tropicalis* were resistant to fluconazole, itraconazole, and voriconazole, respectively. In contrast, Shokohi et al. did not find resistance species in their study. Also Zhang et al. and Aher et al. obtained 10.7% and 4.8% and 52% and 56% of isolates which were resistant to fluconazole and itraconazole, respectively [26, 27, 38]. However *C. tropicalis* isolates were highly susceptible to caspofungin and amphotericin B (100%, 83.3%). Therefore these antifungals seem to be the most active drug for candidiasis treatment. In our study MIC$_{90}$ of fluconazole, itraconazole, and voriconazole for *C. parapsilosis* were 2, 0.5, and $0.25\,\mu g/mL$ whereas Zhang et al., Tay et al., and Bonfietti et al. obtained 2, 0.062, and $0.25\,\mu g/mL$, 4, 0.19, and $0.047\,\mu g/mL$, 2, 0.06, and $0.03\,\mu g/mL$, respectively, as MIC$_{90}$ to mention antifungal drugs [38, 43, 44]. Our results indicated that *C. parapsilosis* isolates from endotracheal tube were highly susceptible to caspofungin and amphotericin B; this data also shows that the concentration of $0.5\,\mu g/mL$ of this medicine is able to inhibit 90% of mentioned isolates.

5. Conclusion

Knowledge of *Candida* species distribution and antifungal resistance pattern of them plays an important role in appropriate therapy. Our results suggest that *Candida* species recovered from endotracheal tube are the most susceptible to caspofungin, followed by amphotericin B, voriconazole, itraconazole, and fluconazole.

Competing Interests

The authors declare no competing interests.

Acknowledgments

The authors are grateful to Dr. Hamid Badali, Mohammad Reza Safari, and Azar Berahmeh for their help in part of the analysis. The authors wish to thank the staff of Imam Khomeini and Golestan Hospitals for help in technical assistance to sampling.

References

[1] R. P. Wenzel, "Nosocomial candidemia: risk factors and attributable mortality," *Clinical Infectious Diseases*, vol. 20, no. 6, pp. 1531–1534, 1995.

[2] S. Khodavaisy, M. Nabili, B. Davari, and M. Vahedi, "Evaluation of bacterial and fungal contamination in the health care workers' hands and rings in the intensive care unit," *Journal of Preventive Medicine and Hygiene*, vol. 52, no. 4, pp. 215–218, 2011.

[3] L. J. Douglas, "Candida biofilms and their role in infection," *Trends in Microbiology*, vol. 11, no. 1, pp. 30–36, 2003.

[4] O. Gudlaugsson, S. Gillespie, K. Lee et al., "Attributable mortality of nosocomial candidemia, revisited," *Clinical Infectious Diseases*, vol. 37, no. 9, pp. 1172–1177, 2003.

[5] P. Afshar, S. Khodavaisy, S. Kalhori, M. Ghasemi, and T. Razavyoon, "Onychomycosis in North-East of Iran," *Iranian Journal of Microbiology*, vol. 6, no. 2, pp. 98–103, 2014.

[6] P. K. Mukherjee and J. Chandra, "*Candida* biofilm resistance," *Drug Resistance Updates*, vol. 7, no. 4-5, pp. 301–309, 2004.

[7] E. M. Kojic and R. O. Darouiche, "Candida infections of medical devices," *Clinical Microbiology Reviews*, vol. 17, no. 2, pp. 255–267, 2004.

[8] M. Aliyali, M. Hedayati, M. Habibi, and S. Khodavaisy, "Clinical risk factors and bronchoscopic features of invasive aspergillosis in intensive care unit patients," *Journal of Preventive Medicine and Hygiene*, vol. 54, no. 2, pp. 80–82, 2013.

[9] G. S. Baillie and L. J. Douglas, "Matrix polymers of *Candida* biofilms and their possible role in biofilm resistance to antifungal agents," *Journal of Antimicrobial Chemotherapy*, vol. 46, no. 3, pp. 397–403, 2000.

[10] J. Chandra, P. K. Mukherjee, S. D. Leidich et al., "Antifungal resistance of Candidal biofilms formed on denture acrylic in vitro," *Journal of Dental Research*, vol. 80, no. 3, pp. 903–908, 2001.

[11] S. A. Yazdanparast, S. Khodavaisy, H. Fakhim et al., "Molecular characterization of highly susceptible *Candida africana* from vulvovaginal candidiasis," *Mycopathologia*, vol. 180, no. 5-6, pp. 317–323, 2015.

[12] N. Jain, R. Kohli, E. Cook, P. Gialanella, T. Chang, and B. C. Fries, "Biofilm formation by and antifungal susceptibility of *Candida* isolates from urine," *Applied and Environmental Microbiology*, vol. 73, no. 6, pp. 1697–1703, 2007.

[13] J.-L. Vincent, E. Anaissie, H. Bruining et al., "Epidemiology, diagnosis and treatment of systemic *Candida* infection in surgical patients under intensive care," *Intensive Care Medicine*, vol. 24, no. 3, pp. 206–216, 1998.

[14] H. Mirhendi, K. Makimura, M. Khoramizadeh, and H. Yamaguchi, "A one-enzyme PCR-RFLP assay for identification of six medically important *Candida* species," *Nippon Ishinkin Gakkai Zasshi*, vol. 47, no. 3, pp. 225–229, 2006.

[15] P. Wayne, "Reference method for broth dlution antifungal susceptibility testing of yeasts fungi," Approved Standard M38-A2, 2008.

[16] S. Khodavaisy, M. Alialy, O. S. Mahdavi et al., "The study on fungal colonization of respiratory tract in patients admitted to intensive care units of sari and babol hospitals," *Medical Journal of Mashhad University of Medical Sciences*, vol. 54, no. 3, pp. 177–184, 2011.

[17] S. H. Fesharaki, I. Haghani, B. Mousavi, M. L. Kargar, M. Boroumand, and M. S. Anvari, "Endocarditis due to a co-infection of *Candida albicans* and *Candida tropicalis* in a drug abuser," *Journal of Medical Microbiology*, vol. 62, no. 11, pp. 1763–1767, 2013.

[18] I. Bitar, R. A. Khalaf, H. Harastani, and S. Tokajian, "Identification, typing, antifungal resistance profile, and biofilm formation of *Candida albicans* isolates from Lebanese hospital patients," *BioMed Research International*, vol. 2014, Article ID 931372, 10 pages, 2014.

[19] A. Bruder-Nascimento, C. H. Camargo, A. L. Mondelli, M. F. Sugizaki, T. Sadatsune, and E. Bagagli, "*Candida* species biofilm and *Candida albicans* ALS3 polymorphisms in clinical isolates," *Brazilian Journal of Microbiology*, vol. 45, no. 4, pp. 1371–1377, 2014.

[20] S. Silva, M. Henriques, A. Martins, R. Oliveira, D. Williams, and J. Azeredo, "Biofilms of non-*Candida albicansCandida* species: quantification, structure and matrix composition," *Medical Mycology*, vol. 47, no. 7, pp. 681–689, 2009.

[21] A. Z. Mahmoudabadi, M. Zarrin, and N. Kiasat, "Biofilm formation and susceptibility to amphotericin B and fluconazole in *Candida albicans*," *Jundishapur Journal of Microbiology*, vol. 7, no. 7, Article ID e17105, 2014.

[22] M. Laal Kargar, S. Fooladi-Rad, M. Mohammad Davoodi et al., "Fungal colonization in patients with cystic fibrosis," *Journal of Mazandaran University of Medical Sciences*, vol. 22, no. 2, pp. 204–218, 2013.

[23] P. Badiee and A. Alborzi, "Susceptibility of clinical *Candida* species isolates to antifungal agents by E-test, Southern Iran: a five year study," *Iranian Journal of Microbiology*, vol. 3, no. 4, pp. 183–188, 2011.

[24] N. Papon, V. Courdavault, M. Clastre, and R. J. Bennett, "Emerging and emerged pathogenic *Candida* species: beyond the *Candida albicans* paradigm," *PLoS Pathogens*, vol. 9, no. 9, Article ID e1003550, 2013.

[25] S. S. Richter, R. P. Galask, S. A. Messer, R. J. Hollis, D. J. Diekema, and M. A. Pfaller, "Antifungal susceptibilities of *Candida* species causing vulvovaginitis and epidemiology of recurrent cases," *Journal of Clinical Microbiology*, vol. 43, no. 5, pp. 2155–2162, 2005.

[26] C. S. Aher, "Species distribution, virulence factors and antifungal susceptibility profile of *Candida* isolated from oropharyngeal lesions of HIV infected patients," *International Journal of Current Microbiology and Applied Sciences*, vol. 3, no. 1, pp. 453–460, 2014.

[27] T. Shokohi, Z. Bandalizadeh, M. T. Hedayati, and S. Mayahi, "In vitro antifungal susceptibility of *Candida* species isolated from oropharyngeal lesions of patients with cancer to some antifungal agents," *Jundishapur Journal of Microbiology*, vol. 4, no. 2, pp. S19–S26, 2011.

[28] S. C. Deorukhkar and S. Saini, "Non albicans Candida species: its isolation pattern, species distribution, virulence factors and antifungal susceptibility profile," *International Journal of Medical Science and Public Health*, vol. 2, no. 3, pp. 533–538, 2013.

[29] S. C. Deorukhkar, S. Saini, and S. Mathew, "Non-albicans *Candida* infection: an emerging threat," *Interdisciplinary Perspectives on Infectious Diseases*, vol. 2014, Article ID 615958, 7 pages, 2014.

[30] M. Arendrup, E. Dzajic, R. Jensen et al., "Epidemiological changes with potential implication for antifungal prescription recommendations for fungaemia: data from a nationwide fungaemia surveillance programme," *Clinical Microbiology and Infection*, vol. 19, no. 8, pp. E343–E353, 2013.

[31] M. A. Pfaller, S. A. Messer, L. N. Woosley, R. N. Jones, and M. Castanheira, "Echinocandin and triazole antifungal susceptibility profiles for clinical opportunistic yeast and mold isolates collected from 2010 to 2011: application of new CLSI clinical breakpoints and epidemiological cutoff values for characterization of geographic and temporal trends of antifungal resistance," *Journal of Clinical Microbiology*, vol. 51, no. 8, pp. 2571–2581, 2013.

[32] L. Wiebusch, D. Lonchiati, L. Rodrigues, C. Dantas, A. Almeida, and K. Oliveira, "Profile susceptibility to fluconazole and voriconazole antifungals by species of *Candida albicans* isolated from urine culture," *BMC Proceedings*, vol. 8, supplement 4, article P34, 2014.

[33] A. L. Njunda, D. S. Nsagha, J. C. Assob, H. L. Kamga, and P. Teyim, "In vitro antifungal susceptibility patterns of *Candida albicans* from HIV and AIDS patients attending the Nylon Health District Hospital in Douala, Cameroon," *Journal of Public Health in Africa*, vol. 3, no. 1, p. 2, 2012.

[34] N. T. Wabe, J. Hussein, S. Suleman, and K. Abdella, "In vitro antifungal susceptibility of *Candida albicans* isolates from oral cavities of patients infected with human immunodeficiency virus in Ethiopia," *Retrovirology*, vol. 9, supplement 1, p. P44, 2012.

[35] R. C. Roy, G. D. Sharma, S. R. Barman, and S. Chanda, "Trend of *Candida* infection and antifungal resistance in a tertiary care hospital of north east India," *Blood*, vol. 100, p. 19, 2013.

[36] A. Al-Mamari, M. Al-Buryhi, M. A. Al-Heggami, and S. Al-Hag, "Identify and sensitivity to antifungal drugs of *Candida* species causing vaginitis isolated from vulvovaginal infected patients in Sana'a city," *Der Pharma Chemica*, vol. 6, no. 1, pp. 336–342, 2014.

[37] A. Awari, "Species distribution and antifungal susceptibility profile of *Candida* isolated from urine samples," *International Journal of Applied and Basic Medical Research*, vol. 18, pp. 228–234, 2011.

[38] L. Zhang, S. Zhou, A. Pan, J. Li, and B. Liu, "Surveillance of antifungal susceptibilities in clinical isolates of *Candida* species at 36 hospitals in China from 2009 to 2013," *International Journal of Infectious Diseases*, vol. 33, pp. e1–e4, 2015.

[39] M. E. Bosco-Borgeat, C. G. Taverna, S. Cordoba et al., "Prevalence of candida dubliniensis fungemia in argentina: identification by a novel multiplex PCR and comparison of different phenotypic methods," *Mycopathologia*, vol. 172, no. 5, pp. 407–414, 2011.

[40] P. Haddadi, S. Zareifar, P. Badiee et al., "Yeast colonization and drug susceptibility pattern in the pediatric patients with neutropenia," *Jundishapur Journal of Microbiology*, vol. 7, no. 9, Article ID e11858, 2014.

[41] S. Silva, M. Negri, M. Henriques, R. Oliveira, D. W. Williams, and J. Azeredo, "*Candida glabrata*, *Candida parapsilosis* and *Candida tropicalis*: biology, epidemiology, pathogenicity and antifungal resistance," *FEMS Microbiology Reviews*, vol. 36, no. 2, pp. 288–305, 2012.

[42] F. C. Bizerra, C. Jimenez-Ortigosa, A. C. R. Souza et al., "Breakthrough candidemia due to multidrug-resistant *Candida glabrata* during prophylaxis with a low dose of micafungin," *Antimicrobial Agents and Chemotherapy*, vol. 58, no. 4, pp. 2438–2440, 2014.

[43] L. X. Bonfietti, M. D. A. Martins, M. W. Szeszs et al., "Prevalence, distribution and antifungal susceptibility profiles of *Candida parapsilosis*, *Candida orthopsilosis* and *Candida metapsilosis* bloodstream isolates," *Journal of Medical Microbiology*, vol. 61, part 7, pp. 1003–1008, 2012.

[44] S. T. Tay, S. L. Na, and J. Chong, "Molecular differentiation and antifungal susceptibilities of *Candida parapsilosis* isolated from patients with bloodstream infections," *Journal of Medical Microbiology*, vol. 58, no. 2, pp. 185–191, 2009.

19

Comparison of Clinical and Radiologic Outcome of Adolescent Idiopathic Scoliosis Treated with Hybrid Hook-Screw Instrumentation versus Universal Clamp System

Ebrahim Ghayem Hassankhani,[1] Farzad Omidi-Kashani,[1] Shahram Moradkhani,[2] Golnaz Ghayem Hassankhani,[3] and Mohammad Taghi Shakeri[4]

[1]Orthopedic Research Center, Orthopedic Department, Imam Reza Hospital, Mashhad University of Medical Sciences, Mashhad, Iran
[2]Orthopedic Department, Imam Reza Hospital, Mashhad University of Medical Sciences, Mashhad, Iran
[3]Orthopedic Research Center, Ghaem Hospital, Mashhad University of Medical Sciences, Mashhad, Iran
[4]Faculty of Medicine, Mashhad University of Medical Sciences, Mashhad, Iran

Correspondence should be addressed to Farzad Omidi-Kashani; omidif@mums.ac.ir

Academic Editor: Panagiotis Korovessis

Background. In surgical treatment of adolescent idiopathic scoliosis (AIS), hybrid universal clamp system has been used by some authors. We aimed to compare the clinical and radiologic outcome of hybrid universal clamp with hybrid thoracic hook lumbar screw. *Methods.* A prospective study was performed on 56 consecutive patients with AIS, who had alternatively undergone a posterior spinal fusion and instrumentation with hybrid thoracic hook lumbar screw system (28 patients: group A) and hybrid universal clamp system (28 patients: group B) between June 2006 and January 2014 at Imam Reza University Hospital and had been followed up for more than two years. The comparison was according to radiographic changes, operative time, intraoperative blood loss, complications, and Scoliosis Research Society (SRS-22) outcome scores. *Results.* The preoperative mean curve Cobb angle was $58° \pm 7°$ $(42°–74°)$ in group A and $60° \pm 9°$ $(46°–75°)$ in group B. The mean final coronal curve correction was 60.4% and 75.5% in groups A and B, respectively ($P = 0.001$). Postoperative SRS outcome scores were also comparable. *Conclusion.* Universal clamp instrumentation had a significantly better curve correction and lower complication rate compared with hybrid thoracic hook lumbar screw. Both instrumentation methods had similar operative time, intraoperative blood loss, and postoperative SRS outcome scores.

1. Introduction

The most common systems nowadays used for surgical correction and instrumentation of adolescent idiopathic scoliosis (AIS) are multisegment fixation systems [1–3]. There are various types of posterior instrumentation systems for idiopathic scoliosis such as all hook, all pedicular screw, or hybrid thoracic hook-lumbar pedicular screw instrumentation [4–6]. These systems allow for deformity correction on the coronal, sagittal, and axial planes [2, 7]. The use of imaging techniques such as fluoroscopy, preoperative computed tomography, and navigation system has been recommended by several authors for insertion of pedicle

screws to reduce the neurovascular complications related to malposition of pedicle screws [8, 9]. These techniques can not only improve proper pedicle screw insertion, but also increase the operating time and irradiation [4, 5, 10].

Recently a modified system comprised of soft sublaminar bands associated with metal jaws (clamps) has been proposed by some authors to provide more deformity correction and decrease the operating time, radiation exposure, and blood loss relative to the previous routine spinal implantation. These clamps strongly reduce the most deformed and deviated vertebrae located at the apical region of scoliosis while being attached to the longitudinal rods (hybrid universal clamp system). These soft sublaminar bands apparently decrease the neurovascular risks associated with pedicular screws or wires insertion, provide immediate stability, anchor around the strongest portion of the neural arch, apply less stress at any given point of the bony surface (relative to metal sublaminar hook or wire), and as a result may reduce the risk of cutout fractures during deformity reduction [11, 12]. The purpose of this study was to compare the clinical and radiologic outcome of the hybrid universal clamp with hybrid thoracic hook-lumbar screw instrumentation in the surgical treatment of adolescent idiopathic scoliosis.

2. Materials and Methods

After local institutional review board approval (record number: 930154), we carried out a prospective study on 56 consecutive AIS patients operated on by two surgeons between June 2006 and January 2014 at Imam Reza University Hospital. We included those patients with Lenke type 1, 2, or 3 who had undergone a single posterior approach with either hybrid thoracic hook and lumbar pedicular screw (group A: 28 cases) or hybrid universal clamp technique (group B: 28 patients). We excluded those cases needing two-stage approaches, with major lumbar curves, with congenital or neuromuscular scoliosis, and with scoliosis with underlying spinal cord disorders and those cases with less than 24 months of follow-up. Standing posterior-anterior and lateral and supine bending radiographs and magnetic resonance imaging (MRI) of the total spine were taken from all the cases. Preoperative flexibility (PF) was calculated as follows: [(preoperative standing Cobb angle – supine bending Cobb angle)/preoperative standing Cobb angle] × 100% [13].

In group A, the classic derotation method was used for curve correction and then arthrodesis was performed by facetectomy, decortication, and bone graft (Figure 1). In this group, we aimed to use more screws relative to hooks, but in difficult situations or when the safety of the screw insertion was questionable, we inserted hooks, instead. In fact, all screw technique was too rare in our patients that were negligible. The construct used in group B (Figure 2) consisted of three parts. The proximal part consisted of hook claws (or hook-screw claws) on the two proximal vertebrae. In middle section, sublaminar universal clamp system was used in the concavity. One level was instrumented on the convex side. At the distal end, pedicle screws were used. Intraoperative fluoroscopic guidance was not used. Pedicle screws were placed using the free-hand technique. A frame was obtained with two precontoured 5.5 mm titanium rods united by three transverse connectors (we used the third connector in the apex due to resistance against deforming forces on the rods). The frame was secured to the proximal and distal end. The reduction of deformity was then begun in the center of curve to distal and proximal direction. When the frame was used to reduce the concavity of the thoracic curves, tension was applied to the UC system progressively. Distal screws were tightened at end of correction. Arthrodesis was performed by facetectomy, decortication, and bone graft. All patients had wake-up test during the operation.

TABLE 1: Coronal preoperative, immediate, and final postoperative Cobb angle measurements and final correction in both groups.

Coronal Cobb angle measurements	Group A	Group B	Significance
Mean preoperative	58° (42–74)	60° (46–75)	NS
Mean immediate postoperative	24.5° (14–28)	15° (12.5–19)	$P = 0.001$
Mean final postoperative	28.1° (15–34)	17.4° (13–24)	$P = 000.1$
Mean final curve correction	60.4%	75.5%	$P = 0.001$

After operation, we took standing posterior-anterior and lateral radiographs of the spine and calculated postoperative curve correction (POC) as follows: [(preoperative standing Cobb angle – postoperative standing Cobb angle)/preoperative standing Cobb angle] × 100% [13].

Comparison between pre- and postoperative curves was analyzed by paired-samples t-tests. We set statistical significance as a P value less than 0.05%. The SRS-22 questionnaire was used as our clinical outcomes' measurement tool. Reliability and validity of the Persian version of this questionnaire have already been confirmed [14].

3. Results

56 consecutive patients (42 female, 14 male) with AIS were included in the original study. None of the patients required anterior release and thoracoplasty. All of the patients with AIS (Lenke type 1, 2, or 3 curves) had posterior spinal fusion and instrumentation. 28 patients (20 female, 8 male) are treated with hybrid thoracic hook lumbar screw technique (group A) and 28 patients (22 female, 6 male) with hybrid universal clamp technique (group B). The mean follow-up period was 31.4 ± 5 months (range: 25–108 months).

In preoperative bending films, the PF of the main curve was $58 \pm 8\%$ in group A and $56 \pm 11\%$ in group B. The mean final coronal curve correction was 60.4% (from $58° \pm 7°$ to $18.3° \pm 5°$) in group A and 75.5% (from $60° \pm 9°$ to $15.7° \pm 9°$) in group B. This correction was highly significant, $P < 0.0001$ (Table 1). The mean improvements in sagittal curves were also depicted in Table 2.

There were no differences in the operative time ($P = 0.25$) and blood loss ($P = 0.45$). Postoperative SRS outcome scores were similar in both groups (group A: 94, and group B: 97, $P = 0.19$). There were 4 pedicle hook failures, 4 screws failures, and 3 superficial wound infections in group A and 2 pedicle hook failures in group B.

4. Discussion

The most important purpose in surgical treatment of idiopathic scoliosis is deformity correction on the coronal, sagittal, and axial planes with an effective fusion, fixation, and lowest possible rate of complications. There are various

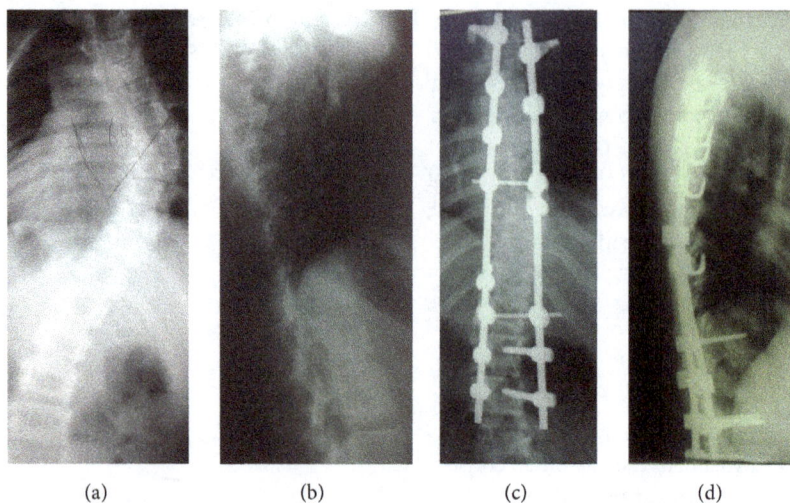

FIGURE 1: (a) and (b) A 17-year-old girl with AIS, with 2-year brace treatment. (c) and (d) After correction, PSF and instrumentation by hybrid thoracic hook lumbar screw technique.

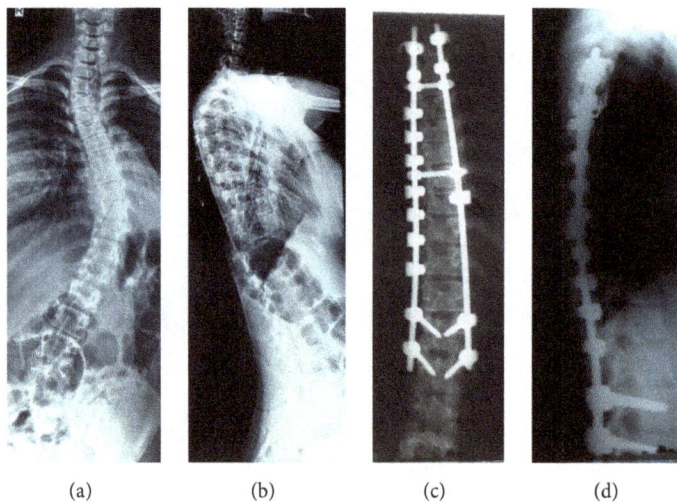

FIGURE 2: (a) and (b) A 16-year-old girl with AIS without brace treatment. (c) and (d) After correction, PSF and instrumentation by hybrid UC technique.

TABLE 2: Sagittal preoperative, immediate, and final postoperative Cobb angle measurements in both groups.

Mean sagittal Cobb angle	Curve	Group A	Group B	Significance
Preoperative	Thoracic	35.2° (3–56)	36.6° (0–68)	NS
	Thoracolumbar	13.8° (−8–22)	14.3° (−11–24)	NS
	Lumbar	−43.6° (−75 to −21)	−42.5° (−68 to −18)	NS
Immediate postoperative	Thoracic	26.6° (15–50)	30.8° (10–58)	NS
	Thoracolumbar	2.9° (−11–3)	2.1° (−13 to 15)	NS
	Lumbar	−42° (−70 to −10)	−40.6° (−61 to −20)	NS
Final postoperative	Thoracic	28.7° (11–55)	27.3° (12–54)	NS
	Thoracolumbar	5.2° (−14–5)	4.8° (−10–15)	NS
	Lumbar	−42° (−73 to −15)	−41.3° (−65 to −18)	NS

types of posterior instrumentation systems for idiopathic scoliosis such as all pedicular hooks, all pedicular screws, lumbar pedicular screws with thoracic hooks (hybrid), hybrid universal clamp, and sublaminar wiring techniques [4, 5, 15].

Many retrospective studies of patients with AIS treated with all-pedicle screw or lumbar pedicular screws with thoracic hooks (hybrid) instrumentation have suggested that conventional all-pedicle screw or lumbar pedicular screws with thoracic hooks (hybrid) constructs tend to worsen flatness of the thoracic spine in AIS [2, 4, 5, 7, 10, 16–18]. Recently Quan and Gibson concluded that in all-pedicle screw constructs the greater the coronal plane correction achieved, the greater the loss of thoracic kyphosis [16]. Vora et al. and Hicks et al. [10, 19] showed in presented series that sagittal balance was more satisfactorily corrected and preserved by hybrid universal clamp technique than by all-pedicle screw technique.

In this study we achieved better correction of coronal and sagittal plans in universal clamp than hybrid techniques. The mean coronal and sagittal curve correction was 75.5% and 80.8% in the universal clamp group while these parameters were 60.4% and 74.3% in hybrid group. To reduce the risk of neurovascular complications related to free-hand insertion of pedicle screws into the thoracic spine specially in all-pedicle screw technique [20, 21], the use of imaging techniques such as fluoroscopy and preoperative computed tomography is needed and recently neuronavigation has been recommended by several authors for safe placement of pedicle screws [8, 9]. These techniques inevitably increase operating time and irradiation exposure. Fluoroscopy is not needed for sublaminar anchorage hybrid universal clamp technique, which can consequently reduce the radiation exposure of the patient, surgeon, and other operating room professionals. In present study we had no significant difference in operation time of both series but irradiation exposure from fluoroscopy was high in all-pedicle screw technique.

There are many reports about the safety of hybrid universal clamp technique. Mazda et al. reported on a group of 75 AIS patients who received hybrid universal clamp technique. There were no complications related to the use of the hybrid universal clamp technique in their report [12].

In pedicle screw technique, screw-related complications may occur due to initial screw malposition or screw pull-out during correction maneuvers resulting in neurological, vascular, or visceral injury [22]. The rate of screw misplacement in the thoracic region has been reported as 5.7 to 50%, and the rate of neurovascular complications varies from 0 to 1% [23–27]. Other complications were infrequent and included pedicle fractures (0.24%), infections (1.9%), screw loosening (0.76%), and a single case of transient paraparesis [28, 29]. Abul-Kasim and Ohlin, in a consecutive series of 81 cases with AIS who had underwent scoliosis surgery, showed in one-third of patients minor screw loosening, 2 years after the intervention, evaluated by low dose CT [30]. We had 12 (5%) misplacements without neurovascular complication, 4 pedicle hook failures, and 4 screws failures in all-pedicle screw or lumbar pedicular screws with thoracic hooks (hybrid) technique but only 2 screws failures in the hybrid universal clamp technique.

Our study has some flaws. One of the most important defects of this study was the heterogeneity of the hybrid group. The ratio of screw to hook was varied but usually this ration was more than 80%, although we did not assess this matter exactly and statistically. We accept this as a flaw in our study and mentioned it in the text. It is recommended that a prospective study would be conducted on three patients groups: all-pedicle screw technique, hybrid hook-screw, and universal clamp, in the future.

5. Conclusion

Universal clamp instrumentation had a significantly better curve correction with lower complication rate compared with hybrid thoracic hook lumbar screw. Both instrumentation methods had similar operative time, intraoperative blood loss, and postoperative SRS outcome scores in the operative treatment of AIS.

Competing Interests

The authors declare that they have no competing interests.

Acknowledgments

The authors thank Orthopedic Research Center Group of Mashhad Medical University for their assistance.

References

[1] J. S. de Gauzy, J.-L. Jouve, F. Accadbled, B. Blondel, and G. Bollini, "Use of the Universal Clamp in adolescent idiopathic scoliosis for deformity correction and as an adjunct to fusion: 2-year follow-up," *Journal of Children's Orthopaedics*, vol. 5, no. 4, pp. 273–282, 2011.

[2] Y. J. Kim, L. G. Lenke, S. K. Cho, K. H. Bridwell, B. Sides, and K. Blanke, "Comparative analysis of pedicle screw versus hook instrumentation in posterior spinal fusion of adolescent idiopathic scoliosis," *Spine*, vol. 29, no. 18, pp. 2040–2048, 2004.

[3] S.-I. Suk, S.-M. Lee, E.-R. Chung, J.-H. Kim, and S.-S. Kim, "Selective thoracic fusion with segmental pedicle screw fixation in the treatment of thoracic idiopathic scoliosis: more than 5-year follow-up," *Spine*, vol. 30, no. 14, pp. 1602–1609, 2005.

[4] I. Cheng, Y. Kim, M. C. Gupta et al., "Apical sublaminar wires versus pedicle screws—which provides better results for surgical correction of adolescent idiopathic scoliosis?," *Spine*, vol. 30, no. 18, pp. 2104–2112, 2005.

[5] J. E. Lowenstein, H. Matsumoto, M. G. Vitale et al., "Coronal and sagittal plane correction in adolescent idiopathic scoliosis: a comparison between all pedicle screw versus hybrid thoracic hook lumbar screw constructs," *Spine*, vol. 32, no. 4, pp. 448–452, 2007.

[6] B. Ilharreborde, J. Even, Y. Lefevre et al., "Hybrid constructs for tridimensional correction of the thoracic spine in adolescent idiopathic scoliosis: a comparative analysis of universal clamps versus hooks," *Spine*, vol. 35, no. 3, pp. 306–314, 2010.

[7] Y. J. Kim, L. G. Lenke, J. Kim et al., "Comparative analysis of pedicle screw versus hybrid instrumentation in posterior spinal fusion of adolescent idiopathic scoliosis," *Spine*, vol. 31, no. 3, pp. 291–298, 2006.

[8] J. J. Carbone, P. J. Tortolani, and L. G. Quartararo, "Fluoroscopically assisted pedicle screw fixation for thoracic and thoracolumbar injuries: technique and short-term complications," *Spine*, vol. 28, no. 1, pp. 91–97, 2003.

[9] Y. J. Kim, L. G. Lenke, K. H. Bridwell, Y. S. Cho, and K. D. Riew, "Free hand pedicle screw placement in the thoracic spine: is it safe," *Spine*, vol. 29, no. 3, pp. 333–342, 2004.

[10] V. Vora, A. Crawford, N. Babekhir et al., "A pedicle screw construct gives an enhanced posterior correction of adolescent idiopathic scoliosis when compared with other constructs: myth or reality," *Spine*, vol. 32, no. 17, pp. 1869–1874, 2007.

[11] M. Takahata, M. Ito, K. Abumi et al., "Comparison of novel ultra-high molecular weight polyethylene tape versus conventional metal wire for sublaminar segmental fixation in the treatment of adolescent idiopathic scoliosis," *Journal of Spinal Disorders and Techniques*, vol. 20, no. 6, pp. 449–455, 2007.

[12] K. Mazda, B. Ilharreborde, J. Even, Y. Lefevre, F. Fitoussi, and G.-F. Penneçot, "Efficacy and safety of posteromedial translation for correction of thoracic curves in adolescent idiopathic scoliosis using a new connection to the spine: The Universal Clamp," *European Spine Journal*, vol. 18, no. 2, pp. 158–169, 2009.

[13] J.-L. Jouve, J. S. de Gauzy, B. Blondel, F. Launay, F. Accadbled, and G. Bollini, "Use of the Universal Clamp for deformity correction and as an adjunct to fusion: preliminary results in scoliosis," *Journal of Children's Orthopaedics*, vol. 4, no. 1, pp. 73–80, 2010.

[14] S. J. Mousavi, B. Mobini, H. Mehdian et al., "Reliability and validity of the persian version of the scoliosis research society-22r questionnaire," *Spine*, vol. 35, no. 7, pp. 784–789, 2010.

[15] R. B. Winter, J. E. Lonstein, and F. Denis, "How much correction is enough?" *Spine*, vol. 32, no. 24, pp. 2641–2643, 2007.

[16] G. M. Y. Quan and M. J. Gibson, "Correction of main thoracic adolescent idiopathic scoliosis using pedicle screw instrumentation: does higher implant density improve correction?" *Spine*, vol. 35, no. 5, pp. 562–567, 2010.

[17] J.-L. Clement, E. Chau, C. Kimkpe, and M.-J. Vallade, "Restoration of thoracic kyphosis by posterior instrumentation in adolescent idiopathic scoliosis: comparative radiographic analysis of two methods of reduction," *Spine*, vol. 33, no. 14, pp. 1579–1587, 2008.

[18] G. P. Vallespir, J. B. Flores, I. S. Trigueros et al., "Vertebral coplanar alignment: a standardized technique for three dimensional correction in scoliosis surgery: technical description and preliminary results in lenke type 1 curves," *Spine*, vol. 33, no. 14, pp. 1588–1597, 2008.

[19] J. M. Hicks, A. Singla, F. H. Shen, and V. Arlet, "Complications of pedicle screw fixation in scoliosis surgery: a systematic review," *Spine*, vol. 35, no. 11, pp. E465–E470, 2010.

[20] R. K. Bergeson, R. M. Schwend, T. DeLucia, S. R. Silva, J. E. Smith, and F. R. Avilucea, "How accurately do novice surgeons place thoracic pedicle screws with the free hand technique?" *Spine*, vol. 33, no. 15, pp. E501–E507, 2008.

[21] H. Senaran, S. A. Shah, P. G. Gabos, A. G. Littleton, G. Neiss, and J. T. Guille, "Difficult thoracic pedicle screw placement in adolescent idiopathic scoliosis," *Journal of Spinal Disorders and Techniques*, vol. 21, no. 3, pp. 187–191, 2008.

[22] A. Sud and A. I. Tsirikos, "Current concepts and controversies on adolescent idiopathic scoliosis: part II," *Indian Journal of Orthopaedics*, vol. 47, no. 3, pp. 219–229, 2013.

[23] K. Abul-Kasim, A. Ohlin, A. Strömbeck, P. Maly, and P. C. Sundgren, "Radiological and clinical outcome of screw placement in adolescent idiopathic scoliosis: evaluation with low-dose computed tomography," *European Spine Journal*, vol. 19, no. 1, pp. 96–104, 2010.

[24] M. Di Silvestre, P. Parisini, F. Lolli, and G. Bakaloudis, "Complications of thoracic pedicle screws in scoliosis treatment," *Spine*, vol. 32, no. 15, pp. 1655–1661, 2007.

[25] B. N. Upendra, D. Meena, B. Chowdhury, A. Ahmad, and A. Jayaswal, "Outcome-based classification for assessment of thoracic pedicular screw placement," *Spine*, vol. 33, no. 4, pp. 384–390, 2008.

[26] U. R. Liljenqvist, H. F. H. Halm, and T. M. Link, "Pedicle screw instrumentation of the thoracic spine in idiopathic scoliosis," *Spine*, vol. 22, no. 19, pp. 2239–2245, 1997.

[27] P. J. Belmont Jr., W. R. Klemme, A. Dhawan, and D. W. Polly Jr., "In vivo accuracy of thoracic pedicle screws," *Spine*, vol. 26, no. 21, pp. 2340–2346, 2001.

[28] G. Li, G. Lv, P. Passias et al., "Complications associated with thoracic pedicle screws in spinal deformity," *European Spine Journal*, vol. 19, no. 9, pp. 1576–1584, 2010.

[29] S.-I. Suk, W.-J. Kim, S.-M. Lee, J.-H. Kim, and E.-R. Chung, "Thoracic pedicle screw fixation in spinal deformities: are they really safe?" *Spine*, vol. 26, no. 18, pp. 2049–2057, 2001.

[30] K. Abul-Kasim and A. Ohlin, "Evaluation of implant loosening following segmental pedicle screw fixation in adolescent idiopathic scoliosis: a 2 year follow-up with low-dose CT," *Scoliosis*, vol. 9, article 13, 2014.

20

Knowledge and Attitude toward Epilepsy of Close Family Members of People with Epilepsy in North of Iran

Narges Karimi[1] and Seyyed Ali Akbarian[2]

[1]Department of Neurology, School of Medicine, Immunogenetics Research Center, Clinical Research Development Unit of
 Bou Ali Sina Hospital, Mazandaran University of Medical Sciences, Sari, Iran
[2]Department of Emergency Medicine, School of Medicine, Mazandaran University of Medical Sciences, Sari, Iran

Correspondence should be addressed to Narges Karimi; drkarimi_236@yahoo.com

Academic Editor: Louis Lemieux

Background. Knowledge and attitudes are required for relatives of people with epilepsy to allow them to better understand and cope with this condition. This study evaluated the knowledge and attitudes of family members of people with epilepsy about the disease. *Methods.* This cross-sectional survey was conducted using a self-administered questionnaire completed by close family members of people with epilepsy at the outpatient clinic of a medical university. The questionnaire included 25 items that determined the demographics and information on the level of knowledge and attitudes about epilepsy. *Results.* The 124 participants had an average age of 36.88 ± 10.68 years. The mean knowledge score was 10.32 ± 2.25 (range: 4 to 15). 87.1% of respondents answered that epilepsy is a brain disorder, 39 (31.5%) said epilepsy is inherited. As a whole, 62 (50%) had good knowledge about the disease. The mean score of attitude was 7.25 ± 1.54 (range: 2 to 10). 83.9% of respondents believed that a person with epilepsy can get married and get pregnant (76.6%). Overall, 15 (12.1%) had negative attitudes and 109 (87.9%) had positive attitudes. *Conclusion.* The main findings of this study indicated good knowledge and a positive attitude about epilepsy among family members of people with epilepsy.

1. Introduction

Epilepsy is a common neurological condition that affects personal and familial behavior and social support [1, 2]. About 50 million people worldwide suffer from epilepsy and the prevalence of active epilepsy in developing countries is 5 to 10 per 100 persons [3]. A prevalence of 0.7–1.8% has been reported in Iran [4]. Individuals with epilepsy may suffer from psychological issues such as depression, anxiety, and psychosis [5]. Accordingly, living with a person with epilepsy will provide some challenges, particularly at home. Studies have reported that relatives of people with epilepsy have an increased risk of anxiety [6]. Epilepsy can inflict an enormous burden on both the people with epilepsy (PWE) and their family caregivers, decreasing their quality of life and daily efficiency [7]. Awareness, knowledge, and attitudes are important qualities for relatives of people with epilepsy to better understand this condition [8]. Studies have shown that people with less awareness and knowledge about epilepsy tend to have negative attitudes toward the

disease and misperceptions such as epilepsy being a form of insanity, untreatable, contagious, and hereditary or a form of mental retardation [9–12]. Cultural beliefs, superstition, and lack of information about epilepsy have perpetuated such misconceptions in developing countries [13–16].

Several factors about people with epilepsy and their caregivers influence the quality of life of patients. These include social disadvantages, family circumstances, seizure frequency, and severity and rate of response to treatment [17]. Studies have demonstrated that people with epilepsy and their relatives do not have adequate basic information about epilepsy including seizure precipitants, types of seizures, and side effects of medications [18]. Misunderstandings and misinformation should be recognized and corrected for optimal care. In Iran, few studies regarding knowledge of people living with epilepsy and their relatives about epilepsy were conducted.

One study in Iran reported that knowledge about epilepsy of relatives of PWE was poor and they tended to have a negative attitude toward the disease [19]. The present study evaluated the level of knowledge and attitudes of family members of people living with epilepsy about the disease.

2. Methodology

This cross-sectional survey was conducted using a self-administered questionnaire completed by adult family members of people with epilepsy at an outpatient clinic of a medical university (Tooba clinic) in Mazandaran province in the city of Sari in northern Iran. The patients have been referred to the clinic from all urban or rural regions of Mazandaran province. This clinic is a tertiary referral center. Approximately 250 neurological patients are seen at the clinic daily.

The participants were the relatives of people with epilepsy who had a close relationship with the patient, lived in the same house, and had heard of epilepsy. The participants were interviewed at the Neurology Outpatient Clinic during patient visits. The respondents included the mothers, fathers, brothers, sisters, or the husband/wife of patients that were over 15 years of age. Iran is a Muslim country with Islamic customs. The populations of Mazandaran province are primarily Shia Muslims.

The questionnaire comprised closed-ended questions to which the responses were either "Yes," "No," or "I do not know." The participants filled out the questionnaire at a prearranged time and location and were not obliged to hurry in their responses. The investigators waited while the questionnaire was completed to offer help if there were any questions. The data was collected from April 2014 through May 2016.

The 25 items were developed after an extensive review of the international literature [20–23]. The questions were translated into Farsi from the English version and then back-translated by psychiatrists and neurologists. Straightforwardness, accuracy, and meaning were carefully checked. A pilot study was conducted with 20 randomly selected family members of people with epilepsy on two separate occasions two weeks apart to determine the feasibility and reliability of the Farsi version of the questionnaire. The reliability of the questionnaire was tested by Cronbach's alpha which resulted in an internal consistency of 0.74.

The questions were divided into three sections. Section 1 requested demographic information including age, gender, marital status, educational level, and occupation. Section 2 investigated the level of knowledge about epilepsy (15 items) and Section 3 explored the attitudes, perception, and beliefs of the respondents toward epilepsy (10 items). Knowledge and attitude were evaluated separately for each participant. Each correct answer was awarded one point and incorrect or "I don't know" responses were awarded scores of zero. For evaluation of total attitude and knowledge of participants, the scores were summed up for each participant. The range for knowledge was 0–15 and for attitude was 0–10. The knowledge score was further categorized as poor (0–5), fair (6–10), or good (11–15). The attitude score was categorized as negative (0–5) or positive (6–10) [21, 24–26].

This project was approved by the ethics committee of the Medical School of Mazandaran University of Medical Sciences. The study was conducted in accordance with the Helsinki declaration on research ethics. Participation was voluntary and the responses were anonymous. After obtaining informed consent, 124 literate subjects were enrolled in the study.

The data was analyzed using SPSS version 20.0. The demographic data and epilepsy knowledge and attitude scores of close relatives were analyzed using descriptive statistics (mean, percentage, and frequency distribution). Chi-square (χ^2) was used to determine the association between variables and demographic data. To assess the relationships between demographic information and the knowledge and attitude scores, regression analysis was conducted. Pearson's correlation was used to determine the association between attitude and knowledge. The results were considered significant at $P < 0.05$.

3. Results

Of the 124 participants, 35.5% ($n = 44$) were males and 64.5% ($n = 80$) were females. The ages ranged from 18 to 58 years with a mean of 36.88 ± 10.68 years. The majority (34.7%) of subjects were 37–47 years of age. Table 1 shows the demographic characteristics of the respondents. There were no differences between males and females regarding age distribution, educational level, or number of family members, but there were differences between gender and marital status and also occupation. The majority of females were married and unemployed.

3.1. Knowledge about Epilepsy. The mean knowledge score was 10.32 ± 2.25 (range: 4 to 15). Of the 124 participants, 4 (3.2%) scored as having poor knowledge; 58 (46.80%) had fair knowledge; and 62 (50%) had good knowledge. The results are summarized in Table 2. When asked about the cause of epilepsy, the majority of participants (108; 87.1%) answered that epilepsy is a brain disorder, 39 (31.5%) said that epilepsy is inherited, 58 (46.8%) said that it is without a specific cause, 54 (43.5%) said that epilepsy is a mental disorder, and also 5 (4%) believed that it is contagious. Of the 124 responders, 10 (8.1%) believed epilepsy to be demonic possession or of supernatural origin. In terms of knowledge about trigger factors for repeated seizures, the responses were as follows: specific foods and drinks (53.5%), sleep deprivation (66.9%), starvation (56.5%), and watching TV or using the computer for a long time (66.1%). In comparison with other disorders, 64 (51.6%) of respondents said that epilepsy is more dangerous than diabetes mellitus but only 17 (13.7%) of participants believed that epilepsy is more violent than malignant carcinoma.

To assess the relationships between demographic information and knowledge, regression analysis was conducted. A significant association was found between the knowledge score and the level of education and larger family size, but not for age, gender, marital status, or occupation.

3.2. Attitudes toward Epilepsy. The mean score for attitude was 7.25 ± 1.54 (range: 2 to 10). Of the 124 responders, 15

TABLE 1: Demographic characteristics of the respondents ($n = 124$).

	Male = 44 (%)	Female = 80 (%)	Total (%)	P value
Age (years)				
15–25	11 (61.2)	7 (38.8)	18 (14.5)	
26–36	11 (26.2)	31 (73.8)	42 (33.9)	0.51
37–47	13 (30.24)	30 (69.76)	43 (34.7)	
≥48	9 (42.9)	12 (57.1)	21 (16.9)	
Marital status				
Single	16 (57.14)	12 (42.86)	28 (22.6)	0.007
Married	28 (29.16)	68 (70.84)	96 (77.4)	
Educational level				
Under diploma	10 (21.73)	36 (78.27)	46 (37.09)	
Diploma	19 (41.31)	27 (58.69)	46 (37.09)	0.134
University education	15 (46.87)	17 (53.13)	32 (25.91)	
Number of members in family				
Small (<3)	9 (31.04)	20 (68.96)	29 (23.4)	
Average (3–5)	30 (40)	45 (60)	75 (60.5)	0.39
Big (>5)	5 (25)	15 (75)	20 (16.1)	
Occupation				
Employed	11 (64.71)	6 (35.29)	17 (13.73)	
Unemployed	33 (63.47)	19 (36.53)	52 (41.92)	0.0001
Housewife	0	55 (100)	55 (45.35)	

TABLE 2: Responses to questions on knowledge of epilepsy.

Questions	Yes %	No %	Don't Know %
(1) Epilepsy is a hereditary disorder	31.5	66.9	1.6
(2) Epilepsy is a disorder of the brain	87.1	12.1	0.8
(3) The cause of epilepsy is unknown	46.8	51.6	1.6
(4) Epilepsy is caused by demon possession or supernatural powers	8.1	88.7	3.2
(5) Malnutrition is the cause of epilepsy	33.1	65.3	1.6
(6) Epilepsy is an infectious disease and contagious	4	96	0.0
(7) Epilepsy is a form of mental illness	43.6	54.8	1.6
(8) Starvation can cause attacks of seizure in epileptic patients	56.5	43.5	0.0
(9) Inadequate sleep can cause attacks of seizure in PWE	66.1	31.5	1.6
(10) Some certain foods or drinks make a seizure	53.2	44.4	2.4
(11) Looking at the TV or computer for a long time is caused of epileptic attacks	66.1	32.3	1.6
(12) Epilepsy is more *violent* than			
(i) Diabetes mellitus	51.6	46	2.4
(ii) AIDS	24.2	73.4	2.4
(iii) Malignant carcinoma	13.7	83.1	3.2
(iv) Stroke	26.6	72.6	0.8

(12.1%) had negative attitudes and 109 (87.9%) had positive attitudes. The results are summarized in Table 3. The majority of responders, 109 (83.9%), believed that a person with epilepsy can get married and get pregnant (76.6%). One hundred and four (83.9%) of the 124 respondents said PWE can have a collage education while thirty-one (25%)

believed PWE have lower intelligence than other people. Three (2.4%) of respondents believed that PWE are insane and 9 (7.3%) of participants believed that magic and religious practices improve epilepsy. In terms of treatment, 74 (59.7%) of respondents believed that PWE require lifelong treatment. Sixty-three (50.8%) believed that it is safe for people with

TABLE 3: Responses to questions related to attitudes toward epilepsy.

Questions	Yes %	No %	Don't Know %
(1) It is possible for a person with epilepsy to get married	83.9	15.3	0.8
(2) PWE can get pregnant	76.6	21.8	1.6
(3) PWE can drive safely	50.8	47.6	1.6
(4) PWE can swim	54.8	44.4	0.8
(5) PWE can get opportunities of appropriate occupation	77.4	22.6	0.0
(6) PWE require lifelong treatment	59.7	40.3	0.0
(7) PWE can have a collage education	83.9	15.3	0.8
(8) PWE are insane	2.4	97.6	0.0
(9) PWE have lower intelligence than other people	25	74.2	0.8
(10) Cure is achievable by magic/religious practices	7.3	92.7	0.0

PWE: people with epilepsy.

epilepsy to drive and 68 (54.8%) believed that they can swim. Regression analysis showed a significant association between a positive attitude score and the female gender and level of education but no association with age, marital status, or occupation.

3.3. Correlation of Knowledge and Attitude toward Epilepsy. 64 (61.5%) of the 83 respondents who said "epilepsy is not hereditary" believed that people with epilepsy can marry. There was significant difference among this groups ($P = 0.014$).

Of the 68 respondents who thought "epilepsy is not a form of mental illness," 66 (97.05%) believed people with epilepsy are not insane ($P = 0.1$), 57 (86.36%) of respondents believed persons with epilepsy can get opportunities of appropriate occupation ($P = 0.017$), and also 60 (88.23%) said persons with epilepsy can have university education (0.039). Of the 110 respondents who said "epilepsy is not caused by demon possession," 106 (92.2%) of them believed that religious practices are not effective in improvement of epilepsy (0.0001).

As a whole, in terms of relationship between knowledge and attitude toward epilepsy, there was no significant difference between knowledge and attitude.

4. Discussion

This study assessed the levels of knowledge and attitudes about epilepsy of close family members of people with epilepsy. Although most people with epilepsy manage their disease on their own, family members play an important role in the follow-up and treatment of patients. The care of people with epilepsy is emotionally overwhelming and relatives are at an increased risk for depression [27]. Few studies have been done in developing countries, especially Iran, on the knowledge and attitudes of relatives of people with epilepsy about epilepsy. The present study showed that close family members of people with epilepsy had strong conceptions and good knowledge about epilepsy. They believed that epilepsy is a brain disorder (87.1%) or an infectious disease or contagious

(96%) and is not of supernatural origin (88.7%). They had less information about triggers of epilepsy. Overall attitudes toward epilepsy among family members were positive. Most respondents believed PWE can marry, hold an appropriate occupation, receive university education, and are as intelligent as nonepileptics. These findings are similar to results of studies among school teachers in Iran [4] and in the UK [28]. Nevertheless, there were negative attitudes in some aspects. One less than positive finding was that persons with epilepsy can swim and drive safely. Singh and Arora found that the majority of people believed that PWE should not swim or drive [20]. The results of the present study suggest that this erroneous belief can be dangerous for the patient and other people. Religious and cultural beliefs influence the treatment and follow-up of persons with epilepsy. In the present study, 8.1% of respondents believed that epilepsy is of supernatural origin and 7.7% believed epileptic patients can be cured by magic/religious practices. Masoud and Kochaki found that 14.4% of respondents believed religious practices can affect the treatment of people with epilepsy [19]. The respondents of the present study also reported supernatural origins as the cause of epilepsy, but this is much lower than other studies and this is a positive finding of our study [20, 29, 30]. In Iran few studies about knowledge of epilepsy in different population groups including teachers, people with epilepsy, general public, and relatives were conducted [4, 19, 31–33]. These studies have shown different results. A previous study in Iran found that knowledge about epilepsy of family members of patients was poor and relatives lacked information about the disease [19]. Also survey on stigma and discrimination experienced by persons with epilepsy in Tehran revealed a moderate level of stigma experiences [33]. Another study in Iran reported poor knowledge of epilepsy and that patients with the disease were thought to have compromised mental health [34]. On the other hand, other studies in between different ethnic groups and school's teachers in Iran indicated that the level of awareness about epilepsy was quite high and teachers had positive attitude about epilepsy [4, 31]. Public awareness of epilepsy in Iran showed similar to studies conducted in high income western countries [32]. There was a significant association between an increase in knowledge score and an increase in family size and educational level in the present study that correlates with the findings of other studies [29, 34]. A higher level of education and larger family size correlated with a higher percentage of correct responses to the knowledge questions. This result is consistent with findings of other study [32]. A relationship was found between increased level of education and the female gender with attitudes about epilepsy. Sidig et al. reported that 26% of respondents had good knowledge and 43% had poor knowledge about epilepsy [30], while, in the present study, only 3.3% of participants showed poor knowledge. In the present study, there was no significant association between attitude and knowledge. Saengsuwan et al. reported a weak and negative correlation between knowledge and attitude toward epilepsy [29]. This finding is different from other studies who found good knowledge to be correlated with more positive attitudes [8, 35].

5. Conclusion

The results of the present study showed that family members of PWE have a high level of knowledge and positive attitude about most aspects of epilepsy. They mostly underlined physical causes of epilepsy and rejected demon possession or supernatural powers which is a metaphysical cause. They had a positive attitude about getting an appropriate occupation and to get married. With respect to their attitudes toward the treatment of epilepsy, one-half of the interviewees believed PWE require lifelong treatment. They also declined spiritual healing as method of treatment for epilepsy. Insufficient information and incorrect beliefs about some issues related to epilepsy remain, however. Almost one-half of respondents thought epilepsy is a form of mental illness and also PWE can drive or swim safely. Family members and relatives require more education and training about epilepsy through community education programs to ameliorate misconceptions and increase understanding about this disease.

Disclosure

This study was Dr. Seyyed Ali Akbarian's dissertate doctorate towards the graduation of general medicine.

Competing Interests

The authors declare that there is no conflict of interests regarding the publication of this paper.

Acknowledgments

This study was supported by Mazandaran University of Medical Sciences (Research Project no. 322). The authors would like to appreciate the Vice Chancellor of Research and Technology of Mazandaran University of Medical Sciences for approval and supporting this study. They wish to thank all the respondents who took the time and complete the questionnaires. They also appreciate all colleagues of Department of Neurology for their assistance in collecting samples.

References

[1] R. Koul, S. Razdan, and A. Motta, "Prevalence and pattern of epilepsy (Lath/Mirgi/Laran) in rural Kashmir, India," *Epilepsia*, vol. 29, no. 2, pp. 116–122, 1988.

[2] R. Kobau and P. Price, "Knowledge of epilepsy and familiarity with this disorder in the U.S. population: results from the 2002 healthstyles survey," *Epilepsia*, vol. 44, no. 11, pp. 1449–1454, 2003.

[3] B. C. Ekeh and U. E. Ekrikpo, "The knowledge, attitude, and perception towards epilepsy amongst medical students in Uyo, Southern Nigeria," *Advances in Medicine*, vol. 2015, Article ID 876135, 6 pages, 2015.

[4] N. Karimi and M. Heidari, "Knowledge and attitudes toward epilepsy among school teachers in West of Iran," *Iranian Journal of Neurology*, vol. 14, no. 3, pp. 130–135, 2015.

[5] J. U. Ohaeri, A. W. Awadalla, and A. A. Farah, "Quality of life in people with epilepsy and their family caregivers. An Arab experience using the short version of the World Health Organization quality of life instrument," *Saudi Medical Journal*, vol. 30, no. 10, pp. 1328–1335, 2009.

[6] C. E. Begley, M. Famulari, J. F. Annegers et al., "The cost of epilepsy in the United States: an estimate from population-based clinical and survey data," *Epilepsia*, vol. 41, no. 3, pp. 342–351, 2000.

[7] M. Shafiq, M. Tanwir, A. Tariq et al., "Epilepsy: public knowledge and attitude in a slum area of Karachi, Pakistan," *Seizure*, vol. 16, no. 4, pp. 330–337, 2007.

[8] M. Saengpattrachai, D. Srinualta, N. Lorlertratna, E. Pradermduzzadeeporn, and F. Poonpol, "Public familiarity with, knowledge of, and predictors of negative attitudes toward epilepsy in Thailand," *Epilepsy and Behavior*, vol. 17, no. 4, pp. 497–505, 2010.

[9] S. S. Hasan, W. W. G. Wei, K. Ahmadi, I. S. Ahmed, A. K. S. Yong, and M. Anwar, "Knowledge and attitudes toward epilepsy among Malaysian Chinese," *International Journal of Collaborative Research on Internal Medicine and Public Health*, vol. 2, no. 11, pp. 361–376, 2010.

[10] M.-K. Kim, I.-K. Kim, B.-C. Kim, K.-H. Cho, S.-J. Kim, and J.-D. Moon, "Positive trends of public attitudes toward epilepsy after public education campaign among rural Korean residents," *Journal of Korean Medical Science*, vol. 18, no. 2, pp. 248–254, 2003.

[11] J. Spatt, G. Bauer, C. Baumgartner et al., "Predictors for negative attitudes toward subjects with epilepsy: a representative survey in the general public in Austria," *Epilepsia*, vol. 46, no. 5, pp. 736–742, 2005.

[12] L. Jilek-Aall, M. Jilek, J. Kaaya, L. Mkombachepa, and K. Hillary, "Psychosocial study of epilepsy in Africa," *Social Science and Medicine*, vol. 45, no. 5, pp. 783–795, 1997.

[13] C. T. Tan and S. H. Lim, "Epilepsy in South East Asia," *Neurological Journal of South East Asia*, vol. 2, pp. 11–15, 1997.

[14] U. Seneviratne, P. Rajapakse, R. Pathirana, and T. Seetha, "Knowledge, attitude, and practice of epilepsy in rural Sri Lanka," *Seizure*, vol. 11, no. 1, pp. 40–43, 2002.

[15] A. F. Ab Rahman, "Awareness and knowledge of epilepsy among students in a Malaysian University," *Seizure*, vol. 14, no. 8, pp. 593–596, 2005.

[16] M. Bishop and C. Allen, "Coping with epilepsy: research and intervention," in *Coping with Chronic Illness and Disability: Theoretical, Empirical and Clinical Aspect*, pp. 241–266, Springer, New York, NY, USA, 2007.

[17] P. L. Lua, K. Nor-Khaira-Wahida, A. A. Zariah, and K. F. Lee, "Caregiving for epilepsy: awareness, knowledge, attitude and health-related quality of life of family caregivers," *Malaysian Journal of Psychiatry*, vol. 23, no. 1, 2014, MJP-01-05-14.

[18] J. W. Wheless, "Intractable epilepsy: a survey of patients and caregivers," *Epilepsy and Behavior*, vol. 8, no. 4, pp. 756–764, 2006.

[19] S. A. Masoud and E. Kochaki, "Surveying the family attitude of a patients with epilepsy hospitalized in Shahid Beheshti Hospital in Kashan, 1999-2000," *Journal of Kashan University of Medical Sciences*, vol. 8, no. 1, pp. 79–86, 1999.

[20] A. Singh and A. K. Arora, "Knowledge, attitude and practices of relatives of epileptic towards epilepsy," *Nursing and Midwifery Research Journal*, vol. 1, no. 2, pp. 77–81, 2005.

[21] M. Kabir, Z. Iliyasu, S. Abubakar, Z. S. Kabir, and A. U. Farinyaro, "Knowledge, attitude and beliefs about epilepsy among adults in a northern Nigerian urban community," *Annals of African Medicine*, vol. 4, no. 3, pp. 107–112, 2005.

[22] A. F. Mustapha, O. O. Odu, and O. Akande, "Knowledge, attitudes and perceptions of epilepsy among secondary school teachers in Osogbo South-West Nigeria: a community based study," *Nigerian Journal of Clinical Practice*, vol. 16, no. 1, pp. 12–18, 2013.

[23] M. G. Devi, V. Singh, and K. Bala, "Knowledge, attitude and practices among patients of epilepsy attending tertiary hospital in Delhi, India and a review of Indian studies," *Neurology Asia*, vol. 15, no. 3, pp. 225–232, 2010.

[24] L. F. Owolabi, N. M. Shehu, and S. D. Owolabi, "Epilepsy and education in developing countries: a survey of school teachers' knowledge about epilepsy and their attitude towards students with epilepsy in Northwestern Nigeria," *Pan African Medical Journal*, vol. 18, p. 255, 2014.

[25] B. Thanavanh, M. Harun-Or-Rashid, H. Kasuya, and J. Sakamoto, "Knowledge, attitudes and practices regarding HIV/AIDS among male high school students in Lao People's Democratic Republic," *Journal of the International AIDS Society*, vol. 16, Article ID 17387, 2013.

[26] Y. Shiferaw, A. Alemu, A. Girma et al., "Assessment of knowledge, attitude and risk behaviors towards HIV/AIDS and other sexual transmitted infection among preparatory students of Gondar town, north west Ethiopia," *BMC Research Notes*, vol. 4, article 505, 2011.

[27] J. Elliott and B. Shneker, "Patient, caregiver, and health care practitioner knowledge of, beliefs about, and attitudes toward epilepsy," *Epilepsy and Behavior*, vol. 12, no. 4, pp. 547–556, 2008.

[28] L. McEwan, J. Taylor, M. Casswell et al., "Knowledge of and attitudes expressed toward epilepsy by carers of people with epilepsy: a UK perspective," *Epilepsy and Behavior*, vol. 11, no. 1, pp. 13–19, 2007.

[29] J. Saengsuwan, W. Laohasiriwong, S. Boonyaleepan, K. Sawanyawisuth, and S. Tiamkao, "Knowledge, attitudes, and care techniques of caregivers of PWE in northeastern Thailan," *Epilepsy & Behavior*, vol. 27, no. 1, pp. 257–263, 2013.

[30] A. Sidig, G. Ibrahim, A. Hussein et al., "A study of knowledge, attitude, practice towards epilepsy among relative of epileptic patients in Khartoum State," *Sudanese Journal of Public Health*, vol. 4, no. 4, pp. 393–398, 2009.

[31] E. Masoudnia, "Awareness, understanding and attitudes towards epilepsy among Iranian ethnic groups," *Seizure*, vol. 18, no. 5, pp. 369–373, 2009.

[32] H. Ghanean, M. Nojomi, and L. Jacobsson, "Public awareness and attitudes towards epilepsy in Tehran, Iran," *Global Health Action*, vol. 6, p. 21618, 2013.

[33] H. Ghanean, L. Jacobsson, and M. Nojomy, "Self-perception of stigma in persons with epilepsy in Tehran, Iran," *Epilepsy & Behavior*, vol. 28, no. 2, pp. 163–167, 2013.

[34] F. Behrouzian and S. Neamatpour, "Parental knowledge and mental health in parents of children with epilepsy," *Pakistan Journal of Medical Sciences*, vol. 26, no. 1, pp. 191–194, 2010.

[35] J. Saengsuwan, S. Boonyaleepan, J. Srijakkot, K. Sawanyawisuth, and S. Tiamkao, "Factors associated with knowledge and attitudes in persons with epilepsy," *Epilepsy & Behavior*, vol. 24, no. 1, pp. 23–29, 2012.

21

Reactive Oxygen Species: A Key Hallmark of Cardiovascular Disease

Nisha Panth, Keshav Raj Paudel, and Kalpana Parajuli

Department of Pharmacy, School of Health and Allied Sciences, Pokhara University, Dhungepatan, Kaski 33701, Nepal

Correspondence should be addressed to Kalpana Parajuli; kalpanaprjl@hotmail.com

Academic Editor: Ezequiel Álvarez Castro

Cardiovascular diseases (CVDs) have been the prime cause of mortality worldwide for decades. However, the underlying mechanism of their pathogenesis is not fully clear yet. It has been already established that reactive oxygen species (ROS) play a vital role in the progression of CVDs. ROS are chemically unstable reactive free radicals containing oxygen, normally produced by xanthine oxidase, nicotinamide adenine dinucleotide phosphate oxidase, lipoxygenases, or mitochondria or due to the uncoupling of nitric oxide synthase in vascular cells. When the equilibrium between production of free radicals and antioxidant capacity of human physiology gets altered due to several pathophysiological conditions, oxidative stress is induced, which in turn leads to tissue injury. This review focuses on pathways behind the production of ROS, its involvement in various intracellular signaling cascades leading to several cardiovascular disorders (endothelial dysfunction, ischemia-reperfusion, and atherosclerosis), methods for its detection, and therapeutic strategies for treatment of CVDs targeting the sources of ROS. The information generated by this review aims to provide updated insights into the understanding of the mechanisms behind cardiovascular complications mediated by ROS.

1. Chemical Characteristics of Reactive Oxygen Species (ROS)

Researchers have been continuously studying the potential role of oxidative damage in cardiovascular diseases (CVDs) for a few decades. In a simple term, the common risk factors for CVDs like diabetes mellitus, smoking, aging, hypercholesterolemia, and nitrate intolerance can further increase the possibility of the generation of ROS. Furthermore, these risk factors can trigger several pathways such as apoptosis of endothelial cells (EC), expression of adhesion molecules, activation of metalloproteinases, induction of proliferation and migration of smooth muscle cells, lipid peroxidation, and change in vasomotor functions, collectively leading to CVDs [1, 2]. ROS are chemically reactive molecules containing oxygen. Several ROS with unpaired electrons, for instance, superoxide anion ($O_2^{\bullet-}$), hydroxyl radical ($OH^{\bullet-}$), and lipid radicals, are considered as free radicals. ROS, such as hydrogen peroxide (H_2O_2), peroxynitrite ($ONOO^-$), and hypochlorous acid ($HOCl$), are not free radicals but possess an oxidizing effect resulting in oxidant stress. A chain reaction leads to the production of many reactive oxygen species from one ROS (Figure 1). For example, the reactions of radicals and fatty acids (polyunsaturated fatty acids, PUFAs) within the cytoplasmic membrane result in a fatty acid peroxyl radical which can attack the adjacent side chain of the fatty acid and commence production of other lipid radicals. Lipid radicals generated in this chain reaction get collected in the plasma membrane and may have an innumerable effect on cell function, including alteration in cell membrane permeability and dysfunction of membrane-bound receptors [1, 3].

2. Potential Sources of ROS for CVDs

In a physiological system, the imbalance between antioxidant defense mechanism and ROS production leads to oxidative stress and subsequent pathological conditions [4]. Most prominent ROS causing toxic insult to the human body are H_2O_2, $O_2^{\bullet-}$, $^{\bullet}OH$, and $ONOO^-$ [5]. In the blood vessel wall, each layer can produce ROS in pathological conditions [6].

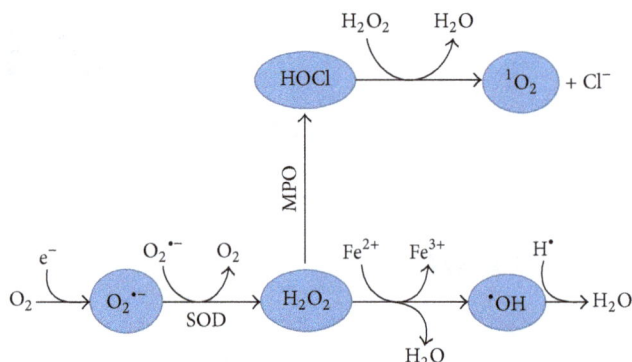

FIGURE 1: Production of ROS. The figure shows the pathway of ROS production in the human body with various enzymes involved. SOD: superoxide dismutase; MPO: myeloperoxidase.

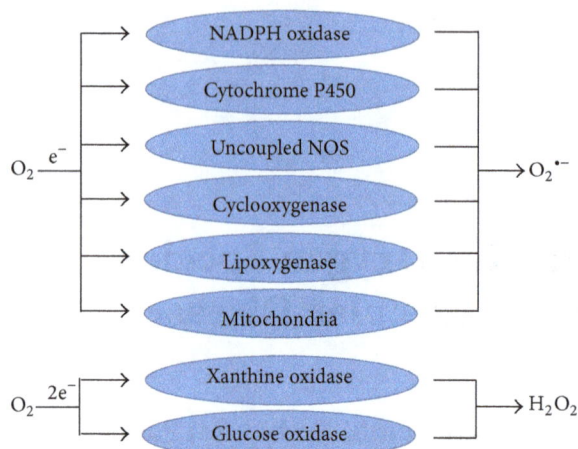

FIGURE 2: Sources of $O_2^{\bullet-}$ and H_2O_2 in cells. The figure shows the enzymatic pathway of superoxide anion ($O_2^{\bullet-}$) and hydrogen peroxide (H_2O_2) generation in cells.

Wattanapitayakul and Bauer reported that, within mitochondria, oxygen is usually utilized for energy production (in the form of ATP) and oxidative phosphorylation. During the mitochondrial electron transport (MET), harmful ROS are formed but they are balanced by antioxidant defense. However, in case of ischemia or hypoxia, MET is imbalanced, leading to ATP depletion, acidosis, mitochondrial depolarization, collection of noxious metabolites, intracellular Ca^{2+} overload, and cell death [7]. For example, approximately 1–3% of molecular oxygen is converted to unstable/reactive $O_2^{\bullet-}$ in mitochondrial complexes I and III through a pathway involving oxidative phosphorylation [8]. In general, cardiac myocytes consume a high level of oxygen due to considerable higher number of mitochondria than other cells [9]. For this reason, cardiac myocytes also release ROS and cause oxidative stress to other cells [10]. But ROS do not have only a negative side, since production of ROS at physiological levels promotes cellular activities, controls the hormone level, maintains chemical balance, strengthens synaptic plasticity, and induces enzymes. Moreover, ROS also helps to fight against invading pathogens and induce an immune response against the pathogenic influence [5]. To a certain extent, ROS are neutralized by intracellular antioxidant enzymes such as glutathione peroxidase (GPx), superoxide dismutase (SOD), and catalase and consumption of other nonenzyme antioxidants like β-carotene, ascorbic acid, and tocopherols as a supplement [7]. In spite of being necessary to carry out cell signaling pathways, overproduction of ROS leads to injury of the cell membrane integrity causing altered permeability, change in proteins expression, and DNA damage [11]. For the majority of CVDs, the enzymatic sources of ROS include NAD(P)H oxidase, lipooxygenase, cyclooxygenase (COX), xanthine oxidase (XO), uncoupled nitric oxide synthases (NOS), cytochrome P450, and mitochondrial respiration [12–14] (Figure 2). The process of increased $O_2^{\bullet-}$ generation, facilitated by XO enzyme, can be antagonized by a therapeutic approach with XO inhibitor, like allopurinol, to ameliorate cardiac conditions [15]. NADPH oxidase (Nox), commonly found on the cellular membrane, is stimulated during phagocytosis leading to increased ROS release [10]. In particular, the overexpression of Nox2 and Nox4 is linked

to the remarkable oxidative stress observed during CVDs. A study done by Kuroda et al. showed that Nox4 knockout mice showed a low level of cardiac O_2^- revealing that Nox4 is a potential source of superoxide in cardiac myocytes. Nox4 overexpression worsened the cardiac function and induced apoptosis and fibrosis in a mouse with response to pressure overload. Thus, Nox4 is a key contributor of oxidative stress in the mitochondrial redox systems leading to cardiac impairment during pressure overload. Therefore, the physiological role of Nox, translocating electrons throughout the membrane, can be deregulated in CVDs leading to cardiac dysfunction [16]. However, some pathways associated with ROS mediated CVDs are yet to be clarified. However, researchers are trying to reveal good, bad, and ugly roles of ROS in the physiological system. In contrast to the good face of ROS on signaling and immune response, at high concentrations, ROS can exhibit the deleterious effect on redox homeostasis leading to intracellular components damage as seen in neurodegenerative diseases, CVDs, and pulmonary disorders [5].

3. Oxidative Stress and Endothelial Dysfunction

Endothelial cells are lining the interior surface of blood and lymphatic vessels cells. Endothelial cells play an important role in homeostasis and immune and inflammatory reactions. EC regulates vascular tone by releasing various vasodilator factors such as nitric oxide (NO) endothelium derived hyperpolarizing factor, prostacyclin or vasoconstrictive factors such as thromboxane (TXA_2), and endothelin-1 (ET-1). Endothelial dysfunction (ED) is a pathological state of the endothelium, which is a predictor of various CVDs, and is caused by imbalance between vasodilating and vasoconstricting substances [17]. ROS are considered as signaling molecules that contribute to ED in experimental and clinical atherosclerosis [3, 18]. NO is a potent vasodilator produced by the endothelium. Besides vasorelaxation, nitric oxide exerts various functions like antiplatelet, antithrombotic, and anti-inflammatory properties and permeability decreasing properties [19]. It is reported that ONOO$^-$ which is formed by the reaction of superoxide and free radical NO can oxidize tetrahydrobiopterin. If formed in a small amount, ONOO$^-$ exerts a similar physiological activity like NO. However, at a high concentration, it shows injurious activity by converting to harmful peroxynitrous acid and causing alteration of protein structure [20]. ED is associated with polymorphisms of various genes which include cytochrome P450, methylene tetrahydrofolate reductase, p22phox, angiotensin convertase enzyme, and glutathione-S-transferase [21]. Excess amount of ROS damages the endothelium, especially the terminal arteries leading to alteration of the intracellular reduction-oxidation homeostasis [22]. In a patient with diabetes mellitus, small vessel disease linked with mitochondrial disorders might also be due to oxidative stress. The result of diabetes mellitus in atherosclerosis is stimulated mainly by oxidative stress [23]. ROS may also activate mitogen activated protein kinase, which regulates the expression of monocyte chemoattractant protein 1 (MCP-1) and favors the chemotaxis of circulating monocyte to the site of atherosclerotic lesion. This demonstrates a potential link between arterial wall strain and atherosclerosis [24].

4. ROS in Ischemia-Reperfusion (I/R) Damage

Several researches support the fact that ROS are involved in ischemic occlusion leading to cardiac damage [39, 40]. Apart from carrying out the function of cellular O_2 storage and supply by oxymyoglobin (Mb), it also acts as a potent preventive source against I/R injury [40]. During the outset of I/R injury, $O_2^{\bullet-}$ release has been observed in an isolated rat heart. Zhu and Zuo speculate that generation of $O_2^{\bullet-}$ is linked with Mb because of the lower myocardium oxygen tension. Results revealed that the rise of fluorescence in the ischemic heart was terminated by a SOD mimic, carbon monoxide (CO), or by Mb gene knockout. Likewise, $O_2^{\bullet-}$ was not formed in intracellular EC but rather from the myocytes, which are considered a potential source of Mb. This suggests that Mb is an important factor responsible for production of $O_2^{\bullet-}$ during ischemia [40]. An enzyme responsive to stress, named sirtuin-6 (SIRT6), displays cardiac protection from I/R injury as revealed in partial SIRT6 knockout mice as well as in vitro cultured cardiomyocyte. SIRT6 is a deacetylase and mono-ADP ribosyltransferase enzyme responsive to oxidative stress and can protect the cell against oxidative stress. This protective activity was achieved by initiating the expression of catalase and manganese SOD antioxidant-encoding gene resulting in reduced cellular oxidative stress [41]. Restoration of the coronary artery blood flow reverse to the ischemic myocardium can have a detrimental effect on the microvascular function, causing arrhythmias [42]. In the endothelium, the rise of ROS release and the opening of mitochondrial permeability transition (MPT) pore play an important role in the protection from I/R damage [43]. However, Kim and Lemasters showed that mitochondrial ROS, accompanied by normalization of pH, stimulate initiation of MPT pore

followed by death of myocytes after reperfusion. However, Ca^{2+} overloading does not promote onset of MPT pore [44]. Research demonstrated that the reason behind the protective effect was the involvement of ROS and potent vasodilator NO in regulating downstream pathways by stimulating adenosine triphosphate sensitive potassium channel in mitochondria [45]. After open cardiac surgery, the I/R injury can influence postsurgical consequences because of the lipid peroxidation mediated by ROS [46]. In comparison to the heart obtained from juvenile rat, the cardiac dysfunction due to I/R was dramatically concealed in the heart obtained from congenital heart disease (CHD) model rats. Moreover, the ratio of n-3/n-6 PUFA was remarkably raised in I/R phase in CHD rats, whereas it was not observed in juvenile rats suggesting that the rise in n-3/n-6 ratio could result in the upregulation of cell defense system against oxidation via n-3 PUFA oxidation product 4-hydroxy-2-hexenal causing higher tolerance to I/R damage [46].

5. ROS and Atherosclerosis

Excess production of ROS plays an important role in inflammation, disturbed blood flow/abnormal shear stress, and arterial wall remodeling. ROS causes remodeling through proliferation of smooth muscle cell and increased inflammation [39]. Repeated continuous exposure to nonstreamline shear stress of arterial regions generates O_2 induced by endothelial Nox resulting in adhesion of monocytes [47]. The upregulation of adhesion molecules including P-selectin, VCAM-1, and E-selectin causes further inflammation by adhesion of white blood cells. Development of inflammatory response increases ROS production by phagocytosis, which is important in the early stage of atherosclerosis [48, 49]. The Nox family of superoxide producing proteins is an important source of ROS in signal transduction. Nox are found to be expressed in phagocytic cells, EC, smooth muscle cells, and fibroblasts. Experiments conducted on arteries from human volunteers with coronary artery disease and animal experimental model with hypertension, diabetes, or atherosclerosis demonstrated that Nox1, Nox2, and Nox5 stimulate endothelial dysfunction, inflammation, and programmed cell death; however, isoform Nox4 protects the vascular system by increasing bioavailability of nitric oxide and stoppage of cell death pathways [50]. Some research presents the controversial role of Nox4 displaying either protective or a deleterious role of Nox4.

Nox4 are found abundantly in kidney, vascular cells, and osteoclasts [16]. Angiotensin II type 1 receptor activation and hypertension are linked to increased expression of Nox1 and Nox4 that could lead to vascular damage during chronic hypertension [51]. MCP-1 is essential for the formation of endothelial cell tumors (hemangioendotheliomas) which is redox sensitive. It was found that only the Nox4 isoform was present in endothelial cell tumors cells whereas knockdown of Nox4 gene remarkably decreased the expression of MCP-1 as well as hemangioendothelioma formation. This was due to the fact that, in hemangioendothelioma cells, Nox4 delivers H_2O_2 to the nuclear compartment causing oxidative alteration of DNA [52]. Inflammation mediates all stages of atherosclerosis and ROS sources might include infiltrated monocytes/macrophages, dysfunctional EC, and smooth muscle cells that migrated from tunica media to tunica intima layers of the wall of an artery. ROS oxidized-LDL is available in the arterial wall and macrophages scavenge it resulting in the formation of foam cells. This is one of the important steps in the progression and development of atherosclerosis [53]. Also, the calcium-dependent zinc containing endopeptidase, matrix metalloproteinase, secreted from EC, foam cells, and vascular smooth cells, is activated during oxidative stress in part due to inflammation and nonlaminar shear stress, resulting in the ruptures of thrombosis [54].

6. Oxidative Stress and Mitochondria

Mitochondria play an important role in cellular signaling pathways, particularly in the modulation of calcium stores within the cell, generation of ROS, respiration, and biogenesis. So, changes in mitochondrial function lead to development of human diseases [55, 56]. Mitochondrial DNA (mtDNA) damage is linked to the atherosclerotic lesions in apolipoprotein E (apoE) knockout mice and also introduces atherogenesis in young apoE knockout mice [57]. Raised levels of mtDNA damage have been seen in the vascular tissue of CVD patients [58]. Mitochondrial dysfunction is due to decreased manganese SOD, increased damage of mtDNA, and increased atherosclerosis in apoE knockout mice [59]. There is excessive mitochondrial damage in atherosclerosis model. Oxidized-LDL stimulates mitochondrial complex I activity which depends on the induction of oxidative stress [60, 61]. Composed of 46 subunits, human mitochondrial complex I is the key enzyme responsible for oxidative phosphorylation. Dysfunction of the mitochondrial oxidative phosphorylation in a physiological system is responsible for occurrence of CVDs in humans, and mitochondrial diseases are linked to mitochondrial respiratory-chain pathologies and mutations of mitochondrial DNA. Studies reported that various stress induced in the cells causes structural and functional disturbance of mitochondria [62, 63]. Dysfunction of mitochondria provokes a signaling pathway for cell death resulting in organ failure and diseases. Mitochondria based pathological conditions including obesity, cancer, stroke, diabetes, neurodegenerative diseases, heart failure, and aging, however, are caused by intrusion of mitochondrial Ca^{2+}, ATP, or ROS metabolism [61, 63]. Myocardial ischemia-reperfusion injury leads to mitochondrial Ca^{2+} overload and consequent generation of ROS and opening of the mitochondrial permeability transition pore [60–62], resulting in apoptosis. Compounds which can reduce mitochondrial Ca^{2+} overload, decrease mitochondrial ROS collection, and prevent mitochondrial energy generation are all potential sources of therapies for preventing disease. Mitochondria produce oxidative stress which plays an important role in mediating programmed cell death (apoptosis) and damage to mtDNA and leads to human aging, cancer, and CVDs. Oxidative damage of the mitochondrial membrane results in depolarization of membrane and uncoupled oxidative phosphorylation and altered cellular respiration. Altered mitochondrial respiratory chain can hinder the pivotal role of providing the energy to the cell as ATP, leading to various disease progression [60–64].

7. Methods for Detection of ROS in CVDs

Since ROS are highly unstable and very reactive, researchers always face the problem of precisely monitoring them in biological systems. One way to find out the possibility of ROS in CVDs subjects involves exploring experimental proof of oxidative reactions. Fluorescent probes and electron spin resonance probes tools for detection of ROS are limited in animal and human experiment due to technical problems [65]. The following list of direct methods can show at least in part indirect evidence of ROS effect in CVDs (Table 1).

7.1. Biomarkers of ROS

7.1.1. Lipid Peroxidation Mediated by ROS. LDL collects in the blood vessels walls and lipid species undergo oxidation in the presence of several ROS [66]. It is reported that oxidative modification of LDL plays an important role in the atherosclerosis process [67]. Macrophages take up oxidized-LDL through scavenger receptor pathways resulting in cholesterol ester-rich foam cells and EC dysfunction, in part, by role of lectin-like oxidized-LDL receptor-1 [68, 69]. In atherosclerotic plaques, the availability of oxidized-LDL has been observed by using immunohistochemical staining for modified primary apolipoprotein B-100, the protein moiety in LDL [38]. Elevated levels of autoantibodies against oxidized-LDL or malondialdehyde-modified LDL particles are linked to atherosclerosis and coronary artery diseases (CADs) including acute coronary syndrome. In healthy people, circulating levels of oxidized-LDL can be identified by techniques such as ultrasound while in diseased subjects it is commonly seen in clinical case of CAD [70–72].

7.1.2. MPO. High levels of the enzyme myeloperoxidase which produces hypochlorous acid (HOCl) are found in human atheroma and are an important predictor of CAD, as well as in patients with unstable angina and mitochondrial infarction (MI). Increased numbers of myeloperoxidase-expressing macrophages are found in eroded or ruptured plaques [73]. Also, MPO and hypochlorite-modified proteins are colocalized in atherosclerotic lesions. Also, in human study research, strong inverse relation occurs between MPO serum concentrations and brachial artery flow-mediated dilation, which is another clinical marker of atherosclerosis [73, 74]. So, lowering MPO levels could lower occurrence of CVDs. Human studies have demonstrated that humans with total or near-total deficiency of MPO have a lower chance of developing CADs [73]. Reduced expression of MPO by its gene promoter polymorphism showed reduced CAD manifestations but increased MPO expression by MPO gene promoter polymorphism demonstrated raised CAD [75]. Since the level of plasma MPO is sensitive to heparin dosing [76], neutrophil activation [77], and the procedure

TABLE 1: Direct methods for detection of ROS in CVDs.

Methods	ROS detected	Applications/mechanism	Reference
Fluorescent protein-based redox probes	Cytoplasmic and mitochondrial H_2O_2	Used to detect redox status and ROS by introducing adenoviruses or plasmids inside cells. Afterwards, cells form chimeric proteins efficient to detect alteration in the redox status or ROS.	[25, 26]
Dihydroethidium (DHE) and mitochondrion-targeted probe mitoSOX	Cellular and mitochondrial $O_2^{\bullet-}$	Can detect mitochondrial $O_2^{\bullet-}$ by adding a triphenylphosphonium group for promoting its collection in the mitochondria. Similar to DHE, mitoSOX reacts with $O_2^{\bullet-}$ to give 2-hydroxy-mito-ethidium (2-OH-Mito-E$^+$) so as to be identified and measured using HPLC.	[27–29]
Cyclic hydroxylamine spin probes	Total cellular and mitochondrial $O_2^{\bullet-}$	Allows measurement of $O_2^{\bullet-}$ in tissue, in in vitro cells, and in vivo.	[30–32]
Boronate-based fluorescent probes	H_2O_2 and $ONOO^{\bullet-}$	As probes have a fluorophore which is secured by boronate, when subjected to H_2O_2, the boronate encounters a nucleophilic attack, followed by its displacement from the fluorophore, thus causing emission of light.	[33, 34]
Immunospin trapping	Free radical adduct formation in the mitochondria, cells, and tissue samples	5,5-Dimethyl-1-pyrroline-N-oxide reacts with protein radicals to form epitopes which can be particularly characterized immunologically.	[35, 36]
In vivo using X- and L-band ESR spectroscopy	Short-lived free radicals in whole living animals	Detection is done in vivo by infusion of cyclic hydroxylamines or nitrone spin traps, followed by ex vivo study of the tissue or blood using X-band (9 GHz) electron spin resonance spectroscopy.	[37, 38]

of collection [78], there is a need for development of an appropriate method for its sampling.

7.1.3. Plasma F_2-Isoprostanes. F_2-isoprostanes are considered as the best biomarkers of oxidative stress status and lipid peroxidation in an in vivo model. F_2-isoprostanes are found in an esterified form in normal biological tissues and are available in free form in biological fluids, demonstrating "physiological" levels of oxidative stress. The F_2-isoprostanes might be produced from membrane phospholipids or circulating LDL [79, 80]. The generation of F_2-isoprostanes can be via the action of several cell types like monocytes which are involved in atherosclerosis and the oxidized products have been restricted to a particular area within foam cells and atherosclerotic plaques individual specimens [81]. Various human studies have demonstrated a link between CAD and isoprostane levels [82]. Raised levels of isoprostanes in urine are an independent risk factor of CAD and are found to be increased in patients having unstable angina. Raised levels of isoprostanes are important markers of ischemic tissue injury, chronic heart failure, congestive heart failure, and cardiac remodeling [79, 82, 83]. Therefore, F_2-isoprostanes could be used for the prediction of cardiovascular events.

8. Molecular Role of ROS in Muscle Contraction

During skeletal muscle contraction, ROS are generated which can affect muscle adaptation and function. Zuo et al. studied whether ROS are generated in the process of muscle contraction in isolated single skeletal muscle fibers (using *Xenopus laevis* muscle), as well as whether these ROS generated by contraction have an impact on fatigue development. To detect the ROS generation, myofibers were loaded with fluorescent probe (dihydrofluorescein-diacetate) which reacts with ROS to form fluorescein. Fluorescein signal was raised remarkably in both the first ($42 \pm 14\%$) and the third periods ($39 \pm 10\%$) of maximal tetanic contraction. However, with the treatment of reference antioxidant compound, ebselen, there was no rise of fluorescein during the second contractile period suggesting that ROS generation is high during contractile activity and antioxidant treatment can halt ROS production without any effect on myofiber contractility [84]. In spite of the various pathways of ROS generation, the study of key pathways of their production is still undergoing. In particular, ROS generation in response to exercise, hypoxia, and heat in the diaphragmatic skeletal muscle (a key muscle during respiration) is a topic of interest [85, 86]. During the state of heat stress, $O_2^{\bullet-}$ is generated by skeletal muscle which can be quantified by cytochrome c reduction as it is correlated with arachidonic acid metabolism. The blockage of enzyme phospholipase A_2 using manoalide remarkably reduced $O_2^{\bullet-}$ release. However, neither the blockage of COX with nonselective COX inhibitor indomethacin nor the blockage of CYP P-450 contingent monooxygenase with SKF-525A reduces $O_2^{\bullet-}$ generation. In contrast, lipoxygenase blockage with common inhibitors cinnamyl-3,4-dihydroxy-α-cyanocinnamate and 5,8,11,14-eicosatetraynoic acid drastically halted the signal. Moreover, $O_2^{\bullet-}$ generation was notably reduced by diethylcarbamazine (5-LOX inhibitor) suggesting that metabolism of arachidonic acid involving LOX is a key mediator of generation of extracellular $O_2^{\bullet-}$ in skeletal muscle [86]. The role of ROS in myocardial I/R injury has been widely studied [87]. Vanden Hoek et al. proposed the generation of a high amount of ROS in case of ischemia before reperfusion by an *in vitro* experiment in isolated cardiomyocyte during simulated I/R. The fluorescent probes $2',7'$-dichlorofluorescein and dihydroethidium (DHE) were significantly oxidized during ischemia, revealing ROS production. After an hour of ischemia, reperfusion leads to further generation of OH^- and H_2O_2. In contrast, treatment of antioxidant compounds (1,10-phenanthroline and 2-mercaptopropionyl glycine) during ischemia injury halted oxidant production, raised the viability of cardiomyocytes, and opposed contraction following ischemia. The ROS production in response to residual O_2 as in case of ischemia causes cellular injury observed in the reperfusion stage [88]. In a similar study on cardiomyocytes model of ischemia performed by Becker et al., an inhibitor of mitochondrial site III (myxothiazol) reduced oxidation. However, the inhibitor of mitochondrial site IV (cyanide) along with NOS inhibitor (nitro-L-arginine methyl ester), XO inhibitor (allopurinol), and Nox inhibitor (apocynin) showed no effect, suggesting that excessive $O_2^{\bullet-}$ production is observed in ischemia prior to reperfusion through ubisemiquinone area of the MET chain [89]. Another study suggests that sublethal H_2O_2 production in isolated cardiomyocytes during the period of simulated ischemia modulates cell death later in reperfusion step, mainly due to the burst of reperfusion oxidant [90].

9. Therapeutic Strategy Targeting ROS Sources in CVD

9.1. Antioxidant. Antioxidants are a prime choice to fight against ROS. Therefore, it is crucial to formulate the strategies to halt abnormal ROS production inside the human body as well as improve innate antioxidant protection capacity. A cross-sectional research performed by Lane et al. reported that dietary supplements of vitamins E, C, and A help to lower occurrence of peripheral arterial disease [91]. Regular consumption of diet rich in vegetables and fruits (as a source of antioxidant vitamins) lowers the prevalence of CVDs, and, globally, it is recommended for enough daily intake of vegetables and fruit [92, 93]. These antioxidants vitamins A, C, and E, CoQ10, lycopene, and quercetin have been studied to explore their therapeutic and/or preventative effects on ventricular remodeling, atherosclerosis, heart failure, myocardial infarction, and ischemia-reperfusion heart injury [94–97]. Various herbal plants such as *Nelumbo nucifera* [98], *Juglans regia* [99], and *Rumex nepalensis* [100] are a rich source of compounds exhibiting remarkable antioxidant activity along with cardioprotective activity. Among the antioxidants, the most commonly used vitamin C and vitamin E as a cardioprotective supplement are discussed in the following section also including the information about their failure to revert the CVDs in some study.

9.1.1. Vitamin C. It is well known that vitamin C helps in regulation of blood pressure. A considerable study favors the notion that vitamin C restores high blood pressure related baroreflex dysfunction [101–103]. Some study revealed that oxidative stress decreases the baroreflex sensitivity leading to the constant hypertensive state. As shown in a hypertensive rat model by Botelho-Ono et al., treatment of vitamin C (150 mg/kg, IV) remarkably lowered heart rate, with improvement in baroreflex sensitivity compared to the untreated hypertensive group. Also, treatment of NADPH oxidase inhibitor apocynin (30 μg/kg, intravenous) maintained baroreflex sensitivity revealing that ROS generated via NADPH oxidase pathway plays a key role in the modification of baroreflex sensitivity in hypertension, whereas treatment of antioxidants (vitamin C) restored this change [102]. Similarly, Nishi et al. [101] also reported that chronic administration of vitamin C at a dose of 150 mg/kg/day drastically lowers the mean arterial pressure (MAP) in a hypertensive rat's model as compared to vitamin C untreated rat. Furthermore, the study also revealed increased expression of angiotensin II type 1 (AT-1) receptor in vitamin C untreated hypertensive rat, with downregulation of AT-1 in the vitamin C-treated group. Likewise, in a human clinical trial, Bruno et al. showed that IV infusion of vitamin C (3 g, over 5 min) significantly reduces both sympathetic nerve activity and blood pressure in essential hypertension patients ($n = 32$) but not in normotensive patients ($n = 20$). This study highlights the notion that the decrease in heart rate and sympathetic nerve activity leading to reduced blood pressure after application with vitamin C was because of makeover of baroreflex function [103]. Endothelial dysfunction, a cause of CVDs, is corrected in a human study ($n = 93$) by treatment with vitamin C (2 g) alone or in combination with vitamin E (600 mg) as shown by Uzun et al. Results showed enhanced vasodilation following an endothelium dependent pathway in the radial artery of a subject with coronary artery disease receiving vitamin C and/or vitamin E [104]. Vitamin C promotes synthesis and deposition of collagen (type IV) in the basement membrane of EC, induces endothelial proliferation, scavenges radicals to prevent EC apoptosis, and increases endothelial NO production. However, there is variation in the beneficial effect of synthetic vitamin C and natural (food-derived) vitamin C on CVDs. One reason may be that, along with dietary vitamin C (from fruits and vegetables), we also consume other phytochemicals which may potentiate its availability to systemic circulation for action. This hypothesis is supported by a study done by Agarwal et al. on a human cohort. The results revealed that although vitamin C supplement did not help to decrease the progression of carotid artery intima-media thickness (IMT) in CVDs like atherosclerosis, dietary vitamin C did [105]. In contrast to the beneficial action of vitamin C to alleviate CVD symptoms, there is some controversy because of the results of the clinical trial which oppose this fact. For instance, a clinical trial done by Ward et al. showed that although monotherapy of vitamin C (for 6 weeks) decreases the systolic blood pressure in hypertensive subjects, combination therapy of vitamin C and grapes seed polyphenol increased it. Moreover, the endothelium independent and dependent vasorelaxation as well as oxidative stress marker were not significantly different from vitamin C/grape seed polyphenol therapy as compared to a hypertensive individual without therapy. This finding recommends that hypertensive individuals on vitamin C and polyphenol supplements therapy should take the necessary precaution [106].

9.1.2. Vitamin E. Various studies have been carried out to examine the beneficial effect of vitamin E on CVDs. Serbinova et al. compared the effect of palm oil vitamin E with tocopherol alone and found that palm oil vitamin E was comparatively more successful in safeguarding the cardiac ischemia-reperfusion damage in the isolated heart [107]. A recent meta-analysis study done by Ashor et al. [108] to observe the potency of vitamins on atrial stiffness in adults disclosed that antioxidant vitamins possess a beneficial effect by reducing arterial stiffness. Moreover, the efficacy was dependent on the duration of treatment and dose supplemented. Those subjects having reduced levels of vitamin E in the blood attained an improved pharmacological effect from this intervention. In another double-blind, placebo-controlled study performed by Stephens et al. [109] on a coronary disease patient, it was found that 400 or 800 IU per day dose of vitamin E notably decreased the incidence of nonfatal myocardial infarction in study subjects.

9.2. Failure of Antioxidant Vitamin Therapy to Revert the CVDs. Although considerable research supports the fact that antioxidants possess therapeutic benefit to fight against disease progression, however, clinical trials are unsuccessful in showing the benefit [110]. Hasty et al. found that vitamin E supplementation for 12 weeks was not successful in alleviating the oxidative damage in western-type diet fed low density lipoprotein receptor knockout (LDLR−/−) mice model of obesity/hyperlipidemia. Although diet was enough to drastically increase the plasma lipid profile like free fatty acid, triglyceride, and total cholesterol (a marker of atherogenesis) in LDLR−/− obese mice with respect to lean mice, there was no beneficial effect observed after supplementation of vitamin E. Furthermore, there was no reduction in the urinary isoprostanes (a biomarker of oxidative stress) levels suggesting that vitamin E does not account for the cardioprotective effect [111]. A human clinical trial done in 730 volunteers (either sex, ≥65 years) for more than 20 years demonstrated that lower vitamin C supplementation was associated with high mortality rate by stroke in elderly people. However, there was no remarkable link between vitamin C diet status and CHD [112]. Similarly, another human clinical trial done in a larger population (6996 men and 2545 women) also showed that vitamin E had no beneficial effect on cardiovascular outcomes in patients who are more prone to cardiovascular events even after treatment for a long period of 4.5 years [113].

9.3. Pharmacological Agent. Various pharmacology agents such as statins and angiotensin-converting enzyme (ACE) inhibitors show pleiotropic effects to halt the oxidative stress. Particularly in the myocardium, oxidative stress and cell signaling proteins like Rac, Rho, and Ras are responsible for the cardiac hypertrophic response [114]. A recent *in vivo* investigation revealed that phagocyte-type Nox could be a potential source of ROS in the myocardium [115]. Nox-dependent ROS production seems to be linked with cardiac hypertrophy mediated by pressure overload [116] and angiotensin II infusion [117]. Even though the principal effect of statin therapy in CVDs is mainly vascular, *in vivo* studies recommend that there are also protective effects on the myocardium. Since Rac1 is essential for Nox function and cardiac hypertrophy resulted to some extent by oxidative stress, probably the statins could reduce cardiac hypertrophy by antioxidant pathway. Particularly, statins were successful in blocking angiotensin II-mediated oxidative injury in a rat model of cardiac hypertrophy [118]. Also, this activity of statins was seen in a clinical trial done in a cardiac hypertrophy subject that presented with hypercholesterolemia [119]. In a patient with heart failure, Nox mediated ROS generation raised in the left ventricular myocardium and associated with the rise in Rac1 GTPase activity, whereas statin therapy was able to reduce Rac1 activity in the heart [120].

9.3.1. Statins. Statins category medicines are not a direct scavenger of ROS; however, they act in an indirect way by hindering the 3-hydroxy-3-methyl-glutaryl-coenzyme A (HMG CoA) reductase pathway involved in cholesterol synthesis. Metabolism with HMG CoA reductase leads to the production of intermediate pyrophosphates, considered as a crucial point for $O_2^{•−}$ formation via Nox. The therapeutic effect of statins to lower the occurrence of CVDs is achieved by their capacity to promote endothelial nitric oxide synthase (eNOS) expression as well as antioxidant nature [118, 121–123]. Factors causing endothelial damage involve ROS such as oxidized-LDL and hypoxia can reduce the expression of eNOS whereas statins group medicine can reverse the eNOS downregulation, highlighting their ability to ameliorate the vessel NO bioavailability and atherosclerotic plaque stability [124–126]. Furthermore, statins also block tumor necrosis factor-α (TNF-α) mediated downregulation of eNOS [127]. Stimulation of angiotensin II hormone will further activate Rac1 and ADP-ribosylation factor 6 (ARF6), a controller of NADPH oxidase function. ARF6 is crucial for ROS production because, in the knocked down situation of this GTPase, angiotensin II cannot stimulate $O_2^{•−}$ (superoxide anion) generation. Likewise, ARF6 also regulates NADPH oxidase 1 (Nox1) expression [128]. A study done by Copaja et al. showed that induction of cardiac myofibroblasts and fibroblasts apoptosis by simvastatin followed a cholesterol synthesis independent pathway but was dependent on Rho GTPases protein isoprenylation. On comparison, cardiac myofibroblasts were less sensitive to apoptosis induction than cardiac fibroblasts by simvastatin. Therefore, it is likely that simvastatin could circumvent harmful cardiac remodeling followed by some fibrotic restoration of the injured tissues [129]. Taken together, the abovementioned beneficial role of statins in prevention of coronary heart disease can promote the development of statin therapy against ROS mediated CVDs.

9.3.2. ACE Inhibitors. ACE is an enzyme that metabolizes angiotensin I to angiotensin II. ACE inhibitors were designed to treat hypertension. During arterial wall remodeling, increased angiotensin II activity leads to thickening of the tunica media and narrowing of the vessel diameter, a key feature of atherosclerosis [130, 131]. In particular, increased angiotensin II level is associated with the proportional release of vascular $O_2^{\bullet-}$ [132]. In a rabbit model of hypercholesterolemia, it was observed that $O_2^{\bullet-}$ bioavailability was decreased in thoracic aorta due to the antioxidative activity of NO [133]. In contrast, NO concentration can decrease after reaction with $O_2^{\bullet-}$, thereby worsening the atheroma plague formation [134]. Although eNOS and neuronal NOS control normal metabolic functions, upregulation of inducible NOS leads to enhanced production of NO displaying deleterious inflammatory responses by forming peroxynitrite by NO and superoxide [135]. Circulating angiotensin II level can be enhanced by angiotensin II type I receptor blocker (ARB) leading to stimulation of angiotensin II type II receptors followed by vasodilation due to NO production [136, 137]. A clinical trial in hypertensive patients undergoing candesartan (a type of ARB) therapy displayed remarkable diminishing of carotid artery intima-media thickness, mainly because of augmented NO production as well as decreased oxidative stress [136]. Likewise, cotreatment of ACE and ARB inhibitor showed a synergistic inhibitory action against oxidative stress in a balloon-injured rat carotid artery [138].

10. Conclusions

The exact mechanism of CVD is complex and is not yet fully understood. ROS plays an important role in the progression and development of CVD. There is a link between ROS and the pathophysiology of CVD. We have developed a greater understanding of production of ROS, detection of ROS, and therapeutic strategy to prevent production of ROS and cardiovascular disease. However, more works to improve the detection and treatment of the ROS mediated dysfunction are necessary in the upcoming days.

Competing Interests

The authors declare that they have no competing interests.

Authors' Contributions

All the authors contributed equally to this review.

References

[1] G. Vogiatzi, D. Tousoulis, and C. Stefanadis, "The role of oxidative stress in atherosclerosis," *Hellenic Journal of Cardiology*, vol. 50, no. 5, pp. 402–409, 2009.

[2] N. Panth, S.-H. Park, H. J. Kim, D.-H. Kim, and M.-H. Oak, "Protective effect of *Salicornia europaea* extracts on high salt intake-induced vascular dysfunction and hypertension," *International Journal of Molecular Sciences*, vol. 17, no. 7, article 1176, 2016.

[3] H. Bayir, "Reactive oxygen species," *Critical Care Medicine*, vol. 33, no. 12, pp. S498–S501, 2005.

[4] T. Heitzer, T. Schlinzig, K. Krohn, T. Meinertz, and T. Münzel, "Endothelial dysfunction, oxidative stress, and risk of cardiovascular events in patients with coronary artery disease," *Circulation*, vol. 104, no. 22, pp. 2673–2678, 2001.

[5] L. Zuo, L. T. Zhou, B. K. Pannell, A. C. Ziegler, and T. M. Best, "Biological and physiological role of reactive oxygen species—the good, the bad and the ugly," *Acta Physiologica*, vol. 214, no. 3, pp. 329–348, 2015.

[6] M. B. Reid, "Redox modulation of skeletal muscle contraction: what we know and what we don't," *Journal of Applied Physiology*, vol. 90, no. 2, pp. 724–731, 2001.

[7] S. K. Wattanapitayakul and J. A. Bauer, "Oxidative pathways in cardiovascular disease: roles, mechanisms, and therapeutic implications," *Pharmacology and Therapeutics*, vol. 89, no. 2, pp. 187–206, 2001.

[8] M. P. Murphy, "How mitochondria produce reactive oxygen species," *Biochemical Journal*, vol. 417, no. 1, pp. 1–13, 2009.

[9] D. B. Zorov, M. Juhaszova, and S. J. Sollott, "Mitochondrial reactive oxygen species (ROS) and ROS-induced ROS release," *Physiological Reviews*, vol. 94, no. 3, pp. 909–950, 2014.

[10] D. E. Handy and J. Loscalzo, "Redox regulation of mitochondrial function," *Antioxidants & Redox Signaling*, vol. 16, no. 11, pp. 1323–1367, 2012.

[11] Y. J. H. J. Taverne, A. J. J. C. Bogers, D. J. Duncker, and D. Merkus, "Reactive oxygen species and the cardiovascular system," *Oxidative Medicine and Cellular Longevity*, vol. 2013, Article ID 862423, 15 pages, 2013.

[12] T. M. Paravicini and R. M. Touyz, "NADPH oxidases, reactive oxygen species, and hypertension: clinical implications and therapeutic possibilities," *Diabetes Care*, vol. 31, supplement 2, pp. S170–S180, 2008.

[13] C. H. Coyle, L. J. Martinez, M. C. Coleman, D. R. Spitz, N. L. Weintraub, and K. N. Kader, "Mechanisms of H_2O_2-induced oxidative stress in endothelial cells," *Free Radical Biology and Medicine*, vol. 40, no. 12, pp. 2206–2213, 2006.

[14] R. Scherz-Shouval and Z. Elazar, "ROS, mitochondria and the regulation of autophagy," *Trends in Cell Biology*, vol. 17, no. 9, pp. 422–427, 2007.

[15] K. Bedard and K.-H. Krause, "The NOX family of ROS-generating NADPH oxidases: physiology and pathophysiology," *Physiological Reviews*, vol. 87, no. 1, pp. 245–313, 2007.

[16] J. Kuroda, T. Ago, S. Matsushima, P. Zhai, M. D. Schneider, and J. Sadoshima, "NADPH oxidase 4 (Nox4) is a major source of oxidative stress in the failing heart," *Proceedings of the National Academy of Sciences of the United States of America*, vol. 107, no. 35, pp. 15565–15570, 2010.

[17] L. Zuo, S. Pasniciuc, V. P. Wright, A. J. Merola, and T. L. Clanton, "Sources for superoxide release: lessons from blockade of electron transport, NADPH oxidase, and anion channels in diaphragm," *Antioxidants and Redox Signaling*, vol. 5, no. 5, pp. 667–675, 2003.

[18] Y. Taniyama and K. K. Griendling, "Reactive oxygen species in the vasculature: molecular and cellular mechanisms," *Hypertension*, vol. 42, no. 6, pp. 1075–1081, 2003.

[19] C. Napoli and L. J. Ignarro, "Nitric oxide and atherosclerosis," *Nitric Oxide*, vol. 5, no. 2, pp. 88–97, 2001.

[20] M. C. Verhaar, P. E. Westerweel, A. J. Van Zonneveld, and T. J. Rabelink, "Free radical production by dysfunctional eNOS," *Heart*, vol. 90, no. 5, pp. 494–495, 2004.

[21] L. C. Jones and A. D. Hingorani, "Genetic regulation of endothelial function," *Heart*, vol. 91, no. 10, pp. 1275–1277, 2005.

[22] M. de la Paz Scribano, M. del Carmen Baez, B. Florencia et al., "Effects of atorvastatin on oxidative stress biomarkers and mitochondrial morphofunctionality in hyperfibrinogenemia-induced atherogenesis," *Advances in Medicine*, vol. 2014, Article ID 947258, 6 pages, 2014.

[23] B. Lipinski, "Pathophysiology of oxidative stress in diabetes mellitus," *Journal of Diabetes and Its Complications*, vol. 15, no. 4, pp. 203–210, 2001.

[24] X.-L. Chen, Q. Zhang, R. Zhao, and R. M. Medford, "Superoxide, H_2O_2, and iron are required for TNF-α-induced MCP-1 gene expression in endothelial cells: Role of Rac1 and NADPH oxidase," *American Journal of Physiology—Heart and Circulatory Physiology*, vol. 286, no. 3, pp. H1001–H1007, 2004.

[25] M. Malinouski, Y. Zhou, V. V. Belousov, D. L. Hatfield, and V. N. Gladyshev, "Hydrogen peroxide probes directed to different cellular compartments," *PLoS ONE*, vol. 6, no. 1, Article ID e14564, 2011.

[26] V. V. Belousov, A. F. Fradkov, K. A. Lukyanov et al., "Genetically encoded fluorescent indicator for intracellular hydrogen peroxide," *Nature Methods*, vol. 3, no. 4, pp. 281–286, 2006.

[27] S. Dikalov, K. K. Griendling, and D. G. Harrison, "Measurement of reactive oxygen species in cardiovascular studies," *Hypertension*, vol. 49, no. 4, pp. 717–727, 2007.

[28] J. Zielonka, S. Srinivasan, M. Hardy et al., "Cytochrome c-mediated oxidation of hydroethidine and mito-hydroethidine in mitochondria: identification of homo- and heterodimers," *Free Radical Biology and Medicine*, vol. 44, no. 5, pp. 835–846, 2008.

[29] A. E. Dikalova, A. T. Bikineyeva, K. Budzyn et al., "Therapeutic targeting of mitochondrial superoxide in hypertension," *Circulation Research*, vol. 107, no. 1, pp. 106–116, 2010.

[30] S. Dikalov, B. Fink, M. Skatchkov, and E. Bassenge, "Comparison of glyceryl trinitrate-induced with pentaerythrityl tetranitrate-induced in vivo formation of superoxide radicals: effect of vitamin C," *Free Radical Biology and Medicine*, vol. 27, no. 1-2, pp. 170–176, 1999.

[31] S. Dikalov, M. Skatchkov, B. Fink, and E. Bassenge, "Quantification of superoxide radicals and peroxynitrite in vascular cells using oxidation of sterically hindered hydroxylamines and electron spin resonance," *Nitric Oxide*, vol. 1, no. 5, pp. 423–431, 1997.

[32] S. I. Dikalov, A. E. Dikalova, and R. P. Mason, "Noninvasive diagnostic tool for inflammation-induced oxidative stress using electron spin resonance spectroscopy and an extracellular cyclic hydroxylamine," *Archives of Biochemistry and Biophysics*, vol. 402, no. 2, pp. 218–226, 2002.

[33] M. C. Y. Chang, A. Pralle, E. Y. Isacoff, and C. J. Chang, "A selective, cell-permeable optical probe for hydrogen peroxide in living cells," *Journal of the American Chemical Society*, vol. 126, no. 47, pp. 15392–15393, 2004.

[34] E. W. Miller, A. E. Albers, A. Pralle, E. Y. Isacoff, and C. J. Chang, "Boronate-based fluorescent probes for imaging cellular hydrogen peroxide," *Journal of the American Chemical Society*, vol. 127, no. 47, pp. 16652–16659, 2005.

[35] S. E. Gomez-Mejiba, Z. Zhai, H. Akram et al., "Immuno-spin trapping of protein and DNA radicals: 'tagging' free radicals to locate and understand the redox process," *Free Radical Biology and Medicine*, vol. 46, no. 7, pp. 853–865, 2009.

[36] R. P. Mason, "Using anti-5,5-dimethyl-1-pyrroline N-oxide (anti-DMPO) to detect protein radicals in time and space with immuno-spin trapping," *Free Radical Biology and Medicine*, vol. 36, no. 10, pp. 1214–1223, 2004.

[37] J. Jiang, K. J. Liu, X. Shi, and H. M. Swartz, "Detection of short-lived free radicals by low-frequency electron paramagnetic resonance spin trapping in whole living animals," *Archives of Biochemistry and Biophysics*, vol. 319, no. 2, pp. 570–573, 1995.

[38] T. Sano, F. Umeda, T. Hashimoto, H. Nawata, and H. Utsumi, "Oxidative stress measurement by in vivo electron spin resonance spectroscopy in rats with streptozotocin-induced diabetes," *Diabetologia*, vol. 41, no. 11, pp. 1355–1360, 1998.

[39] F. He and L. Zuo, "Redox roles of reactive oxygen species in cardiovascular diseases," *International Journal of Molecular Sciences*, vol. 16, no. 12, pp. 27770–27780, 2015.

[40] X. Zhu and L. Zuo, "Characterization of oxygen radical formation mechanism at early cardiac ischemia," *Cell Death & Disease*, vol. 4, no. 9, article e787, 7 pages, 2013.

[41] X.-X. Wang, X.-L. Wang, M.-M. Tong et al., "SIRT6 protects cardiomyocytes against ischemia/reperfusion injury by augmenting FoxO3α-dependent antioxidant defense mechanisms," *Basic Research in Cardiology*, vol. 111, no. 2, pp. 1–19, 2016.

[42] B. Halliwell and M. Whiteman, "Measuring reactive species and oxidative damage *in vivo* and in cell culture: how should you do it and what do the results mean?" *British Journal of Pharmacology*, vol. 142, no. 2, pp. 231–255, 2004.

[43] V. Adam-Vizi and C. Chinopoulos, "Bioenergetics and the formation of mitochondrial reactive oxygen species," *Trends in Pharmacological Sciences*, vol. 27, no. 12, pp. 639–645, 2006.

[44] J.-S. Kim, Y. Jin, and J. J. Lemasters, "Reactive oxygen species, but not Ca^{2+} overloading, trigger pH- and mitochondrial permeability transition-dependent death of adult rat myocytes after ischemia-reperfusion," *American Journal of Physiology—Heart and Circulatory Physiology*, vol. 290, no. 5, pp. H2024–H2034, 2006.

[45] M. Rigoulet, E. D. Yoboue, and A. Devin, "Mitochondrial ROS generation and its regulation: mechanisms involved in H_2O_2 signaling," *Antioxidants & Redox Signaling*, vol. 14, no. 3, pp. 459–468, 2011.

[46] D. Asada, T. Itoi, A. Nakamura, and K. Hamaoka, "Tolerance to ischemia reperfusion injury in a congenital heart disease model," *Pediatrics International*, 2016.

[47] X. Huang, J. Zhang, J. Liu et al., "C-reactive protein promotes adhesion of monocytes to endothelial cells via NADPH oxidase-mediated oxidative stress," *Journal of Cellular Biochemistry*, vol. 113, no. 3, pp. 857–867, 2012.

[48] H.-H. Lee, K. R. Paudel, and D.-W. Kim, "*Terminalia chebula* fructus inhibits migration and proliferation of vascular smooth muscle cells and production of inflammatory mediators in RAW 264.7," *Evidence-Based Complementary and Alternative Medicine*, vol. 2015, Article ID 502182, 10 pages, 2015.

[49] K. R. Paudel, N. Panth, and D.-W. Kim, "Circulating endothelial microparticles: a key hallmark of atherosclerosis progression," *Scientifica*, vol. 2016, Article ID 8514056, 9 pages, 2016.

[50] R. M. Touyz, A. M. Briones, M. Sedeek, D. Burger, and A. C. Montezano, "NOX isoforms and reactive oxygen species in vascular health," *Molecular Interventions*, vol. 11, no. 1, pp. 27–35, 2011.

[51] T. Akasaki, Y. Ohya, J. Kuroda et al., "Increased expression of gp91phox homologues of NAD(P)H oxidase in the aortic media during chronic hypertension: Involvement of the renin-angiotensin system," *Hypertension Research*, vol. 29, no. 10, pp. 813–820, 2006.

[52] G. Gordillo, H. Fang, H. Park, and S. Roy, "Nox-4-dependent nuclear H2O2 drives DNA oxidation resulting in 8-OHdG as urinary biomarker and hemangioendothelioma formation," *Antioxidants and Redox Signaling*, vol. 12, no. 8, pp. 933–943, 2010.

[53] D. Harrison, K. K. Griendling, U. Landmesser, B. Hornig, and H. Drexler, "Role of oxidative stress in atherosclerosis," *The American Journal of Cardiology*, vol. 91, no. 3, pp. 7–11, 2003.

[54] D. G. Harrison, "Cellular and molecular mechanisms of endothelial cell dysfunction," *The Journal of Clinical Investigation*, vol. 100, no. 9, pp. 2153–2157, 1997.

[55] M. Y. White, A. V. G. Edwards, S. J. Cordwell, and J. E. Van Eyk, "Mitochondria: a mirror into cellular dysfunction in heart disease," *Proteomics: Clinical Applications*, vol. 2, no. 6, pp. 845–861, 2008.

[56] L. K. Sharma, J. Lu, and Y. Bai, "Mitochondrial respiratory complex I: structure, function and implication in human diseases," *Current Medicinal Chemistry*, vol. 16, no. 10, pp. 1266–1277, 2009.

[57] E. Yu, P. A. Calvert, J. R. Mercer et al., "Mitochondrial DNA damage can promote atherosclerosis independently of reactive oxygen species through effects on smooth muscle cells and monocytes and correlates with higher-risk plaques in humans," *Circulation*, vol. 128, no. 7, pp. 702–712, 2013.

[58] J. L. Fetterman, M. Holbrook, D. G. Westbrook et al., "Mitochondrial DNA damage and vascular function in patients with diabetes mellitus and atherosclerotic cardiovascular disease," *Cardiovascular Diabetology*, vol. 15, no. 53, pp. 1–7, 2016.

[59] I. Fleming, U. R. Michaelis, D. Bredenkötter et al., "Endothelium-derived hyperpolarizing factor synthase (cytochrome P450 2C9) is a functionally significant source of reactive oxygen species in coronary arteries," *Circulation Research*, vol. 88, no. 1, pp. 44–51, 2001.

[60] N. R. Madamanchi and M. S. Runge, "Mitochondrial dysfunction in atherosclerosis," *Circulation Research*, vol. 100, no. 4, pp. 460–473, 2007.

[61] S. W. Ballinger, C. Patterson, C. A. Knight-Lozano et al., "Mitochondrial integrity and function in atherogenesis," *Circulation*, vol. 106, no. 5, pp. 544–549, 2002.

[62] S. DiMauro and E. A. Schon, "Mitochondrial respiratory-chain diseases," *The New England Journal of Medicine*, vol. 348, no. 26, pp. 2656–2668, 2003.

[63] P. S. Brookes, Y. Yoon, J. L. Robotham, M. W. Anders, and S.-S. Sheu, "Calcium, ATP, and ROS: a mitochondrial love-hate triangle," *American Journal of Physiology—Cell Physiology*, vol. 287, no. 4, pp. C817–C833, 2004.

[64] F. Di Lisa and P. Bernardi, "Mitochondrial function and myocardial aging. A critical analysis of the role of permeability transition," *Cardiovascular Research*, vol. 66, no. 2, pp. 222–232, 2005.

[65] H. Utsumi, K. Yasukawa, T. Soeda et al., "Noninvasive mapping of reactive oxygen species by *in vivo* electron spin resonance spectroscopy in indomethacin-induced gastric ulcers in rats," *Journal of Pharmacology and Experimental Therapeutics*, vol. 317, no. 1, pp. 228–235, 2006.

[66] H.-H. Lee, K. R. Paudel, J. Jeong et al., "Antiatherogenic effect of *Camellia japonica* fruit extract in high fat diet-fed rats ," *Evidence-Based Complementary and Alternative Medicine*, vol. 2016, Article ID 9679867, 8 pages, 2016.

[67] K. R. Paudel, U.-W. Lee, and D.-W. Kim, "Chungtaejeon, a Korean fermented tea, prevents the risk of atherosclerosis in rats fed a high-fat atherogenic diet," *Journal of Integrative Medicine*, vol. 14, no. 2, pp. 134–142, 2016.

[68] S. Mitra, T. Goyal, and J. L. Mehta, "Oxidized LDL, LOX-1 and atherosclerosis," *Cardiovascular Drugs and Therapy*, vol. 25, no. 5, pp. 419–429, 2011.

[69] K. R. Paudel, R. Karki, and D.-W. Kim, "Cepharanthine inhibits in vitro VSMC proliferation and migration and vascular inflammatory responses mediated by RAW264.7," *Toxicology in Vitro*, vol. 34, pp. 16–25, 2016.

[70] M. Y. Jun, R. Karki, K. R. Paudel, B. R. Sharma, D. Adhikari, and D.-W. Kim, "Alkaloid rich fraction from *Nelumbo nucifera* targets VSMC proliferation and migration to suppress restenosis in balloon-injured rat carotid artery," *Atherosclerosis*, vol. 248, pp. 179–189, 2016.

[71] S. Ehara, M. Ueda, T. Naruko et al., "Elevated levels of oxidized low density lipoprotein show a positive relationship with the severity of acute coronary syndromes," *Circulation*, vol. 103, no. 15, pp. 1955–1960, 2001.

[72] C. Meisinger, J. Baumert, N. Khuseyinova, H. Loewel, and W. Koenig, "Plasma oxidized low-density lipoprotein, a strong predictor for acute coronary heart disease events in apparently healthy, middle-aged men from the general population," *Circulation*, vol. 112, no. 5, pp. 651–657, 2005.

[73] S. Baldus, C. Heeschen, T. Meinertz et al., "Myeloperoxidase serum levels predict risk in patients with acute coronary syndromes," *Circulation*, vol. 108, no. 12, pp. 1440–1445, 2003.

[74] F. S. Apple, L. A. Pearce, A. Chung, R. Ler, and M. M. Murakami, "Multiple biomarker use for detection of adverse events in patients presenting with symptoms suggestive of acute coronary syndrome," *Clinical Chemistry*, vol. 53, no. 5, pp. 874–881, 2007.

[75] D. Kutter, P. Devaquet, G. Vanderstocken, J. M. Paulus, V. Marchal, and A. Gothot, "Consequences of total and subtotal myeloperoxidase deficiency: risk or benefit?" *Acta Haematologica*, vol. 104, no. 1, pp. 10–15, 2000.

[76] C. Léculier, N. Couprie, P. Adeleine, P. Leitienne, A. Francina, and M. Richard, "The effects of high molecular weight- and low molecular weight-heparins on superoxide ion production and degranulation by human polymorphonuclear leukocytes," *Thrombosis Research*, vol. 69, no. 6, pp. 519–531, 1993.

[77] G. de Gaetano, C. Cerletti, and V. Evangelista, "Recent advances in platelet-polymorphonuclear leukocyte interaction," *Haemostasis*, vol. 29, no. 1, pp. 41–49, 1999.

[78] J. Shih, S. A. Datwyler, S. C. Hsu et al., "Effect of collection tube type and preanalytical handling on myeloperoxidase concentrations," *Clinical Chemistry*, vol. 54, no. 6, pp. 1076–1079, 2008.

[79] G. L. Milne, E. S. Musiek, and J. D. Morrow, "F_2-isoprostanes as markers of oxidative stress *in vivo*: an overview," *Biomarkers*, vol. 10, pp. 10–23, 2005.

[80] B. Shao and J. W. Heinecke, "HDL, lipid peroxidation, and atherosclerosis," *Journal of Lipid Research*, vol. 50, no. 4, pp. 599–601, 2009.

[81] P. Patrignani, G. Santini, M. R. Panara et al., "Induction of prostaglandin endoperoxide synthase-2 in human monocytes associated with cyclo-oxygenase-dependent F2-isoprostane formation," *British Journal of Pharmacology*, vol. 118, no. 5, pp. 1285–1293, 1996.

[82] C. Vassalle, N. Botto, M. G. Andreassi, S. Berti, and A. Biagini, "Evidence for enhanced 8-isoprostane plasma levels, as index of oxidative stress in vivo, in patients with coronary artery disease," *Coronary Artery Disease*, vol. 14, no. 3, pp. 213–218, 2003.

[83] B. Halliwell and C. Y. J. Lee, "Using isoprostanes as biomarkers of oxidative stress: some rarely considered issues," *Antioxidants & Redox Signaling*, vol. 13, no. 2, pp. 145–156, 2010.

[84] L. Zuo, L. Nogueira, and M. C. Hogan, "Reactive oxygen species formation during tetanic contractions in single isolated *Xenopus myofibers*," *Journal of Applied Physiology*, vol. 111, no. 3, pp. 898–904, 2011.

[85] L. Zuo, T. M. Best, W. J. Roberts, P. T. Diaz, and P. D. Wagner, "Characterization of reactive oxygen species in diaphragm," *Acta Physiologica*, vol. 213, no. 3, pp. 700–710, 2015.

[86] L. Zuo, F. L. Christofi, V. P. Wright, S. Bao, and T. L. Clanton, "Lipoxygenase-dependent superoxide release in skeletal muscle," *Journal of Applied Physiology*, vol. 97, no. 2, pp. 661–668, 2004.

[87] T. Zhou, C.-C. Chuang, and L. Zuo, "Molecular characterization of reactive oxygen species in myocardial ischemia-reperfusion injury," *BioMed Research International*, vol. 2015, Article ID 864946, 9 pages, 2015.

[88] T. L. Vanden Hoek, C. Li, Z. Shao, P. T. Schumacker, and L. B. Becker, "Significant levels of oxidants are generated by isolated cardiomyocytes during ischemia prior to reperfusion," *Journal of Molecular and Cellular Cardiology*, vol. 29, no. 9, pp. 2571–2583, 1997.

[89] L. B. Becker, T. L. Vanden Hoek, Z.-H. Shao, C.-Q. Li, and P. T. Schumacker, "Generation of superoxide in cardiomyocytes during ischemia before reperfusion," *American Journal of Physiology—Heart and Circulatory Physiology*, vol. 277, no. 6, pp. H2240–H2246, 1999.

[90] E. Robin, R. D. Guzy, G. Loor et al., "Oxidant stress during simulated ischemia primes cardiomyocytes for cell death during reperfusion," *The Journal of Biological Chemistry*, vol. 282, no. 26, pp. 19133–19143, 2007.

[91] J. S. Lane, C. P. Magno, K. T. Lane, T. Chan, D. B. Hoyt, and S. Greenfield, "Nutrition impacts the prevalence of peripheral arterial disease in the United States," *Journal of Vascular Surgery*, vol. 48, no. 4, pp. 897–904, 2008.

[92] World Cancer Research Fund/American Institute for Cancer Research, *Food, Nutrition and the Prevention of Cancer: A Global Perspective*, American Institute for Cancer Research, Washington, DC, USA, 1997.

[93] WHO, "Report of the joint WHO/FAO expert consultation. Diet, nutrition and the prevention of chronic diseases," WHO Technical Report Series 916 (TRS 916), 2003.

[94] J. M. Rapola, J. Virtamo, S. Ripatti et al., "Randomised trial of α-tocopherol and β-carotene supplements on incidence of major coronary events in men with previous myocardial infarction," *The Lancet*, vol. 349, no. 9067, pp. 1715–1720, 1997.

[95] R. B. Singh, G. S. Wander, A. Rastogi et al., "Randomized, double-blind placebo-controlled trial of coenzyme Q10 in patients with acute myocardial infarction," *Cardiovascular Drugs and Therapy*, vol. 12, no. 4, pp. 347–353, 1998.

[96] S. Das, H. Otani, N. Maulik, and D. K. Das, "Lycopene, tomatoes, and coronary heart disease," *Free Radical Research*, vol. 39, no. 4, pp. 449–455, 2005.

[97] J.-F. Su, C.-J. Guo, J.-Y. Wei, J.-J. Yang, Y.-G. Jiang, and Y.-F. Li, "Protection against hepatic ischemia-reperfusion injury in rats by oral pretreatment with quercetin," *Biomedical and Environmental Sciences*, vol. 16, no. 1, pp. 1–8, 2003.

[98] K. R. Paudel and N. Panth, "Phytochemical profile and biological activity of *Nelumbo nucifera*," *Evidence-based Complementary and Alternative Medicine*, vol. 2015, Article ID 789124, 16 pages, 2015.

[99] N. Panth, K. R. Paudel, and R. Karki, "Phytochemical profile and biological activity of juglans regia," *Journal of Integrative Medicine*, vol. 14, 2016.

[100] S. R. Devkota, K. R. Paudel, K. Sharma et al., "Investigation of antioxidant and anti-inflammatory activity of roots of Rumex nepalensis," *World Journal of Pharmacy and Pharmaceutical Sciences*, vol. 4, no. 3, pp. 582–594, 2015.

[101] E. E. Nishi, R. Ribeiro Campos, C. Toledo Bergamaschi, V. R. de Almeida, and D. A. Ribeiro, "Vitamin C prevents DNA damage induced by renovascular hypertension in multiple organs of Wistar rats," *Human & Experimental Toxicology*, vol. 29, no. 7, pp. 593–599, 2010.

[102] M. S. Botelho-Ono, H. V. Pina, K. H. F. Sousa, F. C. Nunes, I. A. Medeiros, and V. A. Braga, "Acute superoxide scavenging restores depressed baroreflex sensitivity in renovascular hypertensive rats," *Autonomic Neuroscience: Basic and Clinical*, vol. 159, no. 1-2, pp. 38–44, 2011.

[103] R. M. Bruno, E. Daghini, L. Ghiadoni et al., "Effect of acute administration of vitamin C on muscle sympathetic activity, cardiac sympathovagal balance, and baroreflex sensitivity in hypertensive patients," *American Journal of Clinical Nutrition*, vol. 96, no. 2, pp. 302–308, 2012.

[104] A. Uzun, U. Yener, O. F. Cicek et al., "Does vitamin C or its combination with vitamin e improve radial artery endothelium-dependent vasodilatation in patients awaiting coronary artery bypass surgery?" *Cardiovascular Journal of Africa*, vol. 24, no. 7, pp. 255–259, 2013.

[105] M. Agarwal, P. K. Mehta, J. H. Dwyer et al., "Differing relations to early atherosclerosis between vitamin C from supplements vs. food in the Los Angeles atherosclerosis study: a prospective cohort study," *The Open Cardiovascular Medicine Journal*, vol. 6, no. 1, pp. 113–121, 2012.

[106] N. C. Ward, J. M. Hodgson, K. D. Croft, V. Burke, L. J. Beilin, and I. B. Puddey, "The combination of vitamin C and grape-seed polyphenols increases blood pressure: a randomized, double-blind, placebo-controlled trial," *Journal of Hypertension*, vol. 23, no. 2, pp. 427–434, 2005.

[107] E. Serbinova, S. Khwaja, J. Catudioc et al., "Palm oil vitamin E protects against ischemia/reperfusion injury in the isolated perfused langendorff heart," *Nutrition Research*, vol. 12, supplement 1, pp. S203–S215, 1992.

[108] A. W. Ashor, M. Siervo, J. Lara, C. Oggioni, and J. C. Mathers, "Antioxidant vitamin supplementation reduces arterial stiffness in adults: a systematic review and meta-analysis of randomized controlled trials," *Journal of Nutrition*, vol. 144, no. 10, pp. 1594–1602, 2014.

[109] N. G. Stephens, A. Parsons, P. M. Schofield et al., "Randomised controlled trial of vitamin E in patients with coronary disease: cambridge Heart Antioxidant Study (CHAOS)," *The Lancet*, vol. 347, no. 9004, pp. 781–786, 1996.

[110] K. Goszcz, S. J. Deakin, G. G. Duthie, D. Stewart, S. J. Leslie, and I. L. Megson, "Antioxidants in cardiovascular therapy: panacea or false hope?" *Frontiers in Cardiovascular Medicine*, vol. 2, article 29, pp. 1–22, 2015.

[111] A. H. Hasty, M. L. Gruen, E. S. Terry et al., "Effects of vitamin E on oxidative stress and atherosclerosis in an obese hyperlipidemic mouse model," *The Journal of Nutritional Biochemistry*, vol. 18, no. 2, pp. 127–133, 2007.

[112] C. R. Gale, C. N. Martyn, P. D. Winter, and C. Cooper, "Vitamin C and risk of death from stroke and coronary heart disease in cohort of elderly people," *The British Medical Journal*, vol. 310, no. 6994, pp. 1563–1566, 1995.

[113] S. Yusuf, G. Dagenais, J. Pogue, J. Bosch, and P. Sleight, "Vitamin E supplementation and cardiovascular events in high-risk patients. The Heart Outcomes Prevention Evaluation Study

Investigators," *The New England Journal of Medicine*, vol. 342, no. 3, pp. 154–160, 2000.

[114] J. Thorburn, S. Xu, and A. Thorburn, "MAP kinase- and Rho-dependent signals interact to regulate gene expression but not actin morphology in cardiac muscle cells," *The EMBO Journal*, vol. 16, no. 8, pp. 1888–1900, 1997.

[115] J. K. Bendall, A. C. Cave, C. Heymes, N. Gall, and A. M. Shah, "Pivotal role of a gp91(phox)-containing NADPH oxidase in angiotensin II-induced cardiac hyper-trophy in mice," *Circulation*, vol. 105, pp. 293–296, 2002.

[116] J.-M. Li, N. P. Gall, D. J. Grieve, M. Chen, and A. M. Shah, "Activation of NADPH oxidase during progression of cardiac hypertrophy to failure," *Hypertension*, vol. 40, no. 4, pp. 477–484, 2002.

[117] H. Nakagami, M. Takemoto, and J. K. Liao, "NADPH oxidase-derived superoxide anion mediates angiotensin II-induced cardiac hypertrophy," *Journal of Molecular and Cellular Cardiology*, vol. 35, no. 7, pp. 851–859, 2003.

[118] M. Takemoto, K. Node, H. Nakagami et al., "Statins as antioxidant therapy for preventing cardiac myocyte hypertrophy," *The Journal of Clinical Investigation*, vol. 108, no. 10, pp. 1429–1437, 2001.

[119] T. M. Lee, T. F. Chou, and C. H. Tsai, "Association of pravastatin and left ventricular mass in hypercholesterolemic patients: role of 8-iso-prostaglandin f2alpha formation," *Journal of Cardiovascular Pharmacology*, vol. 40, no. 6, pp. 868–874, 2002.

[120] C. Maack, T. Kartes, H. Kilter et al., "Oxygen free radical release in human failing myocardium is associated with increased activity of racl-GTPase and represents a target for statin treatment," *Circulation*, vol. 108, no. 13, pp. 1567–1574, 2003.

[121] Cholesterol Treatment Trialists' (CTT) Collaborators, "Efficacy and safety of cholesterol-lowering treatment: prospective meta-analysis of data from 90,056 participants in 14 randomised trials of statins," *The Lancet*, vol. 366, no. 9493, pp. 1267–1278, 2005.

[122] M. H. Shishehbor, M.-L. Brennan, R. J. Aviles et al., "Statins promote potent systemic antioxidant effects through specific inflammatory pathways," *Circulation*, vol. 108, no. 4, pp. 426–431, 2003.

[123] K. Node, M. Fujita, M. Kitakaze, M. Hori, and J. K. Liao, "Short-term statin therapy improves cardiac function and symptoms in patients with idiopathic dilated cardiomyopathy," *Circulation*, vol. 108, no. 7, pp. 839–843, 2003.

[124] L. P. Mcquillan, G. K. Leung, P. A. Marsden, S. K. Kostyk, and S. Kourembanas, "Hypoxia inhibits expression of enos via transcriptional and posttranscriptional mechanisms," *American Journal of Physiology—Heart and Circulatory Physiology*, vol. 267, no. 5, pp. 1921–1927, 1994.

[125] M. Endres, U. Laufs, J. K. Liao, and M. A. Moskowitz, "Targeting eNOS for stroke protection," *Trends in Neurosciences*, vol. 27, no. 5, pp. 283–289, 2004.

[126] E. Chavakis, E. Dernbach, C. Hermann, U. F. Mondorf, A. M. Zeiher, and S. Dimmeler, "Oxidized LDL inhibits vascular endothelial growth factor—induced endothelial cell migration by an inhibitory effect on the Akt/endothelial nitric oxide synthase pathway," *Circulation*, vol. 103, no. 16, pp. 2102–2107, 2001.

[127] F. Jantzen, S. Konemann, B. Wolff et al., "Isoprenoid depletion by statins antagonizes cytokine-induced down-regulation of endothelial nitric oxide expression and increases no synthase activity in human umbilical vein EC," *Journal of Physiology and Pharmacology*, vol. 58, no. 3, pp. 503–514, 2007.

[128] M. Bourmoum, R. Charles, and A. Claing, "The GTPase ARF6 controls ROS production to mediate angiotensin II-induced vascular smooth muscle cell proliferation," *PLoS ONE*, vol. 11, no. 1, Article ID e0148097, 2016.

[129] M. Copaja, D. Venegas, P. Aránguiz et al., "Simvastatin induces apoptosis by a Rho-dependent mechanism in cultured cardiac fibroblasts and myofibroblasts," *Toxicology and Applied Pharmacology*, vol. 255, no. 1, pp. 57–64, 2011.

[130] K. M. Schmidt-Ott, S. Kagiyama, and M. I. Phillips, "The multiple actions of angiotensin II in atherosclerosis," *Regulatory Peptides*, vol. 93, no. 1–3, pp. 65–77, 2000.

[131] S. Pushpakumar, S. Kundu, T. Pryor et al., "Angiotensin-II induced hypertension and renovascular remodelling in tissue inhibitor of metalloproteinase 2 knockout mice," *Journal of Hypertension*, vol. 31, no. 11, pp. 2270–2281, 2013.

[132] J. B. Laursen, S. Rajagopalan, Z. Galis, M. Tarpey, B. A. Freeman, and D. G. Harrison, "Role of superoxide in angiotensin II—induced but not catecholamine-induced hypertension," *Circulation*, vol. 95, no. 3, pp. 588–593, 1997.

[133] S. Müller, I. König, W. Meyer, and G. Kojda, "Inhibition of vascular oxidative stress in hypercholesterolemia by eccentric isosorbide mononitrate," *Journal of the American College of Cardiology*, vol. 44, no. 3, pp. 624–631, 2004.

[134] L. J. Ignarro and C. Napoli, "Novel features of nitric oxide, endothelial nitric oxide synthase, and atherosclerosis," *Current Diabetes Reports*, vol. 5, no. 1, pp. 17–23, 2005.

[135] L. Zuo, M. S. Koozechian, and L. L. Chen, "Characterization of reactive nitrogen species in allergic asthma," *Annals of Allergy, Asthma & Immunology*, vol. 112, no. 1, pp. 18–22, 2014.

[136] F. Cosentino, C. Savoia, P. De Paolis et al., "Angiotensin II type 2 receptors contribute to vascular responses in spontaneously hypertensive rats treated with angiotensin II type 1 receptor antagonists," *American Journal of Hypertension*, vol. 18, no. 4, pp. 493–499, 2005.

[137] H. Ono, S. Minatoguchi, K. Watanabe et al., "Candesartan decreases carotid intima-media thickness by enhancing nitric oxide and decreasing oxidative stress in patients with hypertension," *Hypertension Research*, vol. 31, no. 2, pp. 271–279, 2008.

[138] S. Yagi, T. Morita, and S. Katayama, "Combined treatment with an AT1 receptor blocker and angiotensin converting enzyme inhibitor has an additive effect on inhibiting neointima formation via improvement of nitric oxide production and suppression of oxidative stress," *Hypertension Research*, vol. 27, no. 2, pp. 129–135, 2004.

22

An Optimized Injectable Hydrogel Scaffold Supports Human Dental Pulp Stem Cell Viability and Spreading

T. D. Jones,[1] A. Kefi,[1] S. Sun,[1] M. Cho,[1] and S. B. Alapati[2]

[1]*Bioengineering, University of Illinois at Chicago, Chicago, IL 60612-7212, USA*
[2]*Endodontics, University of Illinois at Chicago, Chicago, IL 60612-7212, USA*

Correspondence should be addressed to S. B. Alapati; salapati@uic.edu

Academic Editor: Chiaki Kitamura

Introduction. HyStem-C™ is a commercially available injectable hydrogel composed of polyethylene glycol diacrylate (PEGDA), hyaluronan (HA), and gelatin (Gn). These components can be mechanically tuned to enhance cell viability and spreading. *Methods.* The concentration of PEGDA with an added disulfide bond (PEGSSDA) was varied from 0.5 to 8.0% (w/v) to determine the optimal concentration for injectable clinical application. We evaluated the cell viability of human dental pulp stem cells (hDPSCs) embedded in 2% (w/v) PEGSSDA-HA-Gn hydrogels. Volume ratios of HA : Gn from 100 : 0 to 25 : 75 were varied to encourage hDPSC spreading. Fibronectin (Fn) was added to our model to determine the effect of extracellular matrix protein concentration on hDPSC behavior. *Results.* Our preliminary data suggests that the hydrogel gelation time decreased as the PEGSSDA cross-linker concentration increased. The PEGSSDA-HA-Gn was biocompatible with hDPSCs, and increased ratios of HA : Gn enhanced cell viability for 14 days. Additionally, cell proliferation with added fibronectin increased significantly over time at concentrations of 1.0 and 10.0 μg/mL in PEGDA-HA-Gn hydrogels, while cell spreading significantly increased at Fn concentrations of 0.1 μg/mL. *Conclusions.* This study demonstrates that PEG-based injectable hydrogels maintain hDPSC viability and facilitate cell spreading, mainly in the presence of extracellular matrix (ECM) proteins.

1. Introduction

Endodontics is a specialized dental field concerned with treating infected and traumatized dental tissues. During embryonic tooth development, the cranial neural crest gives rise to developing dental epithelium. Ectomesenchymal cells originate from the dental epithelium and form the dental papilla, an aggregate of differentiated ectomesenchymal cells called odontoblasts. During embryogenesis these highly specialized cells secrete primary dentin, a mineralized tissue surrounding dental pulp. Dental pulp is the soft tissue inside of the tooth core that contains nerve and blood vessels subject to thermal, chemical, mechanical, and bacterial insults.

Dental caries formation is the most prevalent disease affecting human teeth and may result in early tooth loss if left untreated [1]. Root canal therapy (RCT) is an endodontic procedure replacing infected or injured pulp tissue with a biologically inert material to resolve pain and control infection [2–5]. Reinfection of the pulp chamber due to bacterial invasion and susceptibility of tooth fracture may result in failed RCTs that require retreatment [6–8]. The successful design of a biological substitute for dental-pulp tissue will likely require a tissue engineering approach designed to restore, maintain, or improve dental-pulp tissue function applying both regenerative endodontics and engineering principles. Recent advances in these two fields support the regeneration potential of pulp tissue using human dental pulp stem cells (hDPSCs) embedded in bioactive scaffolds [9, 10].

This cell source holds considerable promise for dental engineering applications as they have been shown to differentiate into both avascular mineralizing tissues and the vasculature necessary for adequate nutrient exchange [4]. Despite recent progress in stem cell biology for translational clinical approaches, the scaffolds designed for dental pulp tissue engineering applications must be temporally and spatially optimized to set efficiently in complex geometries such as the root canal [9] while simultaneously facilitating cell attachment and spreading [11].

Cell attachment to a scaffold is likely required for the terminal differentiation of hDPSC into functional dentin-secreting odontoblasts [9]. Several groups have reported successful hDPSC attachment on natural or synthetic scaffolds such as collagen or poly(D,L-lactide-co-glycolide) (PLGA), respectively [12–15], but both scaffold types are limiting when considered independently. Natural scaffolds are biocompatible and biodegradable but may be immunogenic and weak [12]. Although synthetic scaffolds may be mechanically tuned and processed into desired shapes, they do not contain environmental cues for cell attachment found in the natural extracellular matrix (ECM) [10]. In addition to cell attachment, cell spreading on a substrate can greatly influence cell proliferation and death. Although cell-ECM interactions such as mediation with adhesive proteins have been well studied, the effect of early hDPSC spreading both on the surface of and embedded in scaffolds is less established. Interestingly, material properties have been shown to independently influence cell spreading.

Recently, it has been shown that "scaffoldless" constructs engineered from hDPSCs promote pulp vascularization [8], but the high cell density requirement, extensive material handling, and lack of characterization of the cells responsible for a regenerated dentin-pulp complex-like structure do not outweigh the clinical translation of more established injectable scaffold models [16] such as hydrogels. Injectable hydrogels combine the benefit of natural and synthetic scaffolds [17] and are practical for syringe applications. To our knowledge, no commercially available injectable hydrogel has been reported specifically for dental pulp tissue engineering applications.

HyStem-C is a thiol-reactive hyaluronan-based (HA) hydrogel that is cross-linked with synthetic polyethylene glycol diacrylate (PEGDA 3400) and thiol-reactive gelatin (Gn). It has been shown to facilitate tissue regeneration in various organ systems including the regeneration of subchondral bone [18]. The molecular weight of the PEG-based cross-linker and concentrations of HA and Gn can be manipulated to mimic desired tissue characteristics [18]. Another modular feature of the HyStem-C system is the ability to add or substitute ECM proteins with the Gn to better mirror target organ architecture.

In this paper, we chemically altered the HyStem-C components to investigate hDPSC biocompatibility and potential for syringe injection into the root canal lumen. We substituted PEGSSDA 8400 in place of PEGDA 3400 and assessed the hydrogel gelation time as a function of cross-linker concentration to increase the mechanical strength. SS indicates the presence of a disulfide bond that enables nonenzymatic cell recovery [18]. Next, we varied the ratio of HA : Gn to optimize cell spreading. A third goal of this paper was to determine the effect of fibronectin, a native dental pulp EMC protein, on hDPSC spreading. The overall goal of this study was to test the hypothesis that a PEGDA-HA based hydrogel combined with gelatin and fibronectin can support hDPSC

viability and spreading using an in vitro injectable three-dimensional (3D) cell delivery strategy.

2. Materials and Methods

2.1. Cell Culture. Human DPSCs were kindly gifted by Dr. Songtao Shi (University of Southern California) and expanded in vitro as previously reported by Gronthos et al. [19]. Briefly, cells between 3rd and 5th passages were grown in single-cell suspensions and seeded in $25\,cm^2$ culture flasks containing α-MEM medium (Invitrogen, Grand Island, NY, USA) supplemented with 20% fetal bovine serum (FBS), 2 mM L-glutamine, 100 mM L-ascorbic acid 2-phosphate, 100 U/mL penicillin, and 100 μg/mL streptomycin and incubated at 37°C in 5% CO_2.

2.2. Evaluation of Gelation Time as a Function of PEGSSDA Concentration. HyStem-C (BioTime, Inc., Alameda, CA) is a hyaluronan-based hydrogel kit containing a thiolated cross-linker (PEGDA molecular weight 3400), thiol-reactive gelatin (denatured collagen), and thiol-reactive hyaluronan. Thiolated PEGSSDA molecular weight ~8400 (Glycosan Biosystems, Inc., Alameda, CA) was used to cross-link the HA and Gn. HA and Gn were dissolved in phosphate-buffered saline (PBS) pH 7.4 to give 1.0% (w/v) solutions. Next, the HA and Gn solutions were mixed in a 1 : 1 (v/v) ratio. To determine the optimal gelation time of PEGSSDA (Glycosan Biosystems) as a function of concentration, the (w/v) of PEGSSDA was varied from 0.5% to 8%. The following concentrations were prepared in triplicate: 0.5%, 1.0%, 2.0%, 4.0%, and 8.0%. Each concentration was diluted in a 1 : 1 (v/v) ratio of hyaluronic acid : gelatin. The final aqueous solution was passed through a 20-gauge needle to model clinical application. Gelation time as a function of concentration was analyzed using nonlinear regression modeling SPSS software (Chicago, IL, USA). Solution-gel transitions were determined by the test tube transition inversion method at room temperature [20].

2.3. 3D Modeling of hDPSC. Human DPSCs were embedded in 100 μL of PEGSSDA-HA-Gn hydrogels at a density of 3.0×10^4 cells per cell culture tissue insert (Millipore, Billerica, MA, USA) in a 24-well plate. Cell culture insert dimensions were 13 mm in diameter and 10.5 mm in height, with a pore size of 8.0 μm. Briefly, a cell pellet was suspended in a 1 : 1 (v/v) ratio of HA : Gn. One volume of 2% (w/v) PEGSSDA was added to the HA + Gn cell slurry in a 1 : 4 volume ratio. The cell-embedded hydrogels were allowed to gel for one hour at 37°C in 5% CO_2 in the tissue culture inserts. Following gelation, 1.0 mL of cell culture medium was added to each insert-containing well. The medium was changed every other day.

2.4. Variation of Volume Ratio of Thiolated Hyaluronan : Thiolated Gelatin. To encourage cell spreading, the volume ratio of thiolated HA : thiolated Gn (Glycosan Biosystems, Inc., Alameda CA) was varied. A cell pellet (3.0 $\times 10^4$ human dental pulp stem cells) was suspended in each of four volume ratios of 1 : 0, 3 : 1, 1 : 1, and 1 : 3 corresponding to the ratio of HA : Gn. Next one volume of 2.0% (w/v)

PEGSSDA was added to four volumes of each prepared HA : Gn + cell sample. All components were dissolved in sterile PBS pH 7.4 and allowed to gel at room temperature for one hour. Experiments were performed in triplicate wells for each volume ratio mixture. The cells were analyzed for cell viability using a live/dead in vitro cell viability assay (Molecular Probes, Eugene, OR) at days 7 and 14 as per the manufacturer's instructions.

2.5. Addition of Fibronectin to PEGDA-HA-Gn Hydrogels.
To determine the effect of fibronectin on cell viability, proliferation, and spreading, purified human fibronectin (Millipore, Billerica, MA, USA) in phosphate buffer saline pH 7.4 was varied from 0.1 to 10 μg/mL and added to 1:1 (v/v) ratios of thiolated HA and Gn solutions. PEGDA 3400 (2.0% w/v) was added to the HA-Gn-Fn mixture in a 1:4 volume ratio to form 200 μL hydrogels in cell culture inserts of a 24-well plate. Positive control (PEGDA-HA-Gn) and negative control (PEGDA-HA-Fn) hydrogels were prepared in parallel. HDPSCs were serum-starved for 24 hours and seeded on the hydrogel surface at a density of 1×10^4 cells per 200 μL of hydrogel solution. The serum-free media were replaced with regular growth media after 24 hours. Samples were analyzed for cell proliferation, viability, and spreading at days 1 and 4 in triplicate. The cells were analyzed for cell viability using a viability assay (Molecular Probes, Eugene, OR) at days 1 and 4 as per the manufacturer's instructions.

2.6. Analysis of hDPSC Proliferation on PEGDA-HA-Gn-Fn Hydrogels.
Human dental pulp stem cell proliferation as a function of varying fibronectin concentration was assessed using a cell proliferation colorimetric assay (Roche, Indianapolis, IN, USA). At days 1 and 4, both the PEGDA-HA-Gn-Fn experimental and positive and negative control hydrogels seeded with 1×10^4 hDPSCs were transferred to fresh wells of a 24-well plate. The relative hDPSC density was assessed following the addition of 20 μL of WST-1 (2-(4-iodophenyl)-3-(4-nitrophenyl)-5-(2,4-disulfophenyl)-2H-tetrazolium, monosodium salt) reagent per well to achieve a 1:10 final concentration. The samples were incubated for three hours at 37°C in 5% CO_2 to allow the color conversion of the tetrazolium salt due to mitochondrial activity. The absorbance was measured using a microplate reader at 450 nm (BioTek, Winooski, VT, USA). Experiments were performed in triplicate wells per concentration at both days 1 and 4.

2.7. Fluorescent Microscopy.
Cell viability was observed using fluorescent microscopy. All samples treated for cell viability (Molecular Probes, Eugene, OR) were visualized with an E-800 Eclipse Nikon fluorescent microscope with a 20x objective lens and a 16-bit charge-coupled device camera (Photometrics, Tuscan, AZ, USA). Images were pseudocolored with MetaMorph imaging software (Molecular Devices, Sunnyvale, CA, USA). The Image J software bundle (National Institutes of Health, Bethesda, MD, USA) was used to quantify the effect of fibronectin concentration on hDPSC spreading. Red, green, and blue (RGB) images were split into

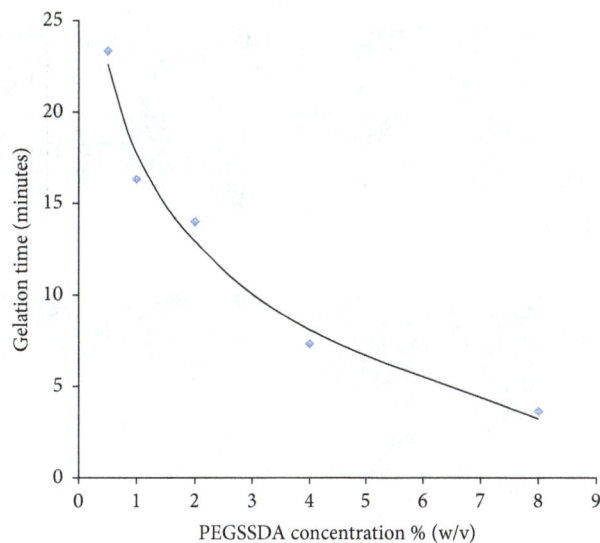

FIGURE 1: Gelation time as a function of PEGSSDA concentration fit to a nonlinear logarithmic regression model. Diamonds represent experimental data. The curved line is theoretical data.

constituent channels, and images were converted to 8-bit greyscale images. The "threshold" command was applied to classify the hDPSC morphology based on cell surface area.

2.8. Analysis of the Effect of Fibronectin Concentration on hDPSC Spreading.
Cell spreading at days 1 and 4 was quantified following the classification of hDPSC morphology into three distinct categories: round, partially spread, and fully spread. Postprocessing imaging using Image J software was used to determine the cell surface area in pixels^2. Cell rounding or spreading was calculated as (average number of round or spread cells/40 cells per field of view) × 100%. Four random fields per hydrogel were chosen for each sample and 10 cells were selected at a time to obtain 40 cells. Three independent samples were tested at both time points.

2.9. Statistical Analysis.
Statistical analysis for all triplicate data was analyzed using the one-way ANOVA followed by Tukey's post hoc test (SPSS, Chicago, IL, USA). A p value < 0.05 was considered significant.

3. Results

3.1. Quantification of Gelation Time as a Function of PEGSSDA Concentration.
Figure 1 shows the average gelation time of the PEGSSDA-HN-Gn hydrogels as a function of varying PEGSSDA concentration. The data represents the average gelation times of experiments conducted in triplicate and fit to a nonlinear logarithmic regression model. Diamonds denote experimental data, while the curved line represents theoretical data. The gelation time decreased as the percentage of (w/v) PEGSSDA concentration increased from 0.5% to 8.0%. The residual sum of squares (RSS) method was used to measure the discrepancy between the experimental and theoretical models and was calculated as 4.482.

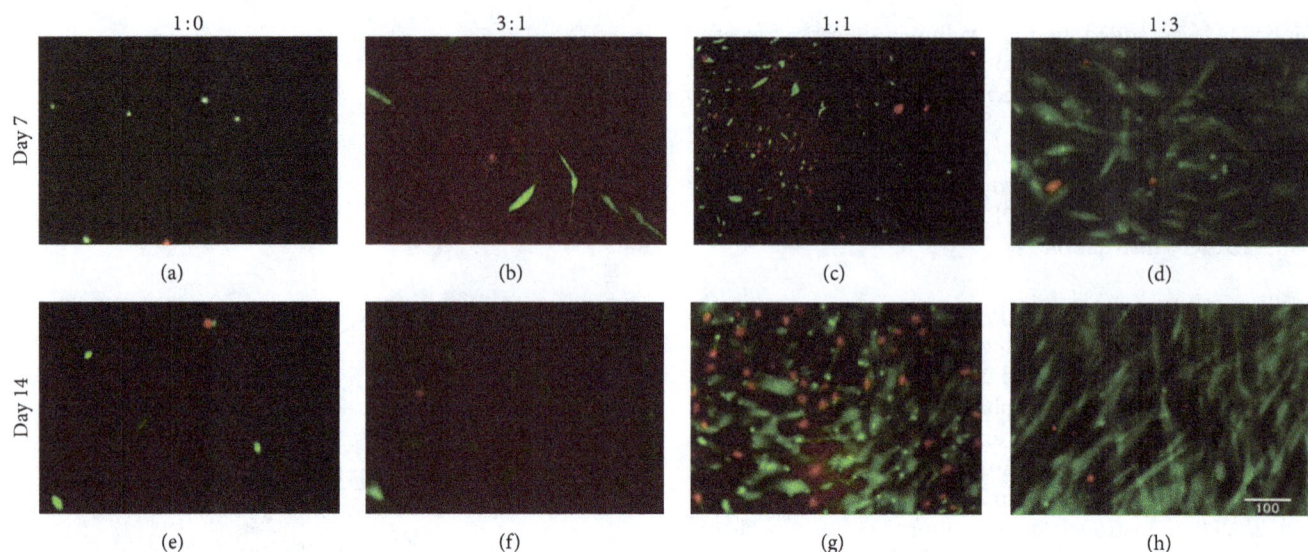

FIGURE 2: Immunofluorescence results for live/dead staining of human dental pulp stem cells embedded in 2.0% (w/v) PEGSSDA and varying (v/v) ratios of HA : GN. Green = live cells. Red = dead cells. Magnification = 20x. Scale bar = 100 μm.

3.2. Variation of Volume Ratio of Thiolated Hyaluronan : Thiolated Gelatin.

Figure 2 shows the hDPSC live/dead viability staining results of varied ratios of HA : Gn while maintaining a 2.0% (w/v) concentration of PEGSSDA. In general, the hDPSCs were more spindle-shaped in the 1 : 1 and 1 : 3 volume ratios of HA : Gn compared to the 1 : 0 and 3 : 1 HA : Gn volume ratios. The average number of live and dead cells per microscopic field of view is shown in Figures 3(a) and 3(b). Based on the limited number of cells in the field of view for the 1 : 0 and 3 : 1 HA : Gn ratios, we calculated the percentage of viable cells based on HA : Gn ratios for the 1 : 1 and 1 : 3 mixtures only (Figure 3(c)). The percentage of viable cells embedded in the 1 : 1 ratio of HA : Gn significantly decreased between days 7 and 14 (Figure 3(c)).

3.3. Analysis of hDPSC Proliferation on PEGDA-HA-Gn-Fn Hydrogels.

The results of the WST-1 assay are shown in Figure 4. The hDPSCs survived in all PEGDA based formulations. There was a significant increase from days 1 to 4 in the PEGDA-HA-Gn hydrogels with 1.0 μg/mL and 10.0 μg/mL of added human fibronectin. The positive control hydrogels lacking fibronectin also showed a significant increase in the relative human dental pulp stem cell density at day 4.

3.4. Human Dental Pulp Stem Cell Viability on PEG-Based Hydrogels.

We observed an increase in cell viability from days 1 to 4 in all PEGDA-HA-Gn hydrogels at all three concentrations of added fibronectin (see Figures 5(a)–5(c) and 5(f)–5(h)). Negative control samples without gelatin (PEGDA-HA) with 10.0 μg/mL of added fibronectin appeared to maintain a round morphology (Figures 5(d) and 5(i)). The positive control samples without added fibronectin were more spindle-shaped with increased spacing between individual cells (Figures 5(e) and 5(j)).

TABLE 1: Classification of hDPSC morphology in pixels^2 based on cell surface area range.

Cell surface area range (pixels^2)	Cell morphology
0–399	Round
400–1599	Partially spread
>1600	Fully spread

3.5. Analysis of the Effect of Fibronectin Concentration on hDPSC Spreading.

Table 1 shows the classification of hDPSC morphology based on the cell surface area range in pixels^2. Three distinct categories were identified based on the cell morphology. The percentage of rounded cells at day 4 in hydrogel samples containing PEGDA-HA-Gn supplemented with 0.1 μg/mL of fibronectin (Figure 6) was significantly less compared to day 1. This data corresponds to a significant increase in the percentage of partial and fully spread hDPSCs at the same hydrogel composition at day 4 (Figure 7).

4. Discussion

The present study builds on the dental tissue engineering triad model for pulp regeneration, combining a cell source, scaffold, and growth factors as possible alternatives to root canal therapy [21]. HDPSCs are an attractive cell source because they are multipotent and capable of differentiating into odontoblasts, vascular endothelial cells, fibroblasts, and neural cells [3]. Although cell differentiation was not a functional aim of this paper, we considered the potential of a single cell source that would maintain viability and spread in an injectable scaffold. Cell-based strategies for regenerative endodontics will require user-friendly cell delivery methods that are capable of gelation in pulp chambers [10].

(a) Volume ratio of hyaluronic acid : gelatin

(b) Volume ratio of hyaluronic acid : gelatin

(c) Volume ratio of hyaluronic acid : gelatin

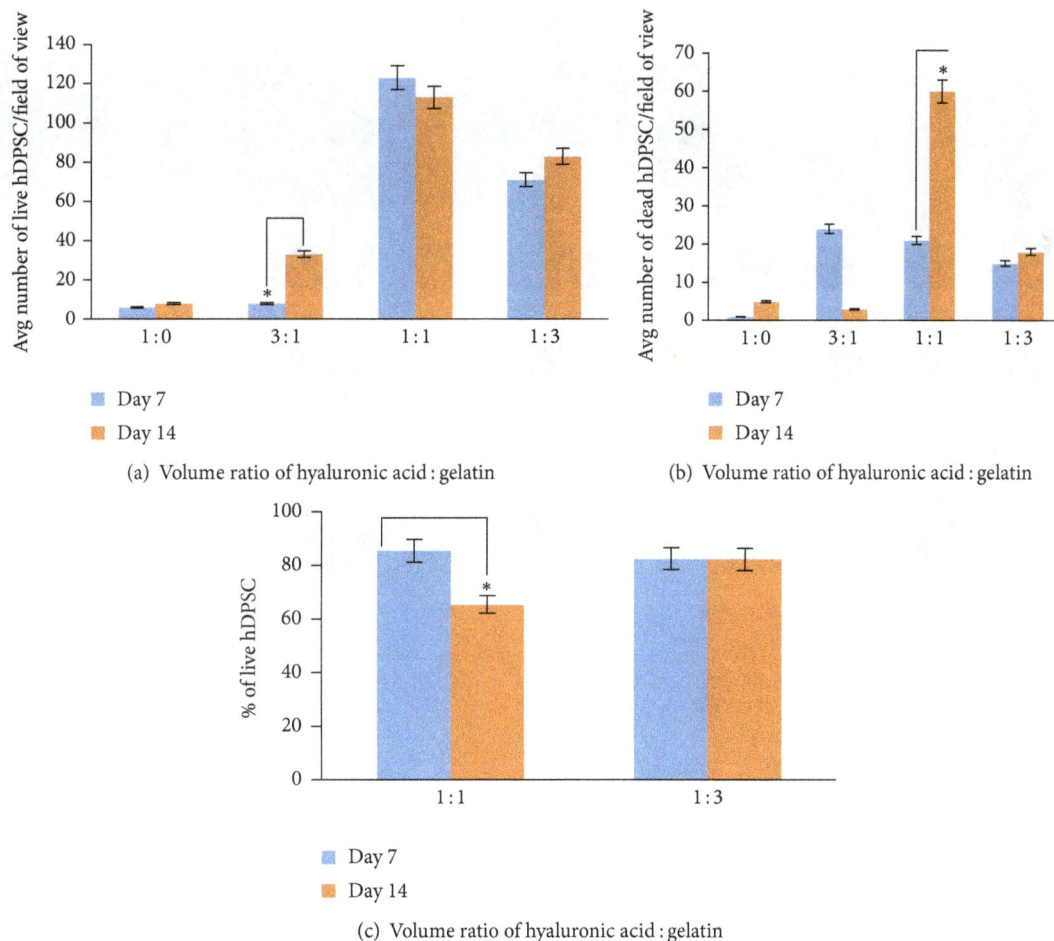

FIGURE 3: (a-b) The average number of live and dead hDPSC per field of view as a function of (v/v) ratio of HA : GN. (c) The percentage of live hDPSC in the 1 : 1 and 1 : 3 (v/v) ratios of HA : GN. $^*p < 0.05$.

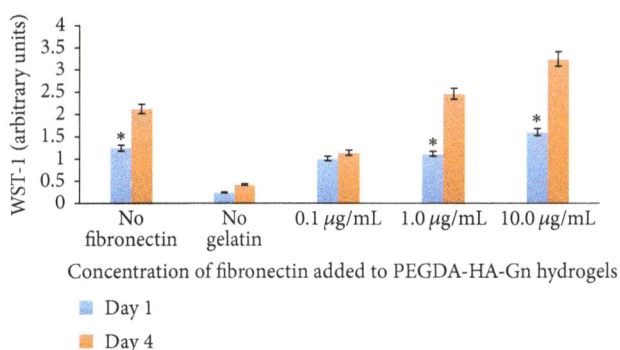

FIGURE 4: Proliferation of hDPSC in PEGDA-HA modified hydrogels with different concentrations of fibronectin. $n = 3$ samples. WST-1 was used to determine the relative cell densities at days 1 and 4. $^*p < 0.05$.

Despite the potential of injectable scaffolds with self-assembling peptides, these hydrogels are limited by poor mechanical strength and lack of pore shape control [22]. To address material and fabrication limitations, we aimed to optimize hDPSC cell viability and spreading by embedding cells in a 3D commercially available injectable scaffold with tunable mechanical properties. We hypothesized that a PEGSSDA (mol wt 8400) cross-linker would be more biocompatible with hDPSCs compared with a PEGDA (mol wt 3400) due to greater mechanical strength. Theoretically, this increased mechanical strength is due to a higher cross-linking density in the PEGSSDA. As such, an early research goal was to determine the relationship between gelation time and the PEGSSDA used in our experiments.

There was an inverse relationship between the gelation time and concentration. Higher PEGSSDA concentrations resulted in lower gelation times. This data is consistent with findings from Gupte and Ma, who suggested that a dense hydrogel network is formed due to an increase in the number of cross-links [23]. Although our experimental findings can be considered as a predictive model for product gelation time for syringe applications, future studies should examine the contribution of the HA and gelatin independently as a function of gelation time to increase the model accuracy. Conducting these experiments may result in a lower residual sum of squares value.

To simulate clinical application, we used a 2% (w/v) PEGSSDA concentration to enable sufficient product gelation time of approximately 14 minutes following extrusion from

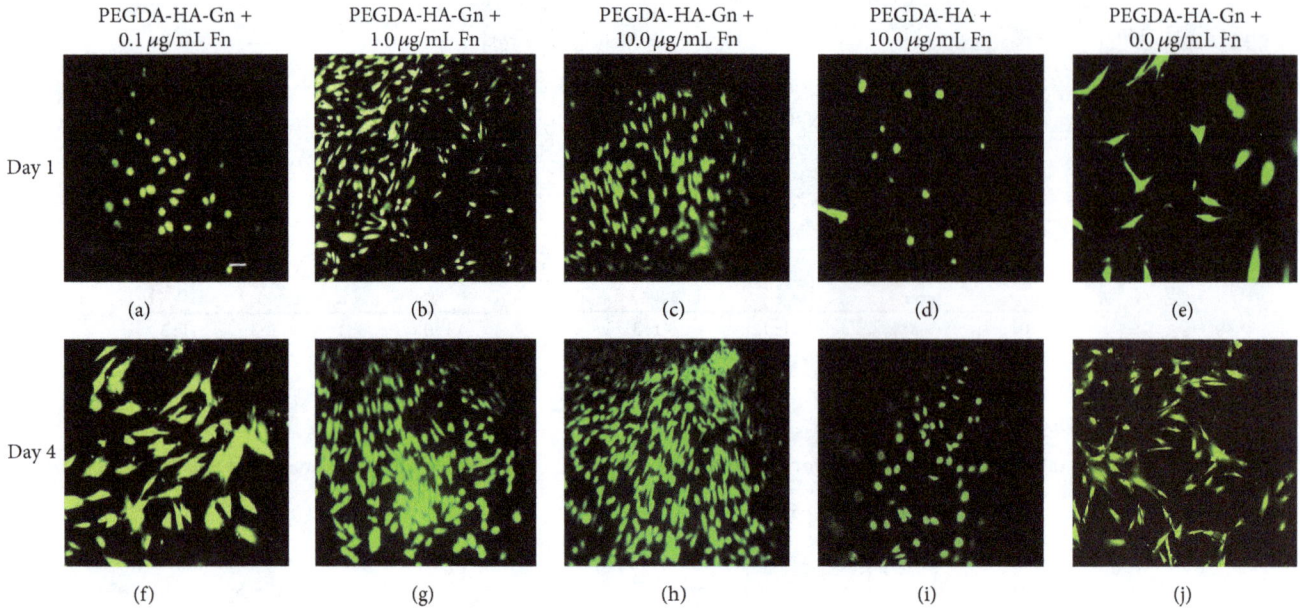

FIGURE 5: (a–j) Immunofluorescence staining results of human dental pulp stem cells seeded on the surface of polyethylene glycol diacrylate-based hydrogels. Data represents a sample of a random field of view from 4 random fields of view per hydrogel. Green = live cells. Magnification = 20x. Scale bar = 50 μm.

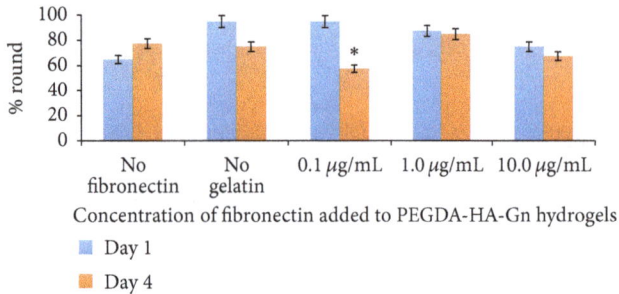

FIGURE 6: Effect of fibronectin concentration on hDPSC rounding. Data represents an average of 40 cells/field of view at 20x magnification. $n = 3$ samples. $^{*}p < 0.05$.

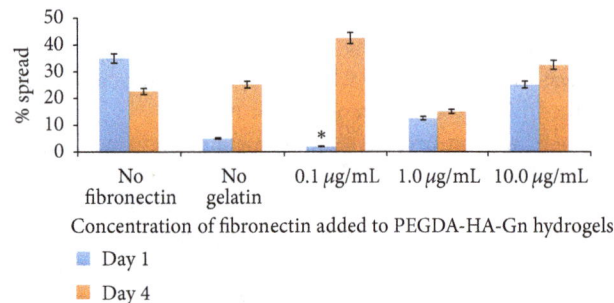

FIGURE 7: Effect of fibronectin concentration on hDPSC spreading. Data represents an average of 40 cells/field of view at 20x magnification. $n = 3$ samples. $^{*}p < 0.05$.

a 20-gauge needle. After maintaining a constant 1% (w/v) of HA and Gn mixed in a 1 : 1 volume ratio with the PEGSSDA, we noted that hDPSCs were viable in the PEGSSDA-HA-Gn hydrogel but exhibited a rounded morphology rather than

a flat spindle shape (data not shown). These results were consistent with a study comparing fibroblast morphology in a PEGDA-HA-Gn product [24]. We then varied the volume ratio of HA : Gn in an effort to increase hDPSC cell spreading.

For the first time, we report an optimal ratio of HA : Gn for cell delivery in an injectable PEG-based hydrogel scaffold. A 1 : 3 ratio of HA : Gn sustained cell viability in the PEGSSDA-HA-Gn scaffolds for up to 14 days in vitro. This could be due to increased gelatin content resulting in increased cell adhesion binding sites [25–27]. The 1 : 1 ratio of HA : Gn significantly increased the percentage of nonviable hDPSCs (data not shown) in the scaffold, which may be attributed to cell culture insert space limitations. Though this is not the aim of this study, PEGSSDA also enables nonenzymatic cell recovery from the hydrogel if desired [28].

The modular inclusion of cell adhesion proteins is a second benefit of using injectable tunable hydrogels for cellular encapsulation [29]. In concert with our long-term goal of fabricating a physiologically relevant hybrid extracellular matrix mimic, we seeded hDPSCs on the surface of PEGDA-HA-Gn scaffolds and varied the concentration of added fibronectin. We selected the PEGDA 3400 as a cross-linking agent for these experiments for two main reasons. Firstly, the viscoelastic properties of PEGDA-HA-Gn scaffolds have been well characterized by Ghosh et al. [30], reporting an elastic modulus of ~550 Pa. More importantly, human dental pulp is a soft tissue; thus we hypothesized that the PEGDA 3400 backbone would be biologically applicable to hDPSCs that were not biochemically induced to differentiate into harder mineralized tissues. These initial 2D experiments are an essential prerequisite to forthcoming 3D studies.

Harumi Miyagi et al. demonstrated that Fn showed the least variation in a study of ECM matrix protein expression in human hDPSC donors [31]. The cell-adhesion signaling cascades mediated by Fn binding allow cells to attach to the ECM and function. We hypothesized that adding Fn to our model would increase cell proliferation, viability, and spreading over time. Despite promising results with our earlier 1 : 3 (v/v) ratios of HA : Gn, we noted that the Fn contains binding domains for gelatin. To account for this, we designed our experiments to include a 1 : 1 volume ratio of HA : Gn. Data from the WST-1 absorbance values suggests that as the concentration of the Fn increases, the hDPSC proliferation increases. This data contrasts the effect of PuraMatrix™ on hDPSC proliferation, which is a self-assembling injectable scaffold [9] that did not demonstrate a concentration dependent relationship.

Interestingly, the biological ligand density on a surface is a major factor that controls both cell attachment and spreading. Our data showed a significant increase in cell spreading based on the Fn concentration of 0.1 μg/mL at day 4. This may have been due to the classification of "spreading" based on our methods. We acknowledge that Figure 7 includes cells that are classified as both partially and fully spread. Although the hDPSCs embedded in the PEGSSDA-HA-Gn hydrogels appeared to spread based on qualitative morphology, hDPSCs seeded on the surface of PEGDA-HA-Gn positive control hydrogels decreased in spreading after four days based on our classification. Thus fibronectin appears to contribute to hDPSC spreading. This hypothesis can be experimentally validated by conducting experiments that quantify the RGD ligand density required for cell spreading [32].

In sum, both collagen and fibronectin are expressed in native dental pulp, and it remains to be seen how the mutual integrin binding sites affect hDPSC fate in injectable hybrid scaffolds. The next step would be to determine how protein modified PEGDA-based injectable hydrogels influence embedded hDPSC attachment and integrin expression.

5. Conclusion

Our results provide new insight for the purposeful design of dental pulp tissue engineering applications. An injectable scaffold with tunable mechanical and biochemical components may facilitate targeted tissue mimicry.

Competing Interests

The authors declare that there is no conflict of interests regarding the publication of this paper.

Acknowledgments

This study is supported by NIH/NIDCR Grant (DE019514-SBA).

References

[1] Y. Zadik, V. Sandler, R. Bechor, and R. Salehrabi, "Analysis of factors related to extraction of endodontically treated teeth," *Oral Surgery, Oral Medicine, Oral Pathology, Oral Radiology and Endodontology*, vol. 106, no. 5, pp. e31–e35, 2008.

[2] S. Friedman, S. Abitbol, and H. P. Lawrence, "Treatment outcome in endodontics: the Toronto Study. Phase 1: initial treatment," *Journal of Endodontics*, vol. 29, no. 12, pp. 787–793, 2003.

[3] V. T. Sakai, M. M. Cordeiro, Z. Dong, Z. Zhang, B. D. Zeitlin, and J. E. Nör, "Tooth slice/scaffold model of dental pulp tissue engineering," *Advances in Dental Research*, vol. 23, no. 3, pp. 325–332, 2011.

[4] J. J. Mao, S. G. Kim, J. Zhou et al., "Regenerative endodontics: barriers and strategies for clinical translation," *Dental Clinics of North America*, vol. 56, no. 3, pp. 639–649, 2012.

[5] Y.-L. Ng, V. Mann, and K. Gulabivala, "Outcome of secondary root canal treatment: a systematic review of the literature," *International Endodontic Journal*, vol. 41, no. 12, pp. 1026–1046, 2008.

[6] V. Rosa, Z. Zhang, R. H. M. Grande, and J. E. Nör, "Dental pulp tissue engineering in full-length human root canals," *Journal of Dental Research*, vol. 92, no. 11, pp. 970–975, 2013.

[7] M. Cvek, "Prognosis of luxated non-vital maxillary incisors treated with calcium hydroxide and filled with gutta-percha. A retrospective clinical study," *Endodontics & Dental Traumatology*, vol. 8, no. 2, pp. 45–55, 1992.

[8] F. N. Syed-Picard, H. L. Ray Jr., P. N. Kumta, and C. Sfeir, "Scaffoldless tissue-engineered dental pulp cell constructs for endodontic therapy," *Journal of Dental Research*, vol. 93, no. 3, pp. 250–255, 2014.

[9] B. N. Cavalcanti, B. D. Zeitlin, and J. E. Nör, "A hydrogel scaffold that maintains viability and supports differentiation of dental pulp stem cells," *Dental Materials*, vol. 29, no. 1, pp. 97–102, 2013.

[10] K. M. Galler, R. N. D'Souza, J. D. Hartgerink, and G. Schmalz, "Scaffolds for dental pulp tissue engineering," *Advances in Dental Research*, vol. 23, no. 3, pp. 333–339, 2011.

[11] K. S. Bohl, J. Shon, B. Rutherford, and D. J. Mooney, "Role of synthetic extracellular matrix in development of engineered dental pulp," *Journal of Biomaterials Science, Polymer Edition*, vol. 9, no. 7, pp. 749–764, 1998.

[12] N. R. Kim, D. H. Lee, P.-H. Chung, and H.-C. Yang, "Distinct differentiation properties of human dental pulp cells on collagen, gelatin, and chitosan scaffolds," *Oral Surgery, Oral Medicine, Oral Pathology, Oral Radiology, and Endodontology*, vol. 108, no. 5, pp. e94–e100, 2009.

[13] G. T.-J. Huang, T. Yamaza, L. D. Shea et al., "Stem/progenitor cell-mediated de novo regeneration of dental pulp with newly deposited continuous layer of dentin in an in vivo model," *Tissue Engineering Part A*, vol. 16, no. 2, pp. 605–615, 2010.

[14] Z. Yuan, H. Nie, and W. Sea, "Biomaterial selection for tooth regeneration," *Tissue Engineering. Part B, Reviews*, vol. 17, no. 5, pp. 373–388, 2011.

[15] M. M. Cordeiro, Z. Dong, T. Kaneko et al., "Dental pulp tissue engineering with stem cells from exfoliated deciduous teeth," *Journal of Endodontics*, vol. 34, no. 8, pp. 962–969, 2008.

[16] V. Rosa, A. Della Bona, B. N. Cavalcanti, and J. E. Nör, "Tissue engineering: from research to dental clinics," *Dental Materials*, vol. 28, no. 4, pp. 341–348, 2012.

[17] Y. Li, J. Rodrigues, and H. Tomás, "Injectable and biodegradable hydrogels: gelation, biodegradation and biomedical applications," *Chemical Society Reviews*, vol. 41, no. 6, pp. 2193–2221, 2012.

[18] G. D. Prestwich, "Hyaluronic acid-based clinical biomaterials derived for cell and molecule delivery in regenerative medicine," *Journal of Controlled Release*, vol. 155, no. 2, pp. 193–199, 2011.

[19] S. Gronthos, J. Brahim, W. Li et al., "Stem cell properties of human dental pulp stem cells," *Journal of Dental Research*, vol. 81, no. 8, pp. 531–535, 2002.

[20] Z. S. Xiao, S. Ahmad, Y. Liu, and G. D. Prestwich, "Synthesis and evaluation of injectable, in situ crosslinkable synthetic extracellular matrices for tissue engineering," *Journal of Biomedical Materials Research Part A*, vol. 79, no. 4, pp. 902–912, 2006.

[21] G. T. Huang, M. Al-Habib, and P. Gauthier, "Challenges of stem cell-based pulp and dentin regeneration: a clinical perspective," *Endodontic Topics*, vol. 28, no. 1, pp. 51–60, 2013.

[22] F. Guilak, M. Cohen, B. Estes et al., "Control of stem cell fate by interactions with the extracellular matrix," *Cell Stem Cell*, vol. 5, pp. 17–26, 2009.

[23] M. J. Gupte and P. X. Ma, "Nanofibrous scaffolds for dental and craniofacial applications," *Journal of Dental Research*, vol. 91, no. 3, pp. 227–234, 2012.

[24] M. A. Serban, Y. Liu, and G. D. Prestwich, "Effects of extracellular matrix analogues on primary human fibroblast behavior," *Acta Biomaterialia*, vol. 4, no. 1, pp. 67–75, 2008.

[25] F. F. Demarco, L. Casagrande, Z. Zhang et al., "Effects of morphogen and scaffold porogen on the differentiation of dental pulp stem cells," *Journal of Endodontics*, vol. 36, no. 11, pp. 1805–1811, 2010.

[26] X. Liu and P. X. Ma, "Phase separation, pore structure, and properties of nanofibrous gelatin scaffolds," *Biomaterials*, vol. 30, no. 25, pp. 4094–4103, 2009.

[27] X. Liu, Y. Won, and P. X. Ma, "Porogen-induced surface modification of nano-fibrous poly(L-lactic acid) scaffolds for tissue engineering," *Biomaterials*, vol. 27, no. 21, pp. 3980–3987, 2006.

[28] J. Zhang, A. Skardal, and G. D. Prestwich, "Engineered extracellular matrices with cleavable crosslinkers for cell expansion and easy cell recovery," *Biomaterials*, vol. 29, no. 34, pp. 4521–4531, 2008.

[29] J. A. Yang, J. Yeom, B. W. Hwang et al., "In situ-forming injectable hydrogels for regenerative medicine," *Progress in Polymer Science*, vol. 39, no. 12, pp. 1973–1986, 2014.

[30] K. Ghosh, Z. Pan, E. Guan et al., "Cell adaptation to a physiologically relevant ECM mimic with different viscoelastic properties," *Biomaterials*, vol. 28, no. 4, pp. 671–679, 2007.

[31] S. P. Harumi Miyagi, I. Kerkis, C. M. da Costa Maranduba, C. M. Gomes, M. D. Martins, and M. M. Marques, "Expression of extracellular matrix proteins in human dental pulp stem cells depends on the donor tooth conditions," *Journal of Endodontics*, vol. 36, no. 5, pp. 826–831, 2010.

[32] S. P. Massia and J. A. Hubbell, "An RGD spacing of 440 nm is sufficient for integrin $\alpha v \beta 3$-mediated fibroblast spreading and 140 nm for focal contact and stress fiber formation," *Journal of Cell Biology*, vol. 114, no. 5, pp. 1089–1100, 1991.

Permissions

The contributors of this book come from diverse backgrounds, making this book a truly international effort. This book will bring forth new frontiers with its revolutionizing research information and detailed analysis of the nascent developments around the world.

We would like to thank all the contributing authors for lending their expertise to make the book truly unique. They have played a crucial role in the development of this book. Without their invaluable contributions this book wouldn't have been possible. They have made vital efforts to compile up to date information on the varied aspects of this subject to make this book a valuable addition to the collection of many professionals and students.

This book was conceptualized with the vision of imparting up-to-date information and advanced data in this field. To ensure the same, a matchless editorial board was set up. Every individual on the board went through rigorous rounds of assessment to prove their worth. After which they invested a large part of their time researching and compiling the most relevant data for our readers.

The editorial board has been involved in producing this book since its inception. They have spent rigorous hours researching and exploring the diverse topics which have resulted in the successful publishing of this book. They have passed on their knowledge of decades through this book. To expedite this challenging task, the publisher supported the team at every step. A small team of assistant editors was also appointed to further simplify the editing procedure and attain best results for the readers.

Apart from the editorial board, the designing team has also invested a significant amount of their time in understanding the subject and creating the most relevant covers. They scrutinized every image to scout for the most suitable representation of the subject and create an appropriate cover for the book.

The publishing team has been an ardent support to the editorial, designing and production team. Their endless efforts to recruit the best for this project, has resulted in the accomplishment of this book. They are a veteran in the field of academics and their pool of knowledge is as vast as their experience in printing. Their expertise and guidance has proved useful at every step. Their uncompromising quality standards have made this book an exceptional effort. Their encouragement from time to time has been an inspiration for everyone.

The publisher and the editorial board hope that this book will prove to be a valuable piece of knowledge for researchers, students, practitioners and scholars across the globe.

List of Contributors

Mehdi Mesri
Office of Cancer Clinical Proteomics Research, National Cancer Institute, NIH, Bethesda, MD 20892, USA

Shimaa Nour Moursi Ahmed
Department of Respiratory Medicine, National Hospital Organization Nagoya Medical Center, Nagoya, Aichi 460-0001, Japan
Department of Respiratory Medicine, Sohag University Hospital, Nasr City Street, Sohag 82524, Egypt

Hideo Saka, Masahide Oki, RieTsuboi and Keiji Sugiyama
Department of Respiratory Medicine, National Hospital Organization Nagoya Medical Center, Nagoya, Aichi 460-0001, Japan

Hamdy Ali Mohammadien and Ola Alkady
Department of Respiratory Medicine, Sohag University Hospital, Nasr City Street, Sohag 82524, Egypt

Yoshimasa Tanikawa and Masahiro Aoyama
Department of Respiratory Medicine and Clinical Immunology, Toyota Kosei Hospital, 500-1 IboharaJosuicho, Toyota-Shi 470-0396, Japan

Matthew M. Hanasono
The University of Texas M.D. Anderson Cancer Center, 1515 Holcombe Boulevard, Unit 443, Houston, TX 77030, USA

Serafino Carta, Mattia Fortina, Alberto Riva, Luigi Meccariello, Enrico Manzi, Antonio Di Giovanni and Paolo Ferrata
Department of Medical and Surgical Sciences and Neuroscience, Section of Orthopedics and Traumatology, University of Siena, University Hospital "Santa Maria alleScotte", Siena, Italy

Ahmet Ali Tuncer and Didem Baskin Embleton
Department of Pediatric Surgery, AfyonKocatepe University Hospital, 03000 Afyonkarahisar, Turkey

Mehmet Fatih Bozkurt
Department of Pathology, Faculty of Veterinary Medicine, Afyon Kocatepe University, 03000 Afyonkarahisar, Turkey

Tulay Koken
Department of Biochemistry, Afyon Kocatepe University Medical Faculty, 03000 Afyonkarahisar, Turkey

Nurhan Dogan
Department of Biostatistics, Afyon Kocatepe University Medical Faculty, 03000 Afyonkarahisar, Turkey

Mine Kanat Pektaş
Department of Obstetrics & Gynecology, Afyon Kocatepe University Hospital, 03000 Afyonkarahisar, Turkey

Lothar Faber
Department of Cardiology, Heart and Diabetes Center North Rhine-Westphalia, University Hospital of the Ruhr University Bochum, Georgstraβe 11, 32545 Bad Oeynhausen, Germany

Olaf Suess
DRK Kliniken Berlin Westend, Zentrumfür Wirbelsäulenchirurgie und Neurotraumatologie, Berlin, Germany
Department of Neurosurgery, Charit'e University Hospital, Berlin, Germany

Markus Schomacher
Department of Neurosurgery, Charité University Hospital, Berlin, Germany
Vivantes Klinikumam Friedrichshain, Neurochirurgische Klinik, Berlin, Germany

Aaron Gipsman, Lisa Rauschert, Michael Daneshvar and Patrick Knott
Chicago Medical School, Rosalind Franklin University of Medicine and Science, 3333 Green Bay Road, North Chicago, IL 60064, USA

Mohammad Hashemi
Cellular and Molecular Research Center, Zahedan University of Medical Sciences, Zahedan 98167-43181, Iran
Department of Clinical Biochemistry, School of Medicine, Zahedan University of Medical Sciences, Zahedan 98167-43181, Iran

Gholamreza Bahari and Maryam Rezaei
Department of Clinical Biochemistry, School of Medicine, Zahedan University of Medical Sciences, Zahedan 98167-43181, Iran

Mahnaz Sandoughi and Seyed Amirhossein Fazeli
Department of Internal Medicine, School of Medicine, Zahedan University of Medical Sciences, Zahedan 98167-43181, Iran

Mathieu Bergeron
Department of Oto-Rhino-Laryngology and Ophthalmology, Faculty of Medicine, Laval University,Quebec City, QC, Canada G1V 0A6

Catherine L. Lorti and Matthieu J. Guitton
Department of Oto-Rhino-Laryngology and Ophthalmology, Faculty of Medicine, Laval University,Quebec City, QC, Canada G1V 0A6
Institut Universitaire en Santé Mentale de Qúebec, Quebec City, QC, Canada G1J 2G3

Argye E. Hillis
Department of Neurology, Johns Hopkins University School of Medicine, Baltimore, MD 21287, USA
Department of Physical Medicine and Rehabilitation, Johns Hopkins University School of Medicine, Baltimore, MD 21287, USA
Department of Cognitive Science, Krieger School of Arts and Sciences, Johns Hopkins University, Baltimore, MD 21218, USA

Donna C. Tippett
Department of Neurology, Johns Hopkins University School of Medicine, Baltimore, MD 21287, USA
Department of Physical Medicine and Rehabilitation, Johns Hopkins University School of Medicine, Baltimore, MD 21287, USA
Department of Otolaryngology-Head and Neck Surgery, Johns Hopkins University School of Medicine, Baltimore, MD 21287, USA

Gita Faghihi and FaribaIraji
Skin Diseases and Leishmaniasis Research Center, Isfahan University of Medical Sciences, Isfahan, Iran

Azam Elahipoor
Department of Dermatology, Qom University of Medical Sciences, Qom, Iran

Shadi Behfar
Department of Dermatology, School of Medicine, Rafsanjan University of Medical Sciences, Rafsanjan, Iran

Bahareh Abtahi-Naeini
Cancer Research Center, Semnan University of Medical Sciences, Semnan, Iran

Mohammad Hossein Rouhani
Food Security Research Center and Department of Community Nutrition, School of Nutrition and Food Science, Isfahan University of Medical Sciences, Isfahan, Iran

Mojgan Mortazavi Najafabadi
Department of Nephrology, Isfahan Kidney Diseases Research Center, Isfahan, Iran

Ahmad Esmaillzadeh
Food Security Research Center and Department of Community Nutrition, School of Nutrition and Food Science, Isfahan University of Medical Sciences, Isfahan, Iran
Department of Community Nutrition, School of Nutritional Sciences and Dietetics, Tehran University of Medical Sciences, Tehran, Iran

Awat Feizi
Faculty of Epidemiology and Biostatistics, Isfahan University of Medical Sciences, Isfahan, Iran

Leila Azadbakht
Food Security Research Center and Department of Community Nutrition, School of Nutrition and Food Science, Isfahan University of Medical Sciences, Isfahan, Iran
Department of Community Nutrition, School of Nutritional Sciences and Dietetics, Tehran University of Medical Sciences, Tehran, Iran
Diabetes Research Center, Endocrinology and Metabolism Clinical Sciences Institute, Tehran University of Medical Sciences, Tehran, Iran

Eli E.Machtei
Department of Periodontology, School of Graduate Dentistry, Rambam Health Care Campus and Faculty of Medicine, Technion (Israel Institute of Technology), Rambam HCC, 8 HáaliaHashnia Street, 31096 Haifa, Israel

Vishnu Kaniyarakkal, Nizamuddin Mundangalam and Anitha Puduvail Moorkoth
Department of Microbiology, Government Medical College Kozhikode, Kozhikode 673016, India

Sheela Mathew
Department of Infectious Diseases, Government Medical College Kozhikode, Kozhikode 673016, India

Desalegne Amare Zelellw
Department of Nursing, College of Medicine and Health Sciences, Bahir Dar University, P.O. Box 79, Bahir Dar, Ethiopia

Teketo Kassaw Tegegne
Department of Public Health, College of Medicine and Health Sciences, Debre Markos University, DebreMarkos, Ethiopia

Girma Alem Getie
Department of Nursing, College of Medicine and Health Sciences, Debre Markos University, Debre Markos, Ethiopia

Lu Bin
Key Laboratory of Environment and Health, Ministry of Education and Ministry of Environmental Protection and State Key Laboratory of Environmental Health (Incubating), School of Public Health, Tongji Medical College, Huazhong University of Science and Technology,Wuhan, Hubei 430030, China

R. Khonde Kumbu
Key Laboratory of Environment and Health, Ministry of Education and Ministry of Environmental Protection and State Key Laboratory of Environmental Health (Incubating), School of Public Health, Tongji Medical College, Huazhong University of Science and Technology,Wuhan, Hubei 430030, China
Department of Pediatrics, Faculty of Medicine, University of Kinshasa, P.O. Box 747, Kinshasa, Democratic Republic of the Congo
Department of Pediatrics, Faculty of Medicine, Catholic University of Bukavu, P.O. Box 285, Bukavu, South Kivu, Democratic Republic of the Congo

K. Mbanzulu Makola
Department of Tropical Medicine, Infectious and Parasitic Diseases, Faculty of Medicine, University of Kinshasa, P.O. Box 747, Kinshasa, Democratic Republic of the Congo

Elham Baghdadi
Department of Microbiology, Faculty of Science, Islamic Azad University, Varamin-Pishva Branch, Tehran, Iran

Farzad Aala
Department of Medical Parasitology and Mycology, Kurdistan University of Medical Sciences, P.O. Box 14155-6446, Sanandaj, Iran

Sadegh Khodavaisy
Department of Medical Parasitology and Mycology, Kurdistan University of Medical Sciences, P.O. Box 14155-6446, Sanandaj, Iran
Division of Molecular Biology, Department of Medical Mycology and Parasitology, School of Public Health, Tehran University of Medical Sciences, Tehran, Iran

Sassan Rezaie
Division of Molecular Biology, Department of Medical Mycology and Parasitology, School of Public Health, Tehran University of Medical Sciences, Tehran, Iran

Sara Abolghasem
Department of Microbiology, Faculty of Science, Islamic Azad University, North Tehran Branch, Tehran, Iran

NedaKiasat
Department of Medical Mycology, Jondishapour University of Medical Sciences, Ahvaz, Iran

Zahra Salehi
Department of Medical Mycology, Tarbiatn Modares University, Tehran, Iran

Somayeh Sharifynia
Clinical Tuberculosis and Epidemiology Research Center, National Research Institute of Tuberculosis and Lung Diseases (NRITLD), Shahid Beheshti University of Medical Sciences, Tehran, Iran

Zahra Zakeri
Department of Internal Medicine, School of Medicine, Shahid Beheshti University of Medical Sciences, Tehran 19857-17443, Iran

Ebrahim Ghayem Hassankhani and Farzad Omidi-Kashani
Orthopedic Research Center, Orthopedic Department, Imam Reza Hospital, Mashhad University of Medical Sciences, Mashhad, Iran

Shahram Moradkhani
Orthopedic Department, Imam Reza Hospital, Mashhad University of Medical Sciences, Mashhad, Iran

Golnaz Ghayem Hassankhani
Orthopedic Research Center, Ghaem Hospital, Mashhad University of Medical Sciences, Mashhad, Iran

Mohammad Taghi Shakeri
Faculty of Medicine, Mashhad University of Medical Sciences, Mashhad, Iran

Narges Karimi
Department of Neurology, School of Medicine, Immunogenetics Research Center, Clinical Research Development Unit of Bou Ali Sina Hospital, Mazandaran University of Medical Sciences, Sari, Iran

Seyyed Ali Akbarian
Department of Emergency Medicine, School of Medicine, Mazandaran University of Medical Sciences, Sari, Iran

Nisha Panth, Keshav Raj Paudel and Kalpana Parajuli
Department of Pharmacy, School of Health and Allied Sciences, Pokhara University, Dhungepatan, Kaski 33701, Nepal

T. D. Jones, A. Kefi, S. Sun and M. Cho
Bioengineering, University of Illinois at Chicago, Chicago, IL 60612-7212, USA

S. B. Alapati
Endodontics, University of Illinois at Chicago, Chicago, IL 60612-7212, USA

Index